Sensation & Perception

SECOND EDITION

FREE ACCESS! Companion Website

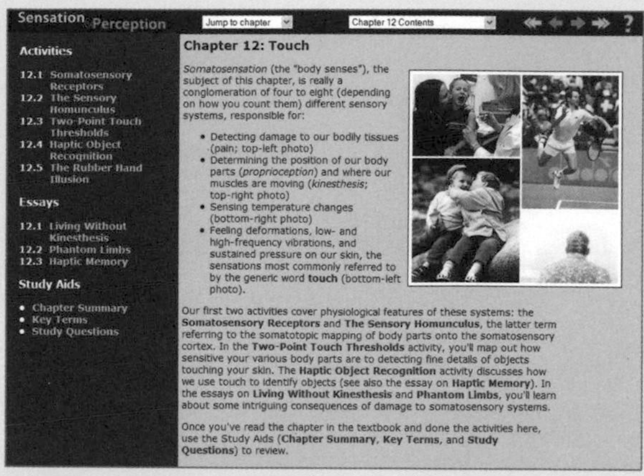

CHAPTER 12 HOME PAGE

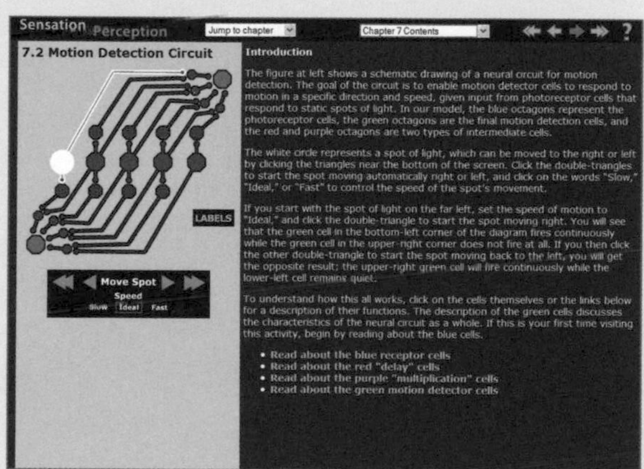

WEB ACTIVITY 7.2 MOTION DETECTION CIRCUIT

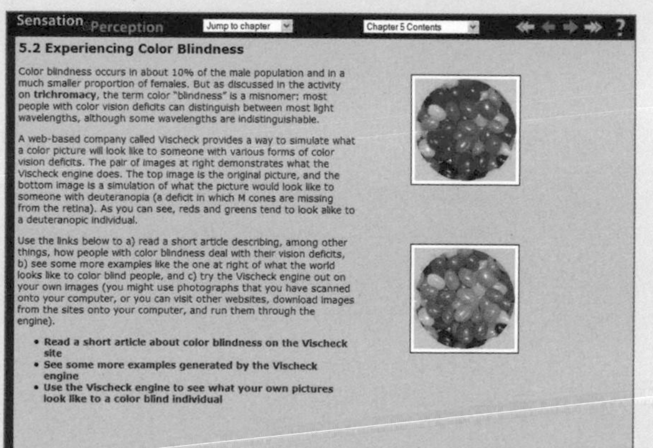

WEB ESSAY 5.2 EXPERIENCING COLOR BLINDNESS

www.sinauer.com/wolfe2e

The **Sensation & Perception** Companion Website is an essential companion to the textbook that can enhance your learning experience with a variety of multimedia resources, all keyed to textbook chapters. The site features interactive activities to help you better understand complex systems and phenomena, essays that provide additional coverage of interesting topics, study questions that help you test your understanding of each chapter, and more. Take advantage of the **Sensation & Perception** Companion Website to help you master the material in your course.

The site features the following resources:

Interactive Activities lead you through important processes, phenomena, and structures. These activities bring to life many of the concepts and examples from the textbook, and give you the opportunity to explore them at your own pace. Topics include perception experiments, illusions that illustrate key concepts, models of cognitive processes, and interactive diagrams of important structures.

Web Essays expand on selected topics from the textbook and provide additional coverage and examples. These essays aid your understanding of textbook material through fascinating descriptions of phenomena, explanations of concepts, and real-world case studies and applications.

Study Questions give you the opportunity to test your mastery of the important concepts, processes, and terminology presented in each chapter. Use these questions as a chapter-by-chapter review after you have read each chapter. Or, work through multiple chapters at once to prepare for exams.

Additional features include **Key Term Quizzes** that help you learn and review the hundreds of terms introduced in the textbook and **Chapter Summaries** that provide a detailed overview of each chapter.

Companion Website activities and essays listed on next page...

Companion Website Activities and Essays

Throughout the textbook, you will see references to the Companion Website in blue text. These refer to specific activities and essays that are relevant to the topic being discussed. Below is the full list of activities and essays, along with the textbook page on which they are first referenced.

Sensation & Perception

SECOND EDITION

Sensation & Perception

SECOND EDITION

Jeremy M. Wolfe *Harvard University Medical School*

Keith R. Kluender *University of Wisconsin, Madison*

Dennis M. Levi *University of California, Berkeley*

Linda M. Bartoshuk *University of Florida*

Rachel S. Herz *Brown University Medical School*

Roberta L. Klatzky *Carnegie Mellon University*

Susan J. Lederman *Queen's University*

Daniel M. Merfeld *Harvard University Medical School*

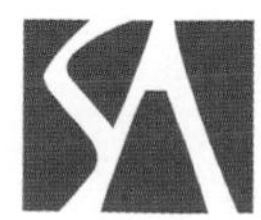

Sinauer Associates, Inc. • Publishers
Sunderland, Massachusetts U.S.A.

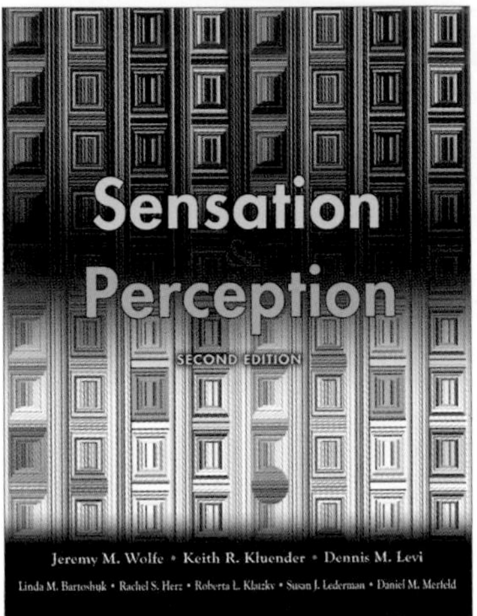

About the cover

FRONT COVER: The Coffer Illusion. Most first time viewers of the cover image see a series of rectangles that they frequently describe as "coffers" or door panels. Eventually, you will see an alternate percept, a grid of circles segmented from the background. If you don't see the circles, the colored ones in the bottom half of the image will serve as a cue. The illusion is an example of an "ambiguous figure" where the visual system entertains more than one interpretation of the same stimulus (see chapter 4). In this case, there appears to be a very strong bias to interpret the image as a series of 3-D structures—coffers—with closed boundaries. The circles almost always take a bit of work to see. However, they come to the fore with extended viewing as if, perhaps, the processes generating the coffer percept become fatigued, allowing the circles to break through. (Image provided and created by Anthony M. Norcia, with the assistance of Mark W. Pettet and Vladimir Vildavski.)

BACK COVER: This illusion combines three different perceptual phenomena. First, it uses bi-stable cubes, which have a long history in perception and relate to the Necker cube, to the art of Vasarely, and even to quilt designs. Second, the faces of the cubes contain a "breathing light" variation of Kanizsa's illusory contours, which raise interesting issues about the nature of form perception. And third, the perspective of the cubes has been altered, giving the impression that we are looking at the surface of cubes from an angle, demonstrating how psychologists have learned so much from artists. (See Simone Gori and D. Alan Stubbs [2006] A new set of illusions—the dynamic luminance-gradient illusion and the breathing light illusion. *Perception* 35: 1573–1577.)

Sensation & Perception

For information, address
Sinauer Associates, Inc., 23 Plumtree Road, Sunderland, MA 01375 USA
Fax: 413-549-1118
E-mail: publish@sinauer.com
Internet: www.sinauer.com

Library of Congress Cataloging-in-Publication Data

Sensation & perception / Jeremy M. Wolfe ... [et al.]. — 2nd ed.
p. cm.
Includes bibliographical references and index.
ISBN 978-0-87893-953-4 (casebound : alk. paper)
1. Senses and sensation. 2. Perception. I. Wolfe, Jeremy M.
QP431.S445 2009
612.8—dc22 2008038731

Printed in China
8 7 6 5 4 3 2

About the Authors

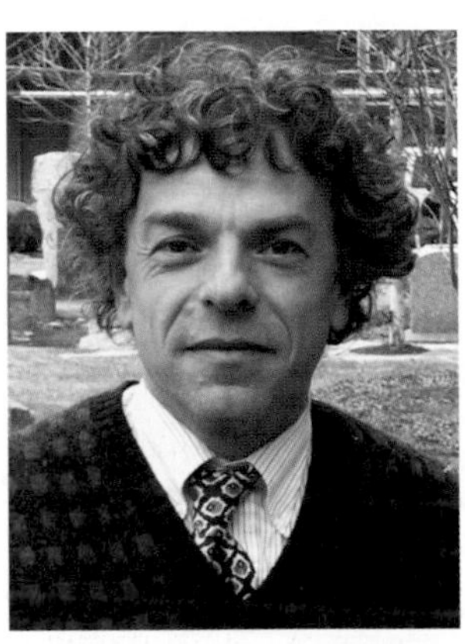

JEREMY M. WOLFE is Professor of Ophthalmology at Harvard Medical School. His early work includes papers on binocular vision, adaptation, and accommodation. Dr. Wolfe was trained as a vision researcher/experimental psychologist and remains one today. The bulk of his recent work has dealt with visual search and visual attention. He has taught Introductory Psychology for over twenty-five years at the Massachusetts Institute of Technology, where he won the Baker Memorial Prize for undergraduate teaching in 1989. He teaches Perception at Harvard.

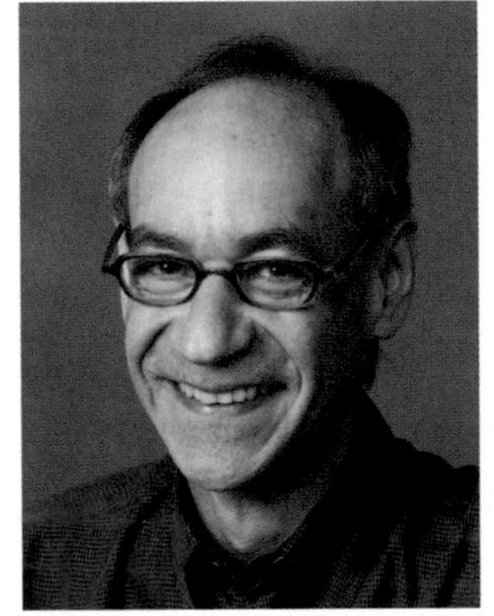

DENNIS M. LEVI has taught at the University of California, Berkeley since 2001. He is Dean/Professor in the School of Optometry and Professor at the Helen Wills Neuroscience Institute. In the lab, Dr. Levi and colleagues use psychophysics, computational modeling, and brain imaging (fMRI) to study the neural mechanisms of normal pattern vision in humans, and to learn how they are degraded by abnormal visual experience (amblyopia).

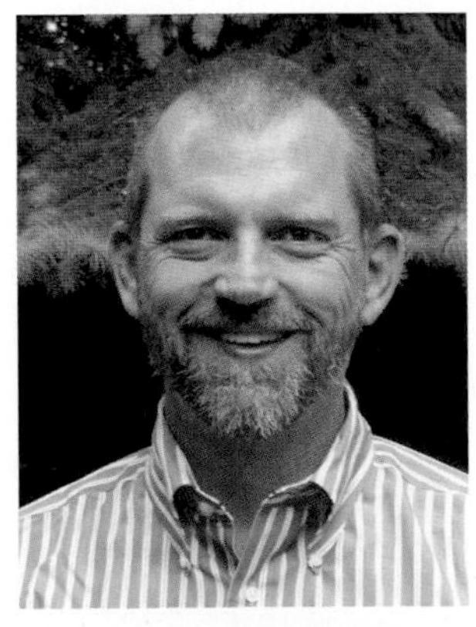

KEITH R. KLUENDER is Professor of Psychology at the University of Wisconsin, Madison. His research encompasses: how people hear complex sounds such as speech; how experience shapes the way we hear; how what we hear guides our actions and communication; clinical problems of hearing impairment or language delay; and practical concerns about computer speech recognition and hearing aid design. Dr. Kluender is deeply committed to teaching, and has taught a wide array of courses—philosophical, psychological, and physiological.

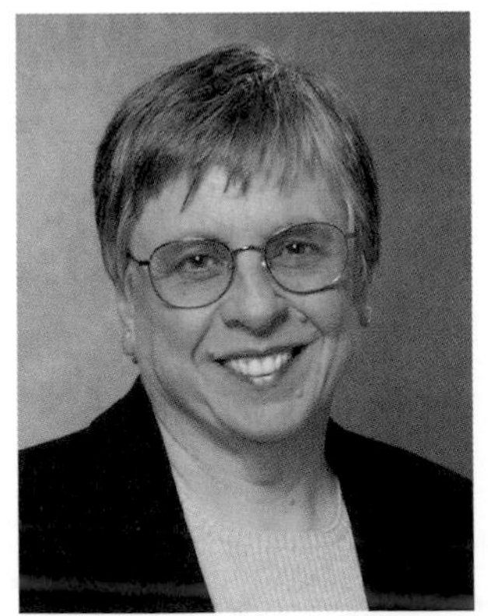

LINDA M. BARTOSHUK is Bushnell Professor, Department of Community Dentistry and Behavioral Science at the University of Florida. Her research on taste has opened up broad new avenues for further study, establishing the impact of both genetic and pathological variation in taste on food preferences, diet, and health. She discovered that taste normally inhibits other oral sensations such that damage to taste leads to unexpected consequences like weight gain and intensified oral pain.

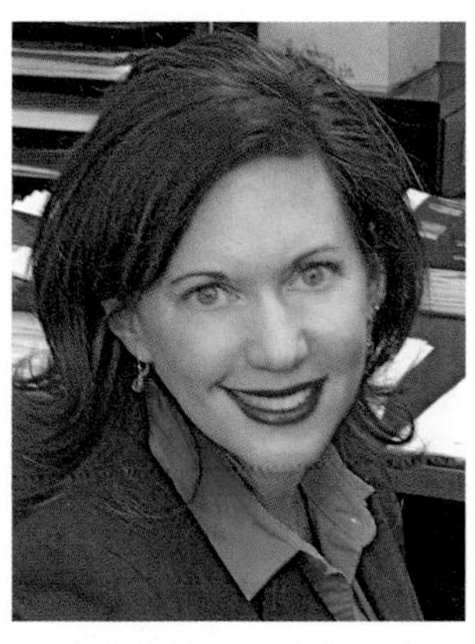

RACHEL S. HERZ is currently a Visiting Assistant Professor in the Department of Psychiatry and Human Behavior at Brown University's Warren Alpert Medical School. Her research focuses on olfactory cognition and perception and the roles and features of emotion, memory, and language. Using an experimental approach grounded in evolutionary theory and incorporating both cognitive–behavioral and neuropsychological techniques, Dr. Herz aims to understand how biological mechanisms and cognitive processes interact to influence perception, cognition, and behavior.

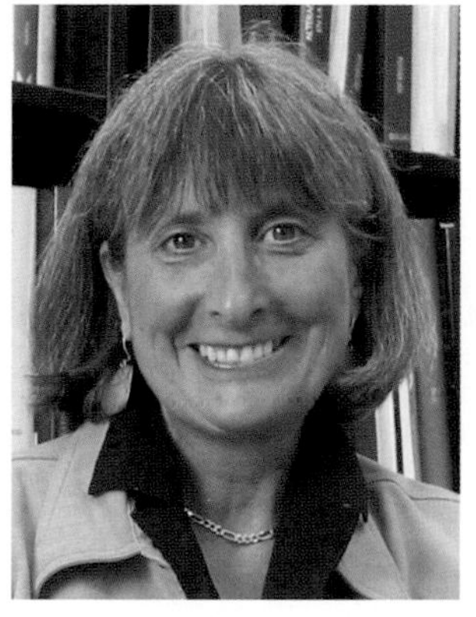

SUSAN J. LEDERMAN is Professor of Psychology at Queen's University, with cross-appointments in the School of Computing and in the Centre for Neuroscience. Her research interests span both perception and cognition, with particular emphases on psychophysics, haptic perception and recognition of objects and their underlying neural processes and representations, multisensory perception, and sensory-guided motor control. She has applied the results of her research to a number of real-world problems, including the design of haptic and multisensory interfaces for virtual environments and teleoperation.

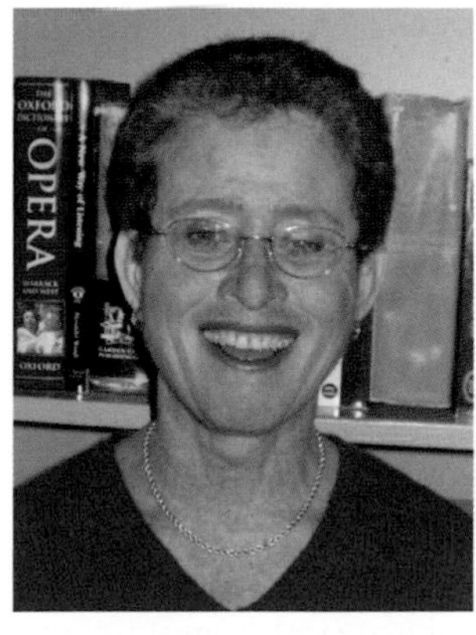

ROBERTA L. KLATZKY is Professor of Psychology at Carnegie Mellon University, where she also holds faculty appointments in the Center for the Neural Basis of Cognition and the Human–Computer Interaction Institute. She has done extensive research on haptic and visual object recognition, space perception and spatial thinking, and motor performance. Her work has application to haptic interfaces, navigation aids for the blind, image-guided surgery, teleoperation, and virtual environments.

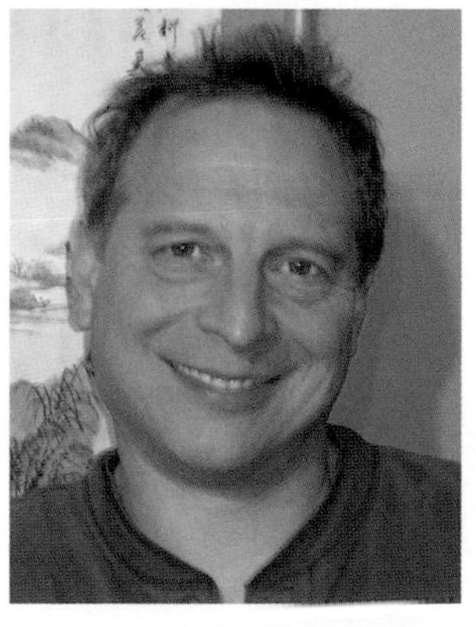

DANIEL M. MERFELD is an Associate Professor of Otology and Laryngology at the Harvard Medical School with cross-appointments at the Harvard-MIT Health, Science, and Technology program and the Harvard Faculty of Arts and Sciences. Most of his research career has been spent studying how the brain combines information from multiple sources, with a specific focus on how the brain processes ambiguous sensory information from the vestibular system. Recent research includes work developing a vestibular implant for patients who have severe problems with their vestibular periphery.

Brief Contents

Contents

CHAPTER 1 *Introduction* 2

CHAPTER 2 *The First Steps in Vision: Seeing Stars* 28

CHAPTER 3 *Spatial Vision: From Stars to Stripes* 50

CHAPTER 7 *Motion Perception* 168

CHAPTER 8 *Attention and Scene Perception* 188

CHAPTER 9 *Hearing: Physiology and Psychoacoustics* 218

Preface to the Second Edition

This is a Sensation and Perception text written by enthusiasts who have spent years working in the field because we think it is fun. Of course, there are other motivations at play as well; we work on problems like oral pain that have medical applications, or issues such as airport security that have broader societal implications. But a good part of what gets us up in the morning is the sheer enjoyment of working to find solutions to these problems.

Our goal in writing an undergraduate textbook is to spread our enthusiasm. How should we go about doing that? Collectively, the authors of this book know a great deal about sensation and perception and we could have created a fat tome simply by stapling together the review chapters we have written for more advanced handbooks. While this may have been quite authoritative, we suspect it would've been more of an undergraduate sleep aid rather than a vehicle for transferring the enthusiasm we feel about sensation and perception. Instead, in each of the 15 chapters of this book, we have tried to tell a coherent and interesting story that will give the reader enough background and exposure to enough current research to understand why these topics are interesting and how they might be further investigated and understood. We are not naïve or immodest enough to believe that you will devour a chapter on "The Perception of Color" or "Perceiving and Recognizing Objects" in the way that you might devour a good novel. However, we do hope that you will find each chapter to be more than a compilation of facts. We hope to be like Cleopatra in Shakespeare's play: while other texts may "cloy the appetites they feed," we want our work to "makes hungry where most it satisfies." We will be satisfied if the book teaches the reader enough to inspire the reader to want to know more.

In service of these goals, we have produced a comparatively brief textbook. You, the student, may not think so at 3:00 a.m. the day before the final exam, but you, the professor, will note that this text is shorter than a number of other current Sensation and Perception texts. The text is not written at a lower level than longer texts. Rather, like many textbook authors, we recognize the futility of trying to get students to learn everything about a topic from a single encounter. We want to present a coherent introduction to the important topics. We hope to leave enough time for the instructor or the interested student to dive into the endless material that lies behind, and to the side of, each point made in the actual text.

Some of that extra material can be found on the text's companion website, www.sinauer.com/wolfe2e. There, in addition to great demonstrations, you will find a number of brief essays on topics that we broken-heartedly removed from earlier and longer versions of our chapters. Given the chance, each of us can talk your ear off on the topics in this book, but we have sincerely tried to avoid doing this.

In trying to convey our enthusiasm for this material, we wanted to create a beautiful book. If we have succeeded, it is in no small part due to our publisher, Sinauer Associates. The people at Sinauer Associates produce beautiful books and we were fortunate enough to have their commitment to a Sensation and Perception text that is full color throughout. We have enjoyed seeing the actual pages as they came to us for proofreading. We hope that you find your experience with the book to be both aesthetically and intellectually appealing.

We were pleased by the reception of the first edition of our textbook and pleased that this reception warranted a second edition. We were very happy with the first edition but there are always parts that could be improved, a few errors to correct, and new science to consider. For the second edition, in addition to editing all the existing chapters, we have added a chapter on the vestibular system and we are pleased to welcome Dan Merfeld of Harvard Medical School to our family of authors. We are also happy to welcome Evan Palmer of the Wichita State University as the guardian of our website, taking over from Pepper Williams.

Acknowledgments

Our editor Graig Donini deserves great credit for tolerating our academic attitude toward deadlines and for nursing this project to completion. Stephanie Hiebert did a fantastic job copyediting and caught our errors, improved the words, and made the text fit for public use. David McIntyre came up with an endless set of clever ideas for better images and photos. Laura Green oversaw the whole production and sent us more FedEx packages than some of us have seen thus far in our lives. We also wish to thank the entire production department at Sinauer Associates: Christopher Small, Jefferson Johnson, who created an elegant book design, and Joanne Delphia, Janice Holabird, and Joan Gemme. Mike Demaray, Craig Durant, and colleagues at Dragonfly Media Group created the beautiful art program of this text. Christian Stilp at the University of Wisconsin provided the color spectrograms for the hearing unit. Rachel Shoup and Ingrid Johnsrude deserve special thanks for their help in making the book more readable and student-friendly. The following colleagues also deserve thanks for their helpful insights and comments: Marianne Dieterich (Ludwig-Maximilians-University of Munich, Germany), Henrik Ehrsson (Karolinska Institute, Sweden), George Gescheider (Hamilton College), and Roland Johansson (Umeå University, Sweden).

The following reviewers read and critiqued drafts of the text, and we are grateful for their expert assistance:

Michael T. Allen (University of Mississippi)

Deborah S. Briihl (Valdosta State University)

Elizabeth Bowering (Mount St. Vincent University, Canada)

Roger Cholewiak (Princeton University)

Walter Jay Dowling (University of Texas, Dallas)

Paula Goolkasian (University of North Carolina, Charlotte)

Lesley Hathorn (Kent State University)

Morton A. Heller (Eastern Illinois University)

Andrew M. Herbert (Rochester Institute of Technology)

Heide D. Island (Pacific University)

Ingrid Johnsrude (Queen's University, Canada)

Barbara J. Juhasz (Wesleyan University)

Zili Liu (University of California, Los Angeles)

Tyler S. Lorig (Washington and Lee University)

Fred Mast (Université de Lausanne, Switzerland)

Eriko Miyahara (California State University, Fullerton)

John Monahan (Central Michigan University)

Patrick Monnier (Colorado State University)

Richard Murray (York University, Canada)

David Peterzell (University of California, San Diego)

Michael Russell (Washburn University)

Lisa Sanders (University of Massachusetts)

Rachel Shoup (California State University, East Bay)

Ruth Spinks (University of Iowa)

Elizabeth Weiss (Ohio State University, Newark)

Finally, many, many colleagues sent us reprints and answered questions about points both specific and general. We gratefully acknowledge their help even if we cannot list all of their names. We are also indebted to the users of the text, students and faculty, who pointed out errors, typos, and other short-comings in the first edition. We hope we caught them all and we hope that the readers of this edition will continue to offer us assistance. If you find a flaw or if you have any other comment...even a positive one, please feel encouraged to let us know. You can use wolfe@search.bwh.harvard.edu as a point of contact for all of us.

Media and Supplements

eBOOK (ISBN 978-0-87893-957-2)

New for the Second Edition, *Sensation & Perception* is available as an online eBook, at a substantial discount off the list price of the printed textbook. The interactive eBook features a variety of tools and resources that make it flexible for instructors and effective for students. For instructors, the eBook offers an unprecedented opportunity to easily customize the textbook with the addition of notes, Web links, images, documents, and more. Students can readily bookmark pages, highlight text, add their own notes, and customize the display of the text. All of the Companion Website's resources are integrated into the eBook, so that students can easily access activities, Web essays, study questions, and more while reading the textbook. For more information, please visit www.sinauer.com/ebooks.

Also available is a **CourseSmart eBook** (ISBN 978-0-87893-937-4). This basic eBook reproduces the look of the printed book exactly, and includes convenient tools for searching the text, highlighting, and notes. For more information, please visit www.coursesmart.com.

FOR THE STUDENT

Companion Website (www.sinauer.com/wolfe2e)
The *Sensation & Perception*, Second Edition companion website provides students with a wealth of study and review materials to help them master the important concepts covered in the textbook. All of the site's content is keyed to textbook chapters, and Web activities and essays are referenced in the textbook. The site is available to students free of charge and includes the following resources:

- *Interactive Activities* lead students through important processes, phenomena, and structures. These exercises give students the opportunity to explore a variety of topics in an interactive, exploratory format, including: perception experiments, illusions that illustrate key concepts, models of cognitive processes, and interactive diagrams of important structures.
- *Web Essays* expand on selected topics from the textbook and provide additional coverage and examples.
- *Study Questions* are designed to give students the opportunity to test their mastery of the important concepts, processes, and terminology presented in the chapter.
- *Key Term Quizzes* help students master the hundreds of new terms introduced in the textbook.
- *Chapter Summaries* provide a detailed overview of each chapter's contents, and include a fill-in-the-blank review feature.

FOR THE INSTRUCTOR

(Available to qualified adopters)

INSTRUCTOR'S RESOURCE LIBRARY

(ISBN 978-0-87893-955-8)
The *Sensation & Perception*, Second Edition Instructor's Resource Library includes a wide range of resources to help instructors in course planning, lecture development, and student assessment. The IRL includes the following:

LECTURE RESOURCES

- *Textbook Figures and Tables*: All of the figures and tables from the textbook, formatted and color-adjusted for optimal legibility when projected. All images are provided as both high- and low-res JPEG files.
- *PowerPoint Presentations*: For each chapter of the textbook, the IRL includes two separate PowerPoint presentations:
  - *Figures & Tables*: All of the figures and tables from the chapter.
  - *Lecture*: A complete lecture presentation that consists of a detailed lecture outline with selected figures and tables inserted.

INSTRUCTOR'S MANUAL

The Instructor's Manual includes a variety of resources to aid in course development, lecture planning, and assessment. The Manual includes the following categories for each chapter of the textbook:

- *Chapter Overview*: The big picture synopsis of what the chapter covers.
- *Chapter Outline*: The outline structure of the chapter, including headings.
- *Chapter Summary*: A detailed breakdown of all the important concepts presented in the chapter.
- *Lecture Outline*: A suggested lecture for each chapter, presented in a slide-by-slide format designed for use in PowerPoint presentations.
- *References for Lecture Development*: A list of references for additional reading and course development on the topics presented in each chapter.

TEST BANK

A complete set of multiple-choice questions for each chapter of the textbook. Questions cover the full range of material covered in each chapter, and include both factual recall and conceptual questions. Some questions also include diagrams. The test bank is provided in several formats:

- *Microsoft Word*
- *Wimba Diploma*: This easy-to-use software allows you to quickly create quizzes and exams using any combination of publisher-provided questions and your own questions.
- *Blackboard* and *WebCT*

Also Available:

PsyCog: Explorations in Perception and Cognition

Robert A. Wyttenbach, *Cornell University*

(ISBN 978-0-87893-950-3)

Available either as a stand-alone or packaged with *Sensation & Perception*, *PsyCog* is a CD-ROM containing over 40 interactive demonstrations and 18 data-generating experiments in sensory and cognitive psychology. The demonstrations include interactive explanatory figures, demonstrations of phenomena, and common visual illusions for which the student can vary many parameters. The experiments generate quantitative data, including data files and graphs that can be saved and printed. Units include: Size and the Retina, Brightness and Contrast, Visual Motion, Depth Perception, Size Illusions, Sound Localization, Pitch Perception, Language, Visual Search, Attention, Iconic Memory, Echoic Memory, Scanning of Working Memory, Implicit Learning, Eyewitness Testimony, Mental Imagery, and more.

Sensation & Perception

SECOND EDITION

CHAPTER 1

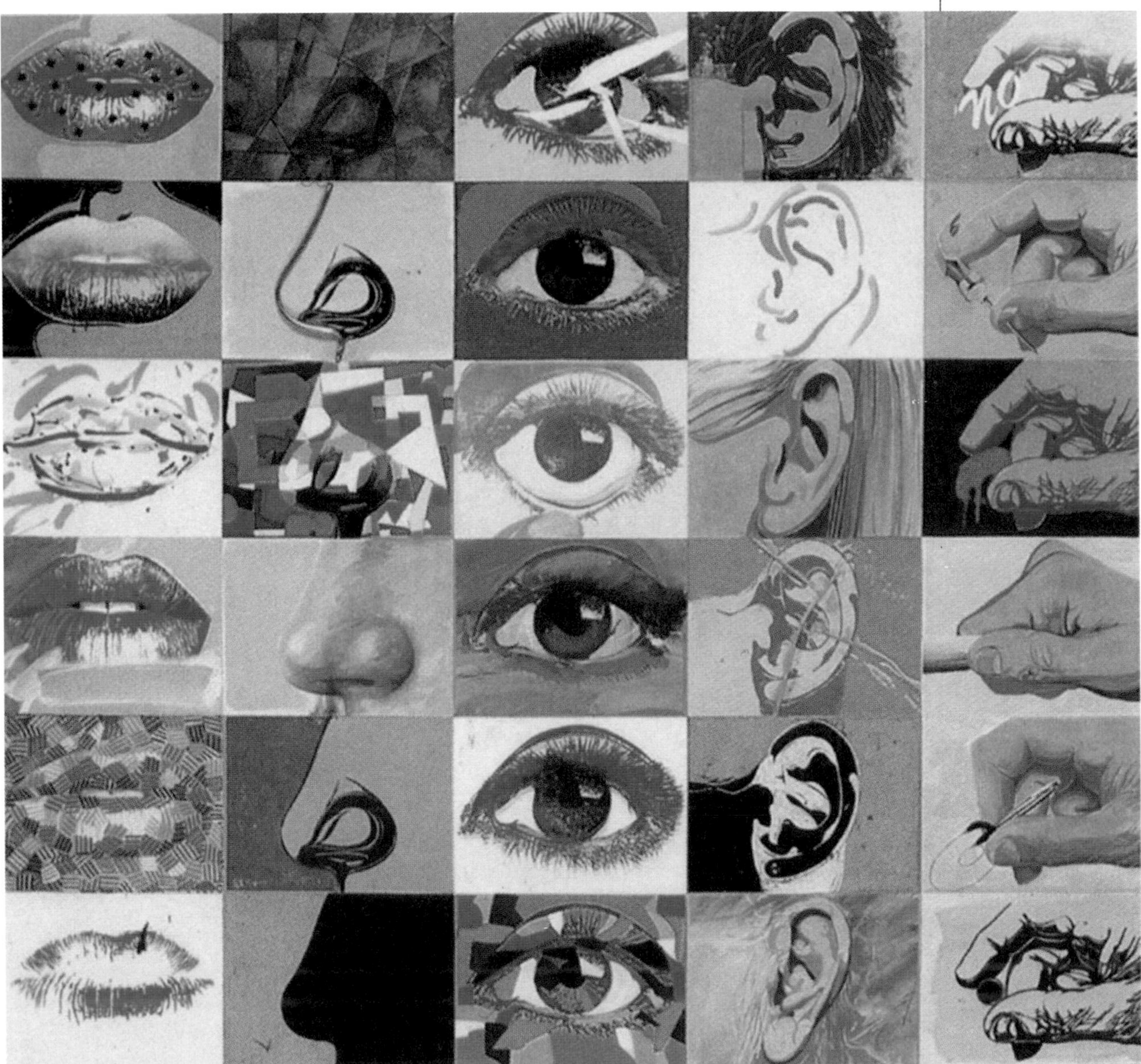

Paul Giovanopoulos, *Five Senses* (detail), 1990

Introduction

"What is real? How do you define real? If you're talking about what you can feel, what you can smell, what you can taste and see, then real is simply electrical signals interpreted by your brain. This is the world that you know." This is Morpheus's answer to Neo in the 1999 movie *The Matrix*, starring Laurence Fishburne and Keanu Reeves (**Figure 1.1**). You are about to embark on a journey to discover how we feel, how we see and hear, and how we smell and taste. Throughout this book, you will learn what has been discovered about how we know what is real—or at least, how we know what we *think* is real.

Early Philosophy of Perception

As you may know or suspect, people have asked these questions for a very long time, perhaps as long as humans have existed. *The Matrix* was actually inspired by "The Allegory of the Cave" in Plato's *Republic*, written in about 380 BCE. In this story, **Plato** (428–348 or 347 BCE) (**Figure 1.2**) compares our ordinary sense of reality to that of prisoners in a cave (**Figure 1.3**). He describes prisoners tethered together since childhood, able to see only the wall in front of them. Far behind them is a fire, and between the fire and the backs of the prisoners are men, sometimes talking and sometimes not, carrying statues and other objects. All the prisoners ever see are shadows on the wall in front of them. This is the prisoners' complete reality.

Plato paints this imaginary picture to emphasize how critically our conception of reality depends on what we can learn about the world through our senses. You do not have to think of yourself as a prisoner tied up in front of a wall, but you should appreciate the fact that almost everything you think is true about the world around you depends on what you can learn through your eyes, ears, nose, tongue, and skin. As you read this book, you will learn how you know what you know about the world around you.

Perception and your sense of reality are the products of evolution. Senses have evolved to help us act in ways that encourage our survival (**Figure 1.4**). If you were an animal moving through the environment, you would be at a great disadvantage if you could not use eyes or ears to gain information about the world around you. In general, our senses have evolved to match just the sorts of energy in the environment that are most important for our survival. For example, human vision is restricted to light in a very narrow band of the electromagnetic energy closely related to the energy that reaches the surface of the Earth from the sun.

Humans sense a subset of the energy that surrounds us (**Figure 1.5**). Other animals can sense energies that we cannot. Bees, for example, can see ultraviolet light that reveals patterns in flowers otherwise invisible to us (see Figure 5.26). Using a special organ in front of each eye (see Figure 1.5*b*), rat-

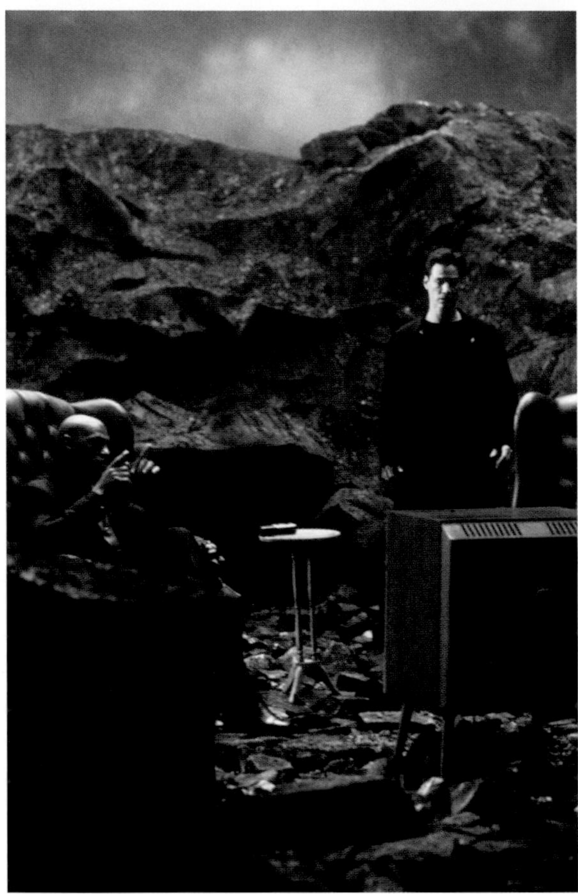

FIGURE 1.1 In the movie *The Matrix*, Morpheus (left) talks to Neo about the nature of reality. ©Warner Brothers.

tlesnakes and other pit vipers sense infrared energy that we cannot see, and they use this sense to locate their prey. Dogs and cats, not to mention bats, can hear sounds with higher frequencies than we can hear. Many birds, turtles, and amphibians are able to use magnetic fields to navigate. Elephants can hear very low-frequency sounds, and they may use this ability to communicate over long distances. As you sit quietly reading this book, you are being bombarded by many types of energy to which you are not sensitive. Although not as limited as the imaginary case of Plato's prisoners in a cave, your understanding of reality, and even your sense of imagination, is restricted to those things that you can perceive through your senses.

More than two millennia before the field of psychology existed and the first formal perception experiments were conducted, philosophers pondered the ways in which our perception of reality depends on our sensory experiences. **Heraclitus** (about 540–480 BCE), a very influential early Greek philosopher, lived about a century before Plato. He is best known for his famous statement, "You can never step into the same river twice." Heraclitus used this metaphor to stress his view that everything is always changing. Because the river flows continually past, the water a person steps into once is not the same water the next time. The same is true of our own perceptual experiences. No two experiences can ever be identical, because experiencing the first event changes the way we experience the same event a second time.

Several important facts follow from Heraclitus's simple observation. Perception does not depend *only* on energy and events that change in the world. Perception also depends on the qualities of the perceiver. Even when exactly the same event happens twice, it will not be perceived the same way twice, because the perceiver has changed following the first event.

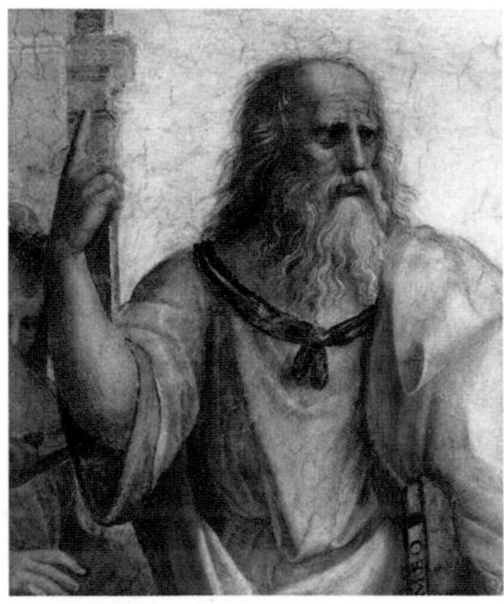

FIGURE 1.2 Plato lived during the golden age of Greece, a time when philosophers often were celebrities. Plato was an especially colorful person. Naked and covered in oil, he competed in the original Olympic Games. (He was younger then!)

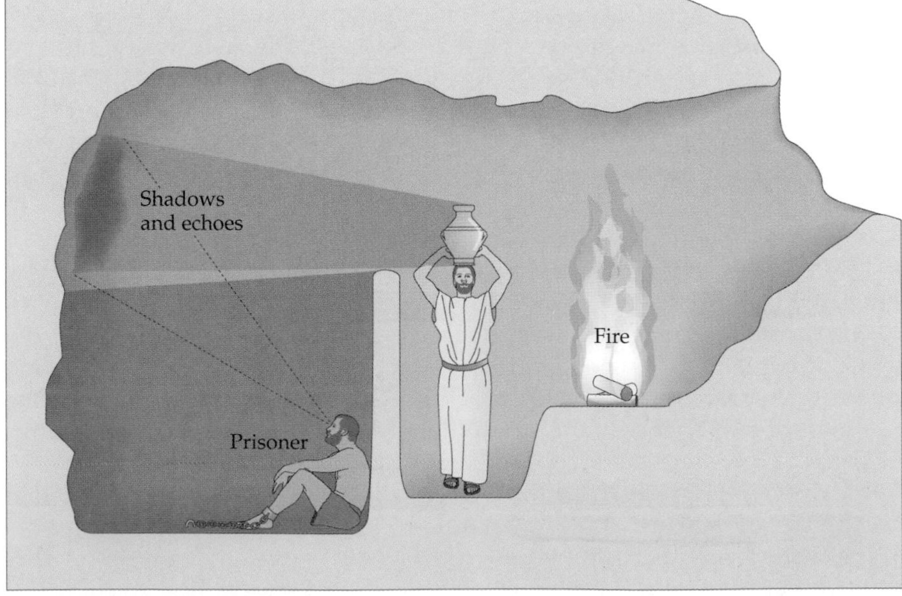

FIGURE 1.3 Prisoners in Plato's imaginary cave could learn about their world only from shadows on and echoes from the wall in front of them.

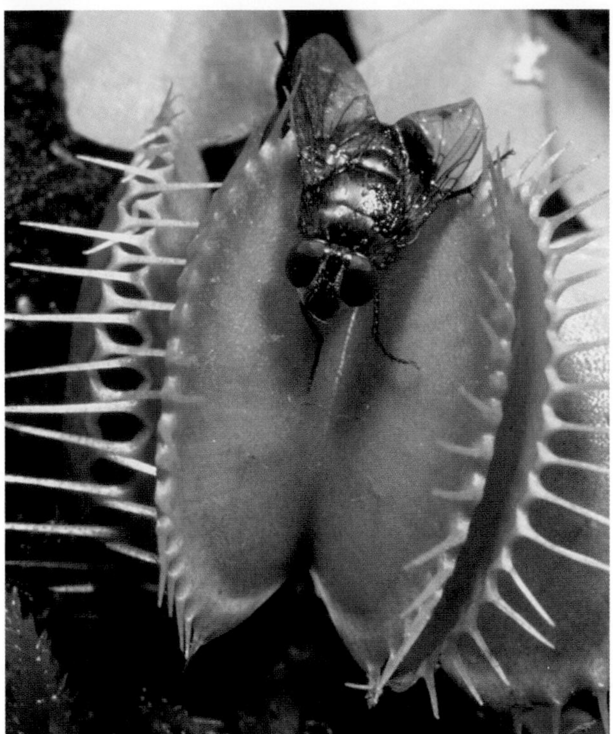

FIGURE 1.4 Sensory systems evolved to guide activity that is essential to survival. The Venus flytrap is one of the rare plants that can sense vibration in order to move quickly to capture prey.

Experience with the world around us plays a very large role in the way perception works, beginning very early in life. Even before birth, the sounds that the fetus hears will shape later listening. The structure of the environment around us, including cultural differences such as the speech and music we hear, molds the way perception works.

The idea that the world is continually changing is important for perception in another way. Perceptual systems are acutely sensitive to change. In

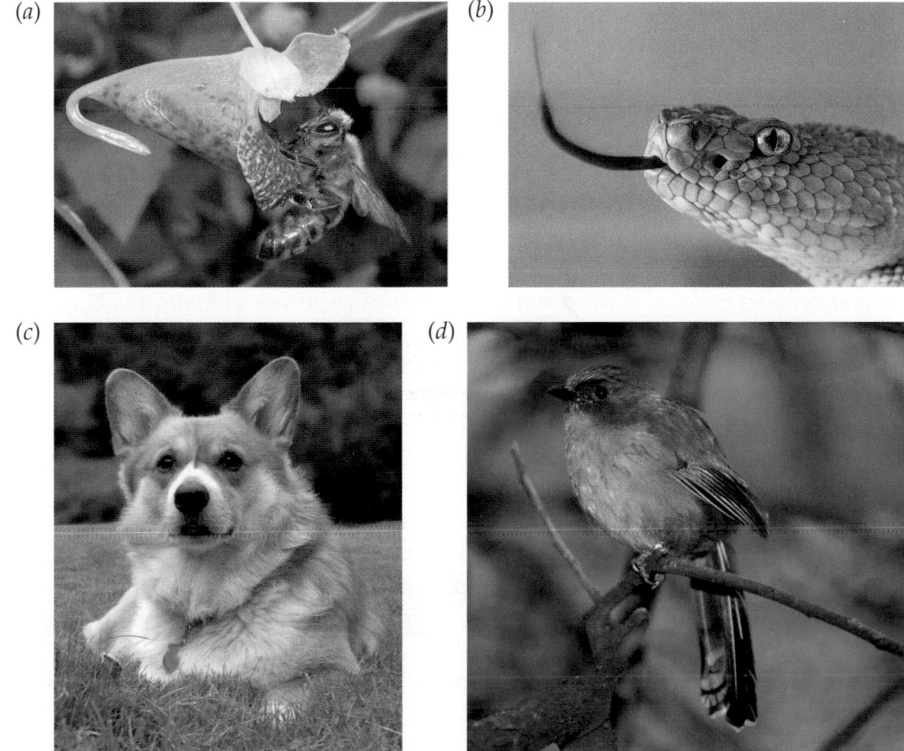

FIGURE 1.5 Our senses are capable of gaining information about only a tiny fraction of the energy and events that occur all around us. Honeybees (*a*), snakes (*b*), dogs (*c*), and birds (*d*) are able to sense a variety of stimuli that humans cannot (see the text for details).

adaptation A reduction in response caused by prior or continuing stimulation.

sensory transducer A receptor that converts physical energy from the environment into neural activity.

many different ways, every sense highlights and emphasizes changes around us. In fact, we tend to be quite unaware of things in our environment that do not change. Things that move draw our attention. Ambulance sirens constantly change in pitch so that drivers are more likely to notice them. The flip side is that perception quickly comes to ignore anything that stays the same for very long. The general mechanism is known as **adaptation**. All of our senses adapt to constant stimulation. For example, when we first arrive at someone's house, we may quickly detect a strong odor—perhaps mothballs, perfume, or dinner. Even though the odor is readily apparent, the olfactory (smell) system soon adapts to it, and we no longer notice it as much, if at all. Adaptation and other perceptual processes render things that are steady or predictable in the environment much less salient than things that are changing.

Unlike his contemporary Plato, the Greek philosopher **Democritus** (about 460–370 BCE) had almost complete trust in the senses. This trust arose from his radical idea that the world is made up of atoms that collide with one another. Of course, Democritus couldn't see these. It would be 2000 years before even simple microscopes were invented to visualize single-cell organisms. Nevertheless, he believed that sensations are caused by atoms leaving objects and making contact with our sense organs. For Democritus, this meant that our senses should be trusted because perception is the result of the physical interaction between the world and our bodies. He thought that the most reliable senses were those that detect the weight or texture of objects, because we are in direct contact with things when we make judgments of weight and texture. Democritus held that all the other qualities were secondary because they have to involve atoms moving from the object to interact with atoms of the perceiver.

Despite being way ahead of his time in suggesting the existence of atoms, Democritus did get some things wrong. It is usually light reflected from an object that allows us to see the object; there are no atomic films peeling off of visible objects. When we hear speech, our ears are detecting sound pressure waves, not atoms from a person's mouth. Taste and olfaction, our sense of smell, come closest to Democritus's theory. In those *chemical senses*, we detect molecules (not isolated atoms, but close enough) binding to receptors on the tongue or deep inside the nose.

Democritus made the distinction between *primary qualities* that can be directly perceived (weight, texture) and *secondary qualities* that require interaction between atoms from objects and atoms in the perceiver. We don't use these terms, but we honor something like this distinction when we talk about sensation and perception (as in the title of this book). The distinction between sensation and perception is not always clear. When we talk about *sensation*, however, we will be concerned with the ways that information from the world is picked up by sense organs and detected by the owners of those organs. Thus, we learn about the **sensory transducers** in eyes, ears, skin, nose, and tongue. A transducer is any substance or structure that changes energy from one form to another form. For every sense, transducers first transform information about the world—whether light, sound, pressure, or chemical composition—into neural signals that can be interpreted by the brain.

Perception deals with the interpretation of those signals. What does a specific pattern of activity in our nervous system tell us about the world outside? Perception is likely to depend more on experience than sensory reception does. For each of the senses discussed in this book, you will learn both about the very early sensory stages, including transducers and neural pathways, and about the complex perceptions that make up our understanding of the world. That said, a division between sensation and perception will not be clearly marked. It can't really be done. If you see a simple patch of red light in the dark, your simple sensation of red will coexist with a perception of red, colored by all the other reds you have ever experienced.

Nativism and Empiricism

Like many realms of psychology, the study of sensation and perception raises the distinction between nature (nativism) and nurture (experience, or empiricism). In this section we explore the two sides of this debate.

Nativism

Plato emphasized the limitations on what our senses can tell us about reality, claiming that the truest sense of reality comes from deep within people's minds and souls. Plato believed that the body and the mind are separate entities, and that certain mental abilities must be innate—a concept known as **nativism**.

Long after Plato, nativist **René Descartes** (1596–1650) (**Figure 1.6**) came to a similar conclusion concerning the relationship between mind and body. He argued that only humans have mind. In his view, similarities between humans and animals would be restricted to body structures and functions. For present purposes, we are interested in Descartes's **dualist** view of the mind. He considered the mind to be quite separate from the body. For Descartes, the mind is unextended (does not take up space) and has no substance. It is distinct from the body and survives the death of the body (like a soul). Like Plato, Descartes thought that all true ideas must come from the mind, and he did not trust his senses. Unlike Plato, who competed in ancient Olympic Games, Descartes was said to have been a very lazy young man. The monks at his church school used to throw buckets of water on young René to get him out of bed, where he would spend much time awake

nativism The idea that the mind produces ideas that are not derived from external sources, and that we have abilities that are innate and not learned.

dualism The idea that both mind and body exist.

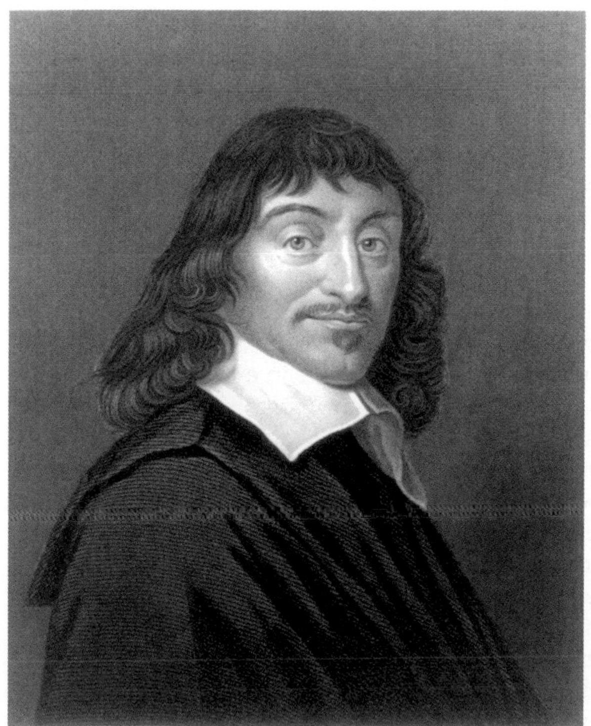

FIGURE 1.6 René Descartes was one of the most important philosophers of all time, and he was equally famous as a physicist, physiologist, and mathematician.

monism The idea that mind and matter are formed from, or reducible to, a single ultimate substance or principle of being.

materialism The idea that physical matter is the only reality, and everything including the mind can be explained in terms of matter and physical phenomena. Materialism is a type of monism.

mentalism The idea that the mind is the true reality and objects exist only as aspects of the mind's awareness. Mentalism is a type of monism.

mind–body dualism Originated by René Descartes, the idea positing the existence of two distinct principles of being in the universe: spirit/soul and matter/body.

empiricism The idea that experience from the senses is the only source of knowledge.

but pondering. Perhaps his attraction to the sedentary life was related to his most famous philosophical statement: *Cogito ergo sum* ("I think, therefore I am"). By this, Descartes asserts that his thinking mind (and not experiences) defines and proves his existence.

Thus far, the distinction between mind and body might seem sensible and consistent with the way you think about yourself and humans in general. People typically think of themselves as having a mind that takes in information about the world through the senses before choosing to act in particular ways on the basis of that information. Indeed, Paul Bloom (2004) believes that children come into the world ready to hold the dualist belief that humans have both material bodies and immaterial minds. The logical alternative to dualism is that humans, and the rest of the universe for that matter, are made up of only one kind of stuff. This position is known as **monism**. Among monists, those who hold that everything is matter embrace **materialism**, and those who hold that everything is mind embrace **mentalism**.

However natural a separation between mind and body may seem, there is a problem with **mind–body dualism**: how does that mind, having no substance and occupying no space, have any effect on the physical body? Philosophers continue to struggle with this problem.

Empiricism

You may ask what, if anything, all this has to do with learning about perception. As it turns out, much of the development of thinking about perception grew out of questions concerning the relationship between mind and body. The British philosopher **Thomas Hobbes** (1588–1679) (**Figure 1.7**) took this problem quite seriously and concluded that, for him, the only sensible answer is that only matter exists. Hobbes rejected the concept of spirit, or God, because such things would have no matter or bodies. Instead, he provided a mechanical model of humans and of society more broadly. In Hobbes's universe of matter alone, he argued that all knowledge must arise from the senses: "For there is no conception in a man's mind, which hath not at first, totally, or in parts, been begotten upon the organs of the Sense" (Hobbes, 1651/1914, p. 3). In short, Hobbes rejected the nativist ideas of Plato and Descartes. Instead, Hobbes was an **empiricist**, meaning that his model of human nature relies entirely on experience.

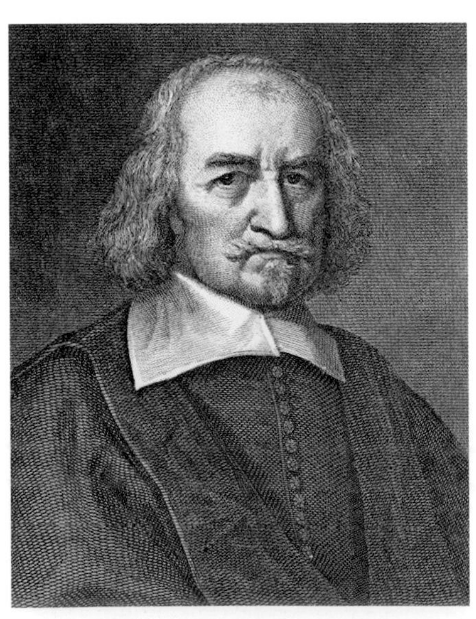

FIGURE 1.7 Thomas Hobbes believed that everything that could ever be known or even imagined had to be learned through the senses.

Because Hobbes viewed all mental activity as a consequence of experience, he had what may seem an especially dim view of memory, thinking, and imagination: he thought memories were simply sensory experiences that were old and faded. And thinking was little more than connections between memories. Because there would be nothing to the mind other than sensory experiences, imagination was not thought to be creative at all. Instead, Hobbes wrote that imagination "is nothing but *decaying sense*" (Hobbes, 1651/1914, p. 5).

John Locke (1632–1704) (**Figure 1.8**), another British philosopher, provided us with empiricism's most vivid image: that of the newborn mind as a *tabula rasa*, or "blank slate," on which experience writes. Like Hobbes, Locke suggested that all ideas must be created through experience. He believed that our rich experiences of the world around us, and our subsequent ideas about that world, all begin when the simple stimulation of our sense organs (eyes, ears, skin, nose, tongue) is conveyed to the mind. These first sensory impressions were called "simple ideas," and they may be thought of as primary qualities. Because they are simple and cannot be divided further, these sensory impressions are not the same as the experiences that we normally have with the world. For example, when we perceive a cat, our experience is the combination of different simple qualities, such as seeing the color, hearing the purr, feeling the fur, and smelling Meow Mix. The combination of these simple qualities comes only through experience.

Locke's ideas led to a famous exchange with the Irish scientist William Molyneux. Locke and Molyneux agreed that people who were born without sight but later gained the ability to see would not be able to recognize objects that they had previously only touched or heard because they had never seen the world with their eyes. To test this speculation, one would need to restore sight to the blind. This doesn't happen frequently. In some cases, however, the optics of the eye are opaque or translucent, and surgery can be performed to remove tissue and restore vision. In the days before anesthesia, operations on such patients were very rare. One famous case was that of a 13-year-old boy, operated on by William Cheselden (1688–1752) in 1728. There have been a modest number of cases since then. Locke and Molyneux probably overstated the visual problems of these individuals. Although such individuals do have real trouble with some aspects of vision (notably, the ability to use cues to depth; Fine et al., 2003), they are able to acquire significant visual abilities over time.

Studies undertaken as part of Project Prakash—a humanitarian and scientific effort to treat congenitally blind children in India and also study their subsequent visual recovery (http://web.mit.edu/bcs/sinha/prakash.html)—demonstrate that children can achieve visual proficiency on many tasks despite several years of blindness (Bouvrie and Sinha, 2007; Ostrovsky, Andalman, and Sinha, 2006). Interestingly, and sadly, many individuals who were treated in late adulthood are not made happier by being able to see, becoming quite depressed with their suddenly new world (Gregory and Wallace, 1963; Sacks, 1993). However, treatment during childhood, as in Project Prakash, does not appear to be accompanied by emotional disturbances.

During the 1700s, the Irish philosopher **George Berkeley** (1685–1753) (pronounced "Barkley") (**Figure 1.9***a*) was inspired by Molyneux's questions

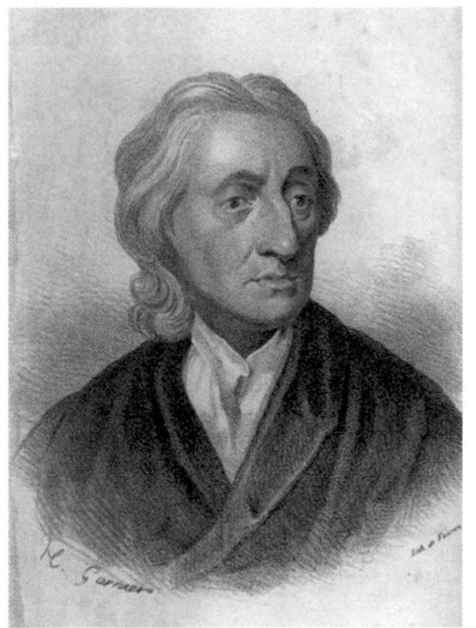

FIGURE 1.8 John Locke sought to explain how all thoughts, even complex ones, could be constructed from experience with a collection of sensations.

(*a*)

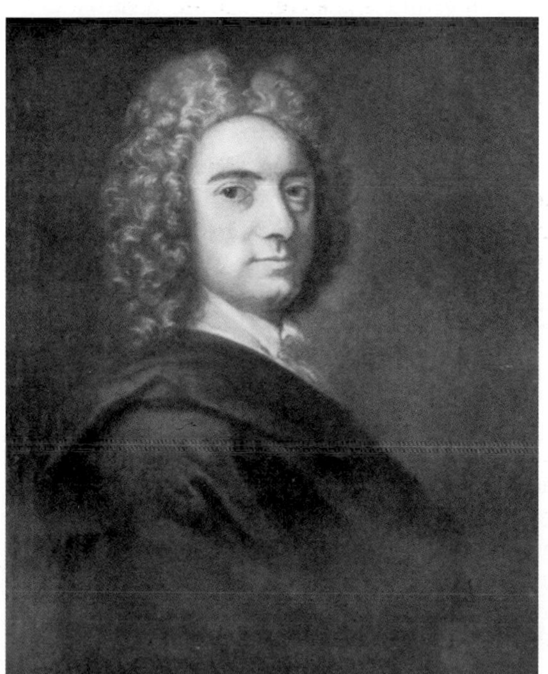

(*b*)

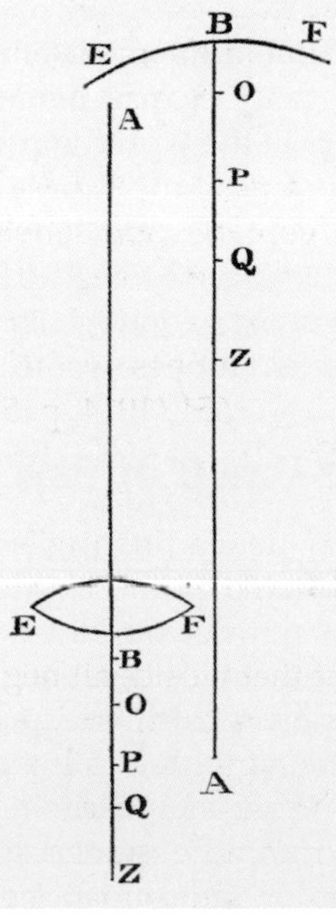

FIGURE 1.9 Berkeley's exploration of how vision works. (*a*) George Berkeley studied ways in which perception, such as perception of distance, is limited by the information available to us through our eyes. Nevertheless, he was convinced that everything we know must come from our sensory experience, no matter how limited it may be. (*b*) One of Berkeley's own drawings illustrating how difficult it is to know the distance of an object on the basis of light entering the eyes. (From Berkeley, 1837 [1709].)

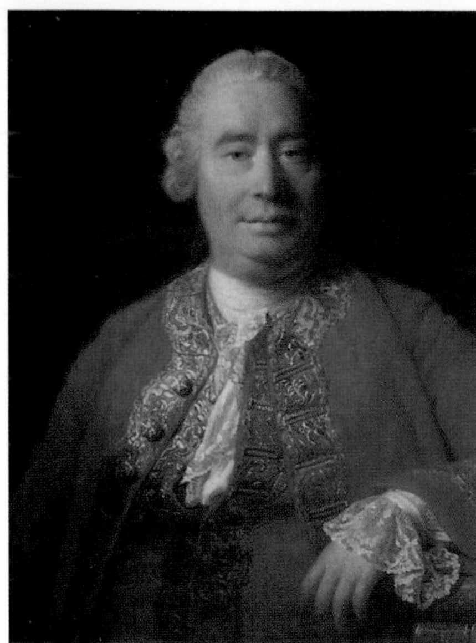

FIGURE 1.10 David Hume believed that we perceive the world as real because our senses are highly reliable, even if limitations on perception do not permit our perception to be completely valid.

about blind people being able to see again, and he was led to think seriously about how vision works. He began by asking the seemingly simple question of how we know how near or far objects are from us when we see them. As will be described in Chapter 6, Berkeley (1837 [1709]) was on the right track when he argued that no single strategy will always tell us how distant something is (Figure 1.9*b*). Instead, observers must use several visual cues to perceive distance. Berkeley concluded that we learn how to perceive distance by experiencing many objects and scenes in the world. When we do this, we learn how different visual cues change together at different distances. Through experience we learn how to use multiple visual cues to arrive at a pretty good estimate of where things are.

When Berkeley thought about perceiving distance, as well as seeing other parts of our visual world, he became convinced that the most important part of perception was experience with the world. Like Plato, Berkeley appreciated that there are limits on perception, no matter how much experience the perceiver has. Like Hobbes and Locke, in contrast, Berkeley concluded that all of our knowledge about the world must come from experience, no matter how limited perception may be. So strong was Berkeley's conviction, that he disagreed with Descartes's "I think, therefore I am," stating instead, *Esse est percipi* ("to be is to be perceived")—the world exists only to the extent that it is perceived. You've no doubt heard the question, "If a tree fell in the forest and no one was there to hear it, did it make a sound?" For Berkeley, if no one was there to hear (or see) it, the tree never existed in the first place.

With all this discussion about the limitations of perception, you may be asking yourself why the world seems so real. If we can see and hear only some wavelengths, and dimensions like size and distance are interpretations by the brain, why does the world around us seem so real and structured? **David Hume** (1711–1776) (**Figure 1.10**), perhaps the most significant of the British empiricists, offered a simple explanation based on the distinction between reliability and validity. *Reliability* refers to the consistency of measurements. Do we get pretty much the same answer every time? *Validity* refers to the relationship of the measurement to what is measured. A measure of your height can be very reliable, but it is not a valid measure of your performance in class. One may hope that exam grades are a more valid measure.

Hume argued that the world, as portrayed through our senses, seems very real because perception is highly reliable. Given the same state of affairs in the world, our senses deliver the same answers. Luckily, evolution has not permitted these answers to vary much from what is necessary for survival. The senses do their job the same way nearly all the time, so they reliably inform our activities in the world. Perceptual illusions are instances in which perception can be very reliable but not an accurate representation of the world. (See, for example, Chapters 3 and 7.)

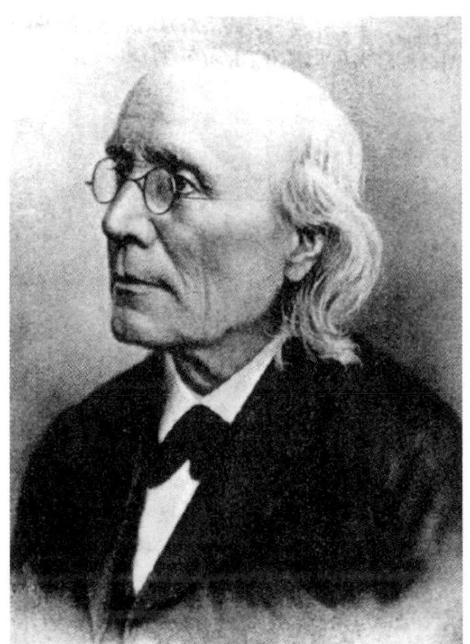

FIGURE 1.11 Gustav Fechner invented psychophysics and is thought by some to be the true founder of experimental psychology. Fechner is best known for his pioneering work relating changes in the physical world to changes in our psychological experiences.

The Dawn of Psychophysics

If you are reading this book as part of a college course, that course is probably offered in the Psychology Department, not in Philosophy. This placement reflects the development, starting in the nineteenth century, of an experimental science devoted to the study of sensation and perception. The position of this topic in psychology (or related fields like cognitive science) can be attributed to the philosophical history sketched in the preceding section. If our mental life relies on information from our senses, then it follows that the place for the study of the senses is within the science of human behavior and human mental life—that is, within psychology. Of course, this placement is not absolute. Researchers studying topics in sensation and perception can be found in biology, computer science, medicine, and many other fields.

To explore the move from philosophy to experimentation, we begin with the very interesting and versatile German scientist-philosopher **Gustav Fechner** (1801–1887) (**Figure 1.11**). Fechner is sometimes considered to be the true founder of experimental psychology (Boring, 1950), even if that title is usually given to Wilhelm Wundt (1832–1920), who began his work sometime later. Before making his first contributions to psychology, Fechner had an eventful personal history. Young Fechner earned his degree in medicine, but his interests turned from biological science to physics and mathematics. Though this might seem an unlikely way to get to psychology, events proved otherwise. Fechner was a very hardworking young scientist. He worked himself to exhaustion. In addition to being overworked, he suffered severe eye damage from gazing too much at the sun while performing vision experiments (a not uncommon problem for curious vision researchers in the days before reliable bright artificial light sources). Fechner fell into deep depression. Not only did he resign from his position at the university; he also withdrew from almost all of his friends and colleagues. For 3 years he spent almost all of his time alone with his thoughts.

Then, Gustav Fechner experienced what he believed to be a miracle when his vision began to recover quickly. His religious convictions deepened, and he became absorbed with the relationship between mind and matter. Fechner the physicist clearly wanted both mind and matter to exist, but he knew the problems with being a dualist. He proposed that the mind, or consciousness, was present in all of nature. This **panpsychism**—the idea that mind exists as a property of all matter—extended not only to animals, but to inanimate things as well. Fechner described his philosophy of panpsychism in a provocative book entitled *Nanna, or Concerning the Mental Life of Plants*. This title alone gives a pretty good idea of what Fechner had in mind.

Inspired by what we might consider to be somewhat unconventional ideas, Fechner took on the job of explaining the relation between the spiritual and material worlds: mind and body. From his experience as a physicist, Fechner thought it should be possible to describe the relation between mind and body using mathematics. His goal was to formally describe the relationship between sensation (mind) and the energy (matter) that gave rise to the sensation. He called both his methods and his theory **psychophysics** (*psycho* for mind, and *physics* for matter).

In his effort, Fechner was inspired by the findings of one of his Leipzig colleagues, **Ernst Weber** (1795–1878) (**Figure 1.12**), an anatomist and physiologist who was interested in touch. Weber tested the accuracy of our sense of touch using a device much like the compass we use when learning geometry. With this device, he could measure the smallest distance between two points that was required for a person to feel two points instead of one. Later, Fechner would call the distance between the points the **two-point touch threshold**. We will discuss two-point touch thresholds, and touch in general, in Chapter 12.

For Fechner, Weber's most important findings involved judgments of lifted weights. Weber would ask people to lift one standard weight (a weight that stayed the same over experimental trials) and one comparison weight that differed from the standard in incremental amounts. He found that the ability of a subject to detect the difference between the standard and comparison weights depended greatly on the weight of the standard. When the standard was relatively light, people were much better at detecting a small difference when they lifted the comparison weight. When the standard was

panpsychism The idea that all matter has consciousness.

psychophysics The science of defining quantitative relationships between physical and psychological (subjective) events.

two-point touch threshold The minimum distance at which two stimuli (e.g., two simultaneous touches) are just perceptible as separate.

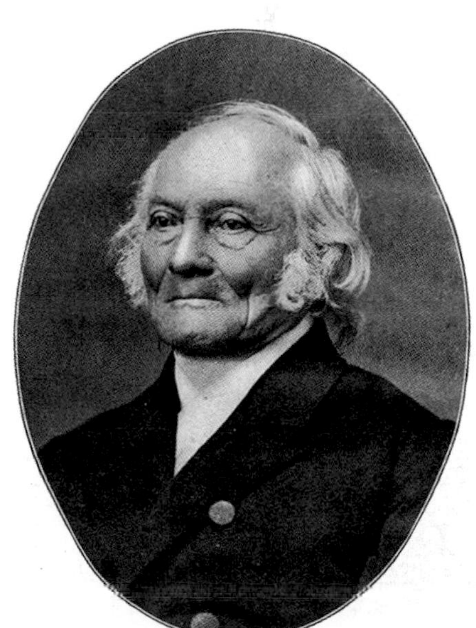

FIGURE 1.12 Ernst Weber discovered that the smallest detectable change in a stimulus, such as the weight of an object, is a constant proportion of the stimulus level. This relationship later became known as "Weber's law."

just noticeable difference (JND) (or difference threshold) The smallest detectable difference between two stimuli, or the minimum change in a stimulus that enables it to be correctly judged as different from a reference stimulus.

Weber fraction The constant of proportionality in Weber's law.

Weber's law The principle that the just noticeable difference (JND) is a constant fraction of the comparison stimulus.

Fechner's law A principle describing the relationship between stimulus and resulting sensation such that the magnitude of subjective sensation increases proportionally to the logarithm of the stimulus intensity.

heavier, people needed a bigger difference before they could detect the change. He called the difference required for detecting a change in weight the **just noticeable difference**, or **JND**. Another term for JND, the smallest change in a stimulus that can be detected, is the **difference threshold**.

Weber noticed that JNDs change in a systematic way. The smallest change in weight that could be detected was always close to one-fortieth of the standard weight. Thus, a 1-gram change could be detected when the standard weighed 40 grams, but a 10-gram change was required when the standard weighed 400 grams. Weber went on to test JNDs for a few other kinds of stimuli, such as judging the lengths of two lines, for which the ratio was only 1:100. For virtually every measure—whether brightness, pitch, or time—constant ratios describe our ability to detect change fairly well, except when intensities are very small or very large, nearing the minimum and maximum of our senses. In recognition of Weber's discovery, Fechner called these ratios, such as 1:40 and 1:100, **Weber fractions**. He also gave Weber's observation a mathematical formula. Fechner named the general rule—that the size of the detectable difference (ΔI) is a constant proportion (K) of the level of the stimulus (I)—**Weber's law**.

In Weber's findings, Fechner found what he was looking for: a way to describe the relationship between mind and matter. Fechner assumed that the smallest detectable change in a stimulus (ΔI) could be considered a unit of the mind because this is the smallest bit of change that is perceived. He then mathematically extended Weber's law to create what became known as **Fechner's law** (**Figure 1.13**), which is

$$S = k \log R$$

where S is the psychological sensation, which is equal to the logarithm of the physical stimulus level ($\log R$) multiplied by a constant k. This equation describes the fact that our psychological experience of the intensity of light, sound, smell, taste, or touch increases less quickly than the actual physical stimulus increases. With this equation, Fechner provided a mathematical expression that formally demonstrated a relationship between psyche and physics (psychophysics). As you learn about the senses when reading this book, you will find that we typically make a distinction between units of physical entities (light, sound) and measures of people's perception. For

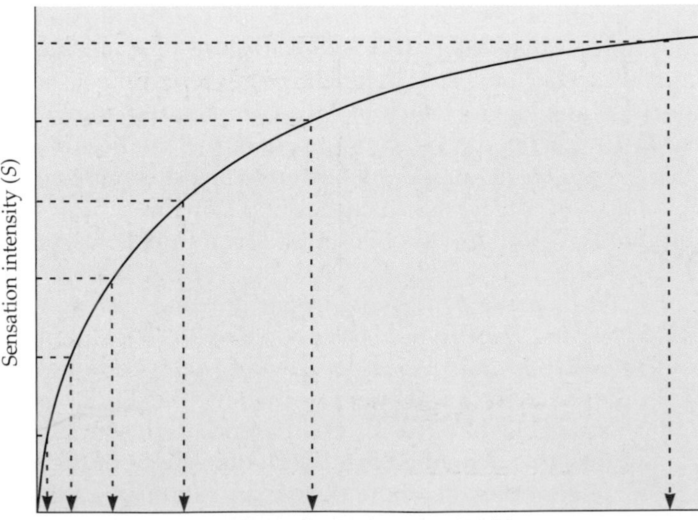

FIGURE 1.13 This illustration of Fechner's law shows that as stimulus intensity grows larger, larger changes are required for the changes to be detected by a perceiver.

TABLE 1.1 Some commonsense absolute thresholds

Sense	Threshold
Vision	Stars at night, or a candle flame 30 miles away on a dark, clear night
Hearing	A ticking watch 20 feet away, with no other noises
Taste	A teaspoon of sugar in 2 gallons of water
Smell	A drop of perfume in three rooms
Touch	The wing of a fly falling on your cheek from a height of 3 inches

Source: From Galanter, 1962.

absolute threshold The minimum amount of stimulation necessary for a person to detect a stimulus 50% of the time.

method of constant stimuli A psychophysical method in which many stimuli, ranging from rarely to almost always perceivable (or rarely to almost always perceivably different from a reference stimulus), are presented one at a time. Participants respond to each presentation: "yes/no," "same/different," and so on.

example, we measure the physical intensity of a sound (sound pressure level) in decibels, but we refer to our sensation as "loudness."

Fechner invented new ways to measure what people see, hear, and feel. All of these methods are still in use today. In explaining these methods here, we will use **absolute threshold** as an example because it is simpler to understand, but we would use the same methods to determine difference thresholds such as ΔI. An absolute threshold is the minimum intensity of a stimulus that can be detected (**Table 1.1**). For example, what is the faintest light, or quietest sound, or softest touch that can be detected? (See **Web Activity 1.1: Psychophysics.**)

Psychophysical Methods

How can we measure an absolute threshold in a valid and reliable manner? One method is known as the **method of constant stimuli**. The method requires creating many stimuli with different intensities in order to find the tiniest intensity that can be detected (**Figure 1.14**). If you have had a hearing test, you may recall having to report when you could and could not hear a tone that the audiologist played to you over headphones. In this test, intensities of all of the tones would be relatively low, not too far above or below the intensity where your threshold was expected to be. The tones, varying in intensity, would be presented randomly, and tones at each intensity would be presented multiple times. As the listener, your task would be to report whether

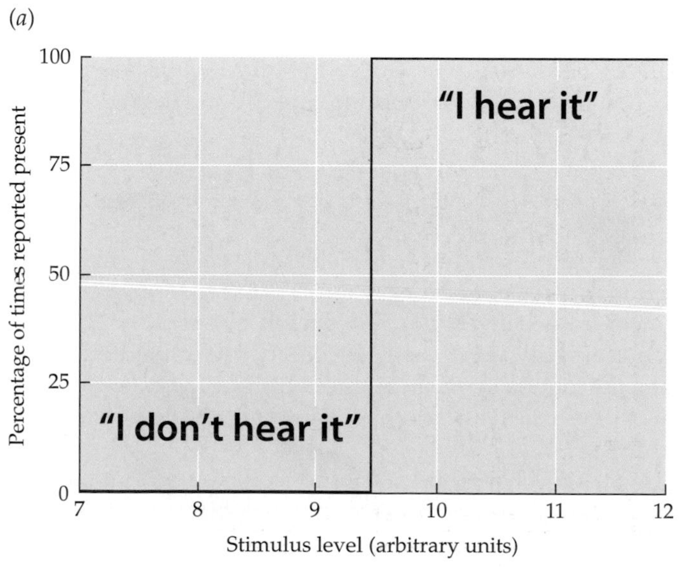

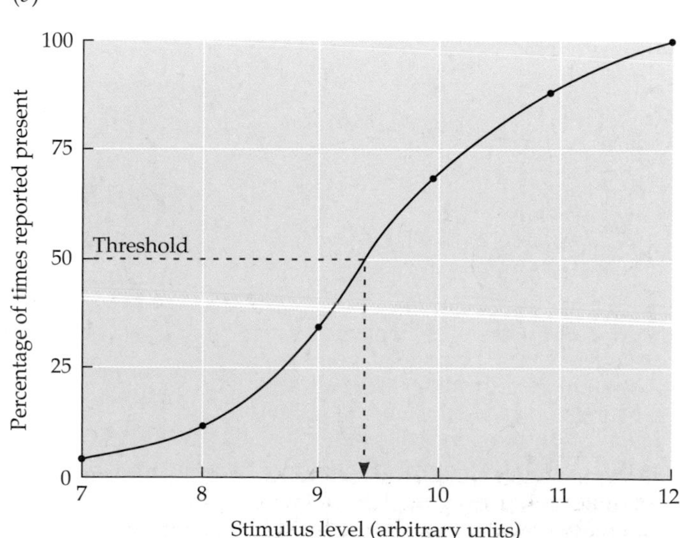

FIGURE 1.14 The method of constant stimuli. (*a*) We might expect threshold to be a sharp change in detection from never reported to always reported but this is not so. (*b*) In reality, experiments measuring absolute threshold produce shallower functions relating stimulus to response. A somewhat arbitrary point on the curve, often 50% detection, is designated as the threshold.

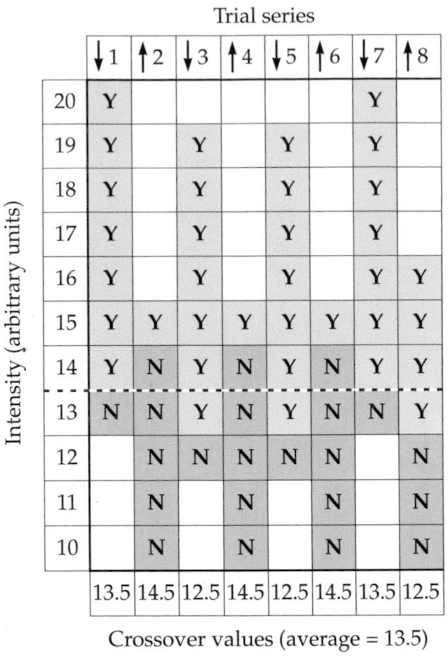

Trial series

Intensity (arbitrary units)	↓1	↑2	↓3	↑4	↓5	↑6	↓7	↑8
20	Y						Y	
19	Y		Y		Y		Y	
18	Y		Y		Y		Y	
17	Y		Y		Y		Y	
16	Y		Y		Y		Y	Y
15	Y	Y	Y	Y	Y	Y	Y	Y
14	Y	N	Y	N	Y	N	Y	Y
13	N	N	Y	N	Y	N	N	Y
12		N	N	N	N	N		N
11		N		N		N		N
10		N		N		N		N
	13.5	14.5	12.5	14.5	12.5	14.5	13.5	12.5

Crossover values (average = 13.5)

FIGURE 1.15 The method of limits. Here the subject attends to multiple series of trials. For each series, the intensity of the stimulus is gradually increased or decreased until the subject detects (Y) or fails to detect (N), respectively, the stimulus. For each series, an estimate of the threshold is taken to be the average of the stimulus level just before and after the change in perception.

you heard a tone or not. You would always report hearing a tone that was relatively far above threshold, and almost never report hearing a tone that was well below threshold. In-between, however, you would be more likely to hear some tone intensities than not hear them, and you would hear other lower intensities on only a few presentations. In general, the point at which a stimulus would be detected 50% of the time is chosen as the threshold.

That 50% definition of absolute threshold is rather interesting. Weren't we looking for a way to measure the weakest detectable stimulus? Using the hearing example, should that be a value below which we just can't hear anything (see Figure 1.14*a*)? It turns out that no such hard boundary exists. Because of variability in the nervous system, stimuli near threshold will be detected some of the time and missed other times. As a result, the function relating the probability of detection with the stimulus level will be more gradual (see Figure 1.14*b*) and we must settle for a somewhat arbitrary definition of an absolute threshold.

The method of constant stimuli is simple to use, but it can be somewhat inefficient in an experiment because much of the subject's time can be spent with stimuli that are clearly well above or below threshold. A somewhat more efficient approach is the **method of limits** (**Figure 1.15**). With this method, the experimenter begins with the same set of stimuli—in this case, tones that vary in intensity. Instead of a random presentation, tones are presented in order of increasing or decreasing intensity. When tones are presented in ascending order, from faintest to loudest, listeners are asked to report when they first hear the tone. With descending order, the task is to report when the tone is no longer audible. The data from an experiment such as this show that there is some "overshoot" in judgments. It usually takes more intensity to report hearing the tone when intensity is increasing, and it takes more decreases in intensity before a listener reports that the tone cannot be heard. We take the average of these crossover points—when listeners shift from reporting hearing the tone to not hearing the tone, and vice versa—to be the threshold.

The third and final of these classic measures of thresholds is the **method of adjustment**. This method is just like the method of limits, except the subject is the one who steadily increases or decreases the intensity of the stimulus. The method of adjustment may be the easiest method to understand because it is much like day-to-day activities such as adjusting the volume dial on a stereo or the dimmer switch for a light. But even though it's the easiest to understand, the method of adjustment is not usually used to measure thresholds. The method would be perfect if threshold data looked like Figure 1.14*a*. However, because reality is closer to Figure 1.14*b*, it is hard to get people to reliably adjust intensity to the same definition threshold across people and time.

Signal Detection Theory

Because thresholds are probabilistic, not really absolute, more sophisticated methods are required if we are to measure how sensitive people are to different stimuli. Let's continue our earlier discussion about why subjects' responses might not necessarily yield clear cutoffs in what they detect and do not detect. Perhaps the fact that people are not entirely consistent in their detection of the same stimulus says something more about the person than about just the stimulus.

One reason why thresholds change from trial to trial may be that subjects change from trial to trial. The stimulus presented to a subject is not the only source of activity in the perceptual system. Our auditory and visual systems

method of limits A psychophysical method in which the particular dimension of a stimulus, or the difference between two stimuli, is varied incrementally until the participant responds differently.

method of adjustment The method of limits for which the subject controls the change in the stimulus.

actually create energy, or "noise." One quick way to demonstrate this is to plug your ears with earplugs, or even just your fingertips. You will notice that you hear a faint rumbling noise generated inside your head. Similarly, if you close your eyes in a dark room, you still see something—a mottled pattern of gray with occasional brighter flashes. When you are trying to detect a faint sound or flash of light, you must detect it above and beyond any activity going on in your head in the first place.

Observers complicate the measurement of thresholds in another way as well: by bringing their own biases to a perception task. They might be more prepared or more motivated to hear or see some things than others. The overshoot that is found with the method of limits is one indicator of such a bias. When subjects are "tuned in" to detecting the stimulus, they are more likely to continue reporting that they detect the stimulus as the intensity of the stimulus is steadily decreased. The exact opposite happens when the subjects begin with stimuli that they cannot detect. It is easy to think of situations in which we would like observers to be especially biased toward detecting something. For example, you would want a radiologist looking at X-rays to be quite biased toward seeing defects when diagnosing whether or not you broke your leg. The cost of missing even a tiny crack could be very high when you tried to walk away from your appointment.

To get a feeling for the interaction of the stimulus and the observer, consider the following situation. You're in the shower. The water is making a noise that we will, imaginatively, call *noise*. Sometimes the noise will sound louder to you. Sometimes it will seem softer. We could plot the distribution of your perception of noise as shown in **Figure 1.16*a***.

Now the phone rings. We will call that the *signal*. Your perceptual task is to detect the signal in the presence of the noise. That signal is added to the noise, so we can imagine that now we have two distributions of responses in your nervous system: a noise-alone distribution and a signal-plus-noise distribution (Figure 1.16*b*).

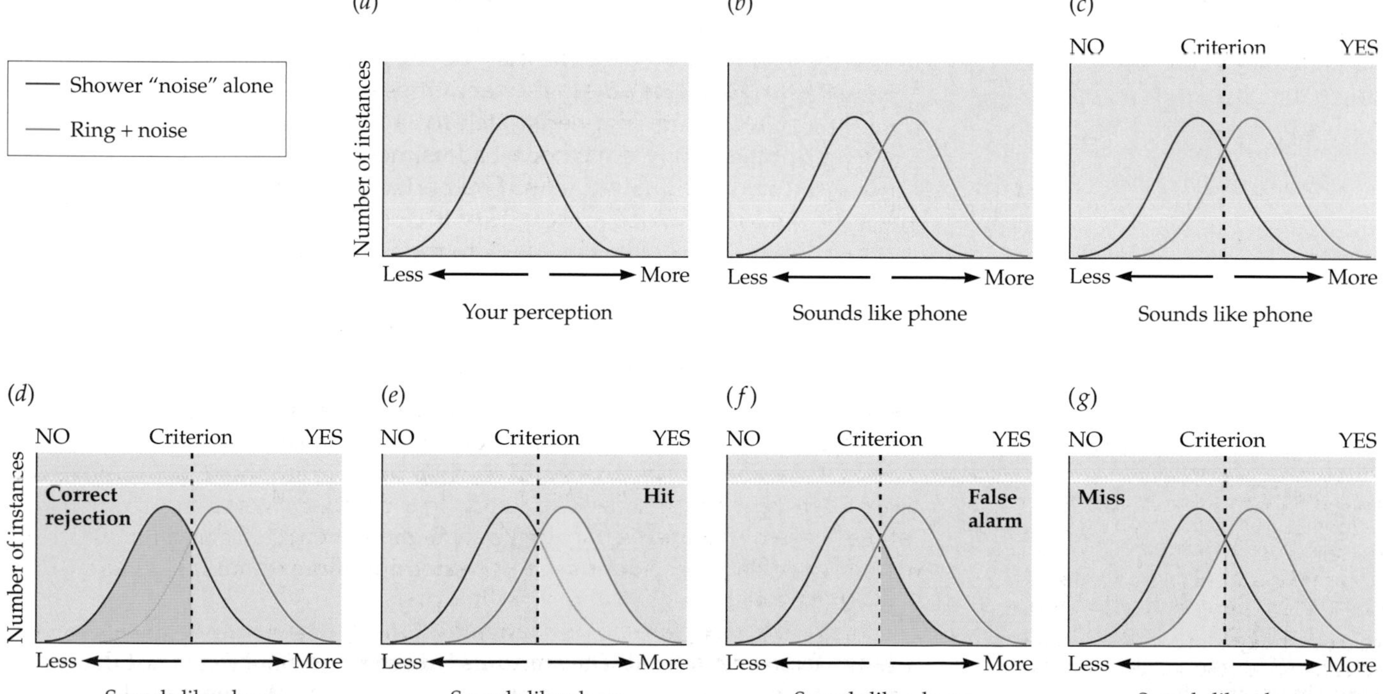

FIGURE 1.16 Detecting a stimulus using the signal detection theory (SDT) approach. (*a*) SDT assumes that all perceptual decisions must be made against a background of noise (the red curve) generated in the world or in the nervous system. (*b*) Your job is to distinguish nervous system responses due to noise alone (red) or to signal plus noise (blue). (*c*) The best you can do is establish a criterion (dotted line) and declare that you detect something if the response is above that criterion. That approach leads to four classes of responses: (*d*) correct rejections (you say "no" and there is, indeed, nothing there); (*e*) hits (you say "yes" and there is a signal); (*f*) false alarm errors (you say "yes" to nothing); and (*g*) miss errors (you say "no" to a real signal).

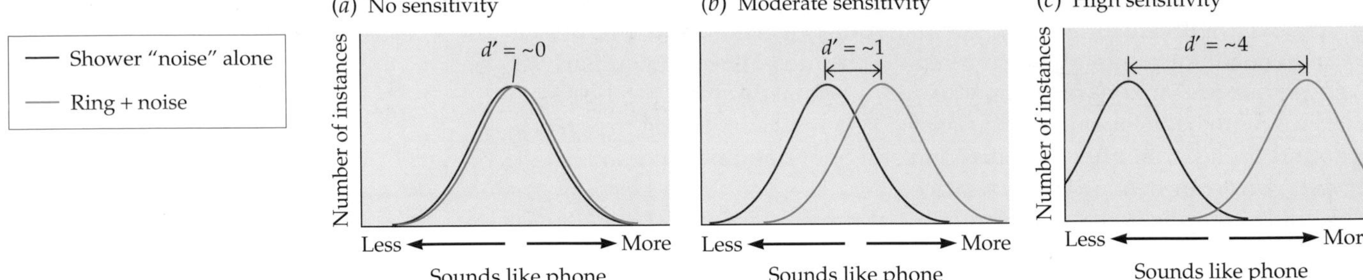

FIGURE 1.17 Your sensitivity to a stimulus is illustrated by the separation between the distributions of your response to noise alone and to signal plus noise. This separation is captured by the measure *d′* (pronounced "*d*-prime"). (*a*) If the distributions completely overlap, *d′* = 0 and you have no ability to detect the signal. (*b*) If *d′* is intermediate, you have some sensitivity but your performance will be imperfect. (*c*) If *d′* is big, then distinguishing signal from noise is trivial.

For the sake of simplicity, let's suppose that more response means that it sounds more like the phone is ringing. So now your job is to decide if it is time to jump out of the shower and answer what might be the phone. The problem is that you have no way of knowing at any given moment whether you're hearing noise alone or signal plus noise. The best you can do is to set up a criterion level of response (Figure 1.16*c*) that you will call a ring and jump out of the shower if the stimulus exceeds that response level. If the level is below the criterion, you will decide that it is not a ring and stay in the shower.

There are four possible outcomes (Figure 1.16*d–g*): You might say "no" when there is no ring; that's a *correct rejection* (1.16*d*). You might say "yes" when there is a ring; that's known as a *hit* (1.16*e*). Then there are the errors. If you jump out of the shower when there is no ring, that's a *false alarm* (1.16*f*). If you miss the call, that's a *miss* (1.16*g*).

How sensitive are you to the ring? In the graphs of Figure 1.16, the sensitivity is shown as the separation between the noise-alone and signal-plus-noise distributions. If the distributions are on top of each other (**Figure 1.17*a***), then you can't tell noise alone from signal plus noise. A false alarm is just as likely as a hit. By knowing the relationship of hits to false alarms, you can calculate a sensitivity measure known as *d′* (*d*-prime), which would be zero in Figure 1.17*a*.

In Figure 1.17*c*, we see the case of a large *d′*. Here you could detect essentially all the rings and never make a false alarm. The situation we have been discussing is in between (Figure 1.17*b*).

Now suppose you're waiting for an important call. You really don't want to miss the call, but you can't make yourself more sensitive. All you can do is move the criterion level of response, as shown in **Figure 1.18*a***.

If you shift your criterion to the left, you won't miss many calls, but you will make lots of false alarms (Figure 1.18*a*). If you shift to the right, you won't make those annoying false alarms, but now you will miss most of the calls (Figure 1.18*c*). For a fixed value of *d′*, changing the criterion changes the

FIGURE 1.18 For a fixed *d′*, all you can do is change the pattern of your errors by shifting the response criterion. If you don't want to miss any signals, you move your criterion to the left (*a*), but then you make more false alarms. If you don't like false alarms, you move to the right (*c*), but then you make more miss errors. In all these cases (*a–c*), your sensitivity, *d′*, remains the same.

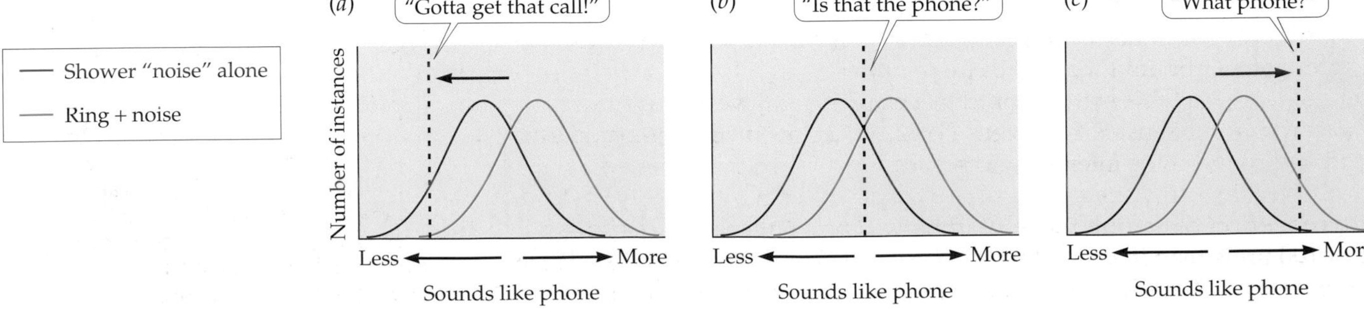

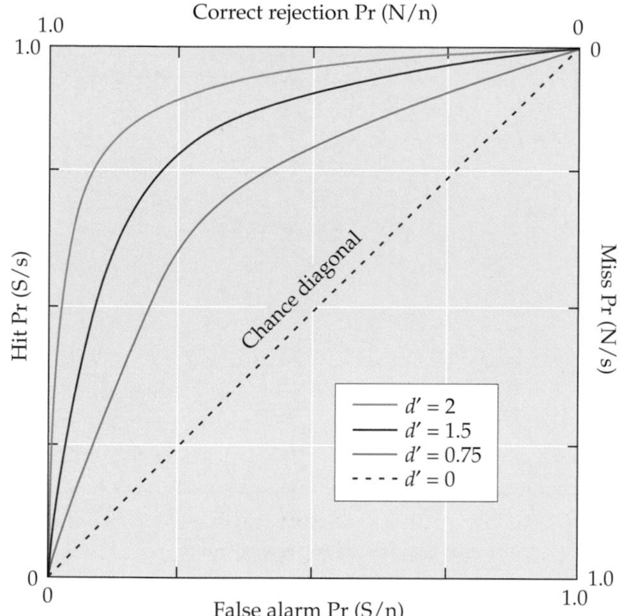

FIGURE 1.19 Theoretical receiver operating characteristics (ROC) curves for different values of d'. Note that $d' = 0$ when performance is at chance. When d' increases, the probability of hits and correct rejections increases, and the probability of misses and false alarms decreases. Pr(N/n), probability of response "no signal present" when no signal is present; Pr(N/s), probability of response "no signal present" when signal is present; Pr(S/n), probability of response "signal present" when no signal is present; Pr(S/s), probability of response "signal present" when signal is present.

hits and false alarms in predictable ways. If you plot hits against false alarms for different criterion values, you get a curve known as a **receiver operating characteristics (ROC) curve** (**Figure 1.19**).

The body of research that studies the detection of signals in noise in this manner is known as **signal detection theory** (D. M. Green and Swets, 1966). To learn about how to calculate d' and about ROC curves, there are many useful websites and numerous texts (e.g., Macmillan and Creelman, 2005).

Before concluding our discussion of psychophysical methods, we should describe one more method. A very straightforward way to address how strong a sensation is would be simply to ask subjects how they rate it. For example, we could play tones with different intensities varying from low to high and simply ask the subject to tell us, in a careful, controlled manner, how loud each tone sounds. One method of doing this is called **magnitude estimation**. When using magnitude estimation, we might ask listeners simply to assign a number of their choice to each sound level. The only requirement is that the numbers make sense for the listener (e.g., they are bigger for louder tones). Although this approach actually works pretty well with subjects choosing their own range of numbers, we can also begin the experiment by playing one tone at an intermediate level and telling the listener to label this level as a specific value—10, for instance. All of the responses should then be sensibly above or below this standard of 10.

One can also use **cross-modality matching** methods to get a measure of the strength of a stimulus. In cross-modality matching, a subject adjusts a stimulus of one sort to match the perceived magnitude of a stimulus of a completely different sort. For example, we might ask the listener to adjust the brightness of a light until it matches the loudness of the tone. It may be surprising to learn that this method produces similar results across subjects.

Harvard psychologist S. S. Stevens (1962, 1975) invented magnitude estimation and found some interesting cases for which Fechner's law would not work. If we have 10 units of stimulus energy, Fechner's law says that the perceptual effect of adding those 10 units will be smaller if we start with a base of 100 units than if we start with a base of 1. Think about candles. If we add the light of 10 candles to 1 candle, that will be a big change in perceived

receiver operating characteristics (ROC) curve In studies of signal detection, the graphical plot of the hit rate as a function of the false alarm rate. If these are the same, points fall on the diagonal, indicating that the observer cannot tell the difference between the presence and absence of the signal. As the observer's sensitivity increases, the curve bows upward toward the upper left corner. That point represents a perfect ability to distinguish signal from noise (100% hits, 0% false alarms).

signal detection theory A psychophysical theory that quantifies the response of an observer to the presentation of a signal in the presence of noise. Measures attained from a series of presentations are sensitivity (d') and criterion of the observer.

magnitude estimation A psychophysical method in which the participant assigns values according to perceived magnitudes of the stimuli.

cross-modality matching The ability to match the intensities of sensations that come from different sensory modalities. This ability enables insight into sensory differences. For example, a listener might adjust the brightness of a light until it matches the loudness of a tone.

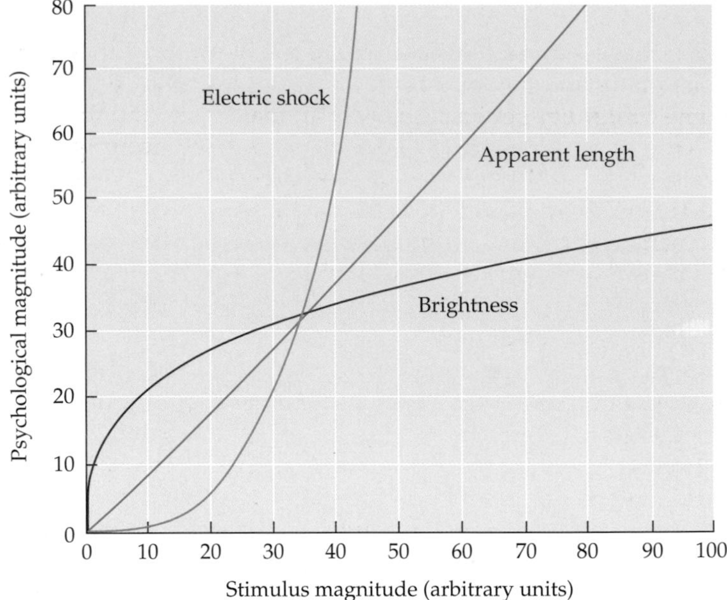

FIGURE 1.20 Magnitude estimation. The lines on this graph plot data from magnitude estimation experiments using electric shocks of different currents, lines of different lengths, and lights of different brightnesses. The exponents that describe these lines are 3.5, 1.1, and 0.33, respectively. For exponents greater than 1, such as for electric shock, Fechner's law does not hold, and Stevens' power law must be used instead. (From S. S. Stevens, 1961.)

Stevens' power law A principle describing the relationship between stimulus and resulting sensation, such that the magnitude of subjective sensation is proportional to the stimulus magnitude raised to an exponent.

brightness. If we add 10 to 100, that will be a modest change. Adding 10 to 10,000 won't even be noticeable.

Stevens found cases in which the sensation grows more rapidly than the physical stimulus. Consider, for example, the pain of electric shock. An increase in electrical current from 1 to 11 would be less dramatic than would an increase from 100 to 110. Stevens proposed what is now known as **Stevens' power law**: $S = aI^b$. It states that the sensation (S) is related to the stimulus intensity (I) by an exponent (b). So, for example, sensation might be intensity squared ($I \times I$). As **Figure 1.20** shows, stimuli like lights that followed Fechner's law quite closely have exponents less than 1 in Stevens' law (about 0.3 for brightness, for example). In the painful case of electric shock, the pain grows with I^3, so an increase of 10-fold in the voltage is 1000-fold in the pain! Properties like length have exponents near 1, so, reasonably enough, a 12-inch-long stick looks twice as long as a 6-inch stick.

At this point in our discussion of psychophysics, it is worth taking a moment to compare the three laws that have been presented: Weber's, Fechner's, and Stevens'. Weber's law involves a clear objective measurement. We know how much we varied the stimulus, and either subjects can tell that the stimulus changed or they cannot. Fechner's law begins with the same sort of objective measurements as Weber's, but the law is actually a calculation based on some assumptions about how sensation works. In particular, Fechner's law assumes that all JNDs are perceptually equivalent. In fact, this turns out to be incorrect and leads to some places where the "law" is violated. Finally, Stevens' law describes rating data quite well, but notice that rating data are qualitatively different from the data for Weber's law. We can record the subjects' ratings and we can check whether those ratings are reasonable and consistent, but there is no way to know whether they are objectively right or wrong.

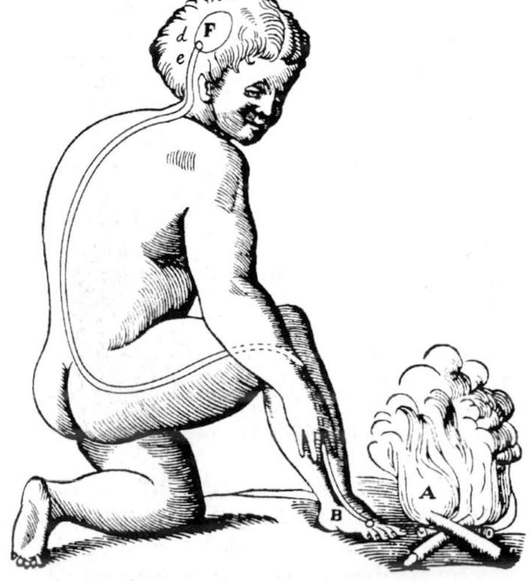

FIGURE 1.21 René Descartes's drawing illustrating his understanding of the reflex of pulling one's foot away from a flame.

The Biology of Perception

During the nineteenth century, when Weber and Fechner were initiating the experimental study of perception, physiologists also were hard at work learning how the senses and the brain operate. Much of this work involved research on animals. It is worth spending a moment on a key assumption here: that studies of animal senses tell us something about human senses. That may seem obvious but the assumption requires the belief that there is some continuity between the way animals work and the way humans work.

One of the intellectual developments that encouraged the study of animals can be attributed to René Descartes. Because of his philosophy of body and mind, Descartes claimed that animals were in most ways very similar to humans. His only distinction between humans and animals was that humans have minds and souls, so he believed that studying animals was a good way to learn about the material parts of humans. Descartes was very interested in learning more about the inner structure of bodies and brains, and he actually dissected both. He proposed that animal spirits (which were matter, not mind—somewhat like mineral spirits or alcoholic beverages) enter the brain and exit through pores that guide this fluid through nerves to muscles (**Figure 1.21**). In effect, he thought of animals as hydraulic machines and humans as machines with the addition of mind and soul.

For anyone who was not a dualist like Descartes, it was a rather short step from Descartes's view of animals to a view that humans, too, are just machines. A famous version of this view can be found in Julien Offray de La Mettrie's (1709–1751) book entitled *Man: A Machine* (La Mettrie, 1912). Étienne Bonnot de Condillac (1715–1780), a French contemporary of La Mettrie, used the metaphor of the *sentient statue* to argue that all forms of thought could be developed through only one's sensations. Both La Mettrie and Condillac suggested that animals would be useful in understanding humans. Even modern researchers who share these strongly *materialist* views are unlikely to think of humans or animals as mindless automatons. Instead, there has been a great deal of work in recent years on humanlike qualities of what could be called the animal mind (Wasserman and Zentall, 2006).

The most powerful argument for a continuity between humans and animals came from Darwin's theory of evolution. During the 1800s, Charles Darwin (1809–1882) proposed his revolutionary theory in *The Origin of Species* (1859). Although many of the ideas found in that book had been brewing for some time, controversy expanded with vigor following Darwin's provocative arguments about how humans evolved from apes, in *The Descent of Man* (1871). If there was continuity between the structure of the bones, heart, and kidneys of cows, dogs, monkeys, and humans, then why wouldn't there be continuity between the structure and function of their respective senses and nervous systems? An inescapable implication of the theory of evolution is that we can learn much about human sensation and perception by studying the structure and function of our nonhuman relatives.

At the same time that Darwin was at work in England, the German physiologist **Johannes Müller** (1801–1858) (**Figure 1.22**) was writing a very influential book, his *Handbook of Physiology* (1838/1912). In this book, in addition to covering most of what was then known about physiology, Müller formulated the **doctrine of specific nerve energies**. The central idea of this doctrine was expressed well in Morpheus's statement to Neo quoted at the beginning of this chapter: we are aware only of the activity in our nerves, and we cannot be aware of the world itself. Further, what is most important is *which* nerves are stimulated, and not *how* they are stimulated. For example, we see because the optic nerve leading from the eye to the brain is stimulated, but it does not matter whether light, or something else, stimulated the nerve. To prove to yourself that this is true, close your eyes and press very gently on the outside corner of one eye through the lid. (This works better in a darkened room.) You will see a spot of light toward the inside of your visual field by your nose. Despite the lack of stimulation by light, your brain interprets the input from your optic nerve as informing you about something visual.

doctrine of specific nerve energies A doctrine formulated by Johannes Müller stating that the nature of a sensation depends on which sensory fibers are stimulated, not on how fibers are stimulated.

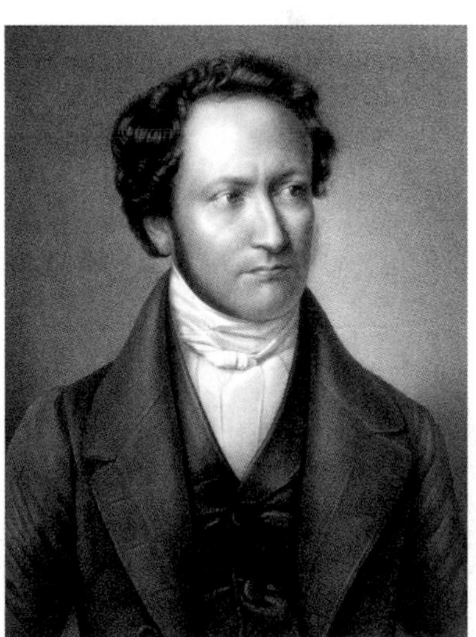

FIGURE 1.22 Johannes Müller formulated the doctrine of specific nerve energies, which says that we are aware only of the activity in our nerves, and we cannot be aware of the world itself. For this reason, what is most important is *which* nerves are stimulated, not *how* they are stimulated.

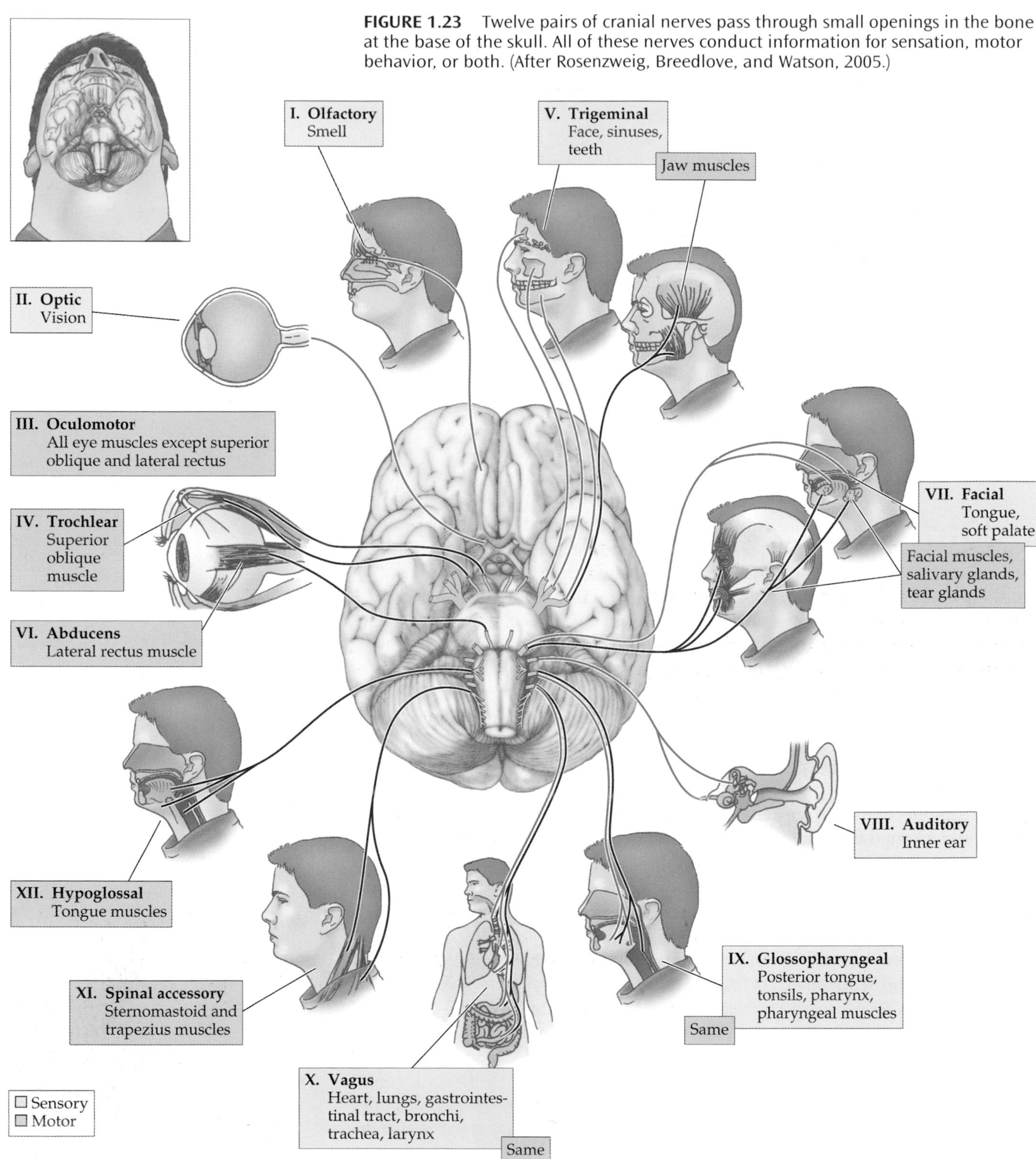

FIGURE 1.23 Twelve pairs of cranial nerves pass through small openings in the bone at the base of the skull. All of these nerves conduct information for sensation, motor behavior, or both. (After Rosenzweig, Breedlove, and Watson, 2005.)

cranial nerves Twelve pairs of nerves (one for each side of the body) that originate in the brain stem and reach sense organs and muscles through openings in the skull.

The **cranial nerves** leading into and out of the skull illustrate the doctrine of specific nerve energies (**Figure 1.23**). The pair of optic nerves is one of 12 pairs of cranial nerves that pass through small openings in the bone at the base of the skull. The cranial nerves are dedicated mainly to sensory and motor systems. Cranial nerves are labeled both by name and by the Roman numeral

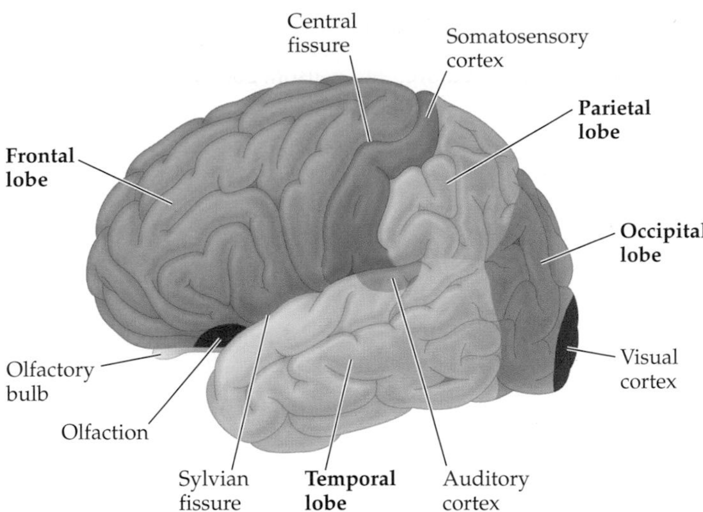

FIGURE 1.24 Cortex of the human brain. The darkened areas are dedicated primarily to processing information for individual senses.

that roughly corresponds to the order of their locations beginning from the front of the skull. Three of the cranial nerves—**olfactory (I)**, **optic (II)**, and **auditory (VIII)**—are exclusively dedicated to sensory information. Three more—**oculomotor (III)**, **trochlear (IV)**, and **abducens (VI)**—are dedicated to muscles that move the eyes. The other six cranial nerves either are exclusively motor (spinal accessory [XI] and hypoglossal [XII]) or convey both sensory and motor signals (trigeminal [V], facial [VII], glossopharyngeal [IX], and vagus [X]). With respect to our study of perception, later we will return to the first six cranial nerves described here, because each one plays an important role in our ability to use our senses to learn about the world around us.

Just as cranial nerves are dedicated to individual sensory and motor tasks, areas of the brain stem and cerebral cortex are similarly dedicated to particular tasks. Areas of the cortex dedicated to perception actually are much larger than the darkened areas in **Figure 1.24**. The areas depicted here are primary sensory areas, and more complex processing is accomplished across cortical regions that spread well beyond these primary areas. For example, visual perception uses cortex that extends both anteriorly (forward) into parietal cortex and ventrally (lower) into regions of the temporal lobe. In addition, as processing extends beyond primary areas, cortex often becomes **polysensory**, meaning that information from more than one sense is being combined in some manner. (See Web Activity 1.2: Sensory Areas in the Brain.)

olfactory (I) nerves The first pair of cranial nerves, which conduct impulses from the mucous membranes of the nose to the olfactory bulb.

optic (II) nerves The second pair of cranial nerves, which arise from the retina and carry visual information to the thalamus and other parts of the brain.

auditory (VIII) nerves The eighth pair of cranial nerves, which connect the inner ear with the brain, transmitting impulses concerned with hearing and balance. The auditory nerve is composed of the cochlear nerve and the vestibular nerve and therefore is sometimes referred to as the "vestibulocochlear nerve."

oculomotor (III) nerves The third pair of cranial nerves, which innervate all the extrinsic muscles of the eye except the lateral rectus and the superior oblique muscles, and which innervate the elevator muscle of the upper eyelid, the ciliary muscle, and the sphincter muscle of the pupil.

trochlear (IV) nerves The fourth pair of cranial nerves, which innervate the superior oblique muscles of the eyeballs.

abducens (VI) nerves The sixth pair of cranial nerves, which innervate the lateral rectus muscle of each eye.

polysensory Blending multiple sensory systems.

Hermann von Helmholtz

Hermann Ludwig Ferdinand von Helmholtz (1821–1894) (**Figure 1.25**), one of the greatest scientists of the nineteenth century, was greatly influenced by Müller at the University of Berlin. Helmholtz really wanted to study physics, but financial constraints led instead to his becoming a surgeon in exchange for having his tuition covered. Following his required service as a surgeon, Helmholtz became a junior professor of physiology at the Univer-

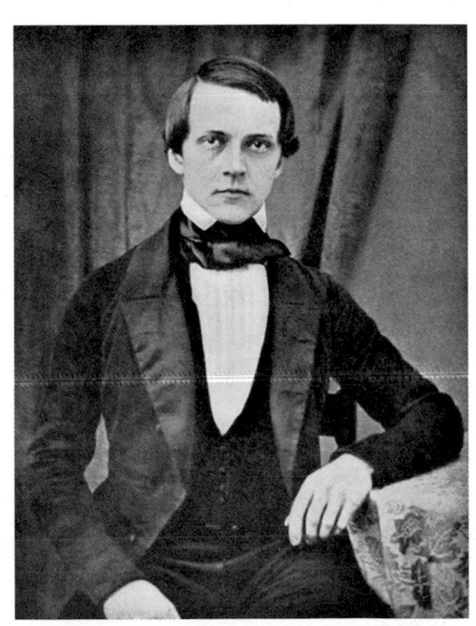

FIGURE 1.25 Hermann von Helmholtz was one of the greatest scientists of all time. He made many important discoveries in physiology and perception.

vitalism The idea that "vital forces" are active within living organisms, and these forces cannot be explained by physical processes of matter more generally.

sity of Königsberg. Although he was initially inspired by Müller, he truly disliked one of Müller's ideas.

Müller believed in **vitalism**, the idea that there is a force in life that is distinct from physical entities. It is easy to see how vitalism fit well with the dualism of Descartes or, perhaps, the panpsychism of Fechner. Remember that Helmholtz really wanted to be a physicist, not a surgeon. He was an empiricist, in the tradition of Hobbes, Locke, Hume, and Berkeley. Like Thomas Hobbes, Helmholtz thought that all behavior should be explained by only physical forces. Vitalism violated the physical law of conservation of energy, and Helmholtz wanted the brain and behavior to obey purely physical laws. He chose a very smart place to begin his attack on vitalism. Müller had claimed that the nerve impulse could never be measured experimentally. So, Helmholtz set out to show that the activity of neurons obeys normal rules of physics and chemistry, by being the first to effectively measure how fast neurons transmit their signals. (See **Web Activity 1.3: Neurons**.)

When thinking about perception, it is very important that we understand how long it takes for our brains to know what is happening in the world, and this requires knowing how fast nerve impulses are. At the time of Helmholtz's work, estimates ranged from 150 feet per second to as fast as 57,600 million feet per second—nearly 60 times the speed of light! Helmholtz thought that the fastest estimates must surely be wrong. If neurons truly were that fast, they would violate normal laws of physics and Müller could be right about vitalism.

In an early effort, Helmholtz estimated that the speed of signal transmission in the nerves in frog legs was only about 90 feet per second. Later he concluded that sensory nerves in people transmitted signals at between 165 and 330 feet per second. In all cases, this transmission was slower than many people believed at the time. Helmholtz emphasized this point when he noted that a "whale probably feels a wound near its tail in about one second, and requires another second to send back orders to the tail to defend itself" (Koenigsberger, 1906/1965, p. 72). As you may already have guessed, not all neurons are equal when it comes to speed; some are faster than others. It's still interesting to realize that you stub your toe a measurable amount of time before you feel that you have stubbed your toe.

When Helmholtz became interested in vision, he invented something completely new to study the eye: the ophthalmoscope. Optometrists use this device to look directly at the retina, the sheet of blood vessels, receptors, and neurons across the back of the eye. In addition to assisting in diagnosing problems with the eye, the ophthalmoscope enables us to see the only part of the central nervous system that is visible from outside the skull. This invention was extremely valuable to physicians, and Helmholtz did financially well selling ophthalmoscopes.

Helmholtz also made major discoveries about hearing. His book *On the Sensations of Tone* (1863/1954) begins as the study of music and perception. True to Helmholtz's love of physics, the text also became the classic book on vibration, particularly vibration in sound. Helmholtz conducted many listening experiments using resonators (**Figure 1.26**), and he was the first to hypothesize that our ability to hear sounds with different pitches depends on where sounds cause the most activity along the cochlea, a tiny snail-shaped structure of the ear that you will learn about in Chapter 9.

Neuronal Connections

During the second half of the nineteenth century, when Helmholtz was making stunning discoveries concerning vision and hearing, other scientists

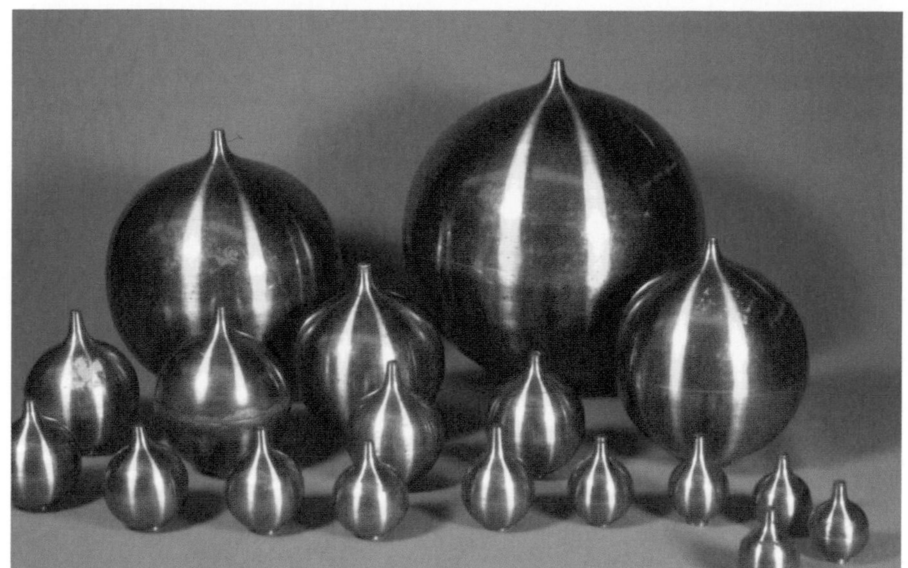

FIGURE 1.26 Helmholtz teamed up with Rudolph Koenig to create these resonators, now known as "Helmholtz resonators." Each resonator is tuned precisely to a certain frequency of vibration, and when the thin end is held at the ear, listeners can pick out a specific frequency from a complex sound. (Courtesy of Thomas B. Greenslade, Jr.)

were learning a great deal about how neurons and brains work. After nearly dying of malaria in Cuba, the Spaniard **Santiago Ramón y Cajal** (1852–1934) (**Figure 1.27***a*) returned to his homeland to develop some of the most painstaking and breathtaking insights into the organization of neurons in the brain. Spending many hours over a microscope, he made the most spectacular detailed drawings of neurons and their connections ever created. Figure 1.27*b* shows an example.

(*a*) (*b*)

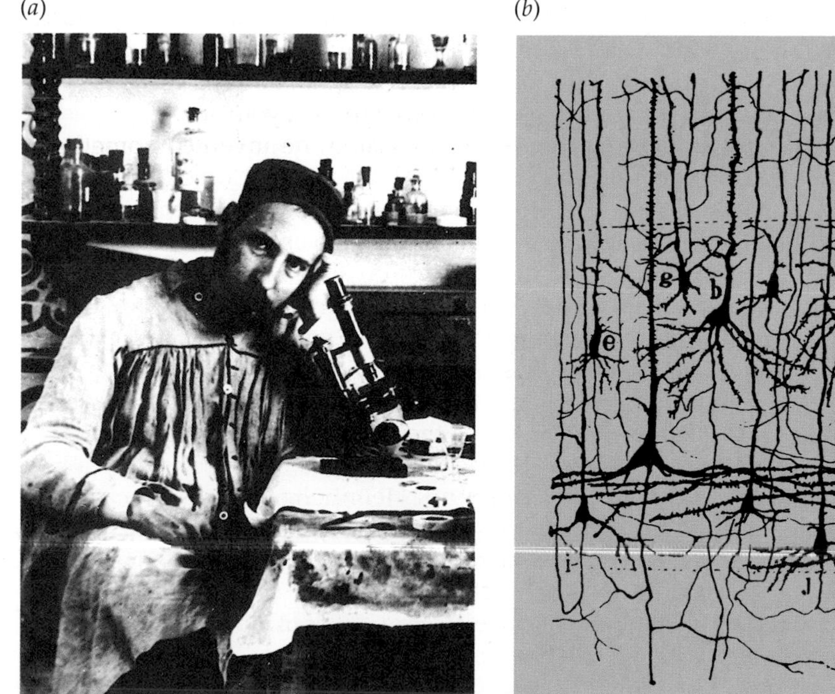

FIGURE 1.27 Santiago Ramón y Cajal (*a*) created these drawings (*b*) of brain neurons while peering into a microscope for many hours. Because of his painstaking care and accuracy, his early drawings are still cited today.

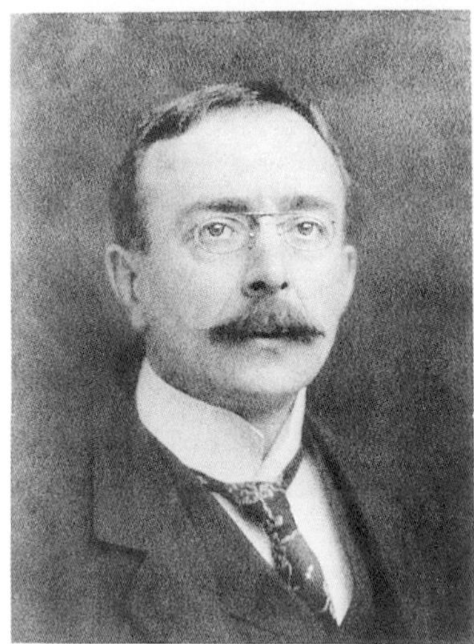

FIGURE 1.28 Sir Charles Sherrington.

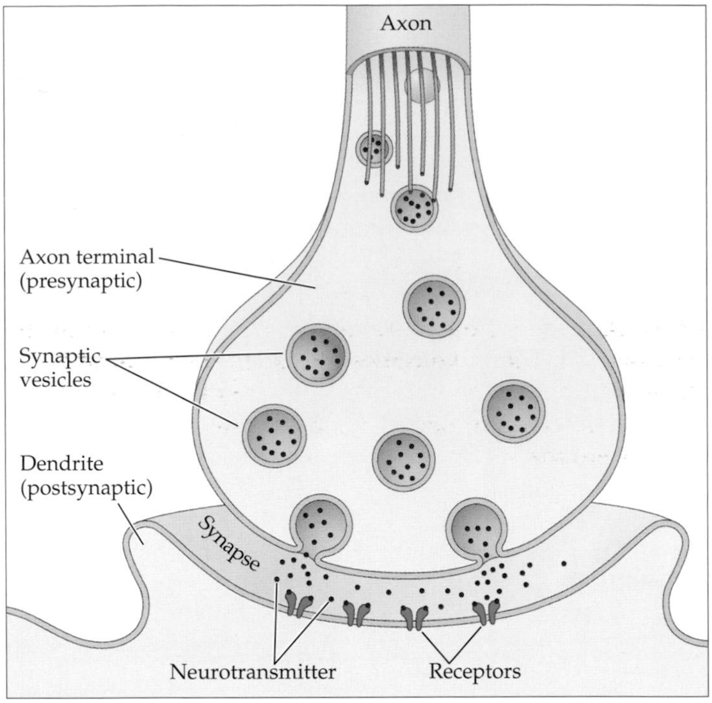

FIGURE 1.29 A synapse. An axon terminal in the presynaptic cell binds to the dendrite of the postsynaptic cell. Neurotransmitters are released by synaptic vesicles in the axon and fit into receptors on the dendrite on the other side of the synapse, thus communicating from the axon of the first neuron to the dendrite of the second neuron.

synapse The junction between neurons that permits information transfer.

Ramón y Cajal's drawings suggested that neurons do not actually touch one another. Instead, he depicted neurons as separate cells with tiny gaps between them. **Sir Charles Sherrington** (1857–1952) (**Figure 1.28**) named the tiny gap between the axon of one neuron and the dendrite of the next a **synapse** (**Figure 1.29**), from the Greek word meaning "to fasten together." Sherrington made very careful measurements demonstrating that the speed of neural transmission decreased at synapses, and this work helped us understand that something special happens at this junction where neurons meet to communicate.

For some time, people thought that some sort of electrical wave traveled across the synapse from one neuron to the next. **Otto Loewi** (1873–1961) (**Figure 1.30**), however, was convinced that this could not be true. One reason is that some neurons increase the response of the next neuron (that is, they are excitatory) but other neurons decrease the response of the next (they are inhibitory). Loewi began thinking that something chemical, instead of electrical, might be at work at the synapse. In the middle of the night before Easter in 1920, he suddenly awoke with an idea for an experimental test of his chemical hypothesis. Unfortunately, the notes that he scribbled then were indecipherable to poor Otto on Easter morning. As luck would have it, at 3:00 a.m. the next morning, he awoke again with the same idea. Not wishing to repeat his mistake, instead of scribbling notes Loewi headed to his laboratory to test his idea.

Loewi's experiment is really quite elegant. He took advantage of the fact that a frog heart continues to beat for some time after being removed from the frog if it is placed in Ringer solution, a mixture of salt water (saline) and other chemicals that preserve tissue function. He took two frog hearts: one with the vagus nerve attached and one with it removed. Stimulating the vagus nerve causes heart muscles to beat more slowly. He stimulated the

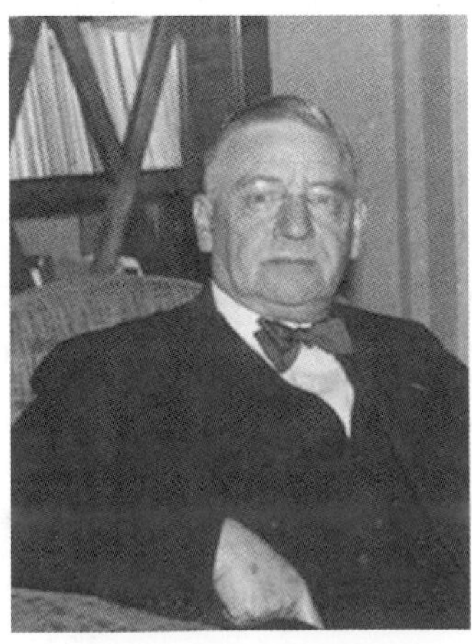

FIGURE 1.30 Otto Loewi.

vagus nerve of the one heart, thus slowing it down. Next he took the Ringer solution from this first heart and poured it over the second heart. The beating of the second heart quickly decreased in frequency, as if the vagus nerve had been stimulated. From this simple, pioneering experiment, Loewi demonstrated that stimulation of the vagus nerve released a chemical that slowed the activity of the heart muscle.

This simple bit of Easter inspiration launched many studies about molecules that travel from the axon across the synapse to the dendrite of the next neuron. These molecules are called **neurotransmitters**. There are many different kinds of neurotransmitters in the brain, and individual neurons are selective with respect to which neurotransmitters excite them or inhibit them from firing. Drugs that are psychoactive, such as amphetamines, work by increasing or decreasing the effectiveness of different neurotransmitters. Today, scientists use chemicals that influence the effects of neurotransmitters in efforts to understand pathways in the brain, including those used in perception.

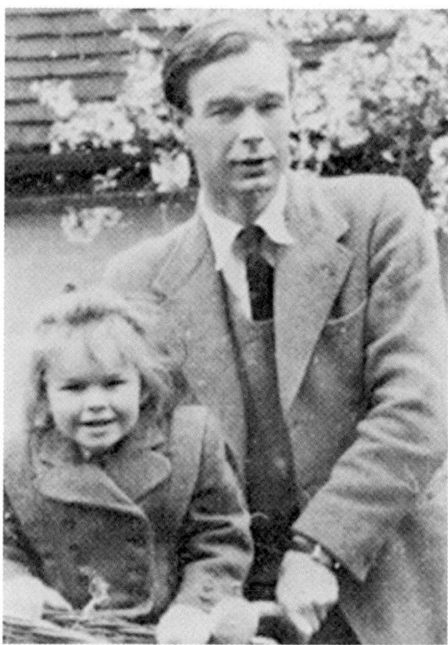

FIGURE 1.31 Sir Alan Hodgkin.

Neural Firing: The Action Potential

Later, scientists learned what it really means to have a neuron "fire." Investigators made the greatest early advances by taking advantage of the fact that some squids have giant neurons as thick as 1 millimeter. **Sir Alan Hodgkin** (1914–1998) (**Figure 1.31**) and **Sir Andrew Huxley** (born 1917) (**Figure 1.32**) conducted experiments in which they could isolate a single neuron from the squid and test how the nerve impulse travels along the axon. With such large axons, they could pierce the axon with an electrode to measure voltage, and they could even inject different chemicals inside. They learned that neural firing is actually electrochemical (**Figure 1.33**). Voltage increases along the axon are caused by changes in the membrane of the neuron that permit positively charged sodium ions (Na^+) to rush very quickly into the axon from outside. Then the membrane very quickly changes again in a way that pushes positively charged potassium ions (K^+) outside the axon, restoring the neuron to its initial resting voltage. All of this—sodium in and potassium out—occurs in about 1/1,000 of a second every time a neuron fires.

neurotransmitter A chemical substance used in neuronal communication at synapses.

By measuring these electrical changes when neurons fire, we have learned a great deal about how our senses work. Because even the biggest axons in mammals are much much smaller than the giant squid axon, it is difficult and even rare to be able to insert an electrode inside a neuron. Usually we measure electrical changes from close outside mammalian neurons (**Figure 1.34**). By measuring the speed and timing of neurons firing, we can learn about how individual neurons encode and transmit information from sense organs through higher levels of the brain.

Modern perception researchers use other tools to understand how thousands of neurons work together within the human brain. For example, electroencephalography (EEG) measures electrical activity through electrodes placed on the scalp. Using EEG, researchers cannot learn what individual neurons are doing and they cannot pinpoint the area of neural activity, but they can measure the activities of whole populations of neurons with very good temporal accuracy. One way to maintain a good measure of the timing of neural activity while providing a better idea of where in the brain neurons are most active is to use magnetoencephalography (MEG). With MEG, researchers use extremely sensitive devices to measure magnetic fields produced by electrical activity in the brain, but superconducting quantum interference devices (SQUIDs) used to measure such tiny changes in magnetic energy are very expensive and are less common than EEG devices.

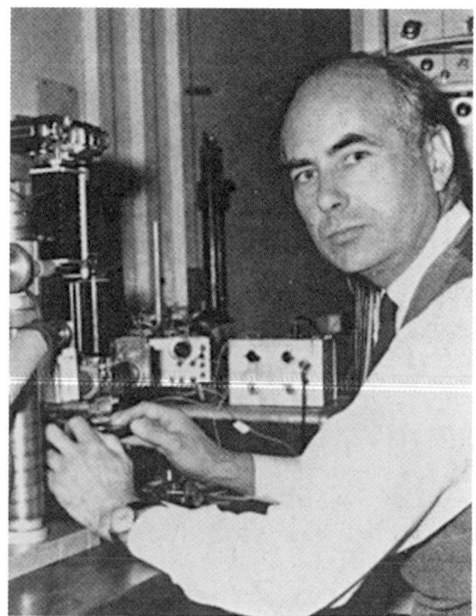

FIGURE 1.32 Sir Andrew Huxley.

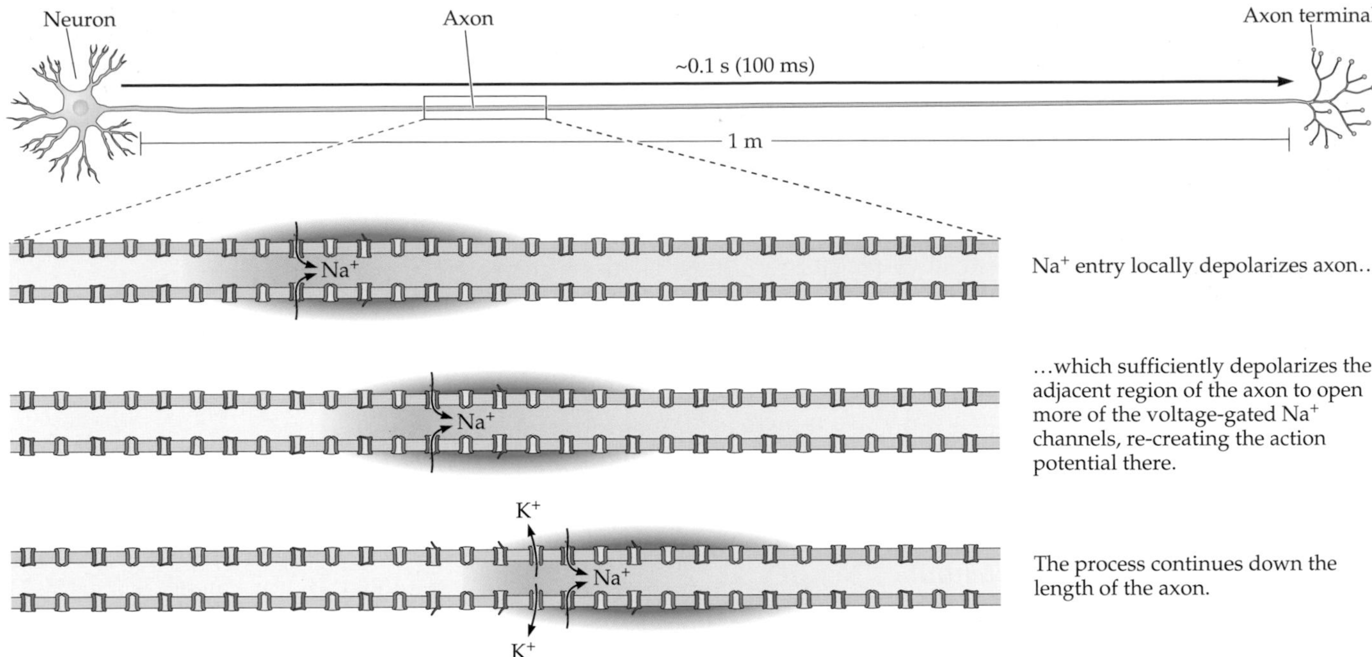

FIGURE 1.33 An action potential (firing) of a neuron is created when the membrane of the neuron permits sodium ions (Na^+) to rush into the cell, thus increasing the voltage. Very quickly afterward, potassium (K^+) flows out of the cell, bringing the voltage back to resting voltage. This process occurs along the length of the axon until the action potential reaches the axon terminal.

FIGURE 1.34 Neuroscientists record activity of single neurons with electrodes close to the axons. Modern techniques permit the insertion of multiple electrodes to measure activity in multiple neurons so that we can better understand how neurons work in concert when encoding sensory information.

Other methods permit investigators to localize neural activity in small regions of the brain, but they cannot be as precise about timing as are EEG and MEG. For example, positron emission tomography (PET) is an imaging technique in which a small amount of a safe, biologically active, radioactive material (tracer) is introduced into the participant's bloodstream, and the PET system detects pairs of gamma rays emitted from brain regions where the tracer is being used most. Although this method is somewhat inconvenient, it has the advantage of being silent, which is helpful in studies of brain activity related to hearing. Much more common, and much noisier, is functional magnetic resonance imaging (fMRI) (**Figure 1.35**). You probably know someone who has been placed in an MRI machine to create images of soft tissue, such as cartilage in the knee. With fMRI, researchers measure changes in magnetic activity in hemoglobin, which carries oxygen to cells. These changes permit us to learn where in the brain neurons are using the most oxygen, which identifies the areas that are most active or involved in whatever task the participant is performing.

With all these methods available, much of modern perception research includes understanding how neurons in the brain work together to learn about the world around us. Or, as Morpheus would say, "If you're talking about what you can feel, what you can smell, what you can taste and see, then real is simply electrical signals interpreted by your brain. This is the world that you know."

Now that you know a little about the very long history and philosophy of thinking and experimenting about perception, it's time to move forward. Just as Neo says at the end of *The Matrix*, "I didn't come here to tell you how this is going to end. I came here to tell you how it's going to begin." We

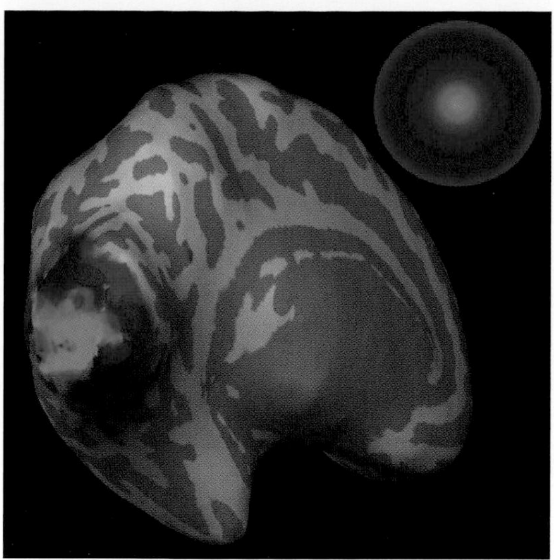

FIGURE 1.35 Modern brain-imaging methods permit researchers to precisely measure activity in the brain where neurons are most active. This image of a brain (left hemisphere inflated, viewed from the back, nose pointing down to the right) shows where a stimulus is represented by neurons in visual cortex (see Figure 1.24). Neural activity is greatest for areas corresponding to where the eyes are fixated (green). (Courtesy of Scott Gorlin.)

hope you enjoy learning how we know what is real, or at least, how we know what we think is real.

Summary

1. Since the time of the earliest writings by philosophers, it has been clear that our perception of reality is limited by what we can learn from our five senses. We are capable of detecting and using only a tiny fraction of the energy and events that occur all around us.
2. Nativists address the limitations on our sensory systems by suggesting that much or most true knowledge is innate within individuals.
3. Empiricists concede that all we can ever know must be learned through our sensory experiences. Part of being an empiricist is acknowledging that some things are simply unknowable because we cannot learn about them through our senses.
4. Another enduring philosophical question that matters for perception is the relationship between mind and body. One common idea is dualism, the assumption that people have material bodies and also immaterial minds. One challenge for dualism is to explain how the immaterial mind, which has no mass and takes up no space, can affect the material body. Gustav Fechner invented psychophysics as part of his efforts to scientifically establish the relationship between mind and matter.
5. Fechner invented several clever methods for measuring the relationship between physical changes in the world and consequent psychological changes in observers. These methods remain in use today.
6. A more recent development for understanding performance—signal detection theory—permits us to simulate changes in the perceiver (e.g., internal noise and biases) in order to understand perceptual performance better.
7. We learn a great deal about perception by understanding the biological structures and processes involved. One early observation—the doctrine of specific nerve energies—expresses the fact that people are aware only of the activity of our nervous systems. For this reason, what matters is which nerves are stimulated, not how they are stimulated. The central nervous system reflects specializations for the senses from cranial nerves to areas of the cerebral cortex involved in perception.
8. The essential activities of all neurons, including those involved in sensory processes, are chemical and electrochemical. Neurons communicate with each other through neurotransmitters, molecules that cross the synapse from the axon of one neuron to the dendrite of the next. Nerve impulses are electrochemical; voltages change along the axon as electrically charged ions (sodium and potassium) pass in and out of the membranes of nerve cells.

Refer to the
Sensation and Perception
website
(www.sinauer.com/wolfe2e)
for activities, essays, study questions, and other study aids.

CHAPTER 2

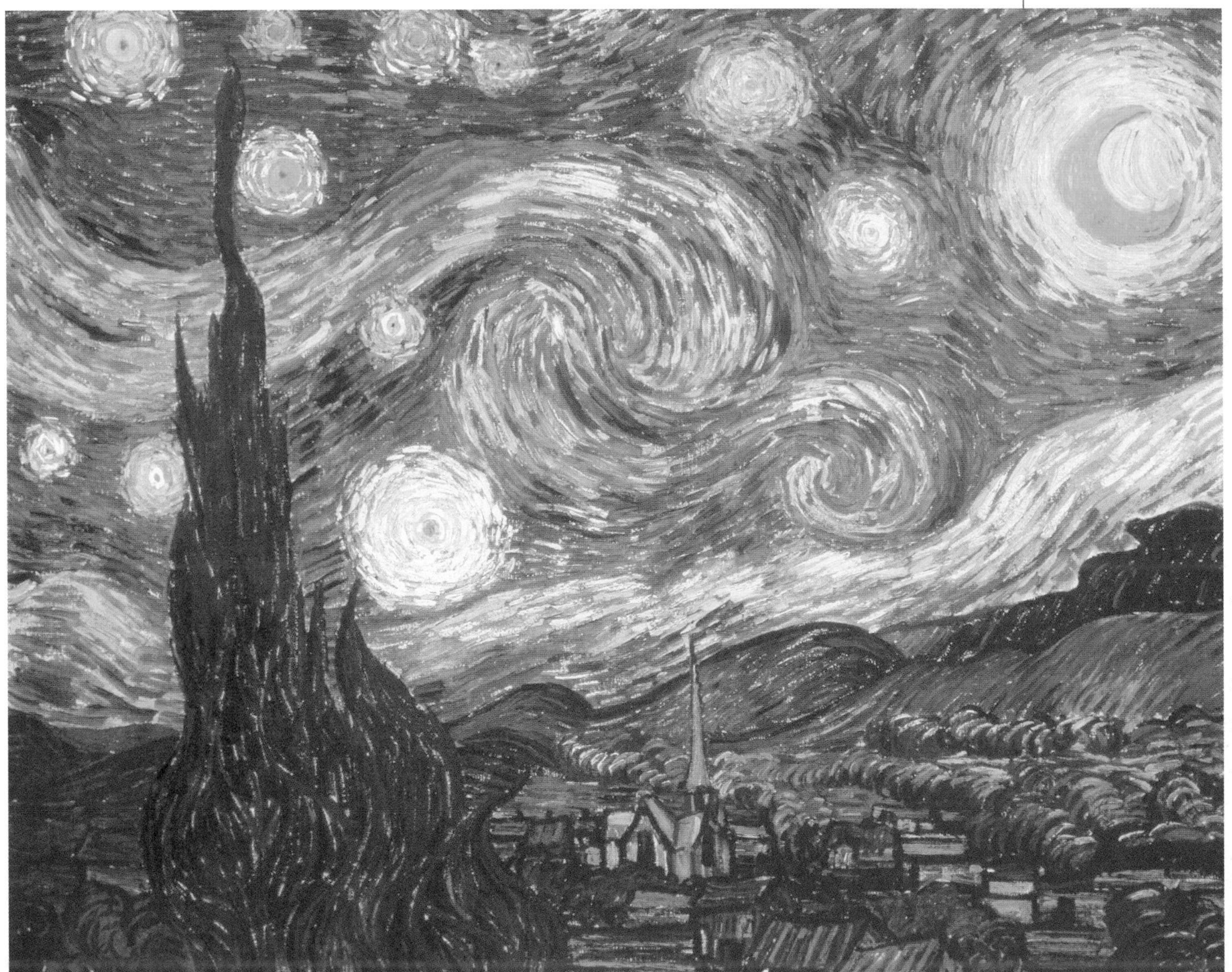

Museum of Modern Art, New York, USA/The Bridgeman Art Library

Vincent van Gogh, *The Starry Night*, 1889

The First Steps in Vision: Seeing Stars

Twinkle twinkle little star
How I wonder what you are
Up above the world so high
Like a diamond in the sky

With the naked eye we can see stars that are up to about 2000 light-years (almost 6 trillion miles) away, and in a dark winter sky far from city lights, the neighboring galaxy, Andromeda, is visible over 2 *million* light-years away! This chapter describes the first steps in seeing stars. To understand how we see stars, we must first consider a little physics and optics, and then we'll look at how the eye is built to capture and begin to process the light from stars.

In subsequent chapters, we'll see how light information gleaned by the eyes travels back through the head to the brain, and how the brain transforms this information into a meaningful interpretation of the outside world. For a preview of the entire visual process, work through **Web Activity 2.1: Visual System Overview**.

A Little Light Physics

Light is a form of electromagnetic radiation—energy produced by vibrations of electrically charged material. There are two ways to conceptualize light: as a **wave** or as a stream of **photons**, tiny particles that each consist of one quantum of energy. This dual nature of light can be confusing to physics and psychology students alike. However, we'll try to avoid confusion as much as possible by treating light as being made up of waves when it moves around the world, and being made up of photons when it is absorbed.

Although the full spectrum of electromagnetic radiation is very wide, light makes up only a tiny portion of this spectrum. **Figure 2.1** illustrates the electromagnetic spectrum from gamma rays (which have very short wavelengths) to radio and television waves (which have very long wavelengths). Visible light waves have wavelengths between 400 and 700 nanometers (nm; 1 nm = 10^{-9} meter), as illustrated on the right-hand side of the figure. Note that as the wavelength varies in the visible spectrum, the color we observe changes from violet at about 400 nm through the whole spectrum of the rainbow up to red at about 650 nm. (As we'll discuss in Chapter 5, however, the light waves themselves are not colored; it is only after our visual system interprets an incoming wave that we perceive the light as "violet" or "red.")

Let's consider what happens to light on its way from a star to an eye. (See **Web Activity 2.2: From Sun to Eye.**) In empty space the electromagnetic radiation from a star travels in a straight line at the speed of light (about 186,000

wave An oscillation that travels through a medium by transferring energy from one particle or point to another without causing any permanent displacement of the medium.

photon A quantum of visible light or other form of electromagnetic radiation demonstrating both particle and wave properties.

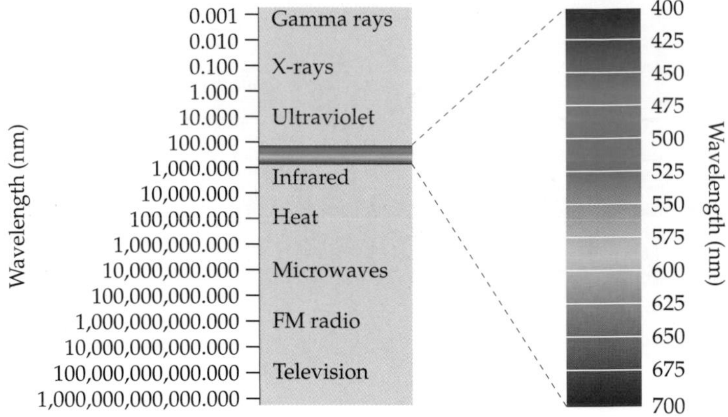

FIGURE 2.1 The spectrum of electromagnetic energy (specified in nanometers), with the visible spectrum (400–700 nm) expanded at right. Note that 1 nm = 10^{-9} m.

miles per second). Once it reaches the atmosphere, some of the starlight's photons will be **absorbed** by encounters with dust, vaporized water, and so on; and some of the light will be **scattered** by these particles. Most of the photons, however, will make it through the atmosphere and will eventually hit the surface of an object.

If the ray of starlight were to strike a light-colored surface, most of the light would be **reflected**. Indeed, the fact that most of the light bounces off the surface accounts for that surface's "light" appearance. On the other hand, most of the light striking a dark surface is absorbed. Light that is neither reflected nor absorbed by the surface is **transmitted** through the surface. If we are gazing at our star through a window, as the light travels from air into the glass some of the light rays will be bent, or **refracted**, as it is transmitted.

Refraction also occurs when light passes from air into water or into the eyeball. In fact, the part of an eye exam in which the eye doctor checks the patient's prescription is often called a "refraction" because the doctor determines how much the light must be bent by eyeglasses for it to be properly focused on the retina. In the next section we'll see how the optical system of our eyes performs this same kind of focusing.

Eyes That See Light

In order to see stars or anything else, we need some type of physiological mechanism for sensing light. Even single-celled organisms such as amoebas respond to light, changing their direction of motion to avoid bright light when it is detected. But eyes go well beyond mere light detection. An eye can form an **image** of the outside world, enabling animals that possess eyes to use light to recognize objects, not just to determine whether light is present and what direction it is coming from.

Before explaining how eyes form images, let's take a tour through the human eye to become familiar with its important parts. **Figure 2.2** shows a front-to-back slice through a human eye, with the most important structures labeled. (See **Web Activity 2.3: Eye Structure**.)

The first tissue that light from the star will encounter is the **cornea**. Contact lenses sit on a thin film of tears in front of the cornea. The cornea provides a window to the world because it is **transparent** (that is, most light photons are transmitted through it, rather than being reflected or absorbed). It is transparent because it is made of a highly ordered arrangement of fibers and because it contains no blood vessels or blood, which would absorb light.

absorb To take up light, noise, or energy and not transmit it at all.

scatter To disperse light in an irregular fashion.

reflect To redirect something that strikes a surface—especially light, sound, or heat—usually back toward its point of origin.

transmit To convey something (e.g., light) from one place or thing to another.

refract 1. To alter the course of a wave of energy that passes into something from another medium, as water does to light entering it from the air. 2. To measure the degree of refraction in a lens or eye.

image A picture or likeness.

cornea The transparent "window" into the eyeball.

transparent Allowing light to pass through with no interruption so that objects on the other side can be clearly seen.

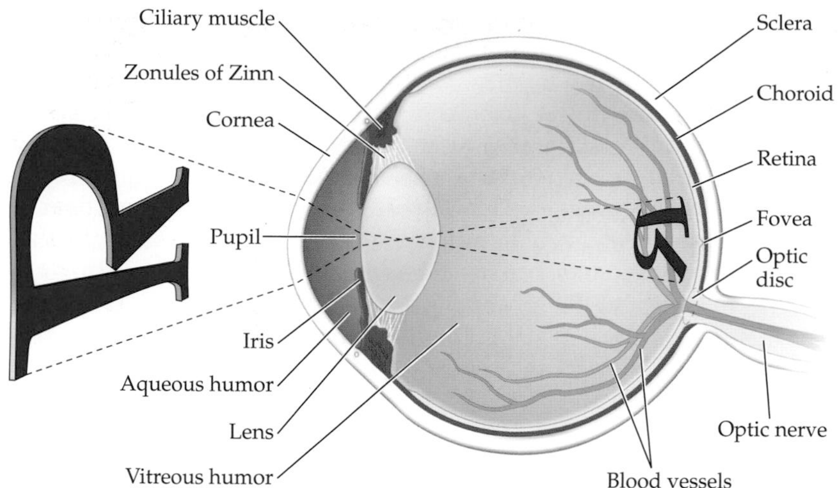

FIGURE 2.2 The human right eye in cross section (viewed from above). Note that the *R* on the retina is reversed right to left, and it is upside down. The "hole" in the retina where the optic nerve leaves the eyeball is the optic disc (where the absence of photoreceptors results in a blind spot). (From Rosenzweig, Breedlove, and Watson, 2005.)

The cornea does, however, have a rich supply of transparent sensory nerve endings, which are there to force the eyes to close and produce tears if the cornea is scratched, preserving its transparency. If you have ever scratched your cornea or worn contact lenses too long, you know exactly how painful this can be! Fortunately, the external layers of the cornea regenerate very quickly, so even when a cornea is scratched, it usually heals within 24 hours.

The **aqueous humor**, a fluid derived from blood, fills the space immediately behind the cornea, supplying oxygen and nutrients to, and removing waste from, the cornea and the **crystalline lens**. Like the cornea, the lens has no blood supply, so that it can be completely transparent, and as we'll see later, the shape of the lens is controlled by the ciliary muscle.

To get to the lens, the light from our favorite star must pass through the **pupil**, which is simply a hole in a muscular structure called the **iris**. The iris gives the eye its distinctive color. The pupil controls the amount of light that reaches the retina, via the pupillary light reflex. When the level of light increases or decreases, the iris automatically expands and contracts to allow more or less light into the eye. When you emerge from a dark room into bright light (e.g., coming out of a movie theater), not only does your pupil constrict, but there's a good chance that you will sneeze. Sneezing in response to being exposed to a bright light—the "photic sneeze reflex"—is not yet understood, even though it has intrigued some of history's greatest minds. Aristotle thought the heat of the sun on the nose might be responsible. However, Francis Bacon (1561–1626) showed that Aristotle was wrong. Bacon stepped into the sun with his eyes closed and did not sneeze; the heat was still there, but the sneeze was not. Bacon guessed that the sun's light makes the eyes water, and that moisture ("braine humour," literally) then seeps into and irritates the nose. We now know that the sneeze takes place too soon after light exposure to be the result of the comparatively slow formation of tears. Current thinking suggests that the photic sneeze reflex is a result of crossed wires in the brain.

After passing through the lens, our starlight enters the vitreous chamber (the space between the lens and the retina), where it will be refracted for the fourth and final time by the **vitreous humor**. This is the longest part of the journey through the eyeball; this chamber comprises 80% of the internal volume of the eye. The vitreous is gel-like and viscous (a bit like egg white), and generally transparent. While staring up at the bright blue sky on a lazy sunny day, however, you may have noticed "floaters," small bits of debris

aqueous humor The watery fluid in the anterior chamber of the eye.

crystalline lens The lens inside the eye that enables changing focus.

pupil The dark circular opening at the center of the iris in the eye, where light enters the eye.

iris The colored part of the eye, consisting of a muscular diaphragm surrounding the pupil and regulating the light entering the eye by expanding and contracting the pupil.

vitreous humor The transparent fluid that fills the vitreous chamber in the posterior part of the eye.

retina A light-sensitive membrane in the back of the eye that contains rods and cones, which receive an image from the lens and send it to the brain through the optic nerve.

accommodation The process by which the eye changes its focus (in which the lens gets fatter as gaze is directed toward nearer objects).

presbyopia Literally "old sight." The loss of near vision because of insufficient accommodation.

cataract Opacity of the crystalline lens.

(biodebris) that drift around in the vitreous. Floaters are quite common, and they are usually not a cause for concern.

Finally, after traveling through the vitreous chamber, the light emitted by our favorite star is (hopefully) brought into focus at the **retina**. To be a bit more precise, only some of the light will actually reach the retina. Much of the light energy will have been lost in space or the atmosphere, because of absorption and scattering, as described already. In addition, a good deal of light becomes lost in the eyeball, so only about half of the starlight that arrives at the cornea actually reaches the retina. The role of the retina is to detect light and "tell the brain about aspects of light that are related to objects in the world" (Oyster, 1999). In other words, the retina is where seeing really begins.

Shining Starlight onto the Retina

Remember that refraction (light bending) is necessary to focus light rays. Because the cornea is highly curved and has a higher refractive index than air (1.376 versus 1), it forms the most powerful refractive surface in the eye. The aqueous and vitreous humors also help refract light. However, the refractive power of these three structures is fixed, so they cannot be used to bring close objects into focus. This job is performed by the lens, which can alter the refractive power by changing its shape—a process called **accommodation**.

Accommodation (change in focus) is accomplished through contraction of the ciliary muscle. The lens is attached to the ciliary muscle through tiny fibers (known as the "zonules of Zinn") (see Figure 2.2). When the ciliary muscle is relaxed, the zonules are stretched and the lens is relatively flat. In this state, the eye will be focused on very distant objects (like our star). But to focus on something closer—say, a wristwatch—the ciliary muscle must contract. This contraction reduces the tension on the zonules and enables the lens to bulge. The fatter the lens is, the more power it has.

Accommodation enables the power of the lens to vary by as much as 15 diopters. If your eyes were corrected for distant vision, 15 diopters of accommodation would enable you to read your watch at a distance of about 6.7 centimeters (cm; the distance in centimeters is equal to 100 divided by the amount of accommodation in diopters—in this case 15). If you can read your watch at 6.7 cm (while wearing your distance correction), you are either very lucky or very young. Our ability to accommodate declines with age, starting from about 8, and we lose about 1 diopter of accommodation every 5 years up to age 30 (and even more after age 30). By the time most people are between 40 and 50 years old, they find that their arms are too short because they can no longer easily accommodate the 2.5 diopters or so needed to see clearly at 40 cm (diopters = 1/distance [in meters]; that is, 1/0.4 = 2.5). This condition is called **presbyopia** (meaning "old sight") and it is, like death and taxes, inevitable! Why do we all have presbyopia to look forward to? The main reason is that the lens becomes sclerotic (harder) and the capsule that encircles the lens (enabling it to change shape) loses its elasticity. Luckily for us, Benjamin Franklin (1706–1790) invented bifocals—lenses that have one power at the top (permitting us to see distant objects) and a different power at the bottom (allowing us to be in focus at a comfortable reading distance).

Like the other optical components of the eye, the lens is normally transparent. It is transparent because the crystallins (a class of proteins that make up the lens) are packed together very densely and therefore are very regular. Anything that interferes with the regularity of the crystallins will result in loss of transparency (areas that are opaque—that is, "opacities"). Opacities of the lens are known as **cataracts**, and they are caused by irregularity of the

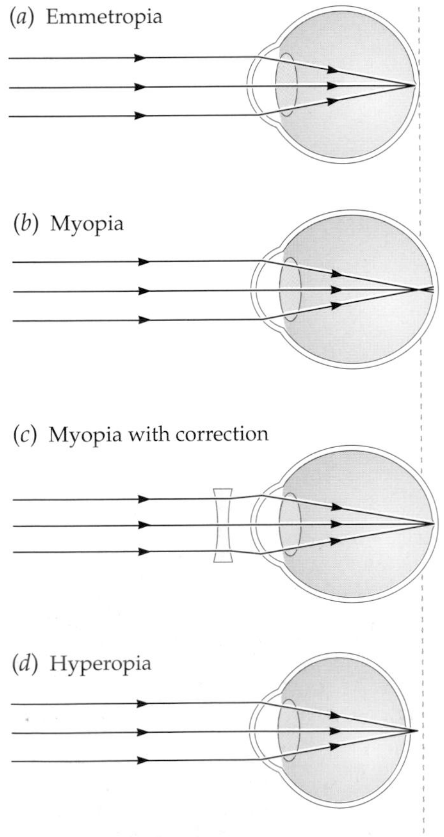

(*a*) Emmetropia

(*b*) Myopia

(*c*) Myopia with correction

(*d*) Hyperopia

FIGURE 2.3 Optics of the human eye. (After Oyster, 1999.)

crystallins. Cataracts can occur at different ages and take many different forms. Congenital cataracts (present at birth) are relatively rare; but if they are dense (and therefore interfere with retinal image quality), they can have devastating effects on normal visual development if not treated as early as possible. Most cataracts are discovered after age 50, and the prevalence of cataracts increases with age so that by 70 almost everyone has some loss of transparency. Cataracts can interfere with vision because they absorb and scatter more light than the normal lens does. Fortunately, treatment of cataracts (in which the opacified lens is extracted and replaced with a plastic or silicone implant) has become quite routine.

To focus our distant star on the retina, the refractive power of the four optical components of the eye must be perfectly matched to the length of the eyeball. This perfect match, known as **emmetropia**, is illustrated in **Figure 2.3***a*. Refractive errors occur when the eyeball is too long or too short relative to the power of the optical components. If the eyeball is too long for the optics (Figure 2.3*b*), the image of our star will be focused *in front* of the retina, and the star will thus be seen as a blur rather than a spot of light. This condition is called **myopia** (or "nearsightedness"). Myopia can be corrected with negative (minus) lenses, which diverge the rays of starlight before they enter the eye (Figure 2.3*c*). If the eyeball is too short for the optics (Figure 2.3*d*), the image of our star will be focused *behind* the retina—a condition called **hyperopia** (or "farsightedness"). If the hyperopia is not too severe, a young hyperope can compensate by accommodating, and thereby increasing the power of the eye. If accommodation fails to correct the hyperopia, the star's image will again be blurred. Hyperopia can be corrected with positive (plus) lenses, which converge the rays of starlight before they enter the eye.

On average, the adult human eye is 24 millimeters (mm) long, about the diameter of a quarter. However, eyeballs can be quite a bit longer or shorter and still be emmetropic because eyes generally grow to match the power of the optical components we're born with. (Most newborns are hyperopic because the optical components of their eyes are relatively well developed at birth compared to the length of their eyeballs.)

As noted earlier, the most powerful refracting surface in the eye is the cornea, which contributes about two-thirds of the eye's focusing power. When the cornea is not spherical, the result is **astigmatism**. With astigmatism, vertical lines might be focused slightly in front of the retina, while horizontal lines are focused slightly behind it (or vice versa). If you have a reasonable degree of uncorrected astigmatism, one or more of the lines in **Figure 2.4** might appear to be out of focus, while other lines appear sharp. Lenses that have two focal points (that is, lenses that provide different amounts of focusing power in the horizontal and vertical planes) can correct astigmatism.

emmetropia The condition in which there is no refractive error, because the refractive power of the eye is perfectly matched to the length of the eyeball.

myopia A common condition in which light entering the eye is focused in front of the retina and distant objects cannot be seen sharply.

hyperopia A common condition in which light entering the eye is focused behind the retina.

astigmatism A visual defect caused by the unequal curving of one or more of the refractive surfaces of the eye, usually the cornea.

The Retina

The preceding discussion covered how the human visual system delivers a focused image of our favorite star onto the retina, which is spread across the back of the eyeball. The optics involved are similar to those in most cameras (see Figure 2.2), which also include a mechanism for regulating the amount of light (the "stop," analogous to the iris in human eyes) and a lens for adjusting focal length so that both near and far objects can be focused on the film spread across the back of the camera. However, this is as far as we can take this analogy, because although the purpose of a camera is simply to record the image projected onto the film, the purpose of the human visual system is to interpret this image. This is the difference between taking a picture and seeing a picture. And the process of seeing begins with the retina,

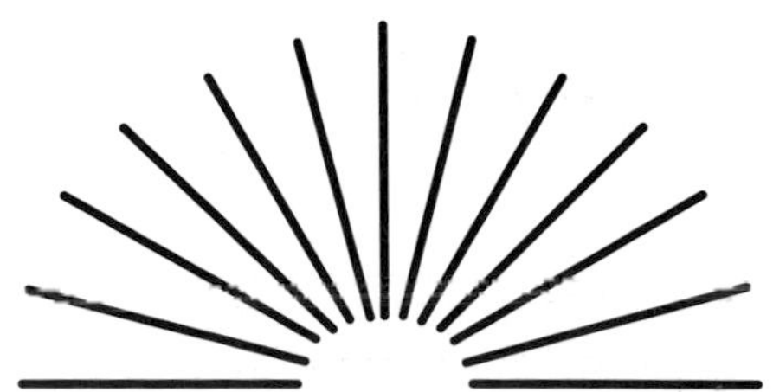

FIGURE 2.4 Fan chart for astigmatism. Take off your glasses (if you wear glasses) and view this "fan." If you have a significant degree of astigmatism, you will notice that one or more of the lines appear to have lower contrast.

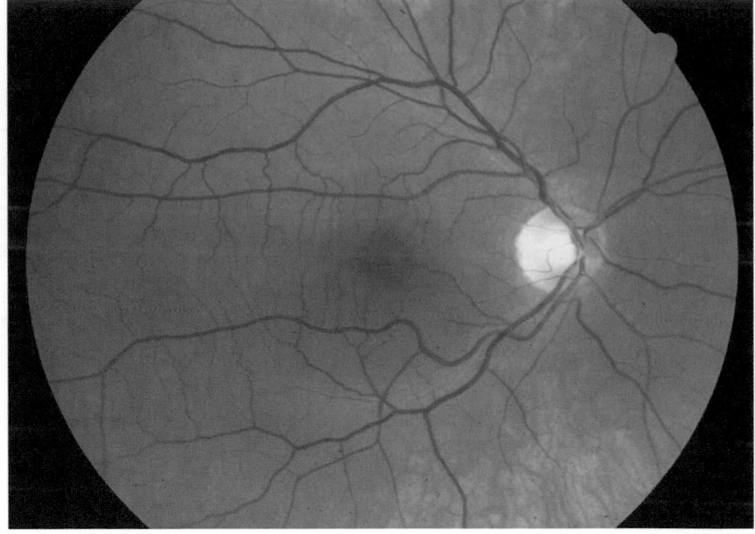

FIGURE 2.5 Fundus of the right eye of a human. (From Rodieck, 1998.)

transduced Referring to the conversion from one form of energy (e.g., light) to another (e.g., electricity).

fundus The back layer of the retina—what the eye doctor sees through an ophthalmoscope.

where the light energy from our star is **transduced** into neural energy that can be interpreted by the brain.

Eye doctors use an instrument called an ophthalmoscope to look at the back surface of their patients' eyes, which is called the **fundus** (plural *fundi*). (You probably remember all too well having that bright light shining into your eye when the doctor examines your fundus.) **Figure 2.5** shows a normal fundus. The white circle is known as the optic disc. This is where the arteries and veins that feed the retina enter the eye, and where the axons of ganglion cells (which we will get to shortly) leave the eye via the optic nerve. This

(*a*)

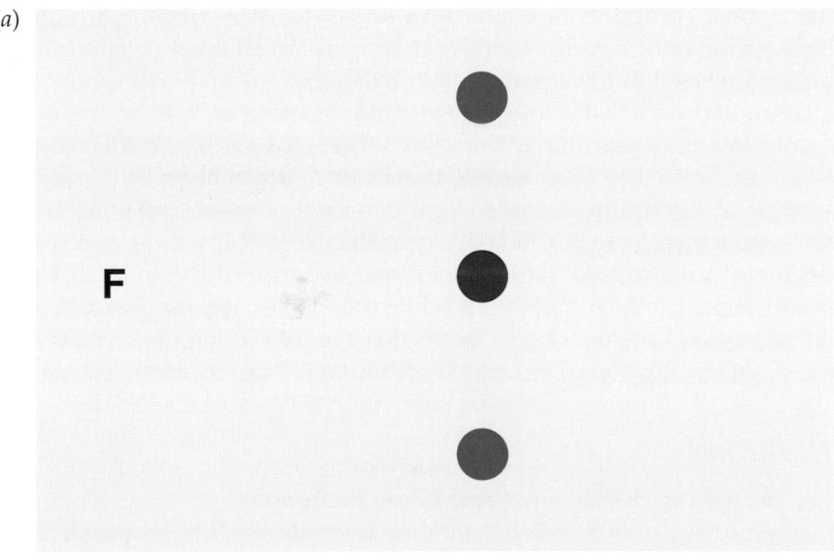

(*b*)

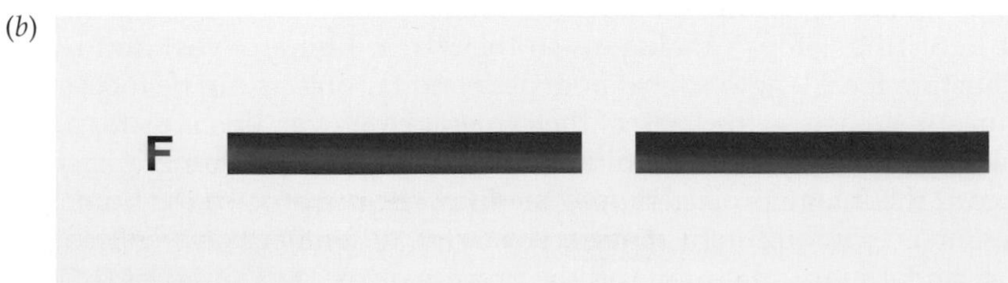

FIGURE 2.6 To experience your blind spot, close your left eye, fixating on the *F* in part (*a*) with your right eye. Hold the book about 15 cm away from your eye, and adjust the distance of the book from your eyes until the red circle disappears. This is your blind spot. Ordinarily you are not aware of it, because the visual system "fills in" the blind spot with information from the surrounding area. If you fixate on the *F* in part (*b*) and again adjust the distance, when the gap in the line falls in your blind spot, it will fill in and you will see a continuous red line.

portion of the retina contains no photoreceptors, and consequently it is blind. You can experience your own blind spot, corresponding to your optic disc, by closing your left eye, fixating on the *F* in **Figure 2.6***a* with your right eye, and adjusting the distance of the book from your eyes until the red circle disappears. The reason you don't normally notice this large blind spot in your visual field is that the visual system "fills it in" with information from the surrounding area (Figure 2.6*b*).

The fundus is the only place in the body where one can see the arteries and veins directly, so it provides doctors with an important window on the well-being of the body's vascular system. The vascular "tree" spreads out across the retina in a characteristic way but stops short of the fovea (the center of the brownish spot near the center of the fundus in Figure 2.5).

To see your own vascular tree, there is a simple trick that requires only a penlight. In a dark room, close your eyes and place the penlight against the outside corner of one eye. Holding the penlight against the eye, gently move the light around (up and down, and back and forth). Within a few seconds you should see the shadows cast by your blood vessels looking like the branches of a tree. We don't normally see them because the blood vessels move with our eyes, so their shadows are stabilized retinal images and, as with the blind spot, the visual system fills in behind them. The motion of the penlight makes the shadows move, enabling you to see them.

Even when viewed through an ophthalmoscope with a lot of magnification, the fundus does not provide a detailed view of the retina. To get a good look at the structure of the retina, we need a photomicrograph (**Figure 2.7**), which reveals that the retina is a layered sheet of clear neurons, about half

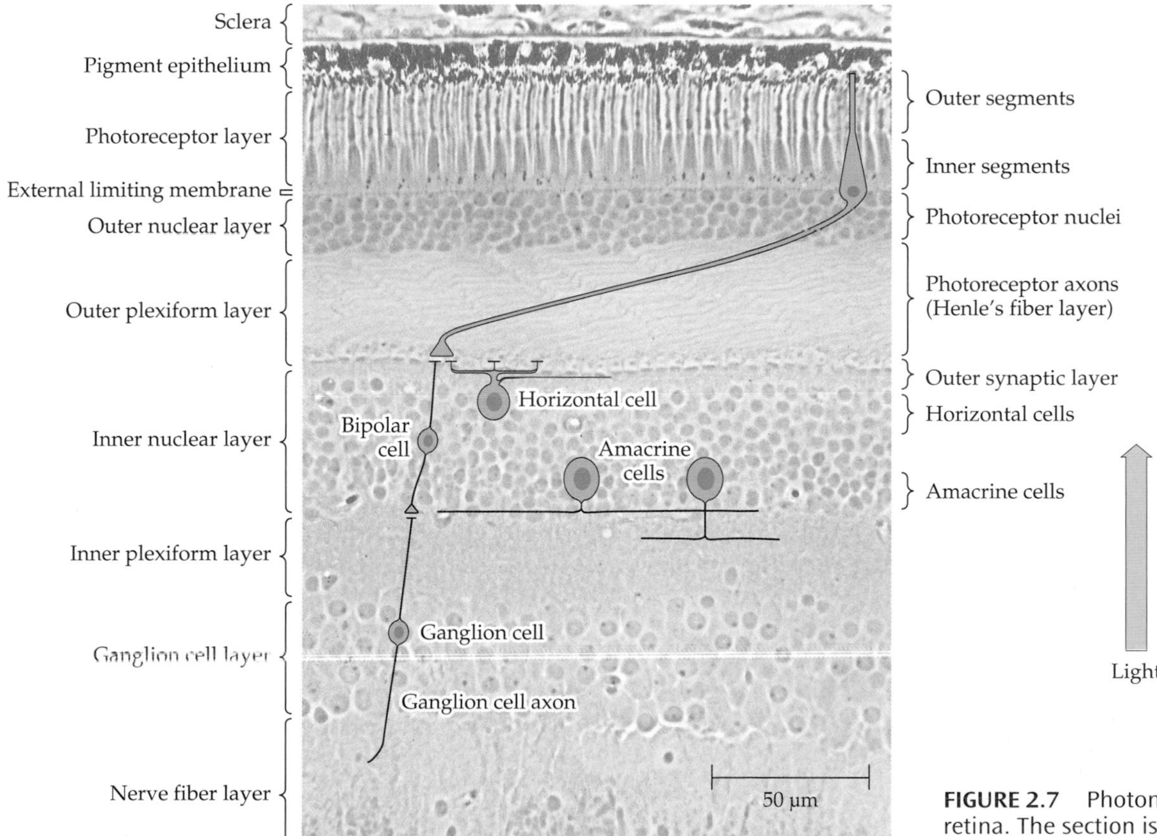

FIGURE 2.7 Photomicrograph of the retina. The section is near the fovea. (From Oyster, 1999; micrograph from Boycott and Dowling, 1969.)

photoreceptors Light-sensitive receptors in the retina.

rods Photoreceptors specialized for night vision.

cones Photoreceptors specialized for daylight vision, fine visual acuity, and color.

duplex In reference to the retina, consisting of two parts: the rods and cones, which operate under different conditions.

outer segment The part of a photoreceptor that contains photopigment molecules.

inner segment The part of a photoreceptor that lies between the outer segment and the cell nucleus.

synaptic terminal The location where axons terminate at the synapse for transmission of information by release of a chemical transmitter.

chromophore The light-catching part of the visual pigments of the retina.

rhodopsin The visual pigment found in rods.

the thickness of a credit card (Rodieck, 1999), with another layer of darker cells, the pigment epithelium, lying behind the final layer.

As we'll see in the next section, together these neurons constitute a minicomputer that begins the process of interpreting the information contained in visual images. The transduction of light energy into neural energy begins in the backmost layer of the retina, which is made up of cells called **photoreceptors**. When photoreceptors sense light, they can stimulate neurons in the intermediate layers, including bipolar cells, horizontal cells, and amacrine cells. These neurons then connect with the frontmost layer of the retina, made up of ganglion cells, whose axons pass through the optic nerve to the brain.

Before we describe the function of these layers, we should address an obvious question regarding the structure of the retina: Why are the photoreceptors at the back—that is, in the last layer? This arrangement requires that light pass through the ganglion, bipolar, horizontal, and amacrine cells before making contact with the photoreceptors. However, these neurons are mostly transparent, whereas cells in the pigment epithelium, which provide vital nutrients to the photoreceptors, are opaque. Once we see that the photoreceptors must be next to both the pigment epithelium and the other neurons, the layering order makes much more sense.

Retinal Information Processing

As noted in the previous section, the retina contains five major classes of neurons: photoreceptors, horizontal cells, bipolar cells, amacrine cells, and ganglion cells (see Figure 2.7). Let's take a closer look at the functions of each of these cell types. (See **Web Activity 2.4: Retinal Structure**.)

Light Transduction by Rod and Cone Photoreceptors

The retina contains roughly 100 million photoreceptors. These are the neurons that capture light and initiate the act of seeing by producing chemical signals. The human retina contains at least two types of photoreceptors: **rods** and **cones**. These two types not only have different shapes (which is how they earned their names; see **Figure 2.8**), but they have different distributions across the retina and serve different functions. Because human retinas have both rods and cones, they are considered to be **duplex** retinas. Some animals, such as rats and owls, have mostly rod retinas; others (e.g., certain lizards) have mostly cone retinas.

Both types of photoreceptors consist of an **outer segment** (which is adjacent to the pigment epithelium), an **inner segment**, and a **synaptic terminal**. Molecules called visual pigments are made in the inner segment (which is like a little factory, filled with mitochondria) and stored in the outer segment, where they are incorporated into the membrane. Visual pigment molecules consist of a protein (an opsin), the structure of which determines which wavelengths of light they absorb, and a **chromophore**, which captures light photons. Each photoreceptor has only one of the four types of visual pigments found in the human retina. The pigment **rhodopsin** is found in the rods, concentrated mainly in the stack of membranous discs in the outer segment. Each cone has one of the other three pigments—which respond to long, medium, and short wavelengths, respectively.

Recent evidence suggests that there may be a third type of photoreceptor—one that "lives" among the ganglion cells, and that is involved in adjusting our biological rhythms to match the day and night of the external world (Baringa, 2002).

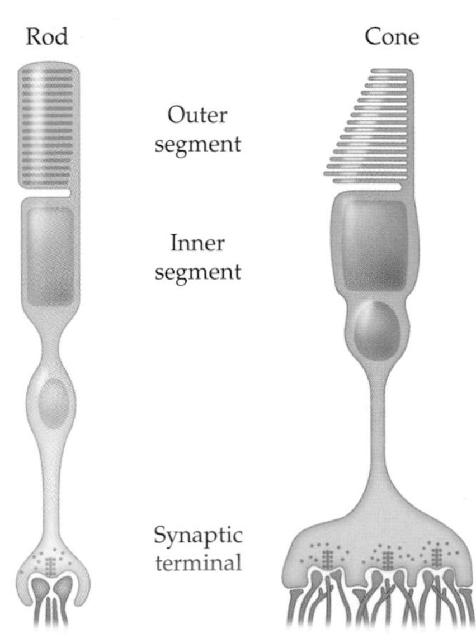

FIGURE 2.8 Rods and cones. (From Rodieck, 1998.)

When a photon from our favorite star makes its way into the outer segment of a rod and is absorbed by a molecule of rhodopsin, it transfers its energy to the chromophore portion of the visual pigment molecule. This process, known as **photoactivation**, initiates a biochemical cascade of events eventually resulting in the closing of channels in the cell membrane that normally allow ions to flow into the rod outer segment. Closing these channels alters the balance of electrical current between the inside and outside of the rod outer segment, making the inside of the cell more negatively charged. This process is known as **hyperpolarization**. Hyperpolarization closes calcium channels at the synaptic terminal, thereby reducing the concentration of free calcium inside the cells. The lowering of the calcium concentration, in turn, reduces the concentration of neurotransmitter (glutamate) molecules at the synaptic terminals, and this change signals to the bipolar cell that the rod has captured a photon. The entire sequence of events takes only a matter of milliseconds. Cones act in a qualitatively similar fashion.

The amount of glutamate present in the photoreceptor–bipolar cell synapse at any one time is inversely proportional to the number of photons being absorbed by the photoreceptor. Thus, unlike most other types of neurons, photoreceptors do not respond in an all-or-nothing fashion. They pass their information on to bipolar cells via **graded potentials** instead of action potentials.

Humans have many more rods (about 90 million) than cones (about 4–5 million), and the two types of cells have very different geographic distributions on the retina (**Figure 2.9**). Rods are completely absent from the center of the fovea, and their density increases to a peak at about 20 degrees, then declines again. The cones are most concentrated in the center of the fovea,

photoactivation Activation by light.

hyperpolarization An increase in membrane potential where the inner membrane surface becomes more negative than the outer membrane surface.

graded potential An electrical potential that can vary continuously in amplitude.

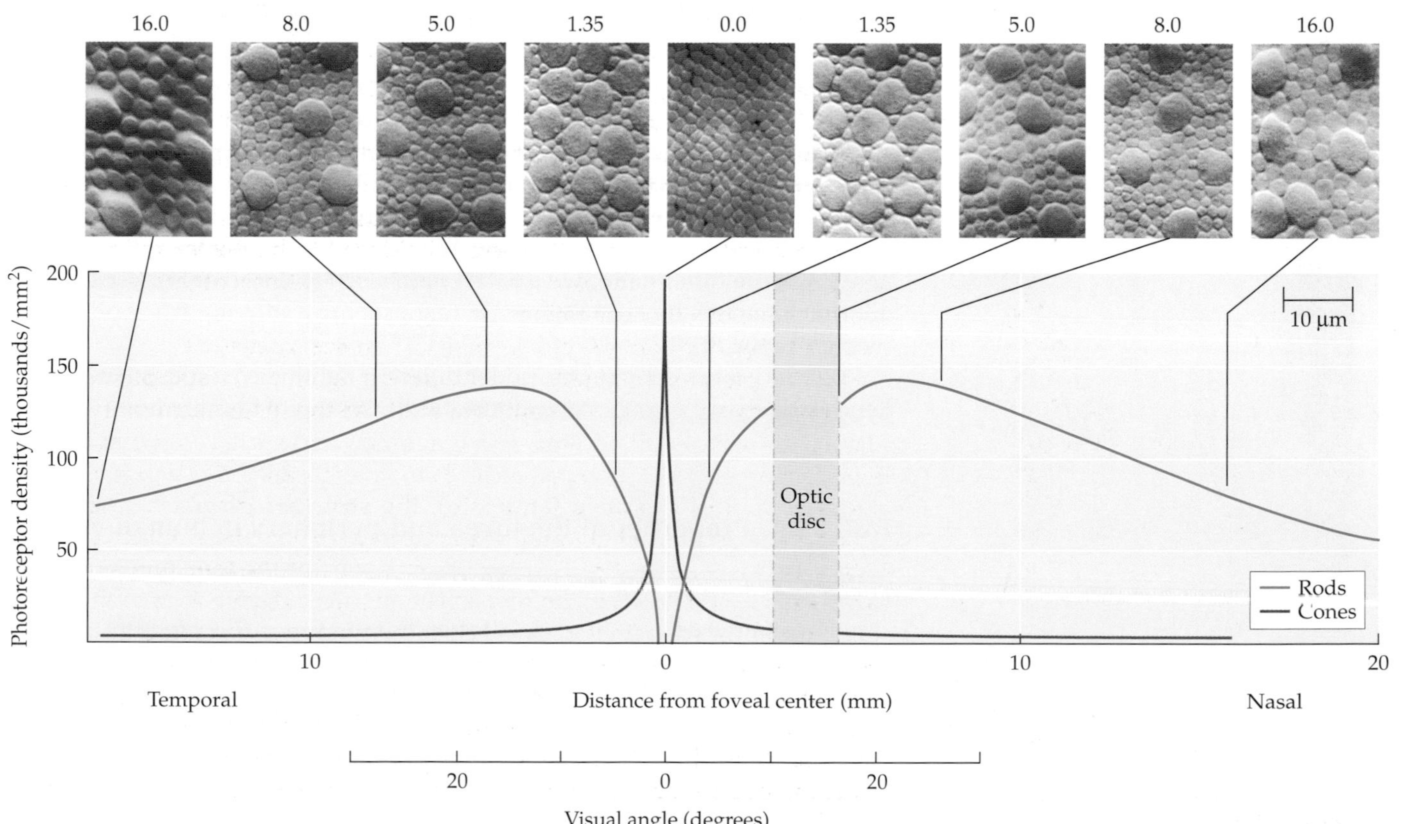

FIGURE 2.9 Photoreceptor density across the retina. The top panels show slices through the photoreceptor inner segments at different eccentricities (distances from the fovea). The graph shows the density of rods and cones plotted as a function of distance from the fovea. Note that in the peripheral slices, the cones are always the larger cells. (After Oyster, 1999; micrographs from Curcio et al., 1990.)

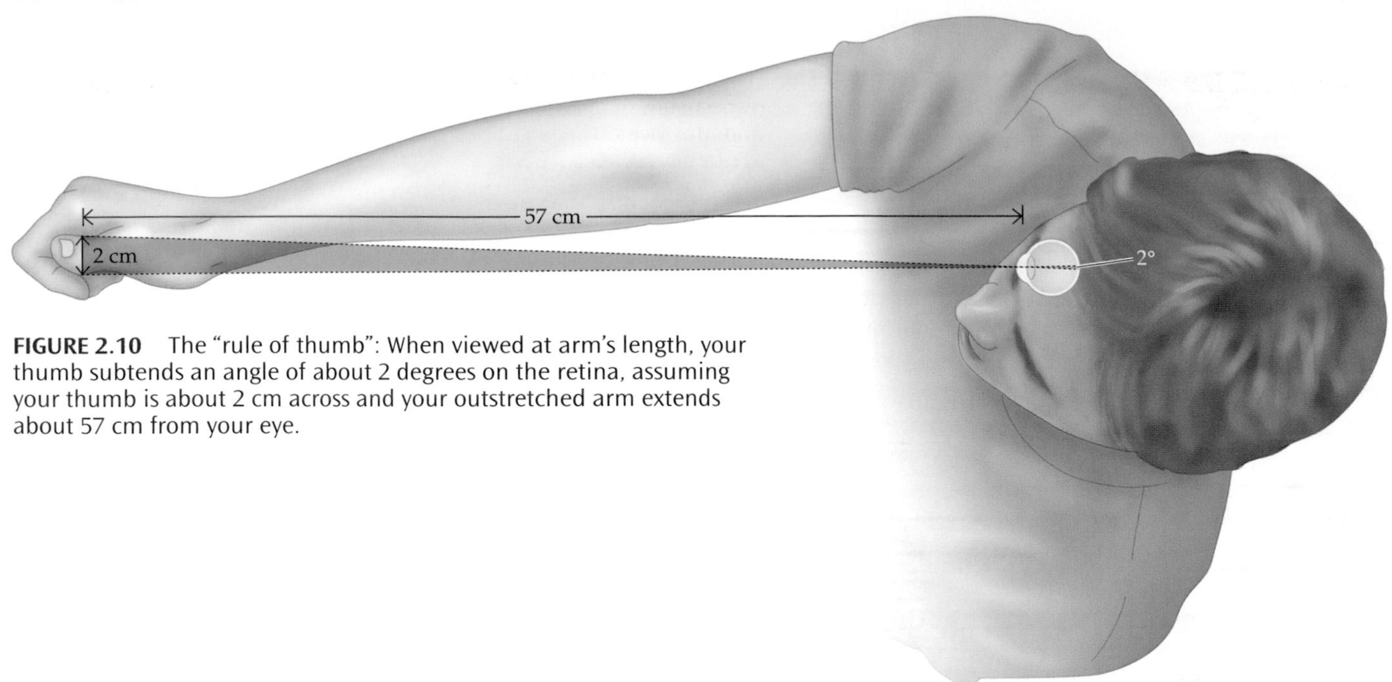

FIGURE 2.10 The "rule of thumb": When viewed at arm's length, your thumb subtends an angle of about 2 degrees on the retina, assuming your thumb is about 2 cm across and your outstretched arm extends about 57 cm from your eye.

eccentricity The distance between the retinal image and the fovea.

and their density drops off dramatically with retinal **eccentricity** (distance from the fovea).

As the photographs of photoreceptors at different eccentricities in Figure 2.9 illustrate, cones are also smaller and more tightly packed in the foveal center. This "rod-free" area (about 300 square micrometers [μm] on the retina) subtends a visual angle of about 1 degree, and it is directly behind the center of the pupil. So if we look directly at an object whose image is smaller than 1 degree, the image will land on a region of the retina that has only cones. (How big is 1 degree? Here's a rule of thumb, illustrated in **Figure 2.10**: Your thumb, when viewed at arm's length, subtends an angle of about 2 degrees on the retina, assuming your thumb is about 2 cm across and your outstretched arm extends about 57 cm from your eye.) **Table 2.1** illustrates some of the fundamental differences in the properties of the fovea compared to the peripheral retina. Most important for us, the fovea has high acuity and we use it to identify objects, to read, and to inspect fine detail. On the other hand, we use the periphery to detect and localize stimuli that we aren't looking at directly (e.g., seeing a moving truck out of the "corner of the eye").

Rods and cones operate best under different lighting conditions: Rods function relatively well under conditions of dim (scotopic) illumination (which is

TABLE 2.1 Properties of the fovea and periphery in human vision

Property	Fovea	Periphery
Photoreceptor type	Mostly cones	Mostly rods
Bipolar cell type	Midget	Diffuse
Convergence	Low	High
Receptive-field size	Small	Large
Acuity (detail)	High	Low
Light sensitivity	Low	High

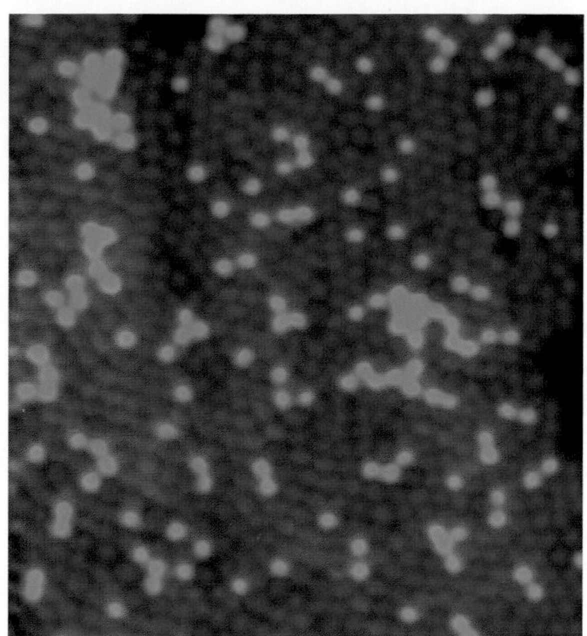

FIGURE 2.11 Blue, green, and red represent the S-, M-, and L-cones, respectively, of a living human being, in a patch of retina at 1 degree from the fovea. The pseudocolor image was made by the use of adaptive optics to measure and bypass the aberrations of the eye, and selective bleaching to isolate the different photopigments. (From Roorda and Williams, 1999; courtesy of Austin Roorda.)

why animals with all-rod retinas are nocturnal), but cones require brighter (photopic) illumination (e.g., sunlight or room lights) to operate efficiently. Having an area at the center of the fovea with no rods means that, under dim illumination, the central 1 degree or so around the fovea is effectively blind! Indeed, practiced stargazers know that it is often easier to spot a dim star by looking out of the corner of one's eye than by looking directly at it.

Rods and cones differ functionally in another important way. Because all rods have the same type of photopigment, they cannot signal differences in color. Each cone, on the other hand, has one of three different photopigments that differ in the wavelengths at which they absorb light most efficiently. Therefore, cones can signal information about wavelength, and thus they provide the basis for our color vision (see Chapter 5). However, the three cone photopigments are not distributed equally among the cones (**Figure 2.11**). Short wavelength–sensitive cones (S-cones) constitute only about 5% to 10% of the total cone population, and they are essentially missing from the center of the fovea. Thus, the foveal center is dichromatic (it has only two color-sensitive cones). We also know that there are more long wavelength–sensitive cones (L-cones) than medium wavelength–sensitive cones (M-cones); it has been estimated that there are, on average, about twice as many L-cones as M-cones, although the ratio of L- to M-cones varies enormously among individuals. **Table 2.2** illustrates some of the fun-

TABLE 2.2 Properties of human photopic and scotopic vision

Property	Photopic system	Scotopic system
Photoreceptors	4–5 million cones	90 million rods
Location in retina	Throughout retina with the highest concentration close to fovea	Outside of fovea
Acuity (detail)	High	Low
Sensitivity	Low	High

damental differences in the properties of the photopic (high illumination) and scotopic (low illumination) visual systems.

When photoreceptors capture light, they produce chemical changes that start a cascade of neural events ending in a visual sensation. Photoreceptors send their signals by way of the synaptic terminals, specialized structures for contacting other retinal neurons. Figure 2.8 shows examples of rod and cone synaptic terminals. The synaptic terminals contain connections from the neurons that photoreceptors "talk to": the horizontal and bipolar cells.

Lateral Inhibition through Horizontal and Amacrine Cells

As the name implies, **horizontal cells** run perpendicular to the photoreceptors, making contacts between nearby photoreceptors. These lateral connections play an important functional role in the form of **lateral inhibition**, which enables the signals that reach retinal ganglion cells to be based on differences in activation between nearby photoreceptors. Lateral inhibition plays an important role in perception, and we will have much more to say about it in the "Center–Surround Receptive Fields" section of this chapter.

Amacrine cells are also part of the lateral pathway. Like horizontal cells, amacrine cells run perpendicular to the photoreceptors in the inner layers of the retina, where they receive inputs from bipolar cells and other amacrine cells and send signals to bipolar, amacrine, and retinal ganglion cells. Amacrine cells come in many flavors, by some estimates as many as 40 (Rodieck, 1998). Although amacrine cells have been implicated in both contrast enhancement and temporal sensitivity (the detection of changes in light patterns over time), their precise function remains unclear.

Convergence and Divergence of Information via Bipolar Cells

If horizontal and amacrine cells form a lateral pathway in the retina, then photoreceptors, bipolar cells, and ganglion cells can be considered to form a vertical pathway. Bipolar cells are the intermediaries. There are various types of bipolar cells, and their wiring determines the information that is passed from the photoreceptors to the ganglion cells. For example, in peripheral vision a **bipolar cell** receives input from as many as 50 photoreceptors, pools this information, and passes it on to a ganglion cell. This convergence of information from many photoreceptors to a single bipolar cell (known as a **diffuse bipolar cell**) is a characteristic of the rod pathway, and the same sort of convergence occurs in the cone pathway in the peripheral retina.

Pooling of information from many photoreceptors is a very important mechanism for increasing visual **sensitivity**. Indeed, the fact that most rods communicate with ganglion cells through diffuse bipolar cells largely accounts for the ability of the rod system to function well in dim lighting conditions. However, convergence wreaks havoc with **visual acuity**: A diffuse bipolar cell may fire at the same rate in response to a single point of bright light or several spots of dim light, so a ganglion cell listening to the diffuse bipolar cell will be unable to tell which pattern of light is present.

In contrast, in the fovea, **midget bipolar cells** receive input from single cones and pass this information on to single ganglion cells. The fact that one-to-one pathways between cones and ganglions exist only in the fovea accounts for why images are seen most clearly when they fall on this part of the retina. The high degree of convergence in peripheral vision ensures high sensitivity to light but poor acuity. The low degree of convergence in the fovea ensures high acuity but poor sensitivity to light. You can explore this trade-off of sensitivity and acuity in **Web Activity 2.5: Acuity versus Sensitivity**.

horizontal cells Specialized retinal cells that contact both photoreceptor and bipolar cells.

lateral inhibition Antagonistic neural interaction between adjacent regions of the retina.

amacrine cells Retinal cells found in the inner synaptic layer that make synaptic contacts with bipolar cells, ganglion cells, and one another.

bipolar cells Retinal cells that synapse with either rods or cones (not both) and with horizontal cells, and then pass the signals on to ganglion cells.

diffuse bipolar cells Bipolar retinal cells whose processes are spread out to receive input from multiple cones.

sensitivity 1. The ability to perceive via the sense organs. 2. Extreme responsiveness to radiation, especially to light of a specific wavelength. 3. The ability to respond to transmitted signals.

visual acuity A measure of the finest detail that can be resolved by the eyes.

midget bipolar cells Small cone bipolar cells in the central retina that receive input from a single cone.

Interestingly, each foveal cone actually contacts two bipolar cells (representing a divergence of information): one responds to an increase in light captured by the cone and is called an **ON bipolar cell**; the other responds to a decrease and is called an **OFF bipolar cell**. The fact that there are both ON and OFF bipolar cells provides information about the sign (or direction) of the change in illumination. This information is important for visual information processing at higher levels in the visual pathway, and as we will see, the ON/OFF distinction built into the anatomical structure of the retina is present at many levels of the visual pathway.

ON bipolar cells Bipolar cells that respond to an increase in light captured by the cones.

OFF bipolar cells Bipolar cells that respond to a decrease in light captured by the cones.

ganglion cells Retinal cells that receive visual information from photoreceptors via two intermediate neuron types (bipolar cells and amacrine cells) and transmit information to the brain and midbrain.

P ganglion cells Small ganglion cells that receive excitatory input from single midget bipolar cells in the central retina and feed the parvocellular layer of the lateral geniculate nucleus.

M ganglion cells Ganglion cells resembling little umbrellas that receive excitatory input from diffuse bipolar cells and feed the magnocellular layer of the lateral geniculate nucleus.

Communicating to the Brain via Ganglion Cells

By the time signals arrive at the final layer of the retina, the ganglion cells, there has already been a lot of information processing. Some information has been pooled through convergence; some has been enhanced by lateral pathways. **Ganglion cells** receive their input from bipolar and amacrine cells, process this input further, and send messages off to the brain through their axons, which gather in the back of the eyeball and emerge together as the optic nerve.

By now you are probably getting the idea that each cell type comes in many varieties, and ganglion cells are no exception. The human retina contains about 1,250,000 ganglion cells, about one-hundredth the number of photoreceptors. Midget bipolar cells send their signals to small ganglion cells, which are widely referred to as **P ganglion cells** because they feed the parvocellular ("small cell") layer of the lateral geniculate nucleus (LGN) (discussed in Chapter 3). P cells constitute about 70% of the ganglion cells in the human retina. Diffuse bipolar cells project to ganglion cells that are known as **M ganglion cells** (Figure 2.12) because they feed the magnocellular ("large-cell") layer of the lateral geniculate nucleus. The dendrites of these ganglion cells spread out much more than those of the P ganglion cells, giving them an umbrella-like appearance. About 8% to 10% of ganglion cells in the human retina are of the M variety. The dendrites of both P and M ganglion cells increase in size with retinal eccentricity, but at all eccentricities the P ganglion cells have much smaller dendritic trees than do the M ganglion cells.

CENTER–SURROUND RECEPTIVE FIELDS Much of what we know about how retinal ganglion cells work comes from painstaking physiological studies in which tiny electrodes are used to study the electrical changes in indi-

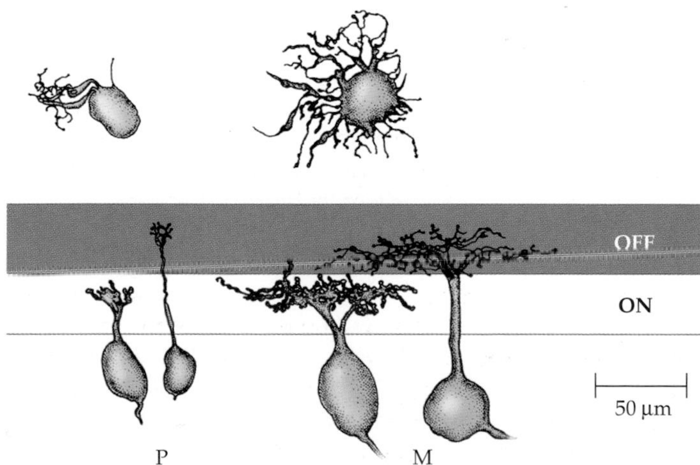

FIGURE 2.12 Different types of retinal P and M ganglion cells. The upper panel shows the cells in the flat-mounted retina; the lower panel shows them in section. (After Oyster, 1999.)

receptive field The region on the retina in which visual stimuli influence a neuron's firing rate.

vidual ganglion cells. Ganglion cells fire action potentials spontaneously, at about one spike per second, even in the absence of visual stimulation. However, each ganglion cell has a small window on the world known as its **receptive field**. The receptive field is the region on the retina in which visual stimuli influence the neuron's firing rate. This influence can be either excitatory, increasing the ganglion's firing rate, or inhibitory, decreasing the ganglion's firing rate.

Work on horseshoe crabs and frogs provided some of our earliest information on the receptive fields of retinal neurons (Hartline, 1940). But it was Stephen Kuffler who first mapped out the receptive fields of individual retinal ganglion cells in the cat, using small spots of light (Kuffler, 1953). **Figure 2.13** illustrates Kuffler's main findings and provides some important insights into how the retina processes visual information. Kuffler's experiments are simulated in **Web Activity 2.6: Ganglion Receptive Fields**.

Let's consider Figure 2.13*a*. Kuffler's visual stimulus was a small spot of light, which he moved about on the retina, turning it on and off while recording impulses from a single retinal ganglion cell. When the spot was placed on a specific small region of the retina, the ganglion cell *increased* its firing rate when the light was turned on (this response is indicated by a plus sign in the figure). This area of the retina is called the "center" of the gan-

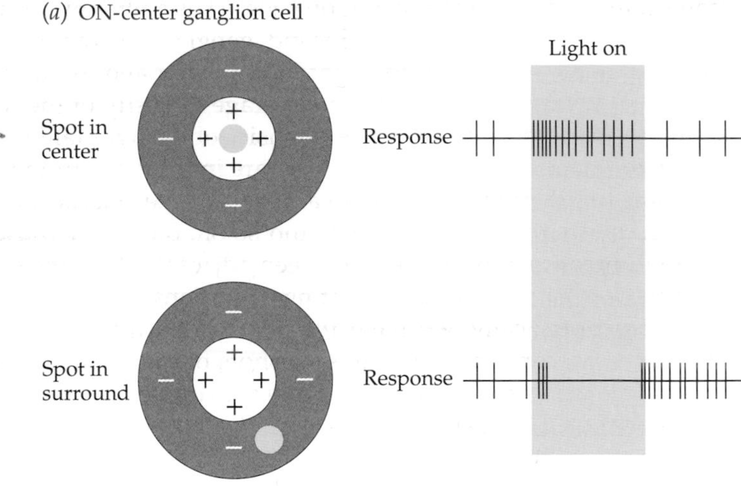

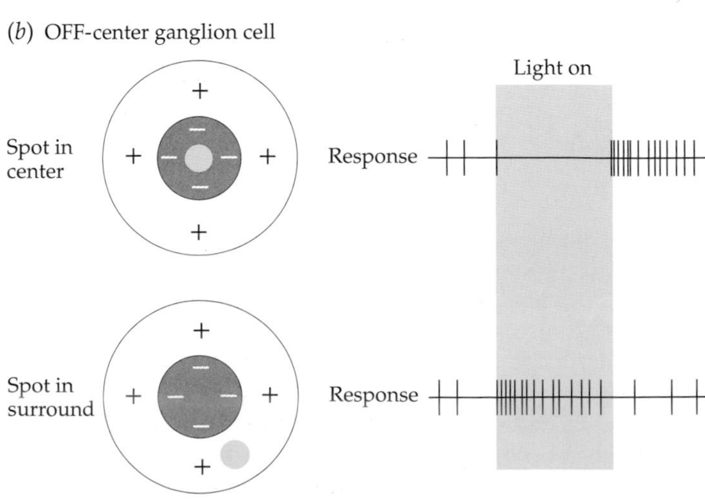

FIGURE 2.13 Retinal ganglion cell receptive fields. (*a*) ON-center field. In each image on the left, the small white circle illustrates the region on the retina where the retinal ganglion cell increased its firing rate when the spot (small yellow circle) was turned on. The large gray circle illustrates the region on the retina where the retinal ganglion cell decreased its firing rate when the spot was turned on and increased its rate when the spot was turned off. The plots on the right illustrate the spikes fired by the retinal ganglion cell. (*b*) OFF-center field. In each image on the left, the large white circle illustrates the region on the retina where the retinal ganglion cell increased its firing rate when the spot was turned on. The small gray circle illustrates the region on the retina where the retinal ganglion cell decreased its firing rate when the spot was turned on and increased its rate when the spot was turned off. The plots on the right illustrate the spikes fired by the retinal ganglion cell.

glion cell's receptive field. But when the spot was moved to an adjacent area of the retina, the ganglion cell *decreased* its firing rate when the light was turned on (indicated by a minus sign). Interestingly, turning the light *off* in this area surrounding the receptive-field center led to a brief surge in the cell's firing rate, after which the cell settled down to its spontaneous rate.

Kuffler found that the spatial layout of the ganglion cell's receptive field is essentially concentric; that is, a small circular area in the center responds to an increase in illumination, and a surrounding annulus responds to a decrease in illumination. The ganglion cell fires fastest when the spot size matches the size of the excitatory center, and it reduces its firing rate when the spot begins to encroach on its inhibitory surround.

The cell just described is known as an **ON-center cell**. It increases its firing rate when a light is turned on in the center of its receptive field, and it decreases its firing rate when the light is turned on in the surround. However, nearly as many ganglion cells do exactly the opposite: their firing rates decrease when a spot in the center of the receptive field is turned on, and increase when the spot is turned on in the surround. These are known as **OFF-center cells** (Figure 2.13*b*). Most retinal ganglion cells have one of these two types of concentric center–surround organization.

This center–surround organization has two important functional consequences. First, it means that each ganglion cell will respond best to spots of a particular size (and will respond less to spots that are either bigger or smaller). In this way, retinal ganglion cells act as a **filter** by editing the information they send on to the brain. Second, ganglion cells are most sensitive to *differences* in the intensity of the light in the center and in the surround, and they are relatively unaffected by the average intensity of the light. This is a useful quality because the average intensity of the light falling on the retina varies a lot, depending on whether you are indoors or outdoors, whether it is daytime or nighttime, how far away you and the objects you're looking at are from the source of illumination, and so on. But the **contrast**—the difference in luminance or brightness between adjacent bits of the scene—will be roughly the same regardless of lighting conditions.

Phenomenologically, we have the impression that our eyes work like video cameras, capturing faithful snapshots of the world around us. Note, though, that the rest of the visual system sees only what the retinal ganglion cells show it, and the ganglion cells are not content simply to pass along the raw images encoded by the photoreceptors. Instead, the ganglion cells, together with the bipolar, amacrine, and horizontal cells, act as an image filter, transforming the raw image into a new representation. This new representation highlights certain important information, such as contrast, and largely discounts other types of less useful information, such as ambient light intensity. In fact, the whole visual system can be considered a long series of filters, with each stage in the system responsible for extracting a particular aspect of the visual world and passing this aspect on to the next stage.

SEEING ILLUSORY STRIPES—MACH BANDS Seeing is not always believing. Sometimes our eyes play tricks on us, and the illusions that we see can be quite informative about the neural operations that the visual system carries out. One well-known visual illusion was described by Ernst Mach (1838–1916), the famous Austrian physicist whose name is attached to the units that describe the speed of sound. **Figure 2.14***a* shows the visual illusion that bears Mach's name. The illusion is known as "Mach bands" because there is an illusory bright stripe in the region marked "B" and an illusory dark stripe in the region marked "D." These bright and dark stripes (Mach bands) are illusions formed by the visual system. The actual intensity distri-

ON-center cell A cell that depolarizes in response to an increase in light intensity in its receptive field center.

OFF-center cell A cell that depolarizes in response to a decrease in light intensity in its receptive field center.

filter An acoustic, electrical, electronic, or optical device, instrument, computer program, or neuron that allows the passage of some frequencies or digital elements and blocks the passage of others.

contrast The difference in luminance between an object and the background, or between lighter and darker parts of the same object.

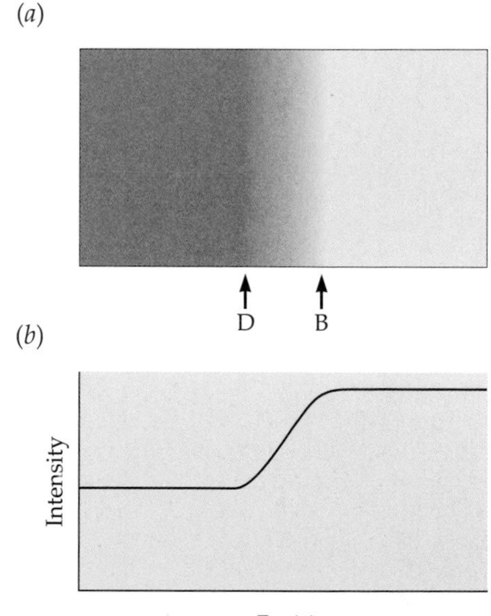

FIGURE 2.14 Mach bands. (*a*) This visual illusion gets its name from the illusory bright stripe in the region marked "B" and the illusory dark stripe in the region marked "D." (*b*) The actual intensity distribution of the Mach pattern illustrates a luminance ramp edge. (*a* from Cornsweet, 1970.)

bution of the Mach pattern, shown in Figure 2.14*b*, is initially constant, increases smoothly over a short distance, and than remains steady at the new (higher) level. This intensity pattern is a luminance ramp edge, which contains no bright or dark stripes. Rather, the vivid perception of bright and dark stripes comes from operations performed by the visual nervous system instead of from the visual stimulus. This is an example where you can't believe your eyes—the perceptual brightness of the pattern varies where its physical intensity does not!

In 1865, when Mach first reported his observations, we had very little direct knowledge about the visual nervous system; however, Mach suggested that the illusory stripes were produced by lateral interactions in the retina. This notion gained wide support following the discovery of center–surround antagonistic receptive fields in the retina. This type of explanation, illustrated in **Figure 2.15**, has been popular for about the last 50 years.

In Figure 2.15*a* the concentric circles represent ON-center retinal (or LGN) receptive fields (RFs). The RF on the left receives less light than the one on the right. If these receptive fields inform the brain about the intensity of light falling within their RFs, the brain will get the message that the left side of the picture is dimmer than the right side. Consider the middle RF in Figure 2.15*a*. Its center falls within the left half of the pattern; however, part of the antagonistic surround falls within the brighter right half. Thus, the middle RF will receive more surround antagonism, and therefore its response will be lower than the response of the RF on the left. The perceptual result will be that the region just to the left of the luminance step will appear as a darker stripe (or Mach band). The bright Mach band would be explained by an RF that had its center just within the bright panel but part of its antagonistic surround in the dimmer left half. The result would be less antagonism compared to the rightmost RF (where the entire surround is in the bright panel), and the perceptual consequence would be a brighter stripe (or Mach band). Figure 2.15*b* shows an alternative way of illustrating the center–surround model of Mach bands. If a luminance ramp edge (left) is filtered by a center–surround (or lateral inhibition) weighting function (middle), the output will have an "undershoot" (a little dip to the left of the ramp) and an "overshoot" (a little bump to the right of the ramp) that seem to correspond to the Mach bands.

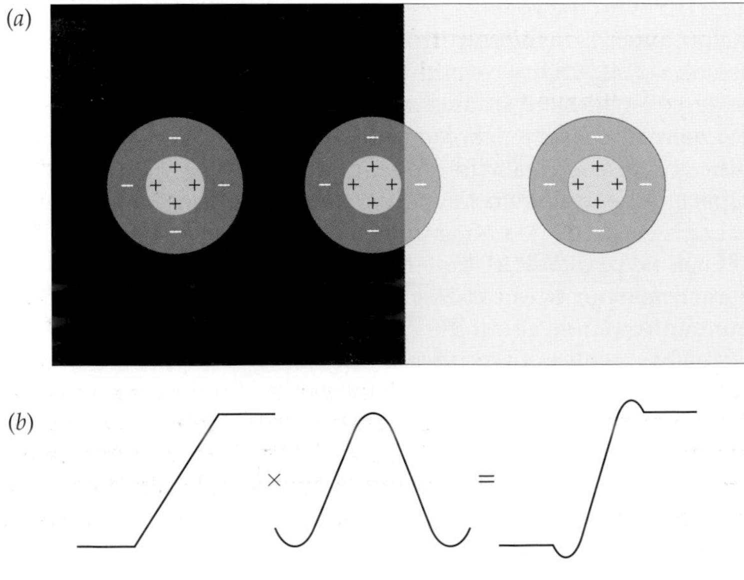

FIGURE 2.15 Neuronal explanation for Mach bands. (*a*) "Cartoon" showing a classic explanation. (*b*) A slightly more modern version.

Although this simple "classic" explanation feels good, it is not the full story, and a complete understanding of Mach bands (and other similar perceptual illusions) will likely require a theory involving stages beyond the retina (for an excellent review, see Pessoa, 1996). For example, this theory fails to explain why Mach bands are less obvious at step edges than they are at ramp edges like the one shown in Figure 2.14*b*. However, the Mach band phenomenon reminds us that our visual system does not simply passively transmit information about the intensities of objects—it acts on that information in ways that often sharpen edges and contours.

P AND M GANGLION CELLS REVISITED As already mentioned, retinal ganglion cells come in several types; for humans, the most important of these are the P and M cells. The receptive fields of these two types of ganglion cells differ in some important ways. First, at all eccentricities P cells have smaller receptive fields than M cells have. This isn't too surprising, because the size of the receptive field is probably determined by the size of its dendritic field (see Figure 2.12): since M cells listen to more photoreceptors (via bipolar, horizontal, and amacrine cells) than P cells do, M cells respond to a larger portion of the visual field.

An additional consequence of the differing sizes of M and P receptive fields is that M cells are much more sensitive—better able to detect visual stimuli—than are P cells under low lighting conditions (e.g., at night). However, the smaller receptive fields of P cells enable them to provide finer resolution (greater acuity) than M cells can, if there is enough light for the P cells to operate. See **Web Activity 2.5: Acuity versus Sensitivity** for more on this trade-off.

P and M ganglion cells also differ in their temporal responses. P cells tend to respond with sustained firing while light shines on their excitatory regions, M cells tend to respond more transiently: an M cell will respond with a brief burst of impulses when the spot is turned on, then quickly return to its spontaneous rate, even if the spot remains lit. Thus, M and P ganglion cells signal different information to the brain. P cells provide information mainly about the contrast in the retinal image, and M cells signal information about how the image changes over time.

Finally, P and M cells differ in what they say to the brain about the color of the light they detect (see Chapter 5).

Whistling in the Dark: Dark and Light Adaptation

If you enter a dark room from bright sunlight, the number of photons of light entering your eye might be reduced by a factor of several billion. Initially you will have trouble seeing anything, but after about 30 minutes in the dark you will be able to detect just a few photons (**Figure 2.16**). And when you reemerge from the dark and return to the sunlight, you will be able to see almost instantly. How does the visual system alter its sensitivity over such a large operating range?

When a flashlight is shone in someone's eye in a dimly lit room, the pupil quickly constricts. The diameter of the pupil can vary by about a factor of 4, from about 2 mm in bright illumination to about 8 mm in the dark (**Figure 2.17**). Because the amount of light entering the eye is proportional to the area of the pupil, the 4-fold increase in diameter accounts for a 16-fold improvement in sensitivity. In other words, 16 times as many quanta can enter the eye when the pupil is completely dilated, compared to when it is constricted. Although this adaptive ability certainly helps, pupil dilation accounts for only a small part of the visual system's overall ability to adapt to light and dark conditions.

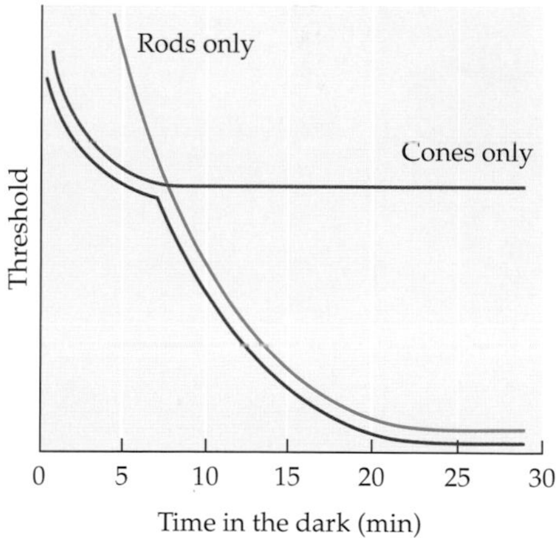

FIGURE 2.16 Dark adaptation curve. The purple curve shows the threshold light intensity required to detect a peripheral spot following several minutes of adaptation to a bright light. The red curve illustrates the rapid adaptation of the cones. The blue curve shows the slower recovery of the rods to much lower threshold intensities (that is, greater sensitivity). The purple curve represents the most sensitive of the two at any given time.

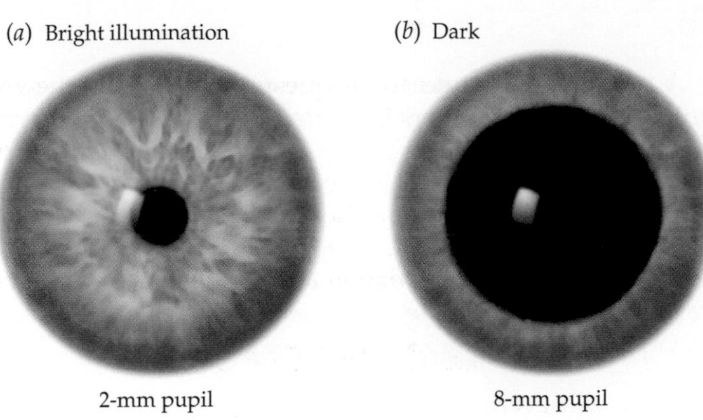

FIGURE 2.17 The black spots in the middle of these two eyeballs show the possible range of pupil sizes as we go from bright illumination (*a*) into the dark (*b*).

A second mechanism for achieving a large sensitivity range is provided by the way photopigments are used up and replaced in receptor cells. In dim lighting conditions, plenty of photopigment is available, and rods and cones absorb and respond to as many photons as they can. As already noted, rods provide better sensitivity in such situations than do cones. Indeed, the rod system is capable of detecting a single quantum of light! (See **Web Essay 2.2: How Many Quanta Does It Take?**) After a photopigment molecule is bleached (used to detect a photon), the molecule must be regenerated before it can be used again to absorb another photon.

As the overall light level increases, the number of photons starts to overwhelm the system: photopigment molecules cannot be regenerated fast enough to detect all the photons hitting the photoreceptors. This slow regeneration is a good thing for increasing our sensitivity range. If photons are scarce, we use them all to see, but if we have an overabundance, we simply throw some of them away and use the leftovers.

This light compensation mechanism is enhanced by humans' duplex retinas. Rods provide exquisite sensitivity at low light levels, but they become overwhelmed when the background light becomes moderately bright, leading to a loss in information quality. Cones are much less sensitive than rods (they function poorly under very dim light), but their operating range is much larger, stretching from about ten photons per second (just enough light to see color) to hundreds of thousands of photons per second (e.g., a snowcapped mountain in bright sunlight). So we use rods to see when the light is low, and the cones take over when there is too much light for the rods to function well. After adapting to a bright light, cones recover sensitivity quickly (red curve in Figure 2.16) and then saturate. They are not very sensitive to very dim light. Rods recover more slowly (blue curve in Figure 2.16), but after 30 minutes or so they are very sensitive to dim light.

However, although pupil size, photopigment regeneration rates, and the rod/cone dichotomy all play a role in dark and light adaptation, the most important reason we are not bothered by variations in overall light levels has to do with the neural circuitry of the retina. As we learned earlier, ganglion cells fire at their maximum rate when the centers of their receptive fields are brightly lit while the surrounds are completely dark (or vice versa) (see Figure 2.13). But the cells will still fire at an above-spontaneous rate when light falls on the entire receptive field, as long as the light is *brighter* in the ON portion than in the OFF portion of the receptive field. Therefore, as long as the photoreceptors feeding the ganglion cells are not completely saturated, the ganglion cells will encode the pattern of relatively light and relatively dark areas in the retinal image. And the pattern of illumination, not the overall light level, is the primary concern of the rest of the visual system.

To sum up, the answer to the question "How does the visual system deal with such large variations in overall light levels?" has two parts. First, we reduce the scale of the problem by regulating the amount of light entering the eyeball, by using different types of photoreceptors in different situations, and by effectively throwing away photons we don't need. Second, by responding to the contrast between adjacent retinal regions, the ganglion cells do their best to ignore whatever variation in overall light level is left over.

The Man Who Could Not See Stars

Imagine not being able to see stars. What follows is the sad story of a man who could not. This man loved to go out at night and look at the sky when he visited the countryside. He used to find his favorite distant star by scanning the northern sky, and when he spotted its faint glow, he would look off to the side so that he could see it out of the corner of his eye. He always found it fascinating that he could see a dim star better with his peripheral vision than when he fixated it directly.

On one visit, his first in 2 years, he was very excited when he spotted his star. To his great dismay, however, when he looked off to the side, as he'd done so many times before, the star disappeared. He had noticed during the preceding year that he had begun experiencing difficulty driving at night. Sometimes he didn't see cars off in the distance, or cars overtaking from the side. And he seemed to be dazzled for a long time by the headlights of oncoming vehicles. Movies were also becoming a problem. It seemed to take forever for his vision to adapt to the darkness of the theater.

He was also beginning to experience other difficulties with his vision. Just in the previous week he had walked into a table in a restaurant, and several times he had tripped over items that he simply hadn't noticed. He hadn't worried too much about these difficulties, because he was having no trouble reading and his vision in bright lights seemed just fine. But not seeing his favorite star out of the corner of his eye really shook him. He was reminded of his father, who in his later years had not been able to drive or read because he had been almost totally blind.

Retinitis pigmentosa (**RP**) is a family of hereditary diseases characterized by the progressive death of photoreceptors and degeneration of the pigment epithelium. In the most common form of RP, exhibited by the man who could not see stars, the rods are affected before the cones. Therefore, people suffering from this form of the disease first notice vision problems in their peripheral vision and under low light conditions—situations in which rods play the dominant role in collecting light. In some cases, vision loss progresses slowly and goes unnoticed until age 20 or later. However, the age of onset and rate of progression vary greatly, probably reflecting complex variations in the genetics of the disease. Eventually, visual loss spreads toward the fovea, often leading to total blindness.

Figure 2.18 shows the fundus of the man who could not see stars. A comparison with the normal fundus pictured in Figure 2.5 shows that the most striking difference is the presence of conspicuous clumps of pigment in the RP fundus that have a characteristic shape and are known as "bone spicules." These bone spicules are the hallmark of retinitis pigmentosa.

When you're reading this book, you direct your gaze (and your fovea) at the words. But if an elephant were to walk up beside you, you would see it out of the corner of your eye (your peripheral field of vision) and make an eye movement to look at it directly. Luckily, the extent of peripheral vision in intact visual systems is pretty big. How big? You can test the extent of your own visual field by closing your left eye, stretching your arms out in front of

retinitis pigmentosa (RP) A progressive degeneration of the retina that affects night vision and peripheral vision. RP commonly runs in families and can be caused by defects in a number of different genes that have recently been identified.

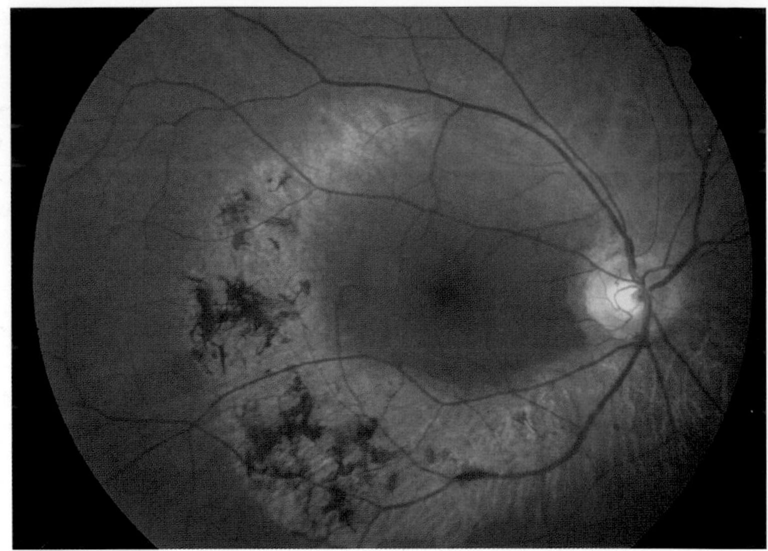

FIGURE 2.18 Fundus of a patient with retinitis pigmentosa. Compare this picture with the normal fundus shown in Figure 2.5. (From Rodieck, 1998.)

you with index fingers raised, and moving your right finger around while you fixate your gaze on the left finger. The points at which you can no longer see the right finger above, below, and to the right and left of the other finger define the limits of your peripheral vision.

Normal visual fields (**Figure 2.19***a*) are limited by anatomy: the upper, lower, and inside edges are set by the prominence of the eyebrows, cheekbones, and nose, respectively; and the outer edge is limited by the abrupt edge of the retina. RP sufferers typically exhibit an overall shrinkage of their visual fields (Figure 2.19*b*), as well as "ring scotomas," bands of blindness between the relatively normal central visual fields and the periphery.

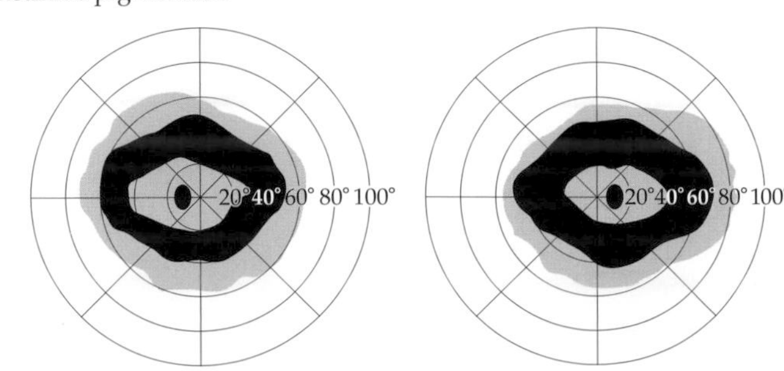

FIGURE 2.19 Visual fields in (*a*) normal individuals and (*b*) the man who couldn't see stars. The fields are pictured as though we were looking through the back of the patient's head at the field limits on the retina. Thus, the right eye is shown on the right, and the left eye on the left. The numbers show the visual angles in degrees. The reddish-shaded area shows the outer limits of vision (the size of the visual field). The small black ovals in the center represent the physiological blind spot (due to the optic nerve head). In part (*b*), note that the outer limits of vision are somewhat shrunken, but more important, a ring of blindness (illustrated by the black ring) occupies the middle of the visual field. This ring scotoma is one of the hallmarks of retinitis pigmentosa.

At present, there is no cure for RP. Large doses of vitamins A and E evidently alter certain electrical potentials that can be measured from the retina and may slow the progression of RP by a very small amount, but it is not clear that these large vitamin doses actually improve either visual fields or dark adaptation. However, there is hope for persons with RP. On June 26, 2000, mapping of the human genome was completed, paving the way for new treatments of genetic diseases. Several genes associated with RP and related diseases have already been identified, and gene replacement therapy has shown promise in mice models.

Summary

1. This chapter provided some insight into the complex journey that is required for us to see stars and other spots of light. The path of the light was traced from a distant star through the eyeball and to its absorption by photoreceptors and its transduction into neural signals. In subsequent chapters we'll learn how those signals are transmitted to the brain and translated into the experience of perception.
2. Light, on its way to becoming a sensation (a visual sensation, that is), can be absorbed, scattered, reflected, transmitted, or refracted. It can become a sensation only when it's absorbed by a photoreceptor in the retina.
3. Vision begins in the retina, when light is absorbed by rods or cones. The retina is like a minicomputer that transduces light energy into neural energy.
4. Retinal ganglion cells have center–surround receptive fields and are concerned with changes in contrast (the difference in intensity between adjacent bits of the scene).
5. The retina sends information to the brain via the ganglion cells, neurons whose axons make up the optic nerves.
6. The visual system deals with large variations in overall light intensity by (a) regulating the amount of light entering the eyeball, (b) using different types of photoreceptors in different situations, and (c) effectively throwing away photons we don't need.
7. Retinitis pigmentosa (RP) is a family of hereditary diseases characterized by the progressive death of photoreceptors and degeneration of the pigment epithelium. In the most common form of the disease, patients first notice vision problems in their peripheral vision and under low light conditions, situations in which rods play the dominant role in collecting light.

Refer to the
Sensation and Perception
website
(www.sinauer.com/wolfe2e)
for activities, essays, study questions, and other study aids.

CHAPTER 3

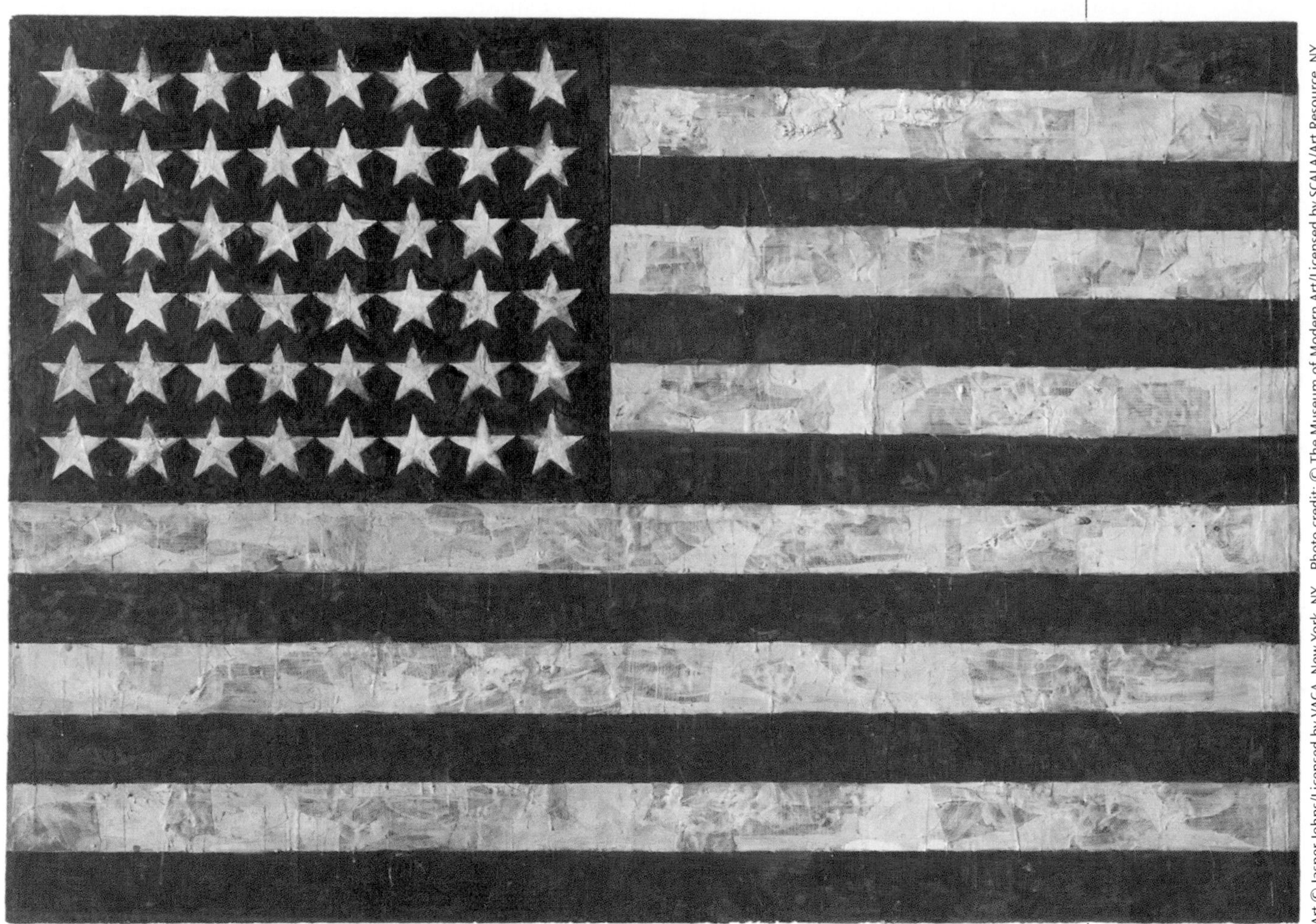

Jasper Johns, *Flag*, 1954–55

Spatial Vision: From Stars to Stripes

In Chapter 2 we learned that the macroscopic structures of the human eye function essentially as a biological camera: the iris regulates the number of light rays entering the eyeball; and the cornea, lens, and aqueous and vitreous humors focus these rays so that a clear image is formed on the retina. The rod and cone photoreceptors capture this image in a way that is roughly analogous to the way the film in a camera captures photographic images.

It is here, however, that the analogy between visual system and camera ends. Cameras take pictures. Visual systems see. How do we get from an image of the world in front of us to an interpretation of that world—what is out there, where it is, and what we can do to it? This process starts in the eyeball itself, where the postreceptor layers of the retina translate the raw light array captured by the photoreceptors into the patterns of spots surrounded by darkness, or vice versa, detected by the ganglion cells (see Figure 2.13). As we discussed in Chapter 2, this retinal translation helps us perceive the pattern of light and dark areas in the visual field regardless of the overall light level (e.g., it enables us to see almost as well at dusk as we can at noon).

In this chapter we follow the path of image processing from the eyeball to the brain (**Figure 3.1**). As we will see, neurons in the cerebral cortex translate the array of stars perceived by retinal ganglion cells into something like an array of stripes. Furthermore, we will see that this portion of visual cortex is organized into thousands of tiny computers, each responsible for determining the orientation, width, color, and other characteristics of the stripes in one small portion of the visual field. In Chapter 4, we will continue this story by examining how other parts of the brain assemble the outputs from these minicomputers to produce a coherent representation of the objects whose reflected light started the photoreceptors firing in the first place.

Visual Acuity: Oh Say, Can You See?

The King said, "I haven't sent the two Messengers, either. They're both gone to the town. Just look along the road, and tell me if you can see either of them."

"I see nobody on the road," said Alice.

"I only wish I had such eyes," the King remarked in a fretful tone. "To be able to see Nobody! And at that distance, too!"

— Lewis Carroll, *Through the Looking Glass*

Since we'll be talking in this chapter about how the visual system codes images in terms of oriented stripes, let's start by determining just how well we see stripes when they are very close together and/or when the difference in illumination between the stripes and the background (the **contrast**) is very

contrast The difference in luminance between an object and the background, or between lighter and darker parts of the same object.

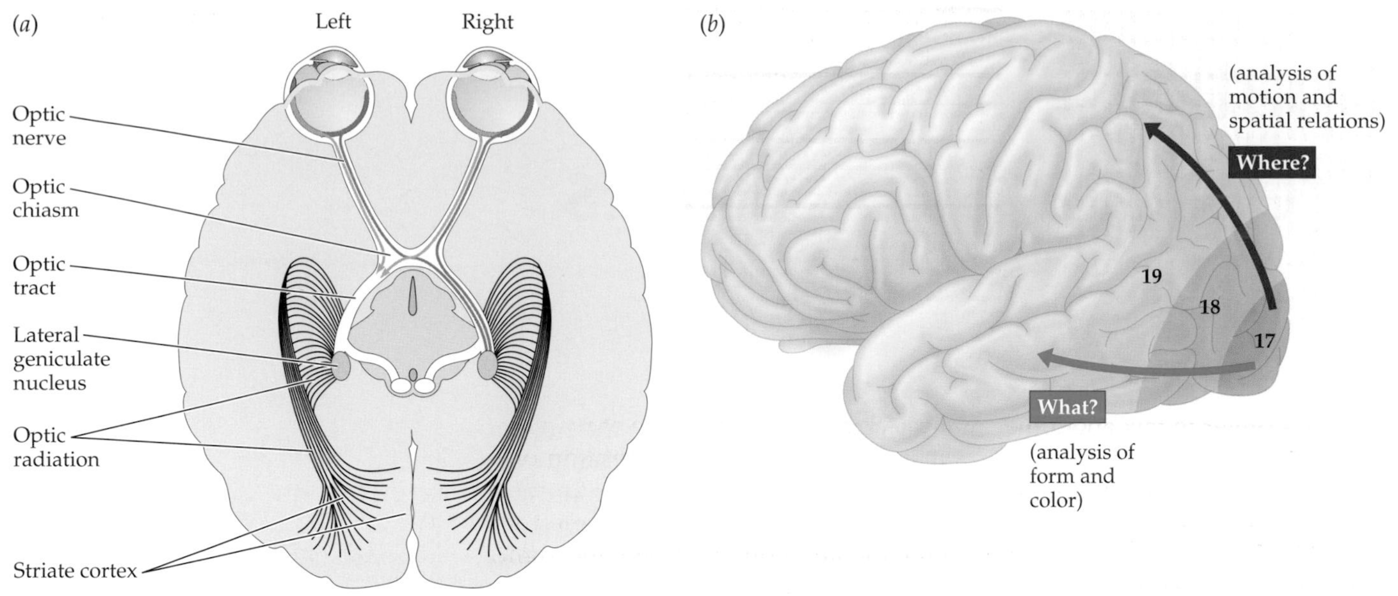

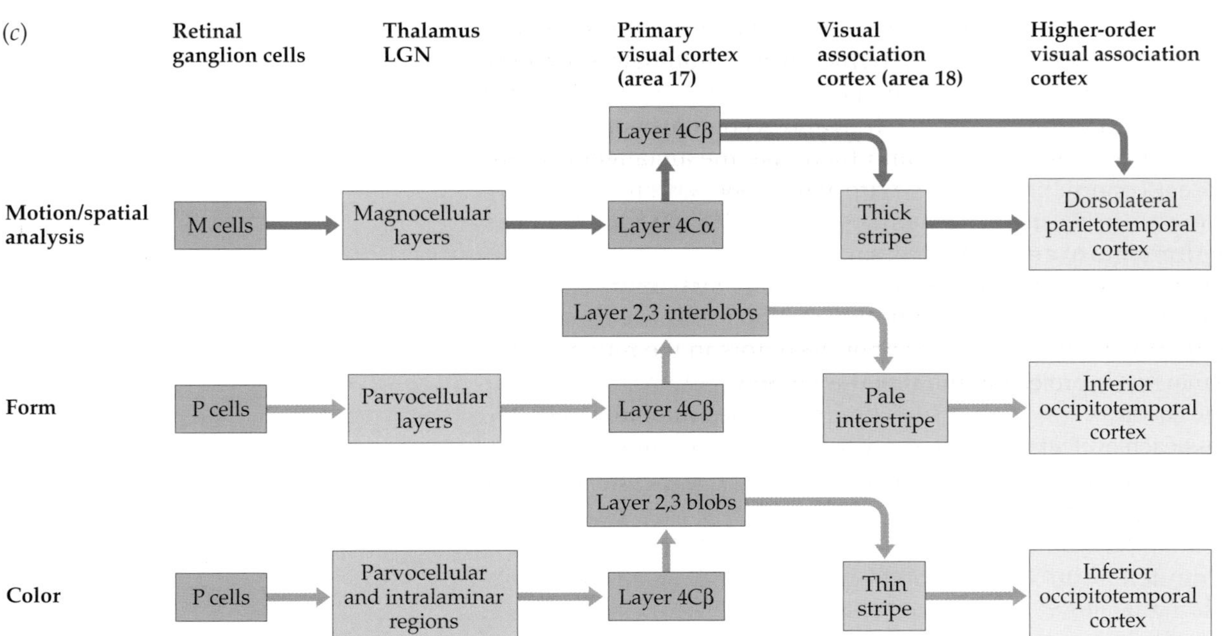

FIGURE 3.1 Cortical visual pathways. (*a*) The basic organization of the primary visual pathway from eyeball to striate cortex, in coronal section. (*b*) A lateral section of the brain, illustrating early visual areas and showing the putative *where* (dorsal) and *what* (ventral) streams. (*c*) The flow of information for motion, form, and color analysis from retinal ganglion cells to higher-order visual association cortex. (Part *a* after Purves et al., 2008; *b* and *c* after Blumenfeld, 2002.)

acuity The smallest spatial detail that can be resolved.

low. In addition to setting the boundary conditions for how well we should expect the visual system to be able to perform, we will use this section to introduce some important jargon that we will need in the rest of the chapter.

Get a tape measure, prop your textbook up, and, while looking at the *X* in the middle of **Figure 3.2**, back up until you cannot tell the orientation of the black and white stripes. Measure how far your eye is from the page. Now walk forward a bit until you're sure you can see which grating includes vertical stripes and which horizontal stripes, and again measure your distance from the page. Congratulations! You just completed a fast (but not terribly accurate) measurement of your own visual resolution **acuity**. Eye doctors specify acuity in terms like *20/20* (more about this in a moment), but vision

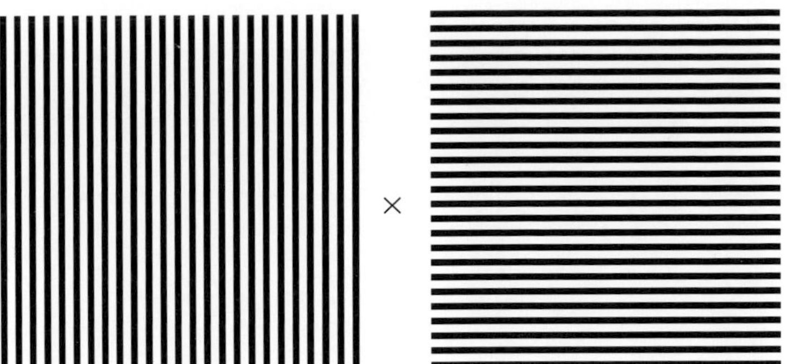

FIGURE 3.2 A visual acuity test. See the text for details.

scientists prefer to talk about the smallest visual angle of a cycle of the grating that we can perceive (**Figure 3.3**). A **cycle** is simply one repetition of a black and a white stripe (both of the gratings in Figure 3.2 have 25 total cycles). **Visual angle**, which we alluded to in Chapter 2, is the angle that would be formed by lines going from the top and bottom (or left and right, depending on the orientation of the stripes) of a cycle on the page, through the center of the lens, and on to the retina. You can learn more about this concept in **Web Activity 3.1: Visual Angle**.

More precisely, to calculate the visual angle of your resolution acuity, divide the size of the cycle in Figure 3.2 (which was 2 millimeters, or 1/16 inch) by the viewing distance at which you could just barely make out the orientation of the gratings (average your first and second measurements to get a rough estimate of this distance), and then take the arctangent of this ratio. Under ideal conditions, humans with very good vision can resolve gratings like those in Figure 3.2 when one cycle subtends an angle of approximately 1 minute of arc (0.017 degree).

This resolution acuity represents one of the fundamental limits of spatial vision: it is the finest high-contrast detail that can be resolved. The limit is determined primarily by the spacing of photoreceptors in the retina. To see why, imagine that we're projecting the **sine wave gratings** shown in **Figure 3.4** onto the retina. The light intensity in such gratings varies smoothly and continuously across each cycle (unlike the gratings in Figure 3.2, in which intensity changes abruptly from black to white and back to black). However, the visual system "samples" the grating discretely, through the array of receptors at the back of the retina (in this respect the eye is more like a digital camera than like a traditional camera that uses film). If the receptors are spaced such that the whitest and blackest parts of the grating fall on separate cones (Figure 3.4*a*), we should be able to make out the grating. But if the entire cycle falls on a single cone (Figure 3.4*b*), we will see nothing but a gray field (or we may experience a phenomenon called **aliasing**, in which we misperceive the cycles to be longer than they actually are).

cycle For a grating, a pair consisting of one dark bar and one bright bar.

visual angle The angle subtended by an object at the retina.

sine wave grating A grating with a sinusoidal luminance profile.

aliasing Misperception of a grating due to undersampling.

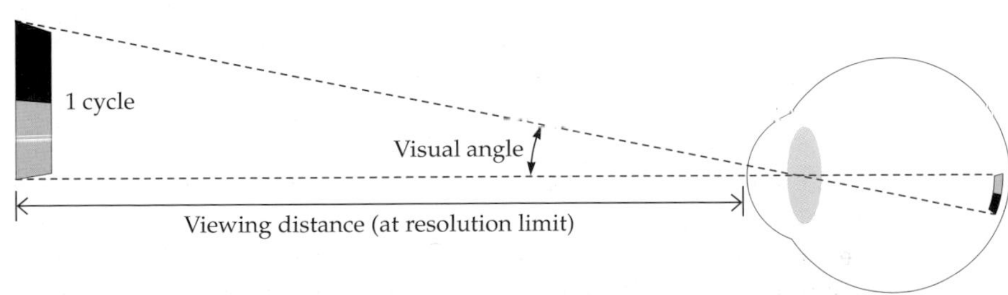

FIGURE 3.3 Visual angle. Shown here is the angle size of one cycle of a grating at the retina.

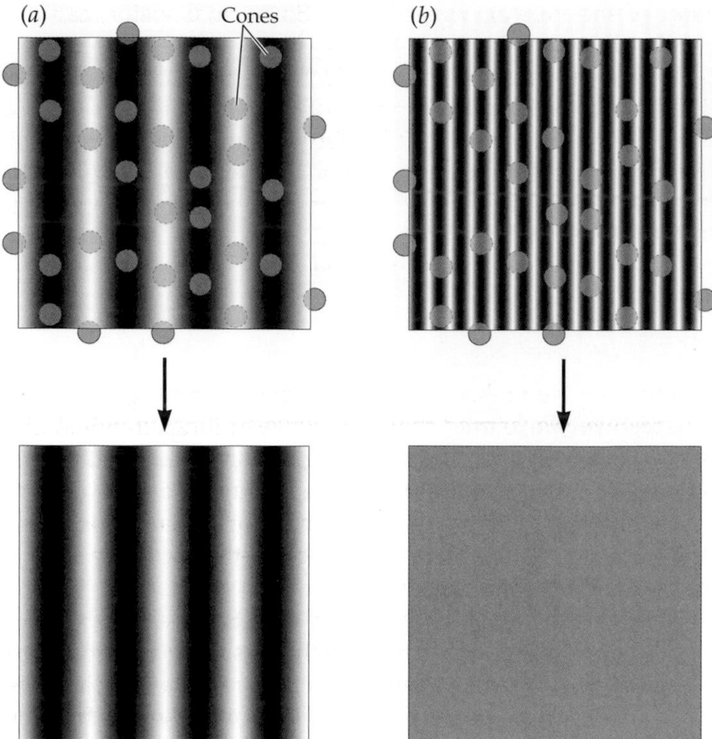

FIGURE 3.4 Sine wave gratings. (*a*) The stripes are wider than the photoreceptors (pink circles in the top panel), and the grating can be reconstructed vertically. (*b*) The stripes are narrower than the photoreceptors, so both black and white bars will fall inside a single receptor (top panel) resulting in a uniform gray field (bottom panel).

Cones in the fovea have a center-to-center separation of about 0.5 minute of arc (0.008 degree), which fits nicely with the observed acuity limit of 1 minute of arc (remember that we need two cones per cycle to be able to perceive it properly). Rods and cones in the periphery are packed together less tightly (recall that rods are physically more tightly packed [denser] than cones), but here many receptors converge on each ganglion cell. As a result, visual acuity is much poorer in the periphery than in the fovea. For a demonstration of the difference between foveal and peripheral vision, see **Web Activity 3.2: Foveal Acuity**. (See also **Web Essay 3.1: Hyperacuity**.)

A Visit to the Eye Doctor

Eye doctors don't describe acuity in terms of visual angles and cycles. The last time you visited your eye doctor, she may have asked you to read letters, decreasing the size of the letters until you made several errors. Then she may have told you that your visual acuity was 20/20 if your vision was good, or 20/30 if you needed glasses, or possibly 20/10 if you could read the smallest letters on the eye chart. This strange method for designating visual acuity was invented in 1862 by a Dutch eye doctor, Herman Snellen (1834–1908). Snellen constructed a set of block letters for which the letter as a whole was five times as large as the strokes that formed the letter (**Figure 3.5**). Note that the resulting patterns are reminiscent of the gratings in Figure 3.2. He then defined visual acuity as follows:

FIGURE 3.5 A Snellen *E*. The letter size is five times the stroke size.

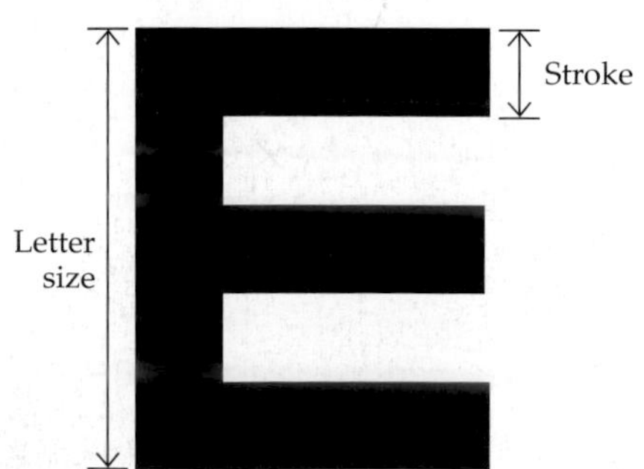

$$\frac{\text{(the distance at which a person can just identify the letters)}}{\text{(the distance at which a person with "normal" vision can just identify the letters)}}$$

In later adaptations of the Snellen test, the viewer was positioned at a constant distance of 20 feet, and the size of the letters, rather than the position of the viewer, was altered. So normal vision came to be defined as 20/20. To relate this back to visual angle, a 20/20 letter is designed to subtend an angle of 5 arc minutes (0.083 degree) at the eye, and each stroke of a 20/20 letter subtends an angle of 1 arc minute (the familiar 0.017 degree). Thus, if you can read a 20/20 letter, you can discern detail that subtends 1 minute of arc. If you have to be at 20 feet to read a letter that someone with normal vision can read at 40 feet, you have 20/40 vision (worse than normal). Although 20/20 is often considered the gold standard, most healthy young adults have an acuity level closer to 20/15.

spatial frequency The number of cycles of a grating per unit of visual angle (usually specified in degrees).

cycles per degree The number of dark and bright bars per degree of visual angle.

contrast sensitivity function (CSF) A function describing how the sensitivity to contrast (defined as the reciprocal of the contrast threshold) depends on the spatial frequency (size) of the stimulus.

Acuity for Low-Contrast Stripes

Up to now we've been discussing the tiniest high-contrast details that we can resolve. We learned that sine wave gratings in which the light stripes are perfectly white and the dark stripes perfectly black can be distinguished from a uniform gray field, as long as adjacent pairs of light or dark stripes are separated by at least 1 arc minute of visual angle. But what happens if the contrast of the stripes is reduced—that is, if the light stripes are made darker and the dark stripes lighter?

This was the question asked by Otto Schade in 1956, when he was working for the RCA Corporation. Schade showed people sine wave gratings with different spatial frequencies and had them adjust the contrast of the gratings until they could just be detected. **Spatial frequency** refers to the number of times a pattern, such as a sine wave grating, repeats in a given unit of space. For example, if you view your book from about 120 centimeters (about 47 inches) away, the visual angle between each pair of white stripes in **Figure 3.6*b*** is about 0.25 degree, so the spatial frequency of this grating is 1/0.25 = 4 **cycles per degree**. Figure 3.6*a* shows a grating with a relatively lower spatial frequency (about 2 cycles per degree), and Figure 3.6*c* illustrates a relatively higher spatial frequency (about 8 cycles per degree). **Web Activity 3.3: Gabor Patches** provides additional illustrations of sine wave gratings at different spatial frequencies.

Intuitively, you might think that the wider the stripes (that is, the lower the spatial frequency), the easier it would be to distinguish the light stripes from the dark stripes. But this is not exactly what Schade found. He, and later Fergus Campbell and Dan Green (1965), demonstrated that the human **contrast sensitivity function (CSF)** is shaped like an upside-down *U*, as shown in **Figure 3.7**. We obtain the units for the y-axis in this graph by taking the recip-

(*a*)

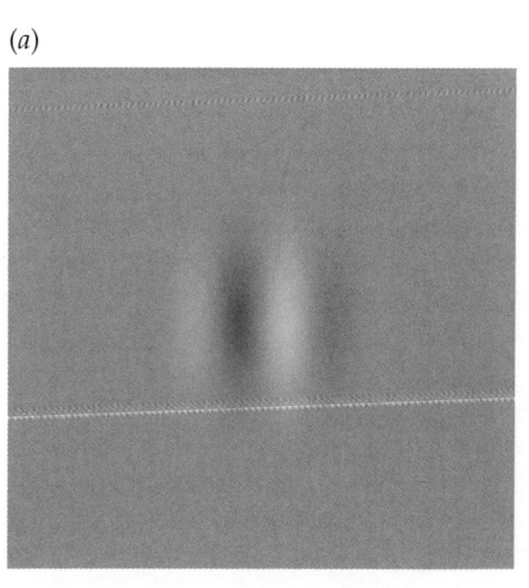

(*b*)

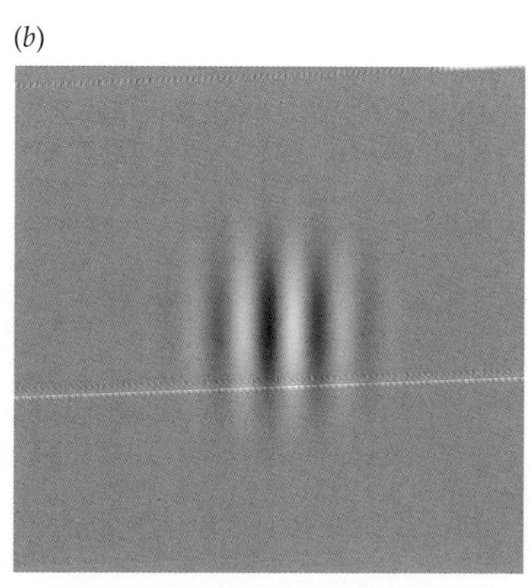

(*c*)

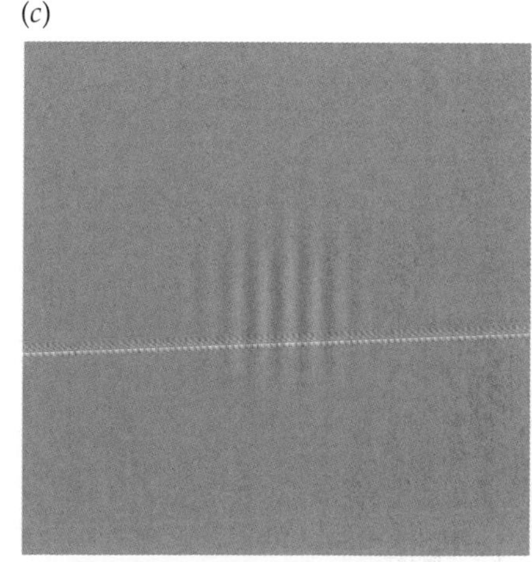

FIGURE 3.6 Sine wave gratings illustrating low (*a*), medium (*b*), and high (*c*) spatial frequencies.

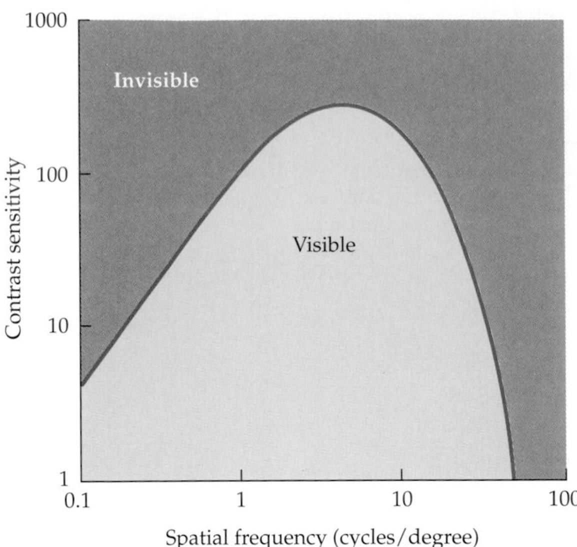

FIGURE 3.7 The contrast sensitivity function (red line): our window of visibility. Any object whose spatial frequencies and contrasts fall within the yellow region will be visible. Those outside the yellow region are outside the window of visibility. The red line delimits the "threshold" between seeing and not seeing.

rocal of the **contrast threshold**. For example, for a 1-cycle/degree grating to be just distinguishable from uniform gray, the dark stripes must be about 1% darker than the light stripes (that is, if a tiny patch of a light stripe reflects 1000 photons, a patch of a dark stripe should reflect 990 photons). The reciprocal of this threshold is 1/0.01 = 100, so this is the point plotted on the red CSF line in Figure 3.7 for this spatial frequency.

Note that a contrast of 100% corresponds to a sensitivity value of 1. The CSF reaches this value on the far right side of the curve in Figure 3.7, at about 60 cycles/degree. Sixty cycles/degree corresponds to a cycle width of 1 minute of arc, the resolution limit we measured previously for high-contrast stripes, which, recall, is determined primarily by cone spacing. The falloff in the CSF on the other side of the curve cannot be explained by cone spacing or by limitations in the optics of the eye. Instead, this part of the function must be due to neural factors, which we will discuss later.

You can visualize your own CSF by using **Figure 3.8**. Here we see a sinusoidal grating whose contrast increases continuously from the top of the figure to the bottom, and whose spatial frequency increases continuously from the left side of the graph to the right side. If you view the figure from a distance of about 2 meters, you will notice the inverted *U* shape where the grating fades from visibility to invisibility. If you bring the book closer to your eye, you should be able to see the stripes on the right side of the figure going farther up, whereas the tops of the stripes on the left side will become less distinct.

contrast threshold The smallest amount of contrast required to detect a pattern.

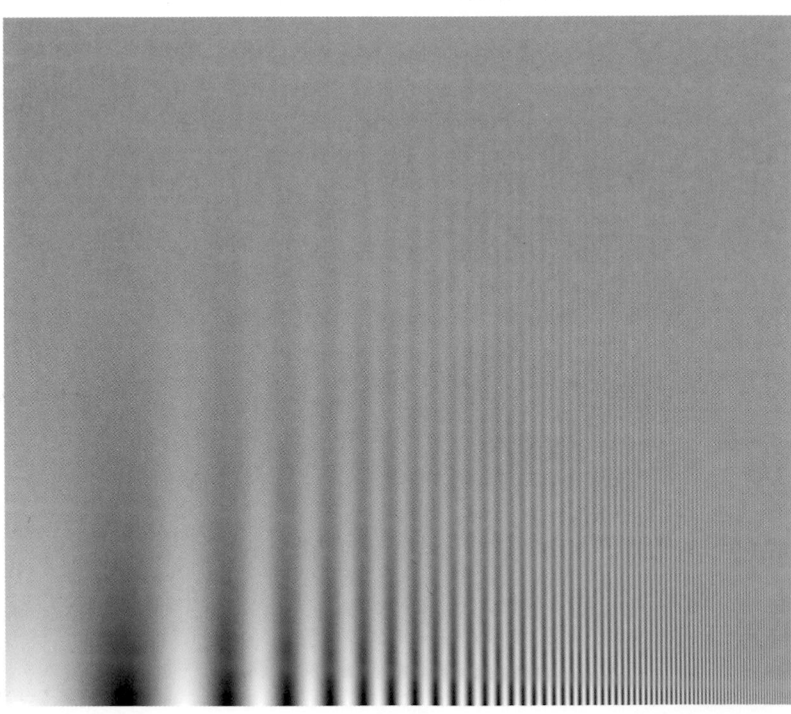

FIGURE 3.8 A grating modulated by contrast (vertically) and by spatial frequency (horizontally). (From Robson and Campbell, 1997; courtesy of Izumi Ohzawa.)

Why Sine Wave Gratings?

Now that we have described the contrast sensitivity function in some detail, one question may be foremost in your mind: Who cares? We don't see sine wave gratings in the real world; we see images of objects and scenes. What does contrast sensitivity for sine wave gratings across different spatial frequencies tell us about how we see real-world images?

One answer to this question is that, although "pure" sine wave gratings may be rare in the real world, patterns of stripes with more or less fuzzy boundaries are quite common: think of trees in a forest, books on a bookshelf, and a map of Manhattan (the latter includes a pattern of horizontal stripes superimposed on a pattern of vertical stripes). Furthermore, the edge of any object produces a single stripe, often blurred by a shadow, in the retinal image.

On a larger scale, the visual system appears to break down real-world images into a vast number of components, each of which is, essentially, a sine wave grating with a particular spatial frequency. This method of processing is analogous to the way in which the auditory system deals with sound and is called Fourier analysis (see Chapter 9). We'll return to this idea later in this chapter. For now, rest assured that scientists don't use sine wave gratings just because they are convenient to manipulate in experiments (although they do make very nice stimuli).

Retinal Ganglion Cells and Stripes

In Chapter 2 we learned that retinal ganglion cells respond vigorously to spots of light. As it turns out, each ganglion cell also responds well to certain types of stripes or gratings. **Figure 3.9** shows how an ON retinal ganglion cell responds to gratings of different spatial frequencies. When the spatial frequency of the grating is too low (Figure 3.9*a*), the ganglion cell responds weakly because part of the fat, bright bar of the grating lands in the inhibitory surround, damping the cell's response. Similarly, when the spatial frequency is too high (Figure 3.9*c*), the ganglion cell responds weakly because both dark and bright stripes fall within the receptive-field center, washing out the response. But when the spatial frequency is just right (Figure 3.9*b*), with a bright bar filling the center and dark bars in the surround, the cell responds vigorously. Thus, retinal ganglion cells are "tuned" to spatial frequency: each cell responds best to a specific spatial frequency that matches its receptive-field size, and it responds less to both higher and lower spatial frequencies.

Christina Enroth-Cugell and John Robson (1984) were the first to record the responses of retinal ganglion cells to sinusoidal gratings. In addition to showing that these cells respond vigorously to gratings of just the right size, these investigators discovered that responses depend on the **phase** of the grating—its

phase The relative position of a grating.

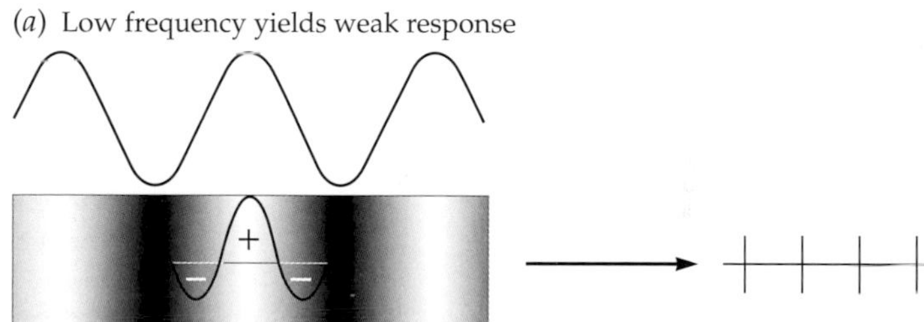

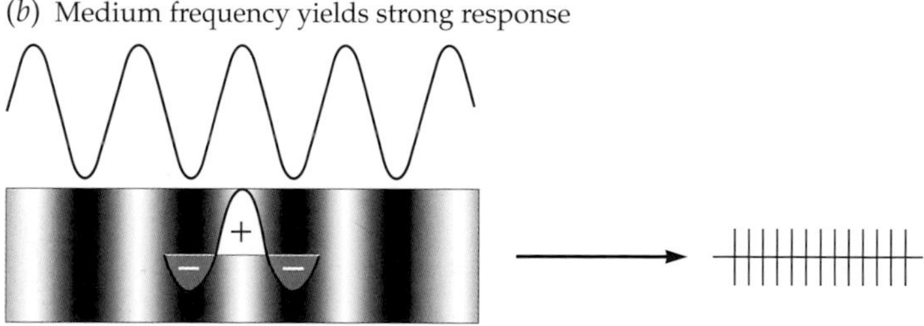

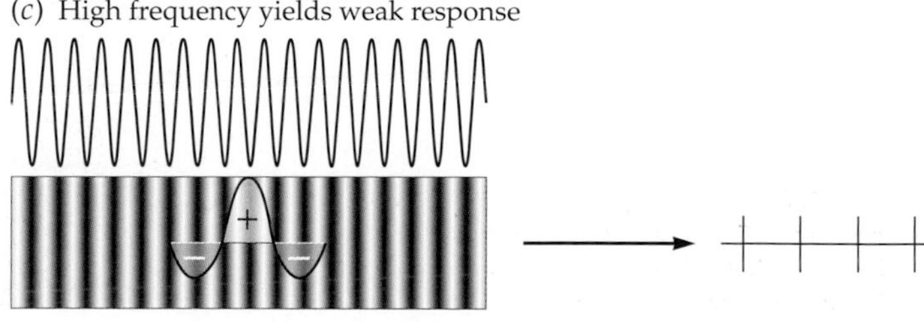

FIGURE 3.9 The response (right) of a ganglion cell to gratings of different spatial frequencies (left): (*a*) low, (*b*) medium, and (*c*) high.

(*a*) 0° – Positive response

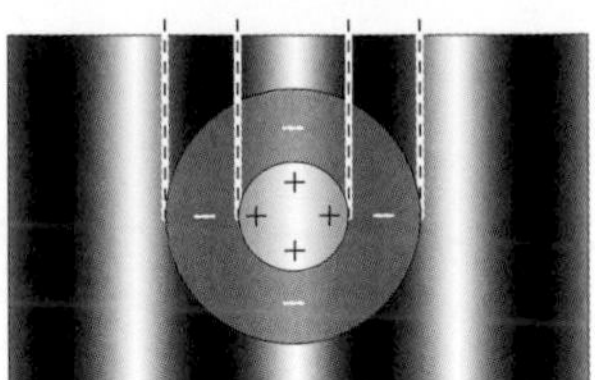

(*b*) 90° – No response

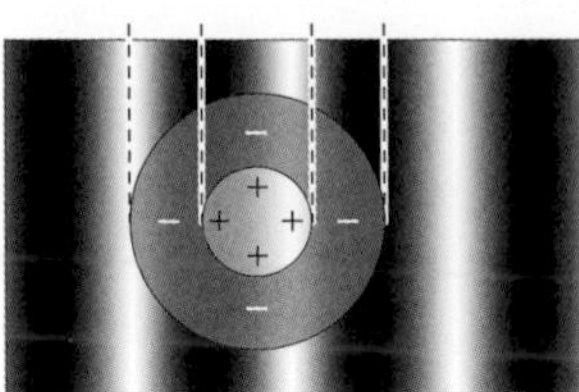

(*c*) 180° – Negative response

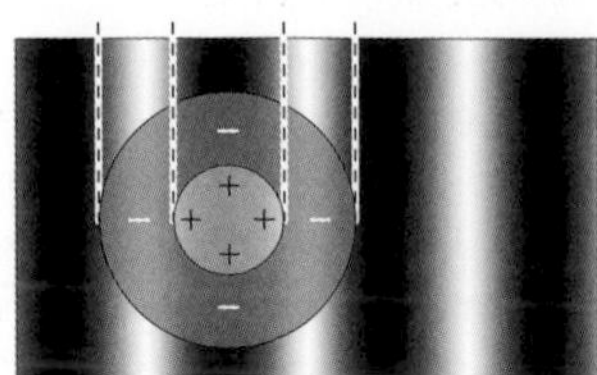

(*d*) 270° – No response

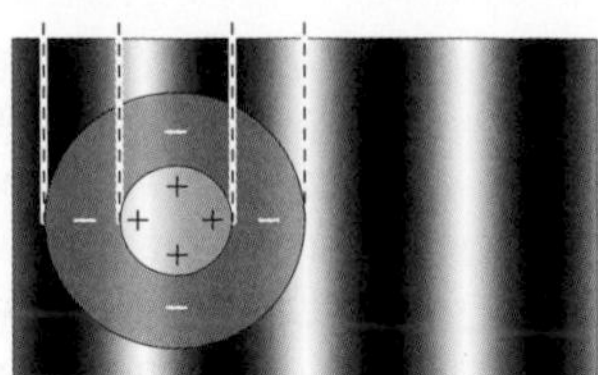

FIGURE 3.10 The response of a ganglion cell to a grating depends on the phase of the grating. This figure illustrates the response of an ON-center retinal ganglion cell to four different phases of an optimally sized grating.

position within the receptive field. **Figure 3.10** illustrates how an ON-center retinal ganglion cell might respond to a grating of just the right spatial frequency (a bar width about the size of the receptive-field center) in four different phases.

When the grating has a light bar filling the receptive-field center and the dark bars in the surround (Figure 3.10*a*), this ON-center cell responds vigorously, increasing its firing rate. If the grating phase is shifted by 90 degrees (Figure 3.10*b*), half the receptive-field center will be filled by a light bar and half by a dark bar, and similarly for the surround. In other words, there will be no net difference between the light intensity in the receptive field's center and its surround. In this case the cell's response rate does not change from its resting rate when the grating is turned on—just what we would predict if the ganglion cell were summing the total amount of light falling on its center and its surround. A second 90-degree shift puts the dark bar in the center and the light bars in the surround, producing a negative response (Figure 3.10*c*) (see Chapter 2); and a third phase shift returns us to the situation after the first shift, with the overall intensities in the center and surround equivalent and the cell therefore blind to the grating (Figure 3.10*d*). (Note that other ganglion cells respond to the 90-degree and 270-degree phases but not to the 0-degree and 180-degree phases, which is why the visual system as a whole is able to see all four phases equally well.)

lateral geniculate nucleus (LGN) A structure in the thalamus, part of the midbrain, that receives input from the retinal ganglion cells and has input and output connections to the visual cortex.

magnocellular layers The neurons in the bottom two layers of the lateral geniculate nucleus, which are physically larger than those in the top four layers.

parvocellular layers The neurons in the top four layers of the LGN, which are physically smaller than those in the bottom two layers.

The Lateral Geniculate Nucleus

The axons of retinal ganglion cells synapse in the two **lateral geniculate nuclei** (**LGNs**), which act as relay stations on the way from the retina to the cortex (see Figure 3.1). **Figure 3.11** shows that the LGN of primates is a six-layered structure, a bit like a stack of pancakes that has been bent in the middle (which is how the *geniculate*, which means "bent," got its name). The neurons in the bottom two layers are physically larger than those in the top four layers; for this reason, the bottom two are called **magnocellular layers** and the top four **parvocellular layers** (*parvo-* is Latin for "small"). The two types of layers also differ in another, more important, way: the magnocellular layers receive input from M ganglion cells in the retina, and the parvocellular layers receive input from P ganglion cells. Functionally, studies in which magnocellular and parvocellular layers are chemi-

Parvocellular layers

Magnocellular layers

FIGURE 3.11 The primate lateral geniculate nucleus. (From Hubel, 1988.)

cally lesioned indicate that the magnocellular pathway responds to large, fast-moving objects, and the parvocellular pathway is responsible for processing details of stationary targets.

The organization of the retinal inputs to the LGN, diagrammed in **Figure 3.12**, provides some important insights into how our visual world is mapped to the brain. First, the left LGN receives projections from the left sides of the retinas in both eyes, and the right LGN receives projections from the right sides of the retinas. Second, each layer of the LGN receives input from one or the other eye. From bottom to top, layers 1, 4, and 6 of the right LGN listen to the left (**contralateral**) eye, while layers 2, 3, and 5 receive input from the right (**ipsilateral**) eye.

Each LGN layer contains a highly organized map of a complete half of the visual field. Figure 3.12 shows schematically how objects in the right visual field (objects to the right of where our gaze is fixated) are mapped onto the different layers of the left LGN (as shown in Figure 3.12, the right side of the world falls on the left side of the retina, whose ganglion cells project to the left LGN). This ordered mapping of the world onto the visual nervous system, which is known as **topographical mapping**, provides us with a neural basis for knowing where things are in space (we will come back to this point a little later).

LGN neurons have concentric receptive fields that are very similar to those of retinal ganglion cells: they respond well to spots and gratings. Given that the LGN cells respond to the same patterns as the ganglion cells that provide their input, you might wonder why the visual system wastes a synapse here. That is, why don't the ganglion cell axons simply travel directly back to the cerebral cortex? One important reason probably has to do with the fact that there are more connections from other parts of the brain to the LGN than there are connections from the LGN to the cortex. In other words, the LGN appears to serve as a staging area where feedback from other parts of the brain modulates input from the eyes.

For example, the LGN is part of a larger brain structure called the "thalamus" (the medial geniculate nucleus, part of the auditory pathway, is another portion of the thalamus); and when we go to sleep, the entire thalamus is inhibited. Thus, even if someone pulls your eyelids open at night, you will not see anything (unless the physical contact awakens you). Input will travel from your retinas to your LGNs, but the neural signals will stop there before reaching the cortex, so they will never be registered. (The thalamic inhibition is not complete, however, which is why loud noises or very bright lights will be perceived, and will cause you to wake up and deal with the stimulus.)

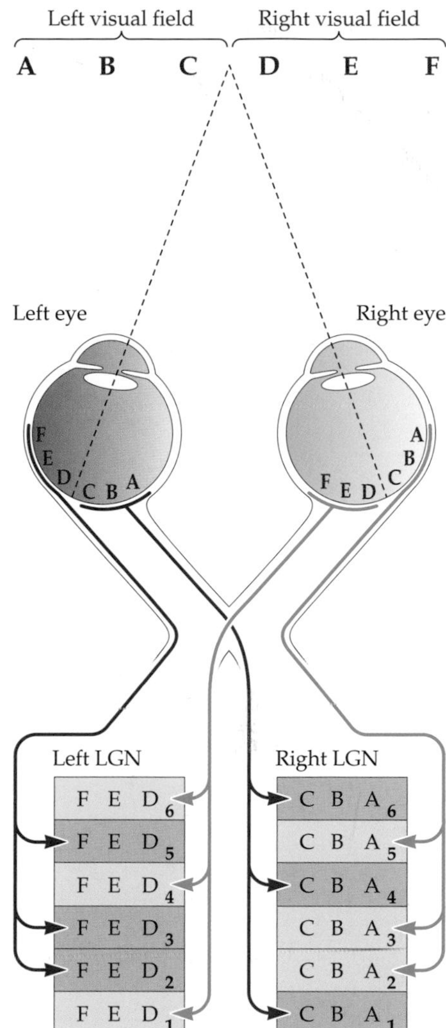

FIGURE 3.12 Input (in this case the letters *ABCDEF*) from the right visual field is mapped in an orderly fashion onto the different layers of the left LGN, and input from the left visual field is mapped to the right LGN. Information from the two eyes is segregated into separate layers. Layers 1 and 2 are the magnocellular layers; layers 3 through 6 are the parvocellular layers.

Striate Cortex

If you place one hand at the back of your head, about an inch or two above the top of your neck, you should be able to feel a small bump known as the "inion." The receiving area for LGN inputs in the cerebral cortex lies below the inion. This area has several names: **primary visual cortex, V1, area 17,** or **striate cortex** (because of the striped pattern it takes on after a certain type of staining procedure). By now you are probably getting the idea that layers are an important property of neural structures in the visual pathway. The striate cortex consists of six major layers, some of which have sublayers (**Figure 3.13**). Fibers from the LGN project mainly (but not exclusively) to layer 4, with magnocellular axons coming in to sublayer 4Cα and parvocellular axons projecting to sublayer 4Cβ. (See **Web Essay 3.2: The Whole Brain Atlas.**)

contralateral Referring to the opposite side of the body (or brain).

ipsilateral Referring to the same side of the body (or brain).

topographical mapping The orderly mapping of the world in the lateral geniculate nucleus and the visual cortex.

primary visual cortex (V1) The area of the cerebral cortex of the brain that receives direct inputs from the lateral geniculate nucleus, as well as feedback from other brain areas, and is responsible for processing visual information. Also called *area 17* or *striate cortex*.

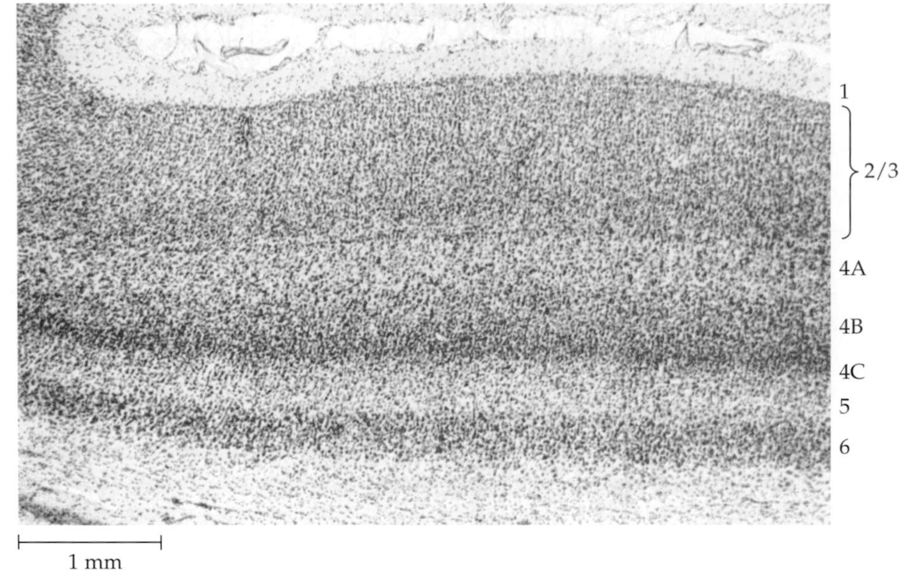

FIGURE 3.13 Striate cortex. (From Hubel, 1988.)

Like the LGN, the striate cortex has a systematic topographical mapping of the visual field. But the striate cortex is not simply a bigger version of the LGN. A major and complex transformation of visual information takes place in the striate cortex. For starters, striate cortex contains on the order of 200 million cells—more than 100 times as many as the LGN has!

Cortical Topography and Cortical Magnification

Figure 3.14 illustrates two important features of the visual cortex. The first is the topographical mapping already noted. The fact that the image of the woman's right eyebrow (*her* right; it appears on the left in Figure 3.14) is mapped onto regions corresponding to the numbers 3 and 4 in the striate cortex, tells the visual system that the eyebrow must be in positions 3 and 4 of the visual field.

The second feature evident in Figure 3.14 is the dramatic scaling of information from different parts of the visual field. Objects imaged on or near the fovea are processed by neurons in a large part of the striate cortex, but objects imaged in the far right or left periphery are allocated only a tiny portion of the striate cortex. This distortion of the visual-field map on the cortex is known as **cortical magnification** because the cortical representation of the fovea is greatly magnified compared to the cortical representation of peripheral vision. (See **Web Essay 3.3: Seeing Images on the Cortex**.)

To gain a sense of the extent of this cortical magnification factor, hold your two arms out in front of you, put up your index fingers, hold them about 10 centimeters (4 inches) apart, close your left eye, and fixate your right finger. In this position, your right fingernail, which is taking up about 1 degree of visual angle on the fovea, is being processed by neurons in about 20 millimeters (mm) of striate cortex. Your left fingernail, which is covering the same amount of visual angle but is falling 10 degrees to the left of the fovea, is being processed by only 1.5 mm of cortex.

One important consequence of cortical magnification is that visual acuity declines in an orderly fashion with eccentricity (distance from the fovea) (Levi, Klein, and Aitsebaomo, 1985)—a phenomenon demonstrated by Hermann Rudolf Aubert well over a century ago (Aubert, 1886). **Web Activity 3.2: Foveal Acuity** allows you to demonstrate this phenomenon yourself, as

cortical magnification The amount of cortical area (usually specified in millimeters) devoted to a specific region (e.g., 1 degree) in the visual field.

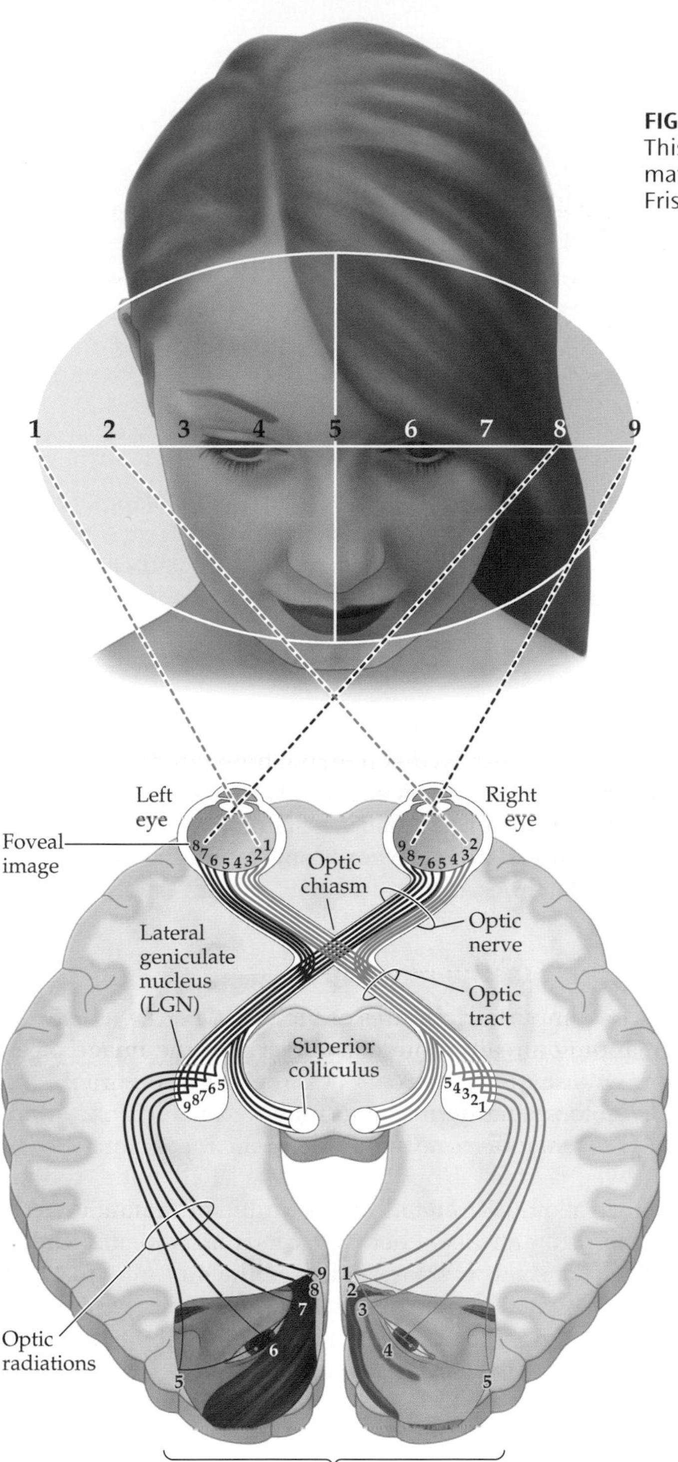

FIGURE 3.14 The mapping of obj[...] This figure illustrates both the topo[...] matic magnification of the foveal re[...] Frisby, 1980.)

does **Figure 3.15**, in which the letters are scaled in size such that each one covers an approximately equal cortical area.

Why is the foveal representation in the cortex so highly magnified? The visual system must make a trade off. High resolution requires a great number of resources: a dense array of photoreceptors, one-to-one lines from photoreceptors to retinal ganglion cells, and a large chunk of striate cortex (not to mention the real estate in other areas of cortex necessary to do something with the visual information coming out of V1). To see the entire visual field with such high resolution, we might need eyes and brains too large to fit in

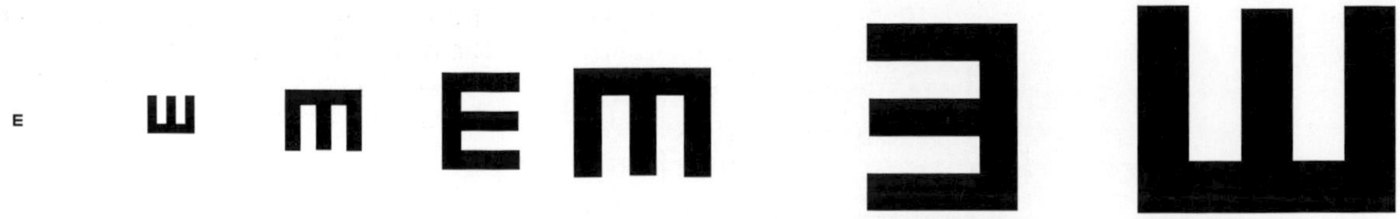

E W m E m ∃ W

FIGURE 3.15 A letter chart in which the letter size increases with eccentricity in proportion to the inverse cortical magnification factor. If you fixate your gaze on the far left side of the figure, all seven letters should be equally easy to see.

our heads! Thus, we have evolved a visual system that provides high resolution in the center and lower resolution in the periphery. If you need to process the details of an object in the corner of your eye, you can simply turn your eye or head so that the object falls on the fovea instead.

Receptive Fields in Striate Cortex

In 1958, David Hubel and Torsten Wiesel began work as postdoctoral students in Stephen Kuffler's laboratory. Their goal was to extend Kuffler's groundbreaking work on retinal ganglion cells to the cortex. So they began trying to map the receptive fields of neurons in striate cortex using spots of light, much as Kuffler (1953) had done earlier (see Chapter 2). To their dismay, however, they found that the cat's cortical cells hardly responded at all to the same spots that made its ganglion cells fire like crazy. To project their stimuli onto the retina, Hubel and Wiesel inserted a glass slide with a black spot into a slot in a special ophthalmoscope (that's the bright light the eye doctor shines in your eye in order to see your retina). One day, they had been recording from a neuron without much luck, when suddenly the cell emitted a strong burst of firing as they inserted the glass slide into the slot. Eventually they realized that the response had nothing to do with the spot itself; instead, the cell had been responding to the shadow cast by the edge of the glass slide as it swept across the ophthalmoscope's light path. And the rest, as they say, is history. Hubel related this story when he and Wiesel received the 1981 Nobel Prize in Physiology or Medicine for uncovering many of the remarkable properties of the visual cortex.

Hubel and Wiesel's most fundamental discovery was that neurons in striate cortex respond to stripes, not stars. More precisely, the receptive fields of striate cortex neurons are not circular, as they are in the retina and LGN. Rather, they are elongated, responding much more vigorously to bars, lines, edges, and gratings than to round circles of light.

Orientation Selectivity

Further investigation by Hubel and Wiesel (1962) uncovered a number of other important properties of the receptive fields of neurons in striate cortex. First, an individual neuron will not respond equivalently to just any old stripe in its receptive field. It responds best when the line or edge is at just the right orientation, and hardly at all when the line is tilted more than 30 degrees away from the optimal orientation (a change equivalent to movement of the minute hand of a clock from 12 to 1). Scientists call this selective responsiveness **orientation tuning**: the cell is tuned to detect lines in a specific orientation in the same way that a piano key is tuned to produce a specific musical note.

orientation tuning The tendency of neurons in striate cortex to respond optimally to certain orientations, and less to others.

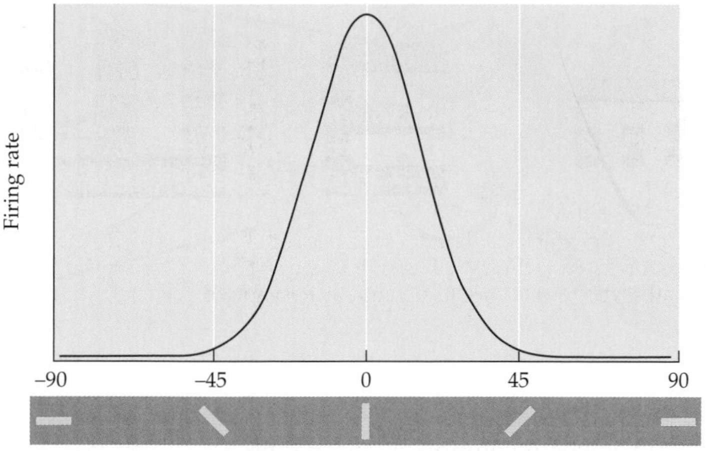

FIGURE 3.16 Orientation tuning function of a cortical cell. The neuron fires vigorously when the line is oriented vertically, but it fires hardly at all when the line orientation is changed by 30 degrees.

A typical orientation tuning function looks like the plot in **Figure 3.16**. The neuron featured here fires vigorously when the line is oriented vertically (at 90 degrees), but the response tapers off rapidly as the line is tilted one way or another, diminishing to close to the cell's resting rate when the line is tilted 45 degrees in either direction. Other cells in striate cortex are selective for 0 degrees (horizontal), 45 degrees, 20 degrees, 62 degrees, and so on, so that the population of neurons as a whole detects all possible orientations. However, more cells are responsive to horizontal and vertical orientations than to obliques (De Valois, Yund, and Hepler, 1982; Li, Peterson, and Freeman, 2003). This physiological finding meshes well with the psychophysical finding that humans have somewhat lower visual acuity and contrast sensitivity for oblique targets than for horizontal and vertical targets.

filter An acoustic, electrical, electronic, or optical device, instrument, computer program, or neuron that allows the passage of some frequencies or digital elements and blocks the passage of others.

How are the circular receptive fields in the LGN transformed into the elongated receptive fields in striate cortex? Hubel and Wiesel suggested a very simple scheme to accomplish this transformation (**Figure 3.17**). Simply put, their idea was that the concentric LGN cells that feed into a cortical cell are all in a row. Later studies (e.g., J. S. Anderson et al., 2000) have shown that the arrangement of LGN inputs is indeed crucial for establishing the orientation selectivity of striate cortex cells. However, other evidence suggests that neural interactions (e.g., lateral inhibition) within the cortex also play an important role in the dynamics of orientation tuning (Pugh et al., 2000).

FIGURE 3.17 Hubel and Wiesel's model of how cortical simple cells get their orientation tuning.

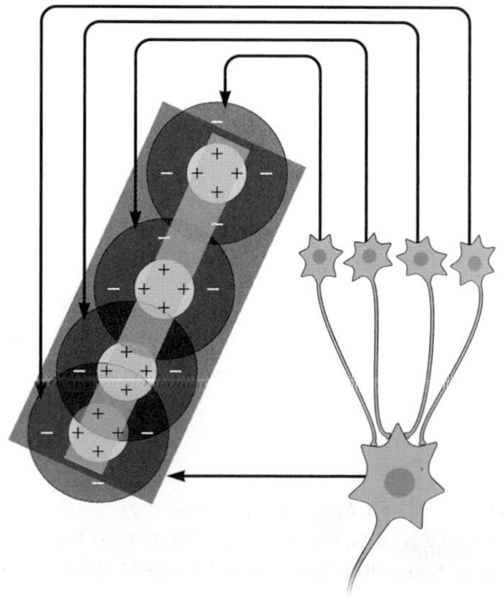

Other Receptive-Field Properties

Cortical cells respond not just to bars, lines, and edges. Like retinal ganglion cells, they also respond well to gratings (which are, after all, collections of lines). And like ganglion cells, they respond best to gratings that have just the right spatial frequency to fill the receptive-field center. That is, each striate cortex cell is tuned to a particular spatial frequency, which corresponds to a particular line width. Indeed, cortical cells are much more narrowly tuned (they respond to a smaller range of spatial frequencies) than retinal ganglion cells (De Valois, Albrecht, and Thorell, 1982). These narrow tuning functions mean that each striate cortex neuron functions as a **filter** for the portion of the image that excites the cell. We will return to the idea of striate cortex as a collection of filters later.

Another important discovery made by Hubel and Wiesel was that many cortical cells respond especially well to *moving* lines, bars, edges, and gratings. Moreover, many neurons respond strongly when a line moves in one

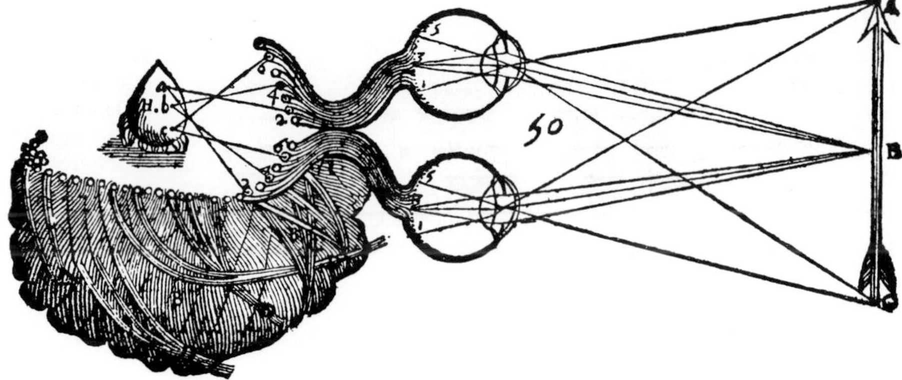

FIGURE 3.18 Drawing by René Descartes, 1664, illustrating the "fusion center." (From Descartes, 1664.)

ocular dominance The property of the receptive fields of striate cortex neurons by which they demonstrate a preference, responding somewhat more rapidly when a stimulus is presented in one eye than when it is presented in the other.

simple cell A cortical neuron with clearly defined excitatory and inhibitory regions.

complex cell A neuron whose receptive-field characteristics cannot be easily predicted by mapping with spots of light.

direction—say, from left to right—but not at all when the same line moves from right to left.

As noted earlier, information from the two eyes is kept separate in the LGN: each LGN cell responds to one eye or the other, but never to both eyes. This arrangement changes dramatically in striate cortex, where a majority of cells can be influenced by input from both the left eye and the right eye. In other words, if a striate cortex neuron responds best to a 5-cycle/degree grating oriented at 45 degrees, it will respond to such a stimulus whether that stimulus is presented in the right eye or the left eye. However, striate cortex neurons often have a preference, responding somewhat more rapidly when a stimulus is presented in one eye than when it is presented in the other. Hubel and Wiesel called this property of striate receptive fields **ocular dominance**.

Given that we see a single, unified world, intuitively it makes sense that information from the two eyes should be brought together at some point. Until Hubel and Wiesel's discovery, however, there were heated arguments about whether the information converged at all, and if so, whether it was in a specialized "fusion center" in the brain—a notion that dates back to Descartes (1664; see Howard and Rogers, 2001) (**Figure 3.18**). We'll describe some of these debates in Chapter 6, when we discuss binocular vision.

Simple and Complex Cells

Like precortical neurons, cortical neurons come in a wide variety of types. Hubel and Wiesel characterized neurons as **simple cells** when those neurons had clearly defined excitatory and inhibitory regions. **Figure 3.19** shows two varieties of simple-cell receptive fields and their preferred stimuli. An edge detector (see Figure 3.19*a*) prefers to see light on one side of its receptive field and darkness on the other side. A stripe detector (see Figure 3.19*b*) responds best to a line of light that has a particular width, surrounded on both sides by darkness. If a grating with the appropriate spatial frequency drifts across the receptive field of this cell, the cell's response will be modulated as dark and bright bars drift across the receptive-field center, in exactly the same way that the response of the retinal ganglion cell shown in Figure 3.10 is modulated.

Other neurons show responses that cannot be simply predicted from their responses to stationary bars of light. Hubel and Wiesel called these **complex cells**. Like simple cells, each complex cell is tuned to a particular orientation

(*a*) Edge detector

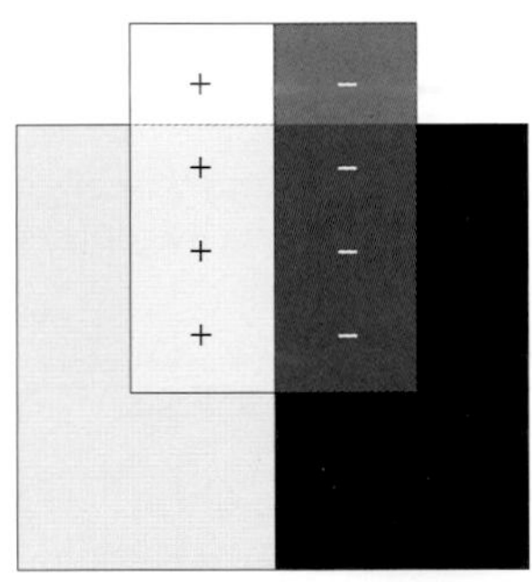

(*b*) Stripe detector

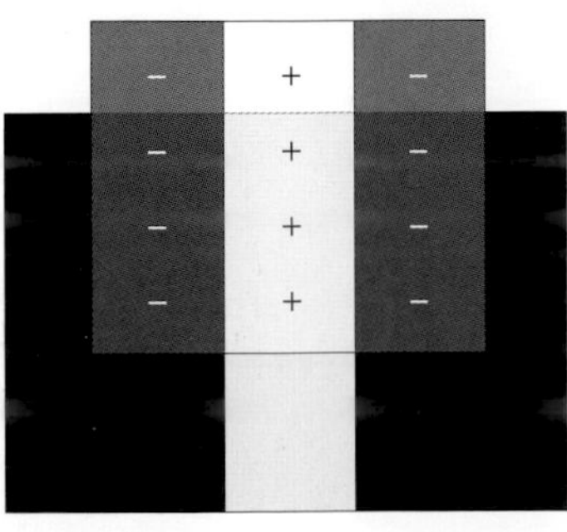

FIGURE 3.19 Two flavors of simple cells: (*a*) an edge detector and (*b*) a stripe detector.

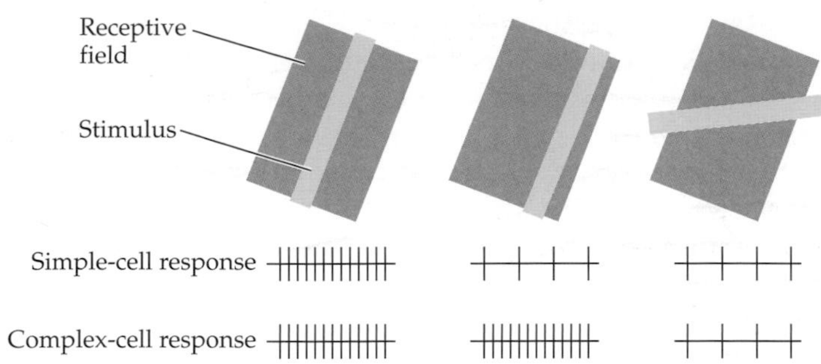

FIGURE 3.20 A simple cell and a complex cell might both be tuned to the same orientation and stripe width (spatial frequency), but the complex cell will respond to that stripe presented anywhere within its receptive field, whereas the simple cell might respond to the stripe in only one position.

and spatial frequency and shows an ocular preference. However, whereas a simple cell might respond only if a stripe is presented in the center of its receptive field, a complex cell will respond regardless of where the stripe is presented, as long as it is somewhere within the cell's receptive field (**Figure 3.20**). When tested with a drifting grating, the complex cell gives a robust response, with little or none of the modulation shown by simple cells (as well as retinal ganglion and LGN cells). Another way of stating this difference is to say that simple cells are "phase-sensitive," and complex cells are "phase-insensitive."

As with all other neurons in the visual system, save retinal photoreceptors, the receptive fields of complex cells represent a pooling of the responses of several subunits. The subunits give the complex cell its spatial frequency and orientation tuning, but the complex pooling operation makes the complex cell insensitive to the precise position of the stimulus within its receptive field. Hubel and Wiesel hypothesized a hierarchy in which LGN cells fed into simple cells, which in turn provided excitatory inputs to complex cells. However, substantial evidence now suggests that complex cells represent a separate parallel pathway (that is, that both simple and complex cells get direct input from LGN neurons).

end stopping The process by which a cell in the cortex first increases its firing rate as the bar length increases to fill up its receptive field, and then decreases its firing rate as the bar is lengthened further.

Further Complications

Hubel and Wiesel described another property of some cells in striate cortex that they called **end stopping**. When they tested an end-stopped cell with bars of increasing lengths, the response rate first increased as the bar filled up its receptive field, and then decreased markedly as the bar was lengthened further (**Figure 3.21**). Hubel and Wiesel called these cells "hypercomplex" cells, although they now appear to be subclasses of the simple and complex cells already discussed here (that is, there are simple end-stopped cells and complex end-stopped cells). End stopping is thought to play an important role in our ability to detect luminance boundaries and discontinuities.

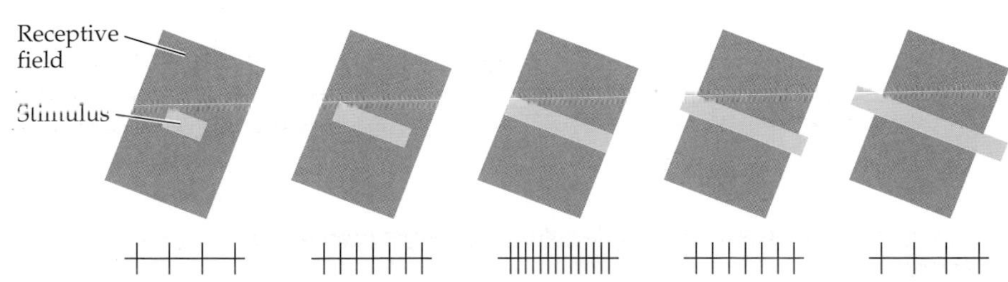

FIGURE 3.21 When the stimulus (bar) does not reach the outside edge of the receptive field or extends beyond the receptive field of an end-stopped cortical neuron, the neuron fires less than when the stimulus is just the right length.

Recent research has revealed further idiosyncrasies in the receptive fields of striate cortex neurons. For example, the size of a particular cell's receptive field appears to vary with target contrast; for instance, the cell might respond to a smaller portion of the visual field when the grating stimulus has a high contrast as opposed to when the difference between light and dark bars is more subtle (Sceniak et al., 1999). And neurons can be influenced by stimuli that fall outside the classic receptive field, via short- or long-range lateral connections and/or via feedback from neurons in other layers (Zipser, Lamme, and Schiller, 1996).

As is the case for most of the visual system, what we don't know about the workings of striate cortex neurons almost certainly dwarfs what we do know. But to review what we do know, spend some time with **Web Activity 3.4: Striate Receptive Fields**, where you can try your hand at determining the receptive field of an unknown virtual neuron.

Columns and Hypercolumns

As we've discussed, each of the approximately 200 million neurons in striate cortex responds to a distinctive set of stimulus properties: stripes, edges, and/or gratings that are oriented at a particular angle, with a particular width or spatial frequency, possibly moving in a particular direction. Some neurons are simple cells and some are complex cells, and each one is end-stopped or not. Most neurons also respond preferentially to stimuli presented in one eye or another. And each neuron responds only when its preferred stimulus is presented in one particular part of the visual field.

Hubel and Wiesel noticed very early on that these various receptive-field properties are not scattered haphazardly around striate cortex. Once they had figured out what the cells were looking for (stripes, rather than spots), they discovered that if they pushed the recording electrode down through the layers of the cortex in a direction perpendicular to the cortical surface, all the cells they encountered showed similar orientation preferences. If they shifted the electrode position over a tiny distance and made another perpendicular penetration, all the cells now responded best to a slightly different orientation, perhaps 10 or 15 degrees from the original orientation. On the basis of these observations, Hubel and Wiesel concluded that neurons with similar orientation preferences are arranged in **columns** that extend vertically through the cortex.

When Hubel and Wiesel made tangential penetrations into striate cortex (inserting an electrode such that it was oriented parallel to the cortical surface, rather than perpendicular), they found a systematic and progressive change in preferred orientation so that essentially all the orientations were encountered in a distance of about 0.5 mm. This finding has been confirmed via alternative physiological techniques. **Figure 3.22***a* shows a small portion of a monkey's striate cortex prepared so that neurons responding to vertically oriented lines are stained black, while other neurons remain white. The distance between the vertical orientation columns revealed by this technique is, sure enough, just about 0.5 mm (LeVay, Hubel, and Wiesel, 1975). The mapping of orientation in the cortex can be appreciated from optical imaging studies (Figure 3.22*c*), where orientation preference is indicated by color.

Orientation is not the only property arranged in columns in the visual cortex. Neurons that share the same eye preference (exhibiting what is referred to as "ocular dominance") also have a columnar arrangement (Figure 3.22*b*). Furthermore, single-cell recording experiments, as well as staining experiments, indicate that eye preference switches (you guessed it) every 0.5 mm or so.

column A vertical arrangement of neurons.

(*a*) Orientation columns

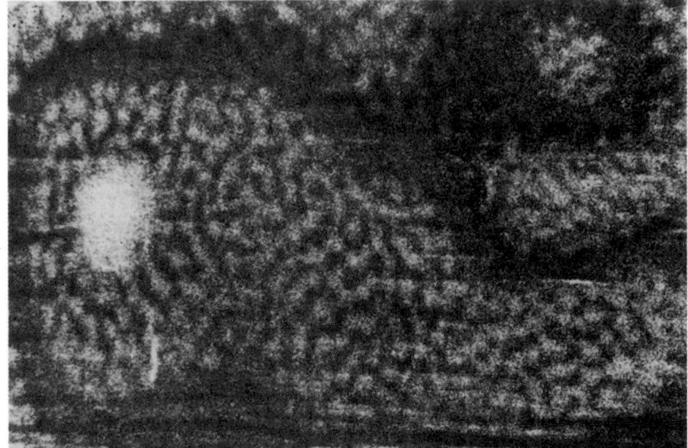

(*b*) Ocular dominance columns

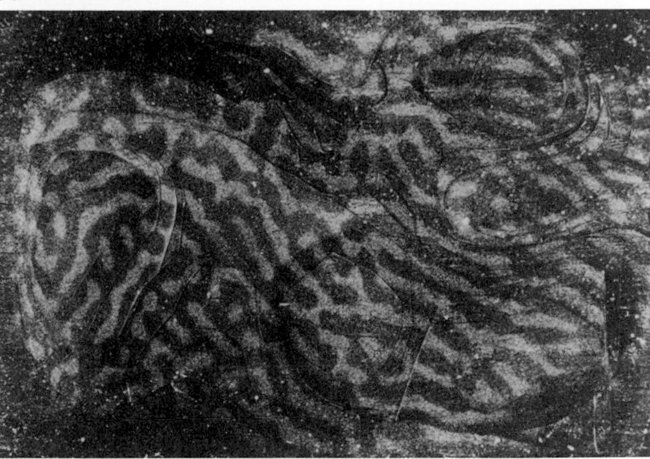

(*c*)

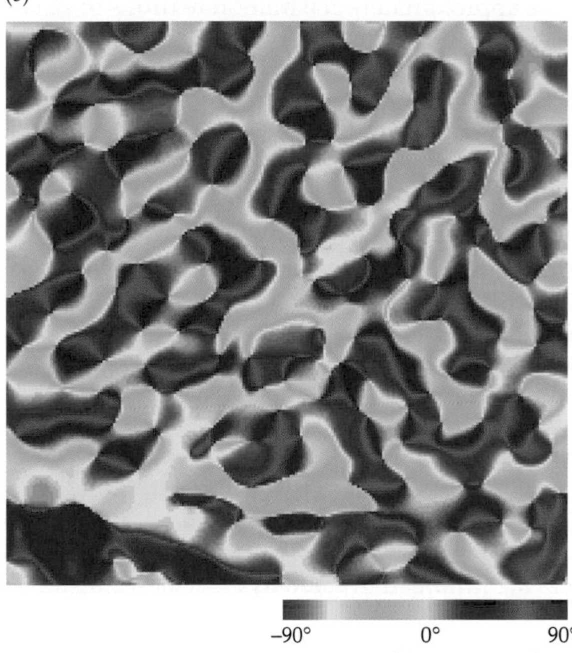

FIGURE 3.22 Orientation (*a*) and ocular dominance (*b*) columns of the striate cortex, revealed by staining. (*c*) Optical imaging of the orientation maps in monkey cortex. (*a* and *b* from Hubel et al., 1978; *c* from Nauhaus et al., 2008.)

Through their studies, Hubel and Wiesel arrived at the model of striate cortical architecture illustrated in **Figure 3.23**. They proposed that a 1-mm block of striate cortex contains "all the machinery necessary to look after everything the visual cortex is responsible for, in a certain small part of the visual world" (Hubel, 1982). Each of these sections of cortex is called a **hypercolumn**. It contains at least two sets of columns, each covering every possible orientation (0–180 degrees), with one set preferring input from the left eye and one set preferring input from the right eye.

Hypercolumns are roughly 1 mm across throughout the striate cortex, but because of the cortical magnification factor discussed earlier, not all hypercolumns see the world at the same level of detail. A hypercolumn in the part of the cortex that represents the fovea may "see" a portion of the visual field that is 0.05 degree of visual angle across; a hypercolumn responding to input 10 degrees to the right of the fovea should cover about 14 times as large an area (0.7 degree across).

hypercolumn A 1-millimeter block of striate cortex containing two sets of columns, each covering every possible orientation (0–180 degrees), with one set preferring input from the left eye and one set preferring input from the right eye.

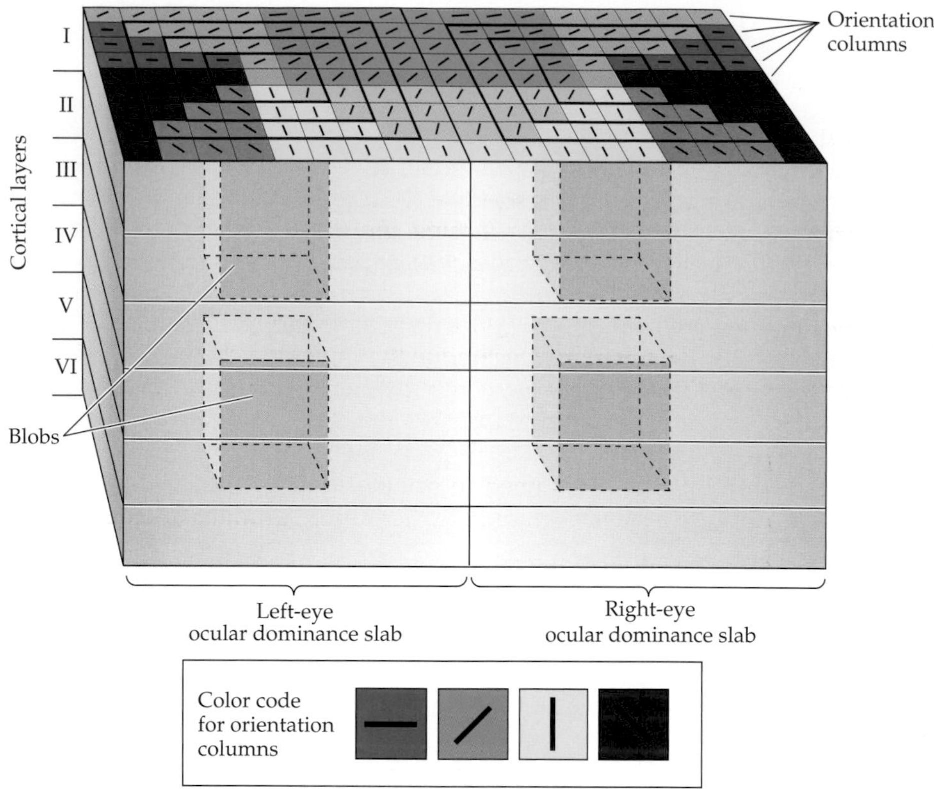

FIGURE 3.23 This model of a hypercolumn shows two ocular dominance columns (one for each eye) and many orientation columns, and illustrates the locations of the cytochrome oxidase (CO) blobs. (From Breedlove et al., 2007.)

cytochrome oxidase (CO) An enzyme used to reveal the regular array of "CO blobs," which are spaced about 0.5 millimeter apart in the primary visual cortex.

Orientation and ocular dominance are probably not the only stimulus dimensions that have a systematic columnar arrangement in the visual cortex. For example, another staining technique, which takes advantage of an enzyme called **cytochrome oxidase (CO)**, has revealed a regular array of "CO blobs" (shown in section in **Figure 3.24**), spaced that magical distance of about 0.5 mm apart (see Figure 3.23). The functional role of these blobs remains unclear, but CO blob columns have been implicated in processing color, with the interblob regions (note the elegant scientific jargon that has developed around this field of study) processing motion and spatial structure (Livingstone and Hubel, 1988). This view is probably too simplistic, but the blob array does suggest some kind of additional organizational layer on top of the orientation and ocular dominance arrays.

In sum, the current state of understanding is that striate cortex is concerned with analyzing the orientation, size, shape, speed, and direction of motion of objects in the world, and that it does so using modular groups of neurons—hypercolumns—each of which receives input from and processes a small piece of the visual world. (You can explore these organizational principles interactively in **Web Activity 3.5: Hypercolumns**.) Combining information from multiple hypercolumns is presumably the job of other portions of cortex farther downstream in the visual system. We will consider some of these portions in Chapter 4, when we discuss the representation and recognition of whole objects.

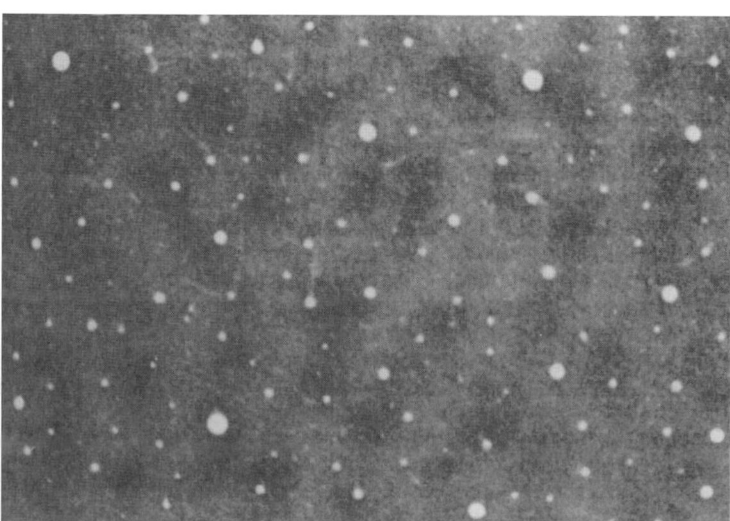

FIGURE 3.24 Cytochrome oxidase (CO) blobs. (From Hubel, 1988.)

Selective Adaptation: The Psychologist's Electrode

adaptation A reduction in response caused by prior or continuing stimulation.

Most of the physiological research reported up to now in this chapter was done using cats, monkeys, or other animals as subjects. Does the human visual system also include neurons selective for orientation, line width, direction of motion, and so on? The difficult thing about answering this question is that we can't normally poke electrodes into a human's brain (which is why Hubel, Wiesel, and their peers had to use cats and monkeys in the first place), so indirect methods of learning about brain function had to be devised. One such method is called **adaptation**, a technique that gives psychologists a noninvasive "electrode" they can use to probe the human brain (Frisby, 1980).

Selective adaptation can provide insights into the properties of cortical neurons, as illustrated in **Figure 3.25**. The green bars in Figure 3.25*a* illustrate the normal firing rates of cells tuned to orientations of 0, 10, –10, 20, –20 degrees, and so on, to a vertical grating. By definition, gratings oriented at 0

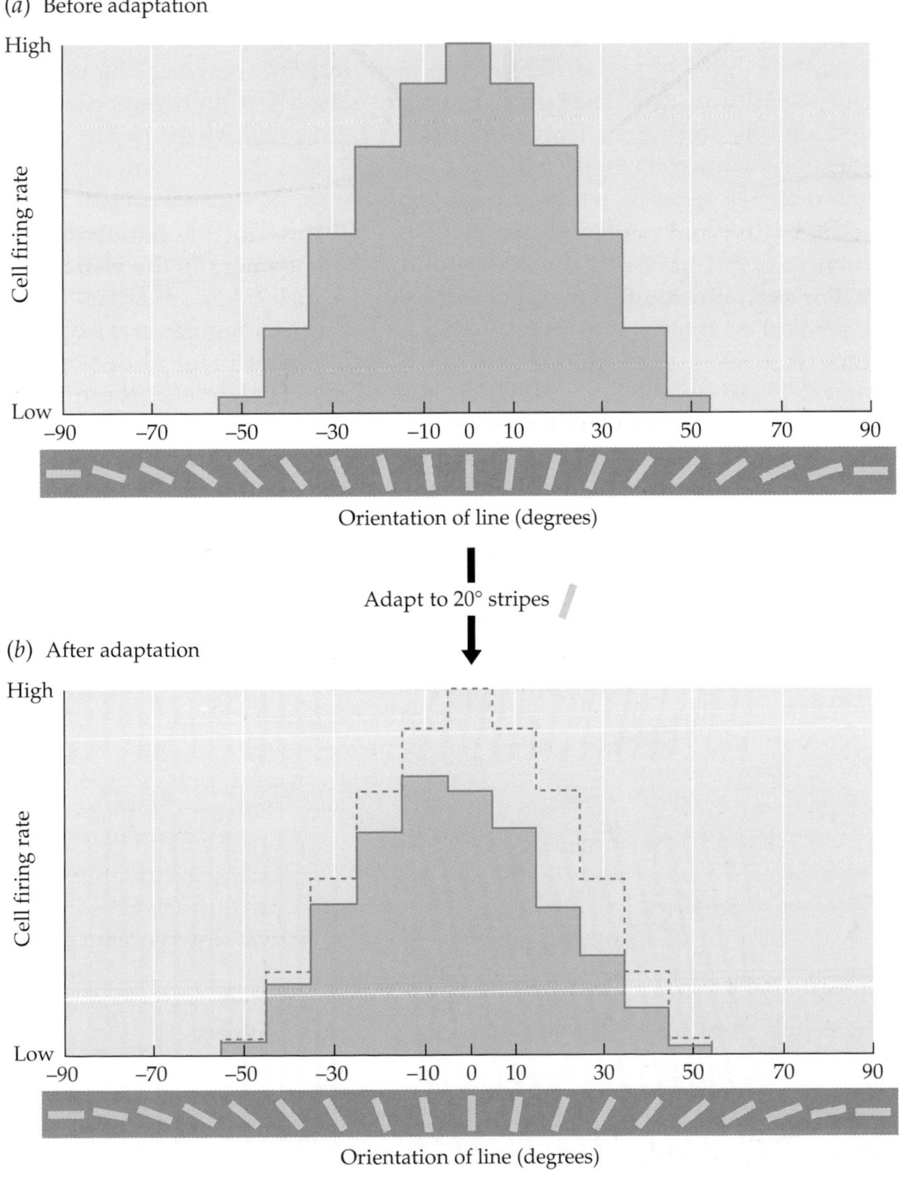

FIGURE 3.25 The psychologist's electrode. This schematic diagram shows how selective adaptation may alter the distribution of neural responses and therefore perception. See the text for explanation.

tilt aftereffect The perceptual illusion of tilt, produced by adaptation to a pattern of a given orientation.

degrees (vertical) elicit the strongest response from the 0-degree cells, followed closely by the 10-degree and –10-degree cells, followed by the 20-degree and –20-degree cells, and so on. Now suppose we expose the visual system that contains these cells to a 20-degree grating for an extended period of time. This adapting stimulus will cause the 20 degree–selective cells to be most active, and the extended activity will fatigue these cells (that is, their maximum firing rate will be reduced for a short period following adaptation). The adaptation procedure will also affect the other cells to some extent: the 10-degree and 30-degree cells will be the next most fatigued, followed by the 0-degree and 40-degree cells, and so on.

Figure 3.25*b* shows what should happen when we present the vertical grating again after adaptation to the 20-degree grating, assuming that our orientation perception is really due to populations of orientation-selective cells like those that Hubel and Wiesel found in the cat cortex. As the dark green bars show, because the 0-degree cells have been fatigued more than the –10-degree cells, the –10-degree cells are now firing fastest. As a result, we should perceive the vertical test stimulus as being oriented 10 degrees to the left.

You can test the validity of this technique yourself using the stimuli in **Figure 3.26**. Start by moving your eyes back and forth along the fixation line between the two gratings in Figure 3.26*a*. After about a minute of this adaptation, look quickly to the right at the fixation point between the vertical stripes in Figure 3.26*b*. The stripes in Figure 3.26*b* should now appear to be tilted slightly from their true vertical orientation (clockwise in the upper panel and counterclockwise in the lower—opposite the orientations in Figure 3.26*a*), just as predicted by the model of the human visual system based on the cat research and diagrammed in Figure 3.25. This **tilt aftereffect** strongly supports the idea that the human visual system contains individual neurons selective for different orientations.

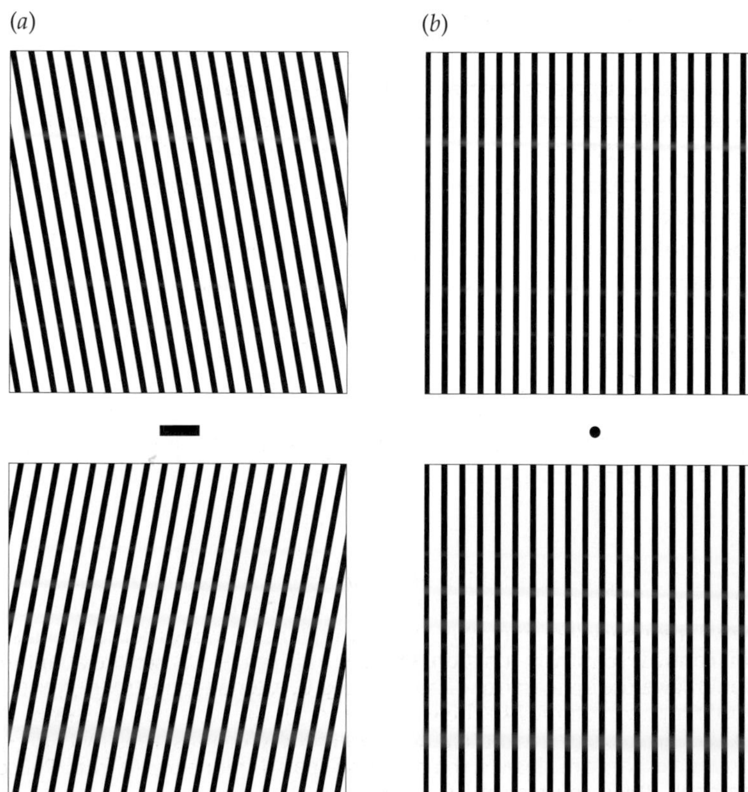

FIGURE 3.26 Stimuli for demonstrating selective adaptation. See the text for details. (After Frisby, 1980.)

Selective Adaptation for Spatial Frequencies

Selective adaptation also provides evidence that the human visual system contains neurons selective for spatial frequency. You can check this with the gratings shown in **Figure 3.27**. First look at Figure 3.27*b*, and make a mental note of your contrast sensitivity function (i.e., the inverted U-shaped area where the gratings fade into the gray background). Now adapt for about 10–20 seconds or so to the grating in Figure 3.27*a* and then quickly shift your gaze back to Figure 3.27*b*, and make a mental note of your contrast sensitivity function now. After repeating this procedure a few times, the outline of your CSF in Figure 3.27*b* should look something like the red curve in Figure 3.27*c*. It should have a notch (indicating reduced contrast sensitivity) for spatial frequencies that are close to the adapting spatial frequency (Figure 3.27*a*). This demonstration shows that adaptation to the high-contrast top panel is selective—resulting in a loss of sensitivity for spatial frequencies close to the adapting frequency, but not for spatial frequencies that are much higher or lower than the adapting frequency.

As noted earlier, selective adaptation causes the neurons most sensitive to the adapting stimulus to become fatigued. In this demonstration, neurons sensitive to the spatial frequency of the adapting stimulus have their contrast sensitivity reduced. That is, higher contrast is needed after adaptation for a test grating to be able to stimulate these neurons. Neurons responsive to much higher or much lower spatial frequencies are not fatigued by the adaptation procedure, so contrast sensitivity for these spatial frequencies is not affected.

Figure 3.28*a* shows more precisely how selective adaptation to a 7-cycle/degree grating produces a selective loss of contrast sensitivity at spatial frequencies of about 7 cycles/degree, with little or no loss at, for example, 1 cycle/degree or at 15 cycles/degree. After adaptation, the contrast sensitivity function has a "notch," as if the detectors sensitive to spatial frequencies near 7 cycles/degree were selectively destroyed (luckily the effects of spatial-frequency adaptation are reversible!). From these measurements of contrast sensitivity before and after adaptation, we can construct the spatial-frequency tuning function shown in Figure 3.28*b*. This function represents the change in contrast threshold (contrast threshold after adaptation, divided by contrast threshold before adaptation) plotted against the spatial frequency of the test grating. This curve represents the spatial-frequency tuning function for a "channel" that is most sensitive to a grating of 7 cycles/degree. The shape and selectivity of this channel are very similar to the spatial-frequency tuning functions for striate cortex neurons of cats and monkeys. Figure 3.28*c* illustrates that the contrast sensitivity function (gray curve) represents the "upper envelope" of the sensitivities of many spatial-frequency channels, each tuned to a different spatial frequency.

(*a*)

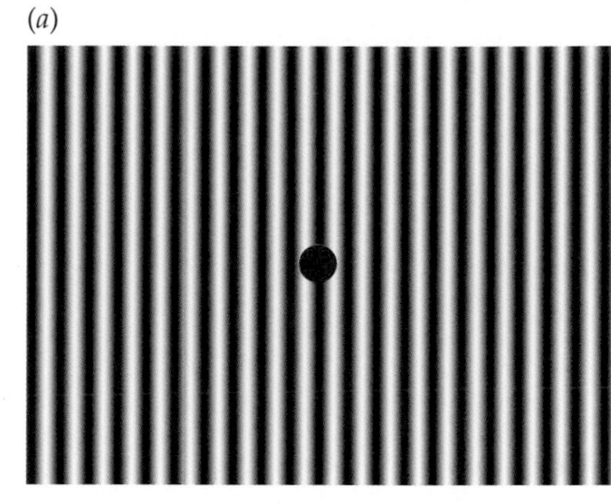

(*b*)

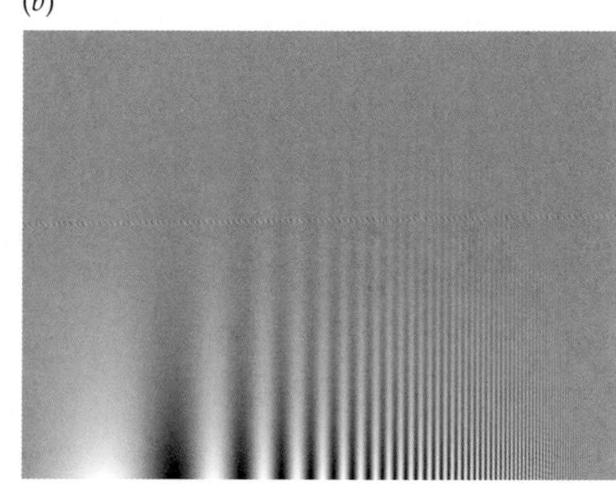

(*c*)

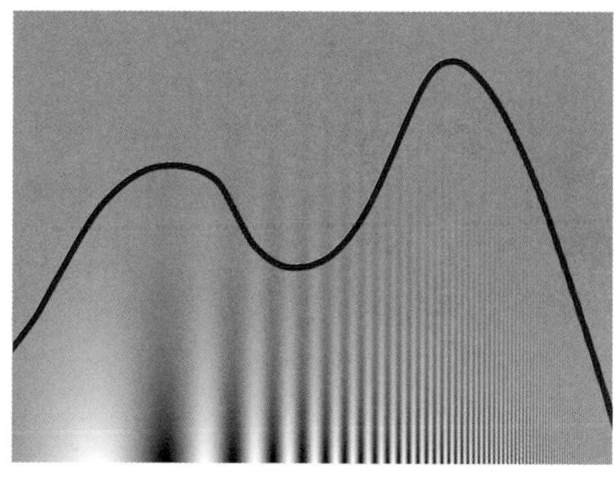

(*d*)

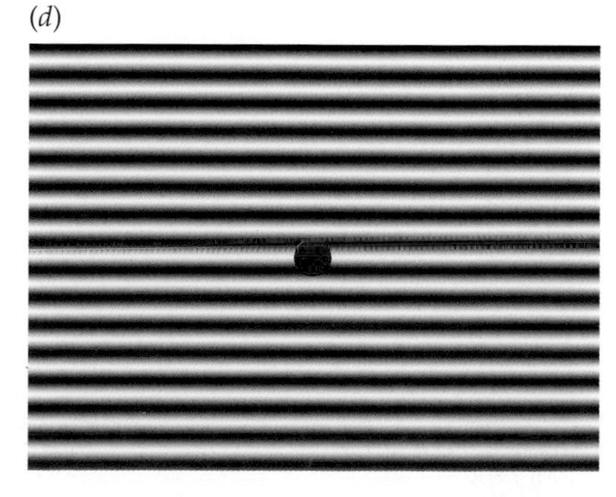

FIGURE 3.27 A demonstration of adaptation that is specific to spatial frequency (SF). (*a*) The adapting grating. (*b*) A grating modulated in contrast (vertically) and spatial frequency (horizontally). This pattern allows the reader to visualize their own contrast sensitivity function (CSF; see also Figure 3.8). Before adaptation it should have the appearance of an inverted U. After adapting to (*a*), your CSF should look something like the red curve in (*c*). The red curve illustrates the effect of adaptation. The notch indicates reduced contrast sensitivity for spatial frequencies that are close to the adapting spatial frequency. (*b* from Robson and Campbell, 1997; courtesy of Izumi Ohzawa.)

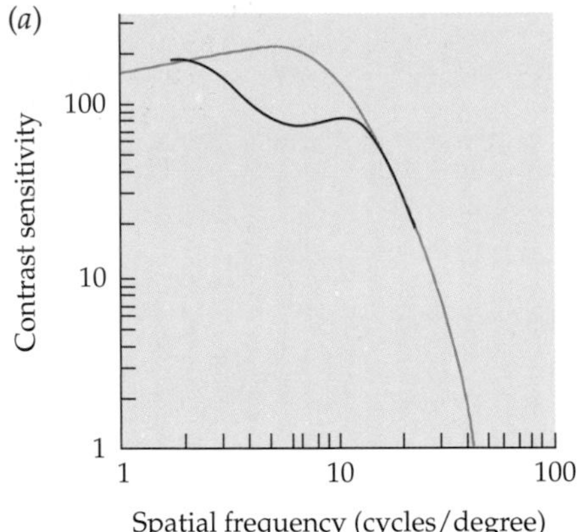

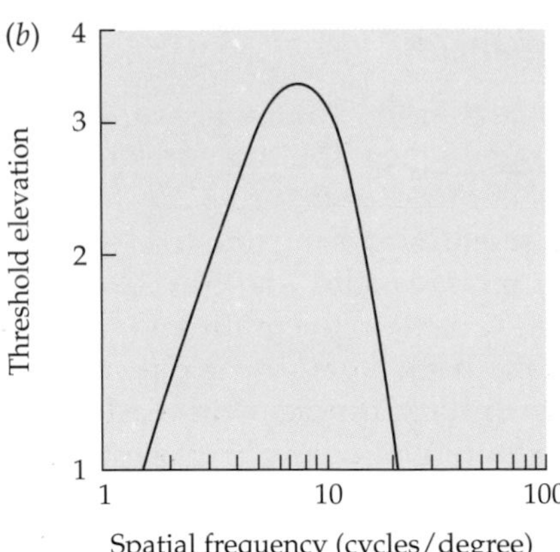

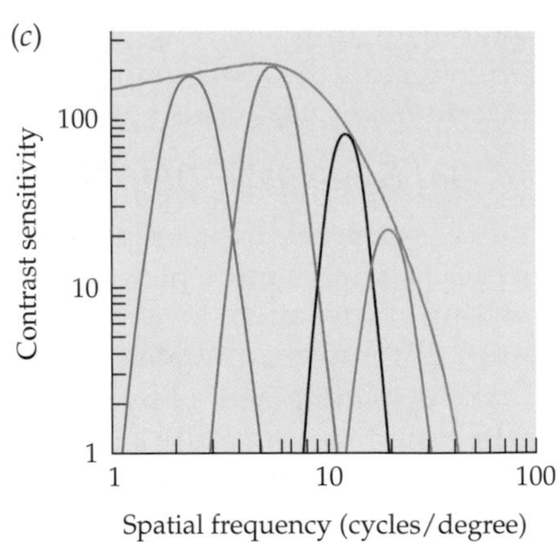

FIGURE 3.28 Spatial-frequency adaptation. (*a*) Selective adaptation to a 7-cycle/degree grating produces a selective loss of contrast sensitivity at spatial frequencies of about 7 cycles/degree, leaving a notch in the contrast sensitivity function. (*b*) Threshold elevation (the change in contrast threshold) following adaptation. (*c*) Physiologically measured spatial-frequency tuning functions for striate cortex neurons in monkeys (colored curves represent different neurons). (*b* after C. Blakemore and Campbell, 1969; *c* after Maffei and Fiorentini, 1973.)

The Site of Selective Adaptation Effects

The adaptation experiments replicated here provide strong evidence that orientation and spatial frequency are coded by neurons somewhere in the human visual system. In cats and monkeys, we know that these neurons are located in striate cortex, not in the retina or LGN. Can we localize the orientation-selective and spatial frequency–selective neurons in humans?

As it turns out, we can do just that with a clever variation on the adaptation experiments. Repeat the orientation (see Figure 3.26) and spatial-frequency (see Figure 3.27) adaptation demonstrations, but this time view the adapting stimuli with your left eye only (keep your right eye closed during the adaptation period), then view the test stimuli with your right eye (close your left eye and open your right eye as you shift your gaze to the test stimuli). You should find that the tilt aftereffect and the decreased contrast sensitivity transfer from one eye to another, although the effect may be somewhat less pronounced than when you did the demonstrations with both eyes open. This transfer of adaptation from the adapted to the nonadapted eye is known as "interocular transfer."

Now recall that information from the two eyes is kept completely separate in the retinas and in the two LGNs; no single neuron receives input from both eyes until the striate cortex. The transfer of adaptation effects from one eye to another thus implies that selective adaptation occurs in cortical neurons, just as we would predict from animal physiology studies.

Combining Spatial Frequency and Orientation Selectivity

Before we leave the selective adaptation paradigm, let's try one more demonstration. Adapt to the grating in Figure 3.27*d* for about a minute, then switch your gaze to the test grating in Figure 3.27*b*. You should find that the contrast sensitivity for this test stimulus is not reduced at all; the test grating should be equally visible both before and after adaptation. What does this result tell us about the coding of orientation and spatial frequency in human cortical neurons?

Remember that in Hubel and Wiesel's studies with cats, each striate cortex neuron was selective for both a particular orientation and a particular spatial frequency. In other words, a cell responded to a test stimulus only if the stimulus was at (or at least near) the cell's preferred orientation *and* close to the cell's preferred spatial frequency. Our selective adaptation findings indicate that human cortical cells operate the same way. The test stimulus in Figure 3.27*b* has the same spatial frequency as the adapting stimulus, but a completely different orientation. Therefore, the two stimuli will stimulate completely different neurons, and we should expect no contrast sensitivity reduction for the test stimulus.

spatial-frequency channel A pattern analyzer, implemented by an ensemble of cortical neurons, in which each set of neurons is tuned to a limited range of spatial frequencies.

Spatial Frequency–Tuned Pattern Analyzers in Human Vision

Selective adaptation to spatial frequency, as well as other evidence, provides strong support for the notion, first suggested by Fergus Campbell and John Robson (1968), that the human contrast sensitivity function actually reflects the sensitivity of multiple individual pattern analyzers. These pattern analyzers are implemented by ensembles of cortical neurons, with each set of cells tuned to a limited range of spatial frequencies and orientations, and they are often referred to as **spatial-frequency channels**. Remember the initially unexplained falloff in the contrast sensitivity function at very low spatial frequencies? Although a number of different explanations have been suggested (e.g., lateral inhibition), the most likely explanation is that we simply have fewer neurons tuned to low spatial frequencies (De Valois, Albrecht, and Thorell, 1982).

The "multiple spatial frequency" model of vision implies that spatial frequencies that stimulate different pattern analyzers will be detected independently, even if the different frequencies are combined in the same image. Consider the compound grating pattern in **Figure 3.29**, made by adding a sine wave with frequency *f* to a sine wave with frequency 3*f*. Graham and Nachmias (1971) found that the contrast sensitivity for this compound pattern was almost the same as the contrast sensitivity for detecting the individual components of the pattern separately. If the two component sine waves had stimulated a common pattern analyzer, then their effects on the analyzer should have been added, so contrast sensitivity should have been greatly improved.

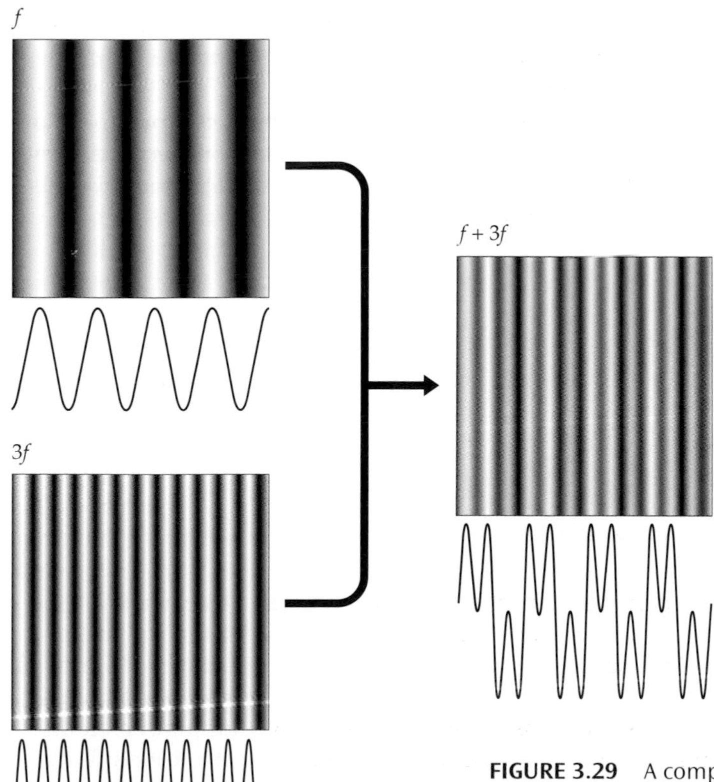

FIGURE 3.29 A compound grating pattern (right), made by the addition of a sine wave of frequency *f* (top left) to one of frequency 3*f* (bottom left). (After Graham and Nachmias, 1971.)

(a)

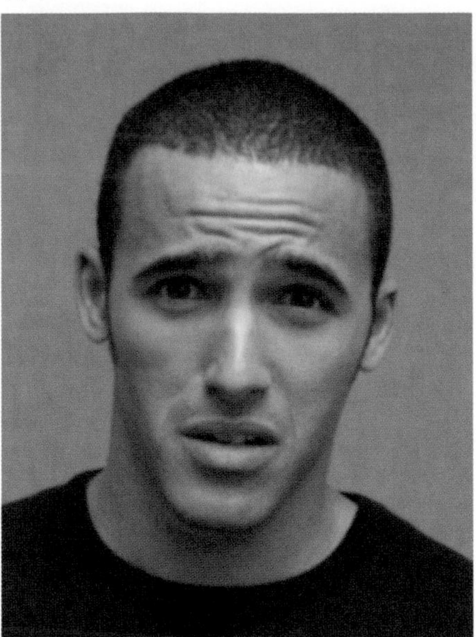

(b)

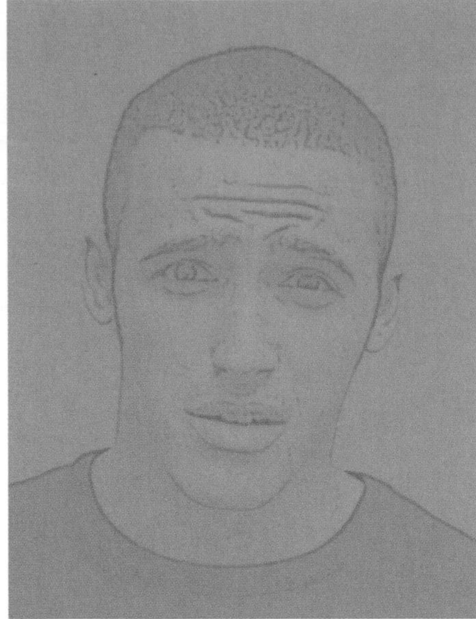

(c)

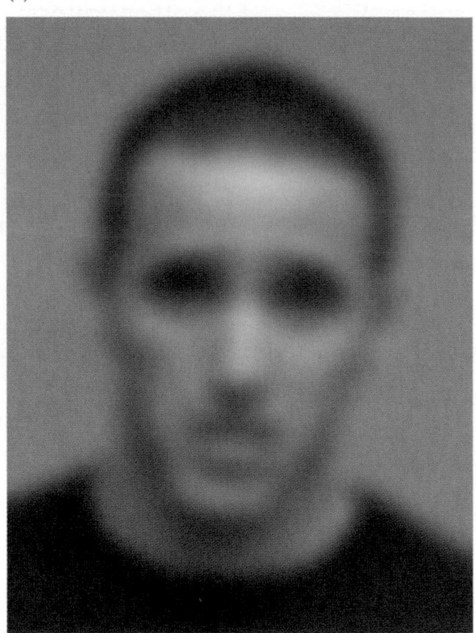

FIGURE 3.30 A complete image (*a*) and simulations of the high-frequency (*b*) and low-frequency (*c*) components of that image.

Why would the visual system use spatial-frequency filters to analyze images? One important reason may be that different spatial frequencies emphasize different types of information. **Figure 3.30** shows a face that has only high-frequency (panel *b*) or low-frequency (panel *c*) components of the face in panel (*a*). These images show that low frequencies emphasize the broad outlines of the face and high frequencies carry information about fine details. If we want to know how many people are in a scene, it is most efficient to consult our low-frequency channels. But if we want to know about the fine details—for example, whether the people are frowning or smiling—we must rely on our high-frequency channels.

FIGURE 3.31 Who is hidden behind the high-spatial-frequency mask in this image?

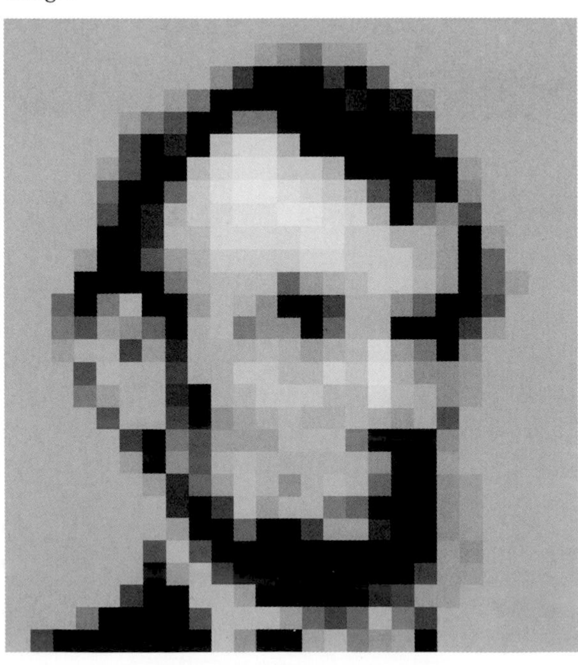

It is widely agreed that at near-threshold contrasts, pattern analyzers operating at different scales of analysis are independent. At high contrasts, however, pattern analyzers do interact. You can experience this for yourself in **Figure 3.31**, where the high spatial frequencies introduced by the small blocks mask the low spatial frequencies that convey an underlying portrait of a famous American. Squinting your eyes will blur the blocks, minimizing the effect of the mask to a point where the face you've seen countless times on the 5-dollar bill will probably show through.

The Development of Spatial Vision

William James (1890) described the infant's world as "a blooming, buzzing confusion." However, studies over the past several decades have shown that the visual system is much more developed at birth than we used to think. One of the difficulties in assessing vision in infants is that we can't simply ask them what they see. Rather, we have to think of tricky ways to coax that information from them. The most widely used method for studying infant vision is based on an observation by Robert Fantz in the early 1960s. What Fantz noticed is that if infants are shown two scenes, they invariably stare at the more complex scene (the scene with the most contours). So, if an infant is shown two patches, one containing stripes, and the other uniform gray, the infant will prefer to look at the stripes. Of course, an infant who couldn't see the stripes would be equally likely to stare at the gray patch as at the striped patch. Thus, preferential looking is one important method used by infant researchers (grown psychologists studying infant vision, not babies in lab coats) to learn what infants can see and respond to behaviorally (**Figure 3.32*a***).

The success of preferential looking depends on the willingness of babies to stare at stimuli near threshold level. An alternative approach, used with considerable success in more recent years, is to measure visually evoked electrical potentials (VEPs) to visual stimuli by attaching electrodes to the scalp and measuring the changes in electrical activity that are elicited by the changing visual stimulus (Figure 3.32*b* and *c*). Using the VEP, we can measure an entire contrast sensitivity function in as little as 10 seconds in a nonverbal infant.

Development of the Contrast Sensitivity Function

The emerging picture suggests that, with increasing age, peak contrast sensitivity increases and the CSF peak shifts toward higher spatial frequencies. Low spatial-frequency sensitivity develops much more rapidly than high

FIGURE 3.32 Assessing vision in infants. (*a*) Forced-choice preferential-looking stimuli (left) and the experimental setup (right). (*b*) Visual evoked potential (VEP) setup. (*c*) Results of a sweep VEP experiment in which the spatial frequency of the stimulus is swept (continuously varied from low to high spatial frequency), illustrating the extrapolated acuity. This particular experiment was done at 80% contrast. (Part *c* after Norcia et al., 1990.)

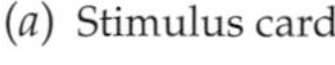

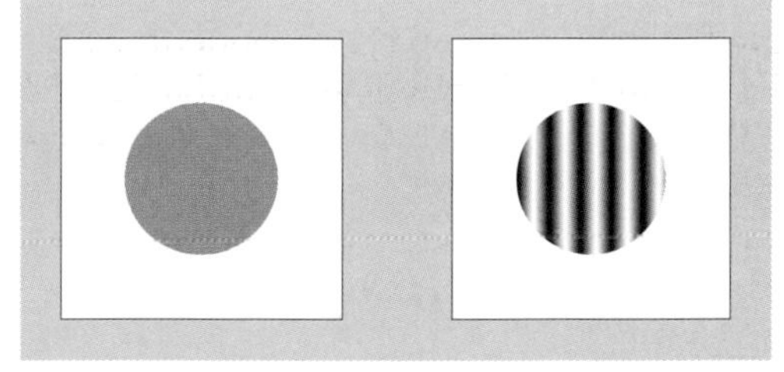

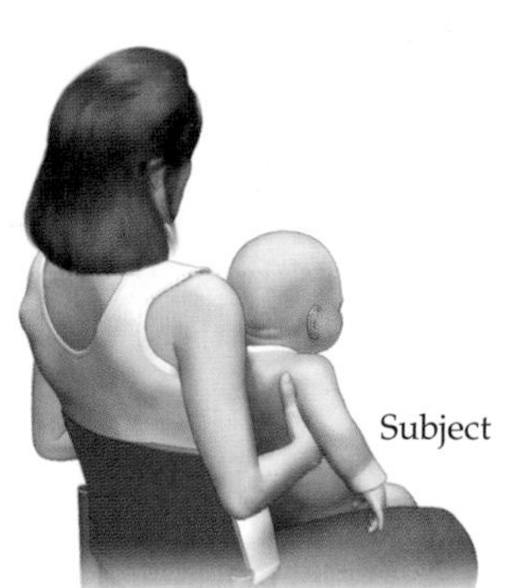

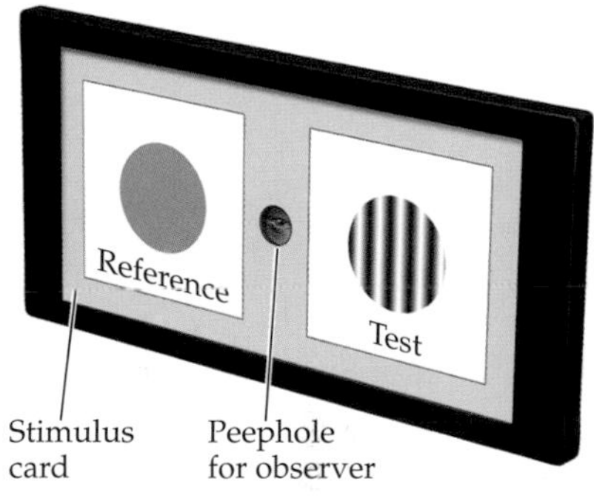

(*b*)

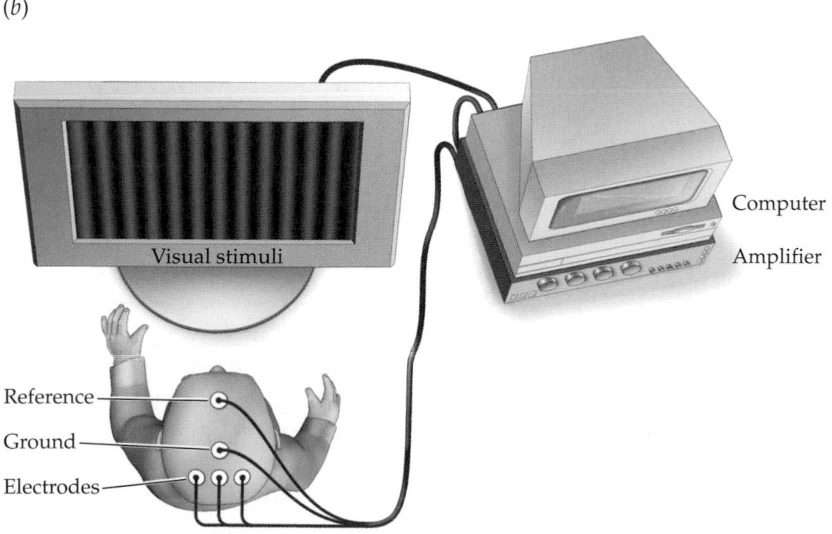

(*c*) Sweep VEP (grating acuity)

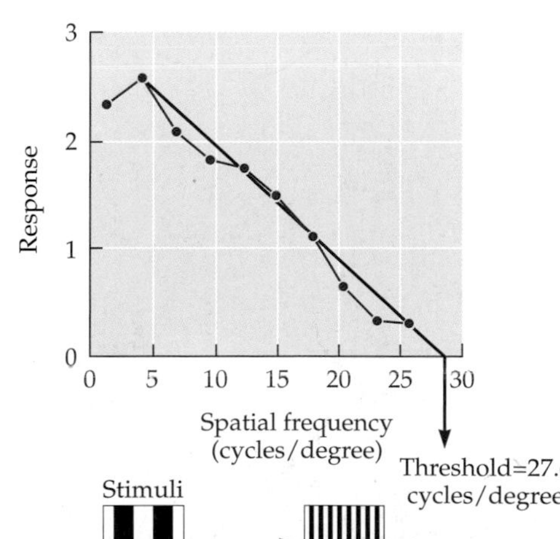

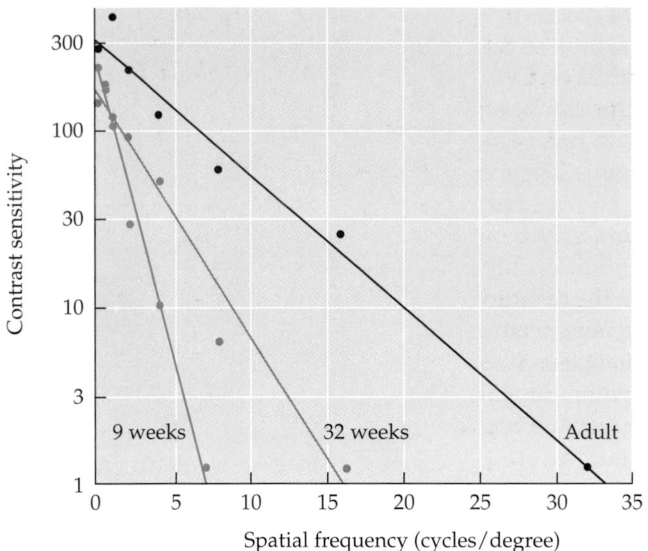

FIGURE 3.33 The development of contrast sensitivity. (After Norcia et al., 1990.)

spatial-frequency sensitivity. Thus, peak contrast sensitivity may reach adult levels as early as about 9 weeks of age, whereas sensitivity at higher spatial frequencies continues to develop dramatically (**Figure 3.33**). There remains a roughly 20-fold difference in the contrast sensitivity of adults and 32-week-olds (Norcia et al., 1990).

What limits the development of acuity and contrast sensitivity? The primary postnatal changes in the retina concern differentiation of the macular region (Boothe, Dobson, and Teller, 1985). After birth, foveal receptor density and cone outer segment length both increase, as foveal cones become thinner and more elongated. There is a dramatic migration of ganglion cells and inner nuclear layers from the foveal region as the foveal pit develops during the first 4 months of life, and not until about 4 years of age is the fovea fully adultlike (Yuodelis and Hendrickson, 1986).

From birth to beyond 4 years of age, cone density increases in the central region, because of both migration of receptors and decreases in their dimensions. Both of these factors result in finer cone sampling (by decreasing the distance between neighboring cones). Alterations in cone spacing and the light-gathering properties of the cones during early development probably contribute a great deal toward the improvements in acuity and contrast sensitivity during the first months of life. The massive migration of retinal cells, and the alterations in the size of retina and eyeball (along with changes in interpupillary distance), may necessitate the plasticity of cortical connections early in life. Interestingly, the peripheral retina appears to develop much more rapidly than the fovea (Yuodelis and Hendrickson, 1986).

The Girl Who Almost Couldn't See Stripes

Normal visual development requires normal visual experience. Abnormal early visual experience can have serious and often permanent consequences for seeing patterns, as illustrated by the story of a girl named Jane. Jane was born with a dense cataract (an opacity of the lens) in her left eye, which prevented clear patterns from forming on her left retina. In addition to causing form deprivation in the left eye, the cataract prevented Jane's two eyes from seeing the same images at the same time.

Studies in cats and monkeys dating back to Hubel and Wiesel in the early 1960s have shown that monocular form deprivation can cause massive changes in cortical physiology that result in a devastating and permanent loss of spatial vision (Wiesel, 1982). Hubel and Wiesel, and many other workers subsequently, demonstrated that there is a critical period of early visual development when normal binocular visual stimulation is required for normal cortical development. In cats and monkeys this critical period covers the first 3 to 4 months of life; in humans it is extended to something on the order of the first 3 to 8 years. During the critical period, cortical neurons are still being wired up to their inputs from the two eyes. This is a period of neural plasticity, when abnormal visual experience can alter the normal neural wiring process. If one eye is not receiving normal stimulation, the neurons that should be destined to respond to that eye do not become properly connected. In fact, some evidence suggests that these neurons are actually co-opted by inputs from the other, normally functioning eye.

If cataracts or other conditions, such as **strabismus**, in which one eye is turned so that it is receiving a view of the world from an abnormal angle, are left untreated during the critical period, the misplaced cortical connections can never be repaired. The result is often **amblyopia** (reduced visual acuity in one eye because of abnormal early visual experience) and an inability to perceive stereopsis (a lack of binocular depth perception; see Chapter 6). Correcting the condition later in life will thus have little effect, because the information from the now-functioning eye can never be properly conveyed to or processed by the cortex.

Luckily for Jane, her pediatrician found the cataract early, and the cataractous lens was surgically replaced by an artificial lens when she was 3 months old. The visual acuity in Jane's left eye just after the contact lens was inserted was 20/1200, about four times worse than the normal value for a 3-month-old. But when tested again 1 month later, acuity in her left eye had already begun to catch up with the acuity in her right eye. In fact, a recent study (Maurer et al., 1999) found significant acuity improvements only an hour after corrective measures had been taken.

strabismus A misalignment of the two eyes such that a single object in space is imaged on the fovea of one eye, and on a nonfoveal area of the other (turned) eye.

amblyopia A developmental disorder that is characterized by reduced spatial vision in an otherwise healthy eye, even with proper correction for refractive error. Often referred to as "lazy eye."

Summary

1. In this chapter we followed the path of image processing from the eyeball to the brain. Neurons in the cerebral cortex translate the array of stars perceived by retinal ganglion cells into the beginnings of forms and patterns. The primary visual cortex is organized into thousands of tiny computers, each responsible for determining the orientation, width, color, and other characteristics of the stripes in one small portion of the visual field. In Chapter 4 we will continue this story by seeing how other parts of the brain combine the outputs from these minicomputers to produce a coherent representation.
2. Perhaps the most important feature of image processing is the remarkable transformation of information from the circular receptive fields of retinal ganglion cells to the elongated receptive fields of the cortex.
3. Cortical neurons are highly selective along a number of dimensions, including stimulus orientation, size, direction of motion, and eye of origin.
4. Neurons with similar preferences are often arranged in columns in primary visual cortex.
5. Selective adaptation provides a powerful, noninvasive tool for learning about stimulus specificity in human vision.
6. The human visual cortex contains pattern analyzers that are specific to spatial frequency and orientation.
7. Normal visual development requires normal visual experience. Abnormal visual experience early in life can cause massive changes in cortical physiology that result in a devastating and permanent loss of spatial vision.

Refer to the
Sensation and Perception
website
(www.sinauer.com/wolfe2e)
for activities, essays, study questions, and other study aids.

CHAPTER 4

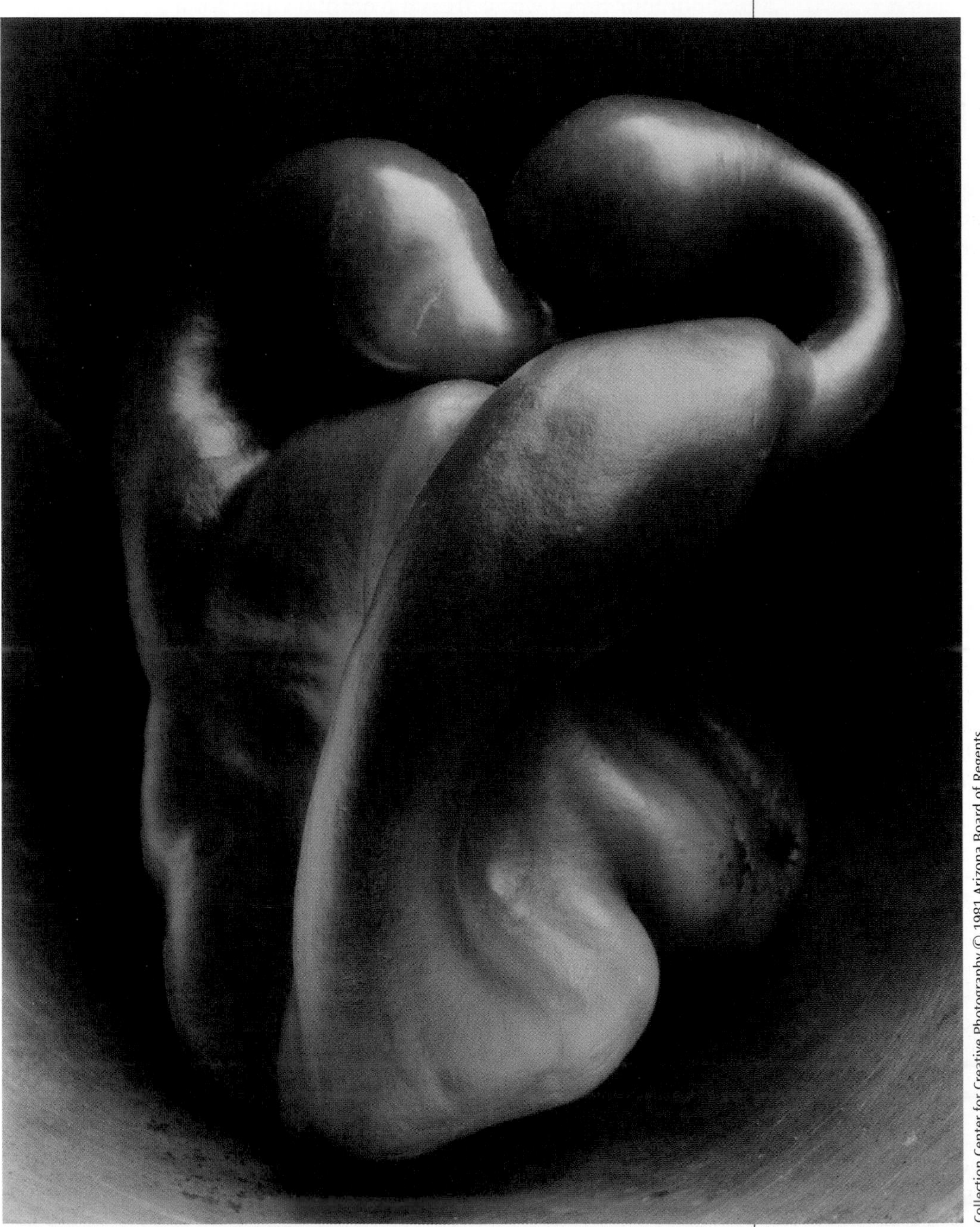
Edward Weston, *Pepper No. 30*, 1930

Perceiving and Recognizing Objects

Figure 4.1*a* is clearly a picture of a house. The image may contain some other things as well, but the chief object of interest is the house. Figure 4.1*b* is pretty clearly a house as well, though in this case the house is part of a more abstract scene painted by the French artist Paul Cézanne in the early twentieth century. This type of the seemingly simple act of object identification is the topic of this chapter. Like many seemingly simple acts, object perception is actually a collection of complex and remarkable accomplishments.

Consider **Figure 4.2***a*. It shows yet another house. How do we recognize it as a house? First we need to gather some basic visual features. The preceding chapters have shown us how single cells in the early visual system respond to stimuli like simple lines. In Figure 4.2*b* each circle is a cartoon of the receptive field of a simple cortical cell. Those cells in striate cortex will respond well to the high-contrast lines in the outline of the house. That limited receptive field is like a window that allows the cell to "see" only a small part of the world. None of these simple cells see a house. They just collect local features like horizontal, vertical, and oblique lines.

At the very least, the local features will need to be assembled into a house. This process could be imagined as the natural extension of a process we have already discussed. One way to "construct" the lines detected by simple cells is to imagine combining a row of dots detected by retinal ganglion cells. Dots could be grouped together into lines. A pair of lines, each collected by a different cell, could be combined by another cell that would sense a corner. This process could go on and on, until we had a house. On closer examination, however, it is clear that this process would not be easy. Consider, for example, Figure 4.2*c*. Again, simple cells would have no problem detecting the lines and edges in this scene, but how do we know which edges go with which objects? How do we avoid considering the snowman part of the house? The house and snowman make corners as do the house and its door and steps. The car and house are separate. None of their lines touch. But this is also true of the outline of the house and its windows.

Clearly we must have processes that successfully combine features into objects. That is one of the tasks that defines **middle** (or **midlevel**) **vision** (as opposed to low-level vision, which was the topic of Chapters 2 and 3). The first part of this chapter looks at some of the processes of middle vision. The second part takes the feature combinations given to us by middle-level vision and asks how we come to know what the object is. The act of recognition must involve matching what we perceive now to a memory of something we perceived in the past. How can we do that? For example, how do we know that all of the images in Figures 4.1 and 4.2 show houses? Without having seen these exact objects before, how do we go about placing them in the "house" category? Furthermore, it's easy to see that Figure 4.1*c* shows

middle (midlevel) vision A loosely defined stage of visual processing that comes after basic features have been extracted from the image (early vision) and before object recognition and scene understanding (high-level vision).

(a)

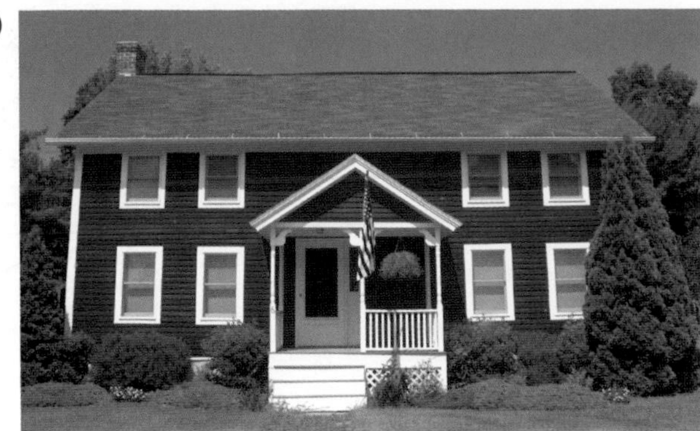

(b)

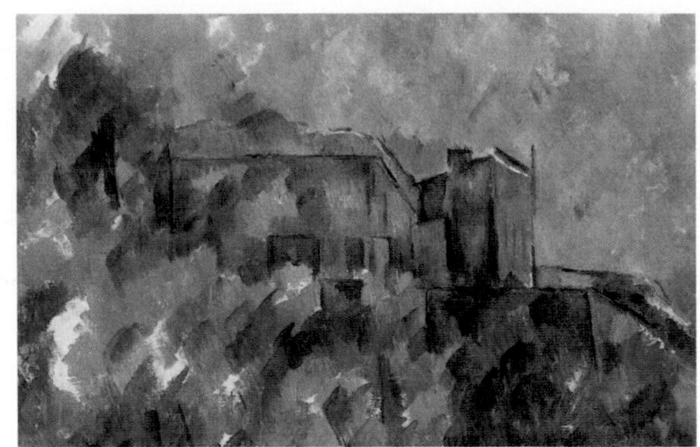

FIGURE 4.1 The problem of object recognition. (*a*) A house. (*b*) Paul Cézanne's *Chateau Noir* (1902–05) looks completely different but it is still a house. (*c*) This image is also very different from the one in (*a*), but it is clearly the same house.

(c)

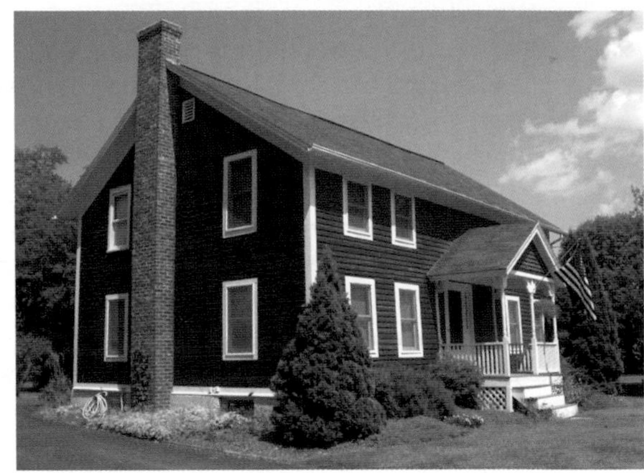

the same house as 4.1*a*. How do we make this connection, given that the images delivered to our retinas in the two figures are radically different? In the second part of this chapter, we'll discuss the high-level visual processes that enable us to recognize familiar objects, novel views of familiar objects, and new instances of familiar object categories.

Middle Vision

The goal of middle vision is to organize the elements of a visual scene into groups that we can then recognize as objects. Let's begin with the simplest case of an object isolated on a simple background. Finding the edges of this object will be a good starting place on the road to recognizing the object.

FIGURE 4.2 The problem continued. (*a*) Another house. (*b*) Cells in primary visual cortex respond well to the local features (circled) of the house. But how do we go from recognizing a collection of local features to perceiving a house? (*c*) A slightly more complicated scene. How do we know which bits belong together?

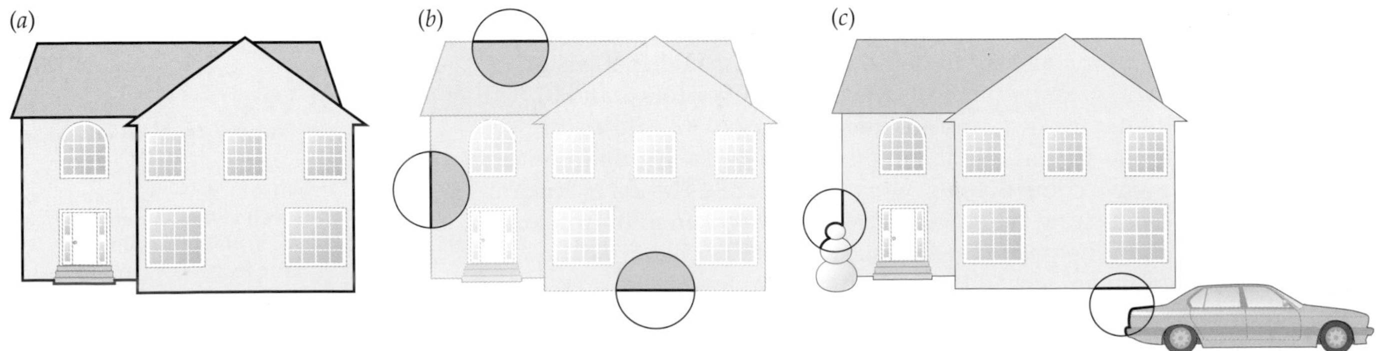

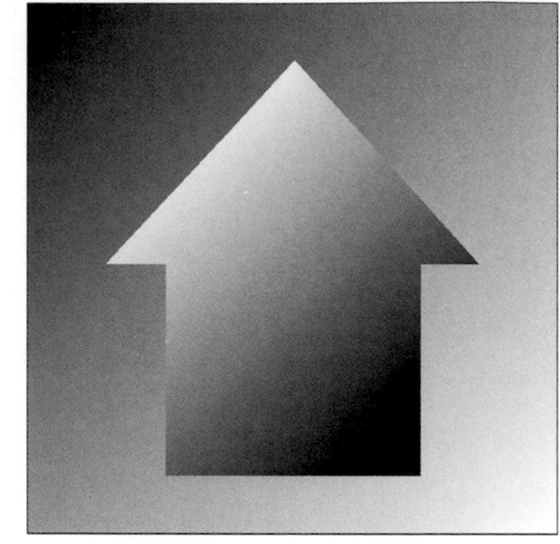

FIGURE 4.3 In some places this object is darker than the background. In other places it is lighter. If the changes are continuous, it follows that there must be places where the edge of this shape simply disappears.

Finding Edges

In Chapter 3, we discussed at length how neurons in striate cortex can detect bits of lines, but how do we decide which bits belong to which objects? We already established that we can't just group all the edges that touch each other into an object. Because objects abut and overlap other objects, simple connectedness will not work. Worse yet, before we can concern ourselves with grouping edges, we need to worry about the quality of the raw edge information. In **Figure 4.3**, part of the house of Figure 4.2 is reduced to a simple, arrow-shaped outline. It is easy to see that arrow. Notice, however, that in some places the object is lighter than the background, while in other places it is darker. This means that, if we trace the edge of the object with a finger, we *must* pass locations where there is no difference between the luminance of the object and the luminance of the background. In other words, at these points the shape has no edge at all.

Interestingly, this occasional lack of an edge doesn't seem to bother our visual system at all. In fact, it may be hard to see the gap. Asking computer graphics software to find the edges in Figure 4.3 yields something like **Figure 4.4***a*. The gaps are there, but the visual system knows that they are accidents of the lighting and fills in the contour. The computer is not so clever. Figures 4.4*b* and *c* show another example. Notice that, in Figure 4.4*c*, the edge-finding software finds all sorts of edges. How do we decide which edges are important?

An even more extreme demonstration of the problems of edge finding and edge quality is shown in **Figure 4.5**. This an example of a "Kanizsa figure"—named after Gaetano Kanizsa (1913–1993), an Italian psychologist who spent many years investigating such stimuli. Here it is easy to see the arrow outline, even though the vast majority of the shape's lines are miss-

(*a*)

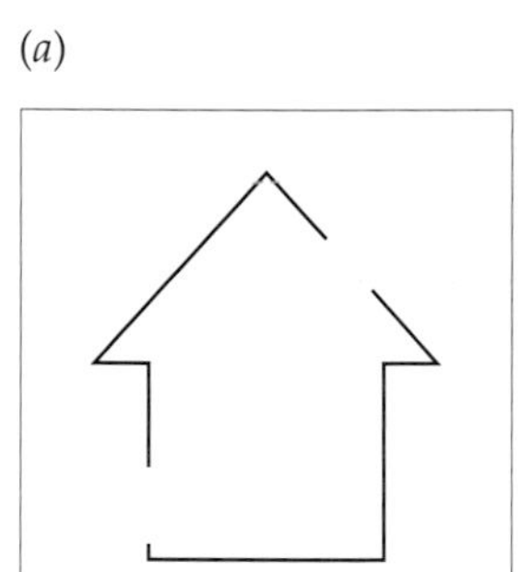

(*b*)

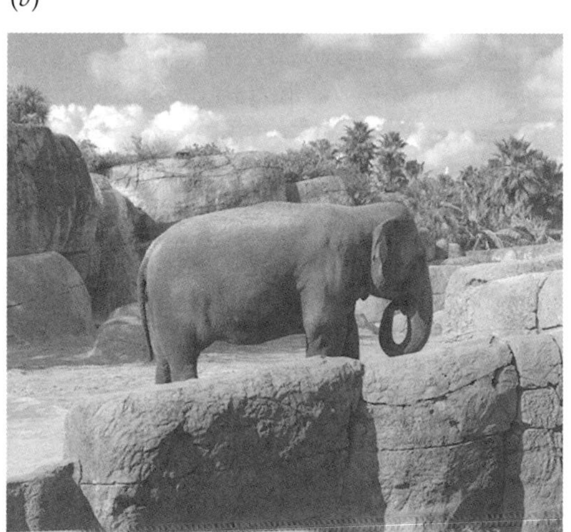

(*c*)

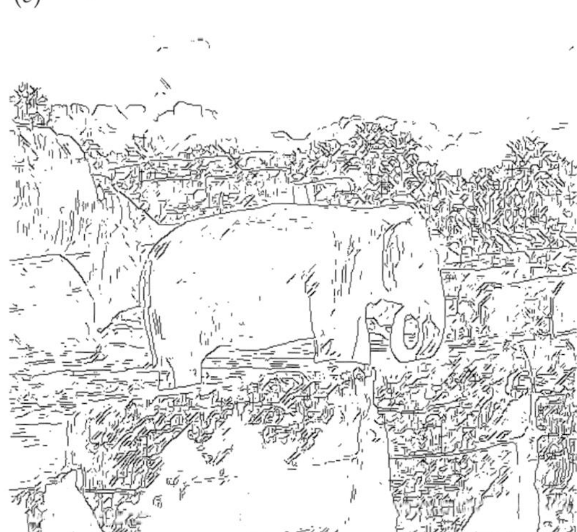

FIGURE 4.4 Finding edges. (*a*) The "find edges" function in a popular graphics program finds gaps in the borders of Figure 4.3—gaps that we do not see. (*b*) When a computer algorithm looks for the edges in this elephant scene, it finds what is shown in (*c*). You can try various edge-finding algorithms at http://marathon.csee.usf.edu/edge/edge_detection.html.

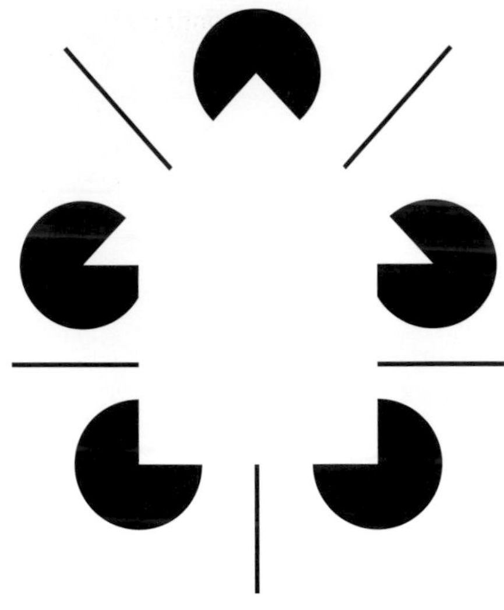

FIGURE 4.5 This "house" outline is constructed from illusory contours. Even though an edge is clearly visible, there is no physical difference between the white background and the white house.

ing. Check it yourself. There really is no border between the white figure and the white background. These edges, which are perceived despite the almost total lack of physical evidence for them, are called **illusory contours**.

RULES THAT MAKE CONTOURS This tendency of the visual system to go beyond the information given was problematic for one of the earliest group of perceptual psychologists, the **structuralists**. Structuralists such as Wilhelm Wundt (1832–1920) and Edward Bradford Titchener (1867–1927) argued that perceptions are the sum of atoms of sensation—bits of color, orientation, and so forth. In the structuralist view, perception is built up of the local sensations the way a crystal might be built up of an array of atoms. An illusory contour challenges this view because an extended edge is seen bridging a gap where no local atom of "edgeness" can be found.

Over time, it became clear that there are many examples where the structuralist argument seems to fail. Inspired by these examples, a second group of psychologists, led by Max Wertheimer (1880–1943), Wolfgang Köhler (1887–1967), and Kurt Koffka (1886–1941), formed the **Gestalt** school. Gestalt theory held that the perceptual whole was more than the sum of its sensory parts. Perhaps the most enduring contribution of this school was to begin the description of a set of organizing principles (sometimes known as **Gestalt grouping rules**) that guide the visual system in its interpretation of the raw retinal image. For example, **Figure 4.6***a* illustrates the tendency of lines of similar orientation to be seen as part of the same contour (Field, Hayes, and Hess, 1992). Such lines "support" each other, in that two visible bits of an edge will actually make it easier to perceive a third, colinear segment that lies between them, even if the middle segment is not actually visible (Polat and Sagi, 1993). If a set of such lines forms a closed shape like the roughly circular contour in Figure 4.6*b*, then the little segments support each other even more strongly (Kovacs and Julesz, 1993).

The Gestaltists called this the principle of **good continuation**, and they illustrated it with examples like the one shown in **Figure 4.7***a*. We tend to see this figure as a pair of intersecting lines (Figure 4.7*b*). There are many other possible organizations (Figure 4.7*c*, for example); but all else being equal, the tendency to see lines continuing in the same direction—in other words, the tendency to group edges that have the same orientation—supports the X-like interpretation illustrated in Figure 4.7*b*.

illusory contour A contour that is perceived, even though nothing changes from one side of the contour to the other in the image.

structuralism A school of thought believing that complex objects or perceptions could be understood by analysis of the components.

Gestalt In German, literally "form." In perception, the name of a school of thought stressing that the perceptual whole could be greater than the apparent sum of the parts.

Gestalt grouping rules A set of rules describing which elements in an image will appear to group together. The original list was assembled by members of the Gestalt school of thought.

good continuation A Gestalt grouping rule stating that two elements will tend to group together if they seem to lie on the same contour.

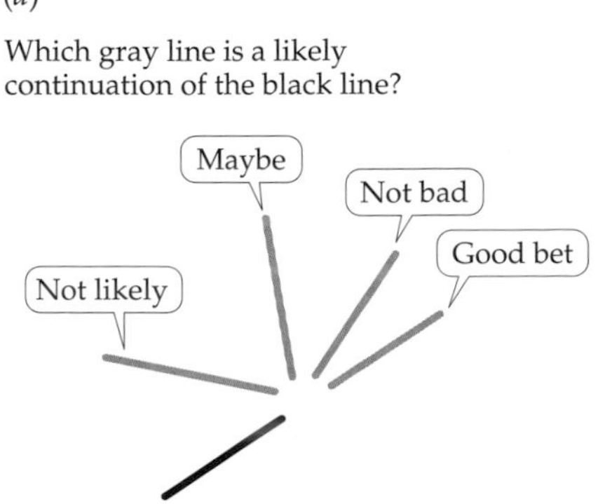

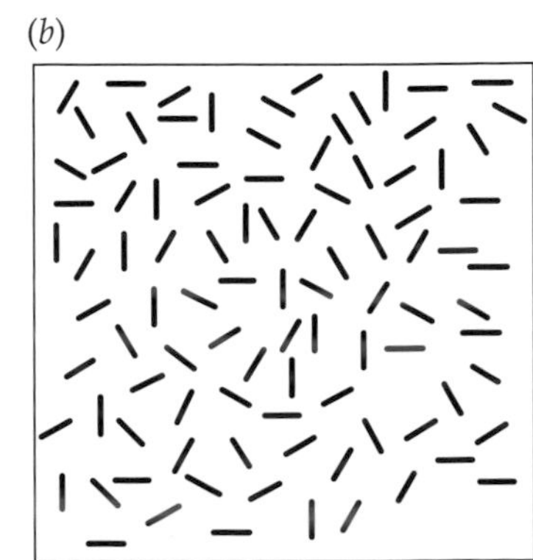

FIGURE 4.6 Contour completion. (*a*) Lines are more likely to be seen as continuous with lines of similar orientation. (*b*) The visual system's application of this rule produces the roughly circular contour shown in the center of this diagram.

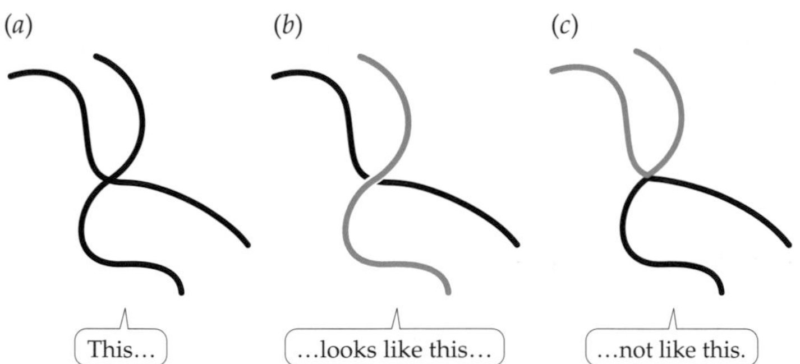

FIGURE 4.7 The Gestalt principle of good continuation.

PERCEPTUAL "COMMITTEES" The "all else being equal" phrase is important. As the Gestalt psychologists knew, and as we will see, a host of rules, principles, and good guesses contribute to our organized perception of the world. These seem to operate on a sort of committee model. Everyone gets together and voices opinions about how the stimulus ought to be understood. Sometimes the opinions collide, and the results in such cases are somewhat unpredictable (in Figure 4.7*c*, for example, color trumps good continuation as an organizing principle). Somehow, though, a consensus view almost always quickly emerges and we settle on a single interpretation of the visual scene. This committee metaphor is very useful and will recur throughout this chapter.

OCCLUSION If an edge suddenly stops in an image, *why* does it stop? One reasonable guess might be that it stops because something else gets in the way, hiding it from our view. So, returning to the Kanizsa figure of Figure 4.5, we can imagine the visual system asking why that vertical line at the bottom of the figure suddenly stops. The answer that the visual system seems to come up with is that there is another contour *occluding* the vertical line, with the occluding edge oriented perpendicularly to the occluded edge.

This guess, combined with a guess that the notches in the circles represent contours that can be extended, leads to the inference of an illusory contour (**Figure 4.8***a* and *b*). (Note that we also interpret the notches as places where one object is occluding another.) Figure 4.8*c* shows another example. If each black line generated weak illusory contours at right angles to its endpoint,

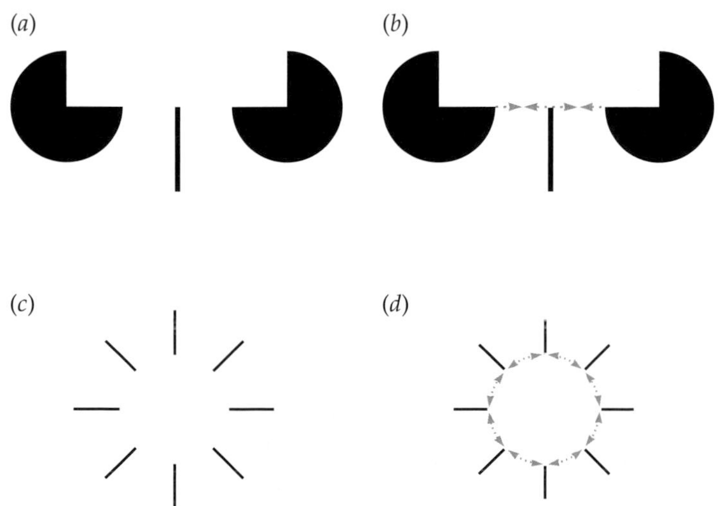

FIGURE 4.8 The making of illusory contours. (*a*) The little arrows in (*b*) and (*d*) represent the visual system's best guess about what is going on in (*a*) and (*c*). The illusory disk in (*c*) arises when the visual system combines a whole collection of guesses about the line terminations as shown in (*d*).

then this figure would contain a set of roughly colinear line segments (Figure 4.8*d*) that could be grouped together to form a convincing circle in the manner of Figure 4.6*b*. (By the way, illusory contours make excellent doodles when you would rather be doing informal perception experiments than paying attention.)

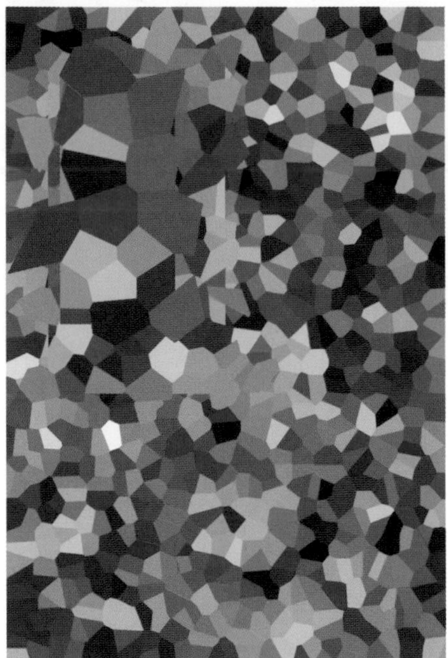

FIGURE 4.9 The problem of texture segmentation. How do we know that the upper left region is different from the rest of the image?

Texture Segmentation and Grouping

Connecting little pieces of line segments will get us only so far in dividing the raw image into objects. In **Figure 4.9** we can see that something is different about the upper left quadrant of the image. An edge detector like the one described in Figure 4.4 will easily find the small, randomly shaped polygons that make up the image, but it will be oblivious to the difference between the larger-grain and smaller-grain textures.

Because the edge-finding members of the "image-parsing committee" are of little use, Figure 4.9 is parsed instead by the visual system's sophisticated mechanisms for **texture segmentation** (Beck, 1982; Bergen and Adelson, 1988; Malik and Perona, 1990). The portion of the image with a coarser texture (the part made up of larger polygons) is separated from the rest of the image.

Texture segmentation is closely related to the Gestalt grouping principles that we have been discussing. **Figure 4.10*a*** illustrates two of the strongest principles: similarity and proximity. **Similarity** means that image chunks that are similar to each other will be more likely to group together. Similar in what ways? Texture grouping can be based on similarity in a limited number of features: color, size, orientation, and, as illustrated here, aspects of form. Combinations ("conjunctions") of features do not work well (Treisman, 1986b). Thus, in Figure 4.10*b* the texture segmentation is not clear, even though the left side contains orange diamonds and green squares and the right side contains green diamonds and orange squares.

The principle of **proximity** holds that items near each other are more likely to group together than are items more widely separated. Proximity grouping gives Figure 4.10*a* its horizontally striped appearance. The original descriptions of these Gestalt principles did not involve extensive experimentation. Illustrative demonstrations, like those of Figure 4.10, seemed to make the point. Since that early Gestalt work, careful experiments have confirmed and quantified what the demonstrations illustrated. For example, Kubovy and his colleagues (Kubovy and Cohen, 2001) have quite precisely measured the strength of the proximity effect.

Figure 4.11 illustrates two somewhat weaker grouping principles: **parallelism** and **symmetry**. Most people see the *parallel* pair of contours (2 and 3) as a group and the *symmetrical* pair (7 and 8) as another group.

Have we identified all the grouping rules? Probably not. In recent years, Steve Palmer (1992) added a couple of grouping principles to the classic list. The black dots in **Figure 4.12** are spaced in exactly the same way in all three

texture segmentation Carving an image into regions of common texture properties.

similarity A Gestalt grouping rule stating that the tendency of two features to group together will increase as the similarity between them increases.

proximity A Gestalt grouping rule stating that the tendency of two features to group together will increase as the distance between them decreases.

parallelism A rule for figure–ground assignment stating that parallel contours are likely to belong to the same figure.

symmetry A rule for figure–ground assignment stating that symmetrical regions are more likely to be seen as figure.

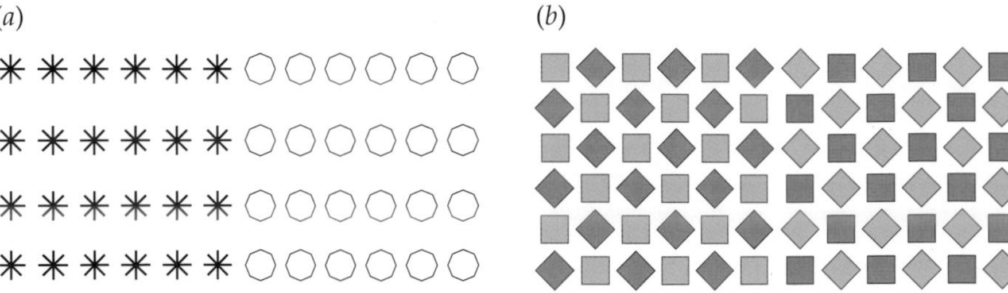

FIGURE 4.10 Similarity and proximity. (*a*) Grouping by similarity and by proximity is useful. (*b*) Grouping by a conjunction of color and form does not work.

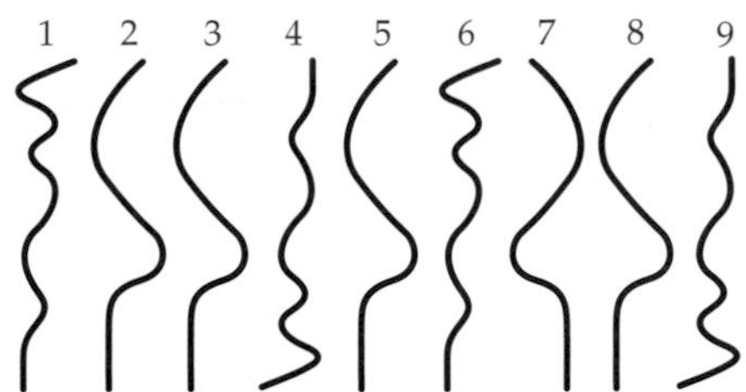

FIGURE 4.11 Parallelism and symmetry. Which pairs of lines go together?

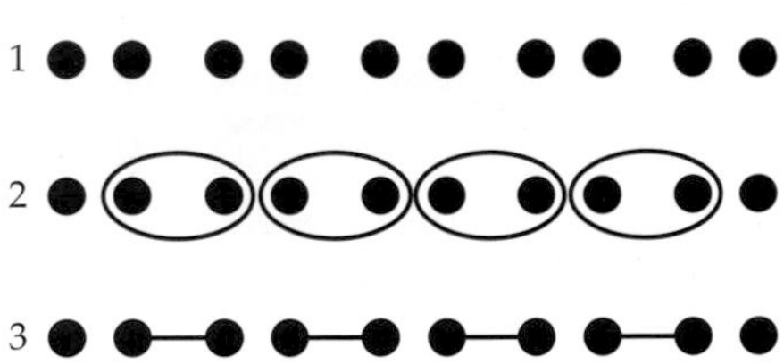

FIGURE 4.12 Proximity grouping (line 1) can be overruled by grouping by common region (line 2) or grouping by connectedness (line 3).

rows. In the first row, they group by proximity into five pairs. In the second row, proximity is overruled by what Palmer called the "principle of **common region**," which states that if two features appear to be part of the same larger region, they will group together. In the third row, the dots are grouped by a similar principle that Palmer dubbed **connectedness**: if two items are connected, then they probably belong together.

Some of the grouping principles are dynamic and thus harder to illustrate on the page. See **Web Activity 4.1: Gestalt Grouping Principles**, for examples of grouping by common fate and synchrony (S.-H. Lee and Blake, 1999).

CAMOUFLAGE The same principles that are normally used to help us find objects in the world can also be exploited to hide them. The art of camouflage is, to a great extent, the art of getting your features to group with the features of the environment so as to persuade an observer that your features do not form a perceptual group of their own. **Figure 4.13** shows some examples from the animal kingdom. The exercise for you is to determine which principles of grouping are at work, hiding the camouflaged animal in each case.

Perceptual Committees Revisited

Now that we've seen some of the problems the visual system has to deal with in parsing an image, let's go back and flesh out the notion of perceptual committees in middle vision. Low-level visual processes deliver fairly straightforward bits of information about a line here and a color there. However, that collection of information needs to be interpreted before we know what we're seeing. Middle vision behaves like a collection of specialists, each with a specific area of expertise and individual opinions about what the input might mean. The goal is to have a single answer emerge out of this diversity of opinions.

common region A Gestalt grouping rule stating that two features will tend to group together if they appear to be part of the same larger region.

connectedness A Gestalt grouping rule stating that two items will tend to group together if they are connected.

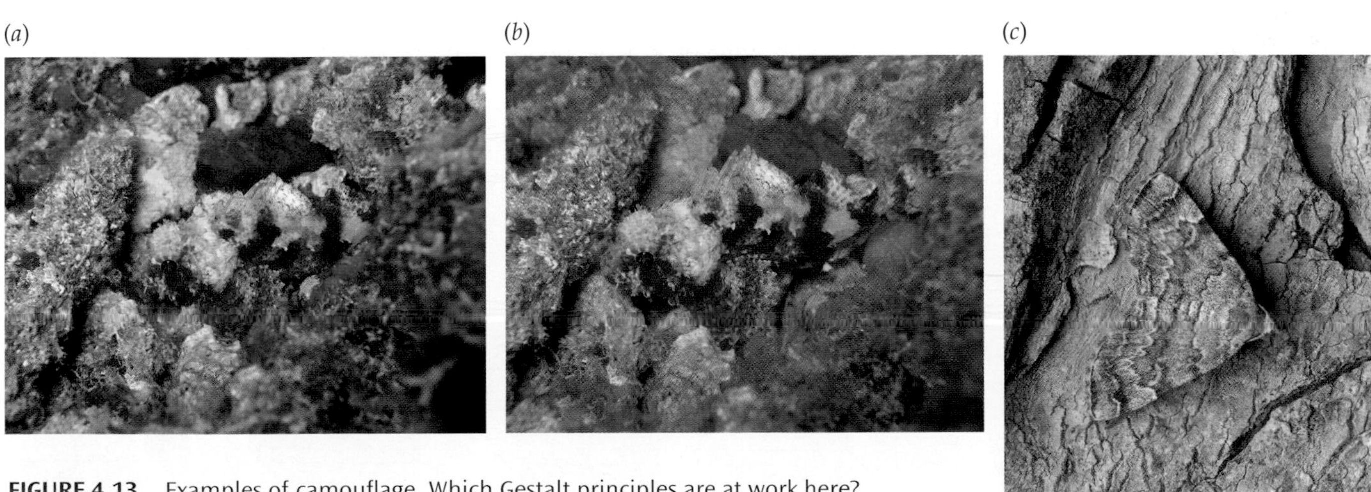

FIGURE 4.13 Examples of camouflage. Which Gestalt principles are at work here?

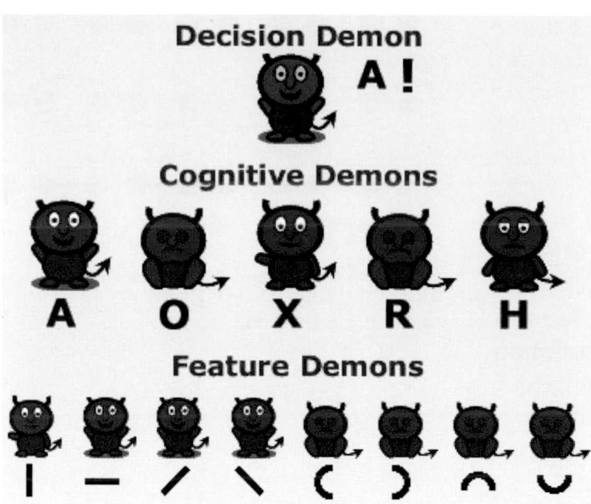

FIGURE 4.14 The Pandemonium model for recognizing an *A*. See **Web Activity 4.2: Pandemonium** to view this in action.

The idea of perception by committee has a long history, though the specific metaphor takes different forms at different times. One early version was Oliver Selfridge's (1959) Pandemonium model for letter recognition (a relatively simple subset of the object recognition problem). Selfridge called his committee members "demons." (Indeed, the word *pandemonium*, which we define as "noise and chaos," was originally John Milton's [1608–1674] word for the abode of all demons in *Paradise Lost*.) Selfridge's theologically neutral feature demons found vertical lines, acute angles, and so forth. Cognitive demons, one for each letter, had ideas about the features of their letters. A cognitive demon looked at the work of the feature demons and made noise proportional to the evidence for its letter. A decision demon listened to the committee of cognitive demons and identified the letter on the basis of the loudest yell. **Figure 4.14** shows a screen shot from **Web Activity 4.2: Pandemonium**. Visit the book's website to experience perception by committee in action.

Of course, no one really thinks that object recognition is accomplished by demons or committees in any literal sense. The physical substrate of a "committee" is probably a massively interconnected set of neurons that takes input and, by virtue of its specific connections, produces an output that can be read as the committee decision by other processes elsewhere (Mozer, 1991). The details of how this might come to pass are beyond the scope of this book. Still, in the next section we can identify some of the working assumptions of these committees.

COMMITTEE RULES: HONOR PHYSICS AND AVOID ACCIDENTS Though we usually come to a single coherent interpretation of the current contents of the sensory world, the decisions made by perceptual committees need not be final. An **ambiguous figure** is one that generates two or more plausible interpretations. For example, **Figure 4.15***a* shows the famous **Necker cube**. Middle-vision committees of the visual system are willing to entertain either of the two solids shown in Figure 4.15*b* and *c* as interpretations of the wire frame pictured in Figure 4.15*a*. However, the system is unwilling to readily consider any of the infinite number of other possible interpretations of the wire image—for example, the flat one in Figure 4.15*d*. **Figure 4.16** shows another classic ambiguous figure, now pressed into the service of commerce.

ambiguous figure A visual stimulus that gives rise to two or more interpretations of its identity or structure.

Necker cube An outline that is perceptually bi-stable. Unlike the situation with most stimuli, two interpretations continually battle for perceptual dominance.

Necker cubes and duck-rabbits are really the exceptions that prove the rule. *Every* image is, in theory, ambiguous, but the perceptual committees almost always agree on a single interpretation. Consider, for example, **Figure**

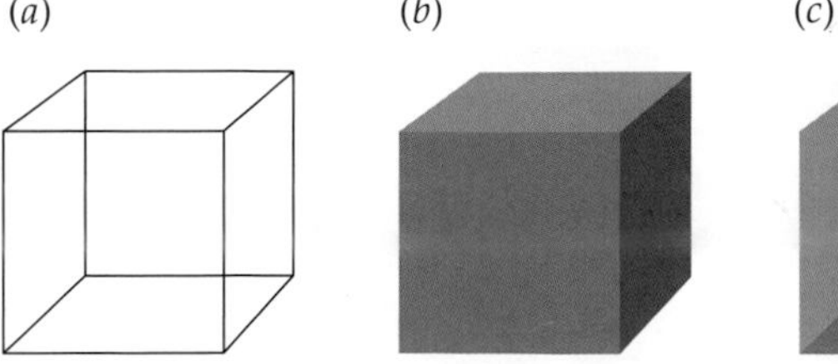

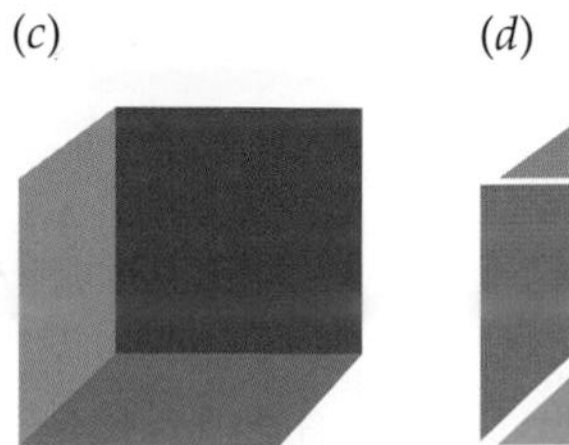

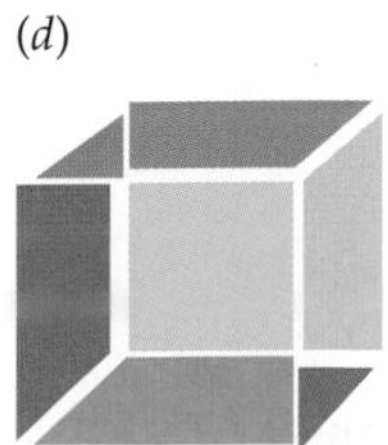

FIGURE 4.15 The wire-frame Necker cube (*a*) can look like either of the solids shown in parts (*b*) or (*c*). It is much less likely to be seen as a collection of flat regions on the page (*d*), even though that is really what it is!

4.17*a*. This pattern might represent the retinal image projected by the scene depicted in Figure 4.17*b*: four surfaces with different shapes, arranged in different orientations, and at different distances. For you to see this as a single shape divided into four square regions, you would have to be viewing the scene from exactly one, very precise location—what object recognition researchers call an **accidental viewpoint**. Any slight shift in viewpoint—say, moving a hair to the left—would destroy the illusion of the four equidistant square regions. (**Web Activity 4.3: Object Ambiguity** illustrates this situation with an animation that makes the relationship between Figure 4.17*a* and *b* clearer.)

The perceptual committees know about accidental viewpoints. More specifically, they know enough not to bet on them. The chances that Figure 4.17*a* is the two-dimensional representation of the three-dimensional scene in Figure 4.17*b* are so slim that the visual system refuses even to consider this possibility. Nor do the perceptual committees care to assume other unlikely accounts of the perceptual input. Thus, unless it has very good reason to do so, the visual system will not conclude that Figure 4.7 represents the meeting, nose to nose, of four snakes.

A second set of assumptions made by the visual system involves an implicit understanding of some aspects of the physics of the world. For example, returning to the Kanizsa figure (see Figure 4.5), we infer the arrow-shaped object, in part, because of our *implicit* understanding that solid objects block light. This understanding of opacity causes us to infer that the lines disappear because something is blocking our view of them. Calling this understanding "implicit" means that we need not be able to verbalize the rule in order to use it. Monkeys seem to see the subjective contours without benefit of instruction in physics (von der Heydt, Peterhans, and Baumgartner, 1984), and we may assume that similar abilities extend far into the animal kingdom. We and our visual systems know this and other physical principles in the same way that a ball "knows" about gravity.

These principles and assumptions may seem so obvious as to be meaningless. But remember that an image has no meaning whatsoever until middle- and high-level visual processes dig into them. One committee uses the knowledge that opaque objects occlude other objects behind them to generate plausible interpretations of image elements like the notched circles and dead-end edges in Figure 4.5. Another committee considers all the possibilities and discards any that involve accidental viewpoints, reducing what is initially a theoretically unsolvable problem (finding the one correct interpretation out of the infinite number of possible ones) to a potentially solvable one. And so we proceed further and further into the visual system, until a single, generally correct interpretation emerges.

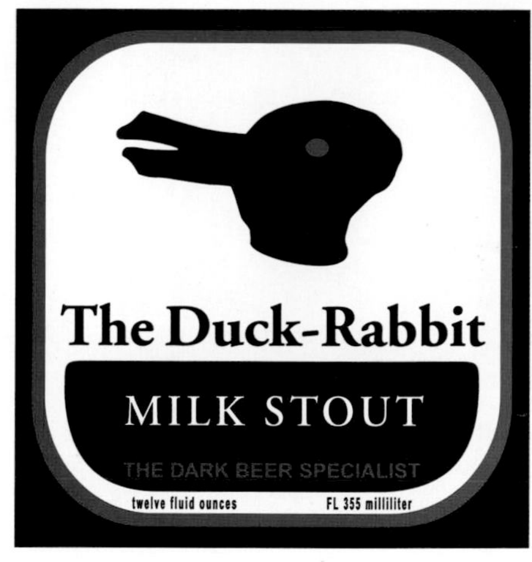

FIGURE 4.16 A classic ambiguous figure gets a new role.

accidental viewpoint A viewing position that produces some regularity in the visual image that is not present in the world (e.g., the sides of two independent objects lining up perfectly).

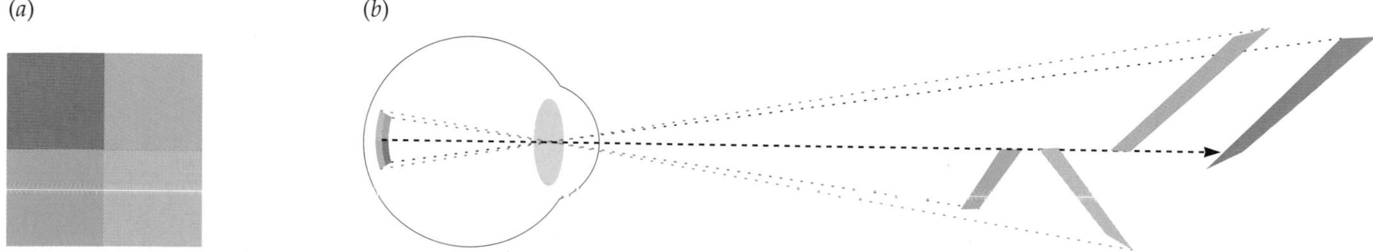

FIGURE 4.17 Accidental viewpoint. (*a*) Why do we see these four squares? (*b*) Maybe the eye just happens to be in the right position to see four arbitrary shapes at arbitrary depths line up to form the pattern. That would be quite a coincidence. That would be an accidental viewpoint.

FIGURE 4.18 What is figure and what is ground?

Figure and Ground

Armed with this understanding of the ground rules of committee deliberation, we can continue with the effort to go from simple features to recognizable objects. The edge- and region-finding mechanisms, discussed earlier, would divide **Figure 4.18** into blue and green regions without much difficulty. But how should those regions be understood? It is extremely likely that we would interpret the illustration as two green figures on a blue background. That is, we would infer that the blue would continue behind the green objects if we could lift them up to check. That need not be the case, however. We could be looking at blue and green puzzle pieces, cut to fit each other perfectly. Or we could be looking at two blue objects, a smaller one on the left and a larger one with a squiggly hole on the right, both sitting on top of a green background.

The ability to distinguish figures (objects in the foreground) from ground (surfaces or objects lying behind the figures) is a critical step on the path from image to object recognition. Like the finding of edges and regions, it is a process governed by a collection of principles acting together, as if in another of these perceptual committees, to decide how the visual world should be understood. As before, the governing goal is to determine the most likely reality behind the image on the retina.

Like the grouping principles, the topic of **figure–ground assignment** became important in visual perception because of the work of the Gestalt psychologists. **Figure 4.19** shows the classic vase/face figure introduced in the 1920s by the Danish psychologist Edgar Rubin (1886–1951). It must be the best-known illustration from the Gestalt school, and it is analogous to the Necker cube, in that it illustrates one of those rare cases in which a perceptual committee has a difficult time reaching consensus. All visual stimuli may be inherently ambiguous, but the processes that determine figure and ground almost always manage to come to a single conclusion, as they do in Figure 4.18. We are surprised when the process fails and delivers two or more interpretations. The surprise we register when the Rubin vase "flips" to a pair of faces reminds us of the perceptual stability that we usually take for granted.

figure–ground assignment The process of determining that some regions of an image belong to a foreground object (figure) and other regions are part of the background (ground).

surroundedness A rule for figure–ground assignment stating that if one region is entirely surrounded by another, it is likely that the surrounded region is the figure.

What principles are at work in the assignment of regions to figure or ground? We can list some of them:

- *Surroundedness.* If one region is entirely surrounded by another, it is likely that the surrounded region is the figure. This **surroundedness** is a factor for the green region on the right in Figure 4.18.
- *Size.* The smaller region is likely to be figure. The cow is smaller than the field in which she stands. These letters that you are reading are smaller than the page.
- *Symmetry.* A symmetrical region is more likely to be seen as figure. How likely is it that the two blue regions in Figure 4.18 just happen to have the symmetrical contours facing each other over what would be the green gap on the left?
- *Parallelism.* Regions with parallel contours are more likely to be seen as figure (thus, purple appears to be figure in **Figure 4.20**?) Again, how likely is it that two contours would be parallel with one another if they did *not* belong to the same object?
- *Extremal edges.* Figure–ground calculations are intended to answer the question "Is region A in front of region B?" In the upper left panel of **Figure 4.21**, the edge of the white disk has shading suggesting that the edge is curving away from the viewer and toward the gray texture. The viewer concludes that it must be closer and must be the figure. In the upper right

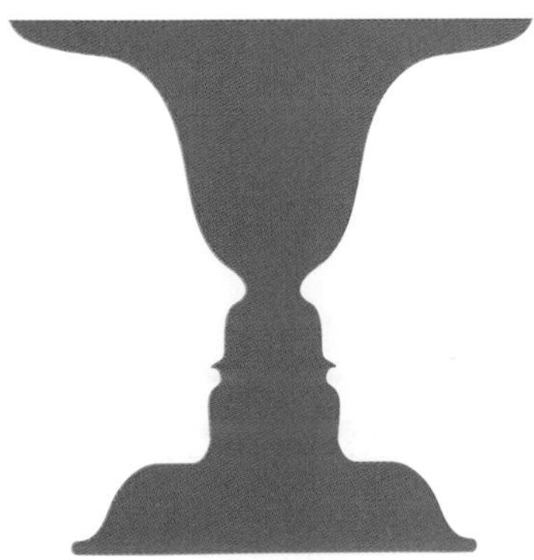

FIGURE 4.19 The Rubin vase/face figure. Do you see a vase or two faces in profile?

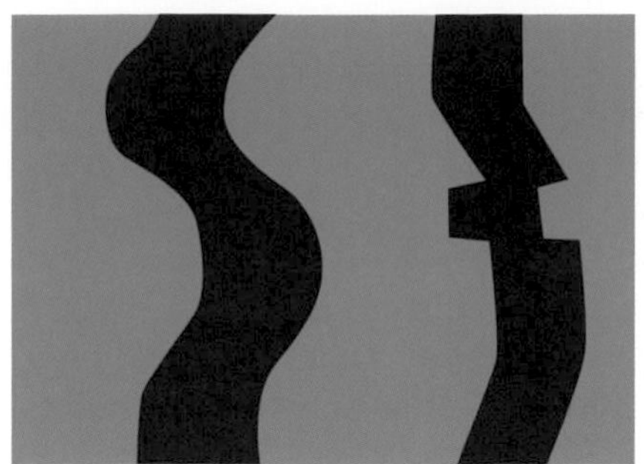

FIGURE 4.20 What is figure here? Parallel contours are often taken to belong to the figure. That is one reason why the purple regions appear to be figure here.

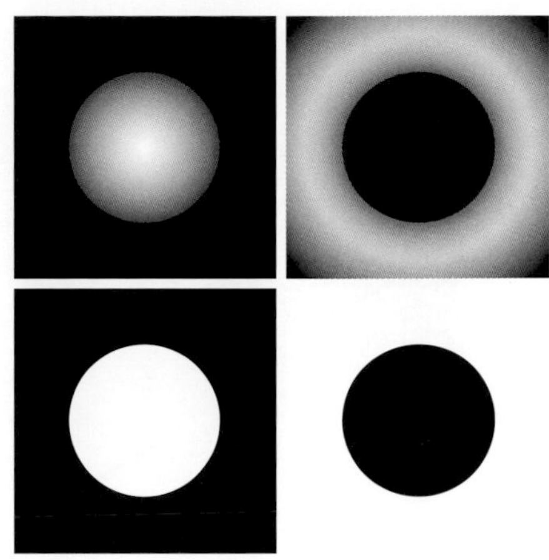

FIGURE 4.21 On the top left, the "extremal edge" cue makes the image look like a sphere on a background. The surrounding region on the top right looks like a doughnut figure and the hole looks like ground. On the bottom, without the edge cue, the figure–ground relations are reversed. (After Palmer and Ghose, 2008.)

panel, the white annulus has this "extremal edge" cue and it becomes the figure. Note that the cue is strong enough to overwhelm cues like surroundedness and size (Palmer and Ghose, 2008), which seem to flip the figure–ground assignment in the bottom panels of the figure.

- *Relative motion.* How surface details move relative to an edge can also determine which portion of a display is the foreground figure and which is the background (Yonas, Craton, and Thompson, 1987). (See **Web Activity 4.1: Gestalt Grouping Principles.**)

A COMPLICATED BUSINESS Although the assignment of figure and ground is governed by rules, it is not a simple process. Consider, for example, **Figure 4.22**. The surroundedness, size, symmetry, and parallelism rules combine to firmly establish the black rectangle as a figure on the blue background. But what about the three circles? These are all smaller than the black rectangle and are completely surrounded by it. Moreover, they are perfectly symmetrical. Yet only the middle circle is perceived as being a separate object (figure); the outer circles are seen as holes in the black rectangle.

You can (and should) speculate about what factors determine whether a circle is seen as a hole or a spot (C. Yin, Kellman, and Shipley, 1997). On the right in Figure 4.22, the answer has something to do with the fact that we interpret those three isolated patches of checkerboard as a vertical rectangle, occluded by the horizontal black rectangle. Apparently, as part of the journey from image to object, we need to understand something about how one object can occlude another. (See **Web Essay 4.1: The Role of Knowledge in Figure–Ground Assignment.**) Indeed, the path to object recognition is not a simple one-way street. Information about object recognition influences figure–ground assignment too (Peterson and Skow, 2008).

FIGURE 4.22 Which circles are figures? Which are holes?

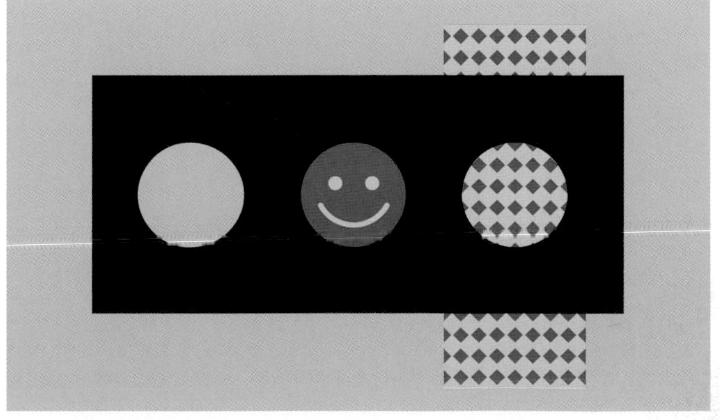

Dealing with Occlusion

Objects are rarely kind enough to present themselves to us in splendid isolation on blank backgrounds. In the real world, objects are often partially hidden by other objects. Indeed, three-dimensional objects often hide parts of themselves. We've already discussed how edge-finding processes can fabricate illusory contours on the basis of the physics of occlusion. We will now need yet another committee to connect the visible pieces of occluded objects by inferring the presence of hidden pieces of the object when necessary.

In their quest to understand the rules governing the completion of occluded objects, Philip Kellman

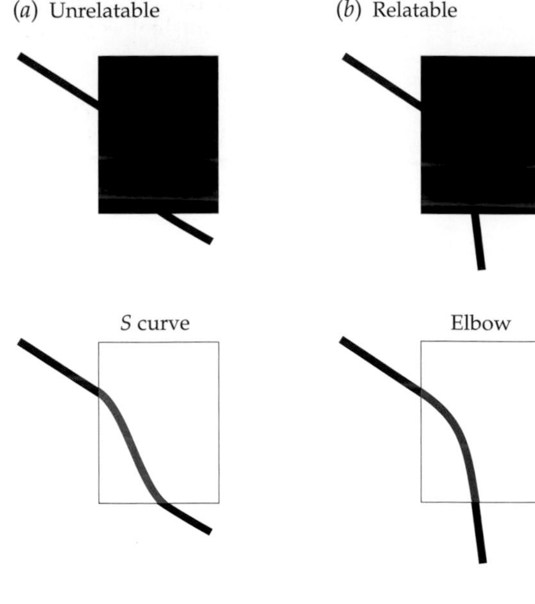

FIGURE 4.23 Two edges are relatable if they can be connected with a smooth, convex or concave curve (*b*), but not if the connection requires an *S* curve (*a*). (After Kellman, 1998.)

and Thomas Shipley (1991) stressed the ways that edges can *relate* across gaps. This concept of **relatability** is illustrated in **Figure 4.23**. Do the two black line segments in each part look like they belong to the same curve, occluded by the black square? In Figure 4.23*a*, the answer is "no." In Figure 4.23*b*, the answer is "yes." Kellman and his colleagues argue that the critical difference is that the lines in Figure 4.23*b* can be related by a simple curve like an elbow or a bend in the road. The lines in Figure 4.23*a* require a more complex *S* curve to make a smooth connection between them. The visual system is unwilling to guess so elaborate a relation, so it concludes that the lines are not actually related at all (that is, they are not parts of the same object). Like the figure–ground rules, this **heuristic** (mental shortcut) is not infallible (after all, some objects really do have *S*-shaped contours). The occlusion committee is apparently willing to accept a few missed completions in order to reduce the vast number of possible completions we would have to consider if we connected every pair of occluded edges. For more on dealing with occlusion, see **Web Essay 4.2: Dynamic Occlusion** and **Web Activity 4.4: Infant Object Perception**.

Additional heuristics emerge when we move from two dimensions to three, as **Figure 4.24** shows. Here we see a pair of box-shaped objects, one partially occluding the other. The overlap of the boxes produces a variety of different line junctions, all of which can be classified as *Y*, *T*, or arrow junctions. *T* junctions almost always occur when one surface occludes another; *Y* and arrow junctions almost always correspond to corners and thus don't signal occlusions. These rules fail to hold true only when we are viewing the scene from an accidental viewpoint. Hence, the various junction types are known as **nonaccidental features** (Lowe, 1985), and they provide another potential tool for use by the perceptual committees charged with dividing the scene into objects and deciding what is occluding what.

relatability The degree to which two line segments appear to be part of the same contour.

heuristic A mental shortcut.

nonaccidental feature A feature of an object that is not dependent on the exact (or accidental) viewing position of the observer.

Parts and Wholes

Glance quickly at **Figure 4.25** and decide whether you see an *H*. Now glance back and look for a *U*. Which of these tasks took longer? Using stimuli like these, David Navon (1977) found that the big letters interfere with the naming of the little letters more than the little letters interfere with recognition of the big letters.

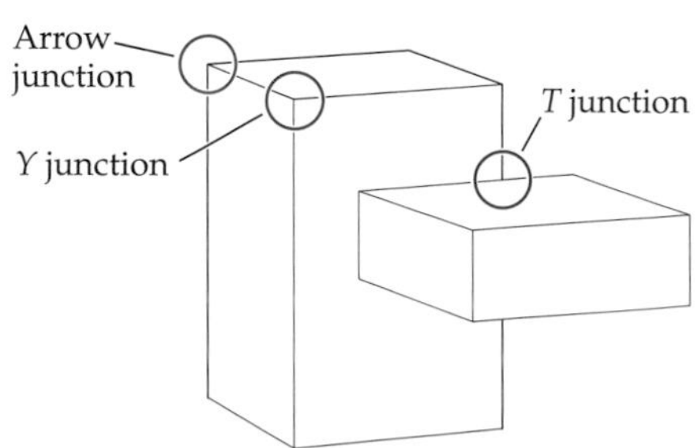

FIGURE 4.24 Different sorts of line junctions have different meanings. *T* junctions indicate occlusion of one region by another. *Y* and arrow junctions indicate corners.

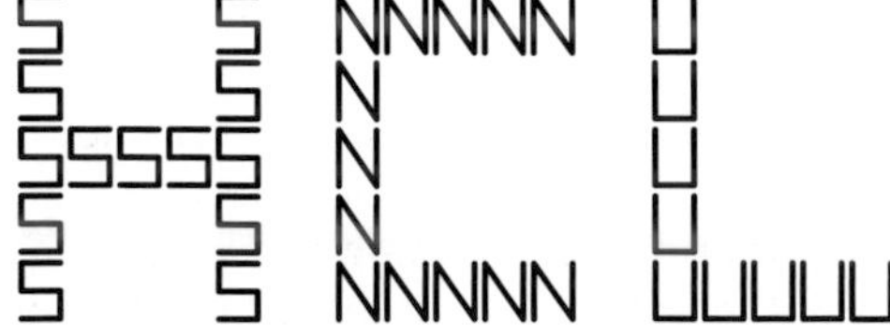

FIGURE 4.25 Global letters composed of local letters. David Navon argued that perceptual processes work from the global to the local.

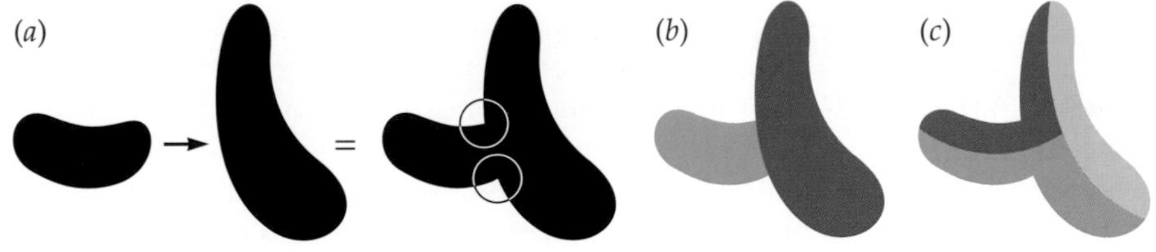

FIGURE 4.26 Finding parts from object boundaries. (*a*) When one blob is pushed into another, a pair of concavities is created. We know this (implicitly, of course), and we work backward from this fact to carve this figure into the two parts shown in (*b*) rather than according to a different scheme, such as the one shown in (*c*).

This **global superiority effect** is consistent with an implicit assumption we've been making throughout our discussion of middle vision: that the first goal is to carve the retinal image into large-scale objects. But as these stimuli also remind us, most objects are composed of parts, and we can recognize these individual parts as well. Indeed, many recognition models (to be discussed shortly) posit that segmenting an object into its constituent parts is a crucial step in deciding what type of object it is.

One heuristic that might be used by perceptual committees when dividing objects into parts is illustrated in **Figure 4.26**. Don Hoffman and Whitman Richards (1984) noted that when one blob is pushed into another, a pair of concavities is created in the silhouette of the resulting two-part object (Figure 4.26*a*). A process that embodied this bit of physics would conclude that valleys, rather than bumps, should be used to mark part boundaries. Thus, we are inclined to parse the object into two parts as shown in Figure 4.26*b*, not into three parts as shown in Figure 4.26*c*.

Summarizing Middle Vision

We have gone from the image and its simple features to objects with parts. It now makes sense to talk about recognizing the object, possibly on the basis of these parts. Before moving on, though, it is worth briefly reviewing how we got here. The goals of the middle-vision processes discussed so far in this chapter might be summarized in five principles:

1. *Bring together that which should be brought together.* We have the Gestalt grouping principles (similarity, proximity, parallelism, symmetry, and so forth), and we have the processes that complete contours and objects even when they are partially hidden behind occluders (e.g., the relatability heuristic).
2. *Split asunder that which should be split asunder.* Complementing the grouping principles are the edge-finding processes that divide regions from each other. Figure–ground mechanisms separate objects from the background.
3. *Use what you know.* Two-dimensional edge configurations are taken to indicate three-dimensional corners or occlusion borders, and objects are divided into parts on the basis of an implicit knowledge of the physics of image formation.
4. *Avoid accidents.* Avoid interpretations that require the assumptions of highly specific, accidental combinations of features or accidental viewpoints.
5. *Seek consensus and avoid ambiguity.* Every image is ambiguous. There are always multiple, even infinite physical situations that could generate a given image. Using the first four principles, the "committees" of middle vision must eliminate all but one of the possibilities, thereby resolving the ambiguity and delivering a single solution to the perceptual problem at hand. This solution serves as the input for processes that will recognize—that is, attach meaningful labels to—the objects that are actually out there in the world. It is to these recognition processes that we turn next.

global superiority effect The finding in various experiments that the properties of the whole object take precedence over the properties of parts of the object.

Object Recognition

In 2005, Quiroga et al. published an amazing result. They recorded from single cells in the temporal lobe of human observers. Normally, we do not put electrodes into the human brain, but these observers were patients being prepared for brain surgery to treat epilepsy. Implanting electrodes was part of the treatment plan and recording visual responses from these cells involved no extra risk to the patient or interference with treatment. In the experiment, the observer just looked at a collection of images while the activity of a cell was monitored. As **Figure 4.27** shows, some of the cells turned out to have very specific tastes. The cell shown in the figure responded to the actress Jennifer Aniston and nothing else presented to the observer. Other cells had preferences for other people. One cell responded to the Sydney Opera House; another, to the Eiffel Tower and the Leaning Tower of Pisa but not to other landmarks (Quiroga et al., 2005).

What is going on here? Could it be that, in listening to the Jennifer Aniston neuron, the researchers were listening in on the act of object recognition? Object recognition is one of the key tasks of visual perception. If the image of Jennifer Aniston falls on your retina, you must be able to take that raw image and generate a description that can be matched to a Jennifer Aniston representation in memory. Of course, if you have no idea who Jennifer Aniston is or what she looks like, you won't recognize her. Even so, you will still recognize her as a woman. How?

This is not a trivial problem and we can quickly dispose of some trivial solutions. You are not matching the "pixels" of the Aniston image with the pixels of an Aniston representation. Figure 4.27 shows that the cell responded to various different images of the actress. Moreover, we know that a detailed,

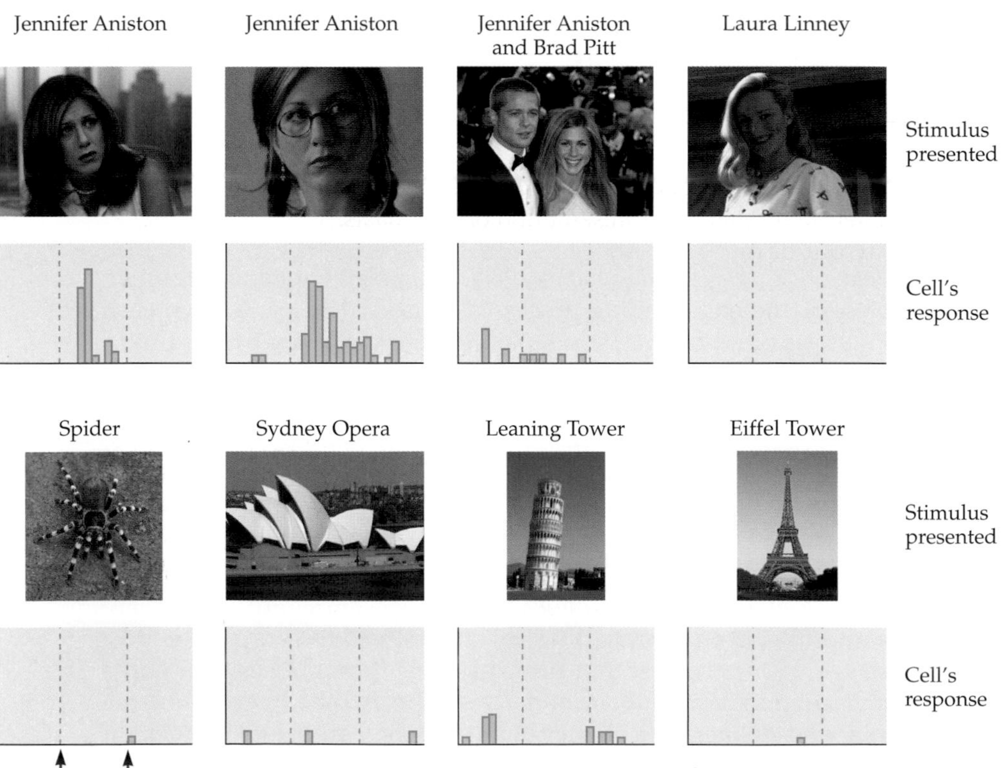

FIGURE 4.27 Results of recording the activity of one cell in the temporal lobe of a human patient. This cell responded to pictures of the actress Jennifer Aniston. The cell did not respond to pictures of anything else, including those of other actresses. (From Quiroga et al., 2005.)

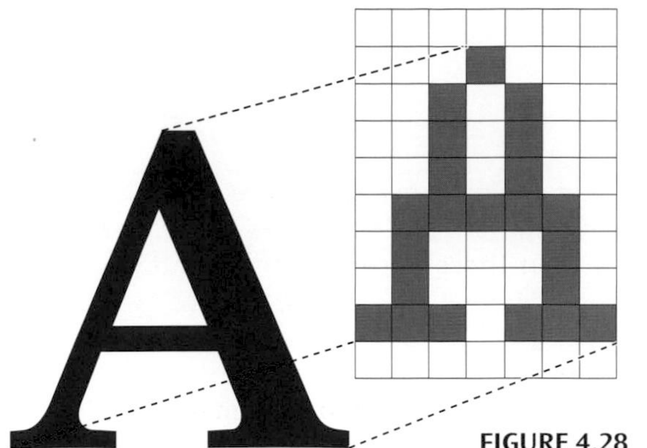

FIGURE 4.28 A basic template.

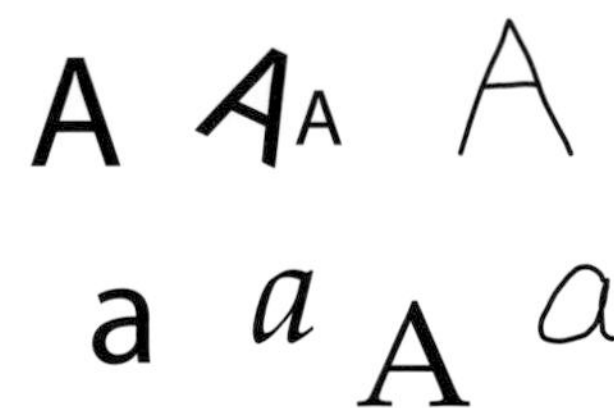

FIGURE 4.29 The problem with templates is that we need a lot of them.

point-by-point representation of objects is not transmitted to the parts of the brain interested in objects. As we've been discussing, the raw image is analyzed by middle-vision processes, and it is the output of those processes that will be available to object recognition processes.

Templates versus Structural Descriptions

The idea that we recognize objects by matching every pixel or even matching every low-level feature of the input to a representation in memory is what might be called **naïve template theory**. It won't even work for simple objects. The basic idea of a template is rather like a lock and key. As we will see in Chapters 13 and 14, locks and keys are quite an apt metaphor in taste and smell where the "key" to be recognized is a molecule like a specific odorant and where that molecular key presents itself in more or less the same shape every time. Figures 4.28 and 4.29 show that recognizable visual objects like the letter *A* are much less well behaved. **Figure 4.28** shows the lock-and-key template idea. A letter *A* stimulus falls on an array of spot detectors. If the *A* falls on the filled detectors and not the empty ones, it is identified as an *A*. Therefore, the array of detectors serves as an *A* template. The difficulty with a naïve template model is that too many templates are required. All of the objects in **Figure 4.29** are *A*s. If we needed a new template for every letter in every position and orientation, we would run out of brain before we ran out of alphabet. And just think about the problem of building a Jennifer Aniston representation on this basis.

One way out of this problem is to notice that all the *A*s—at least all the capital *A*s—share a basic structure. Instead of matching each point in the image to a point in a template, perhaps we perform a more conceptual match. Just about any capital *A* can be described by the relationship of its three lines: the two flanking lines meet, and the third line spans the angle created by those two lines. Now the image of the *A* is being matched to a **structural description** of an *A*, a specification of an object in terms of its parts and the relationships between the parts.

Many versions of structural-description hypotheses have been proposed. A key component of each theory is how object parts are represented in the structural descriptions. Marr and Nishihara (1977) used "generalized cylinders" that could be scaled longer, shorter, fatter, or thinner to represent differently shaped parts. Biederman (1987) proposed a set of **geons** ("geometric ions") (see **Figure 4.30** for examples). Geons are specified as collections of

naïve template theory The proposal that the visual system recognizes objects by matching the neural representation of the image with a stored representation of the same "shape" in the brain.

structural description A description of an object in terms of the nature of its constituent parts and the relationships between those parts.

geons In Biederman's "recognition by components" model, the "geometric ions" out of which perceptual objects are built.

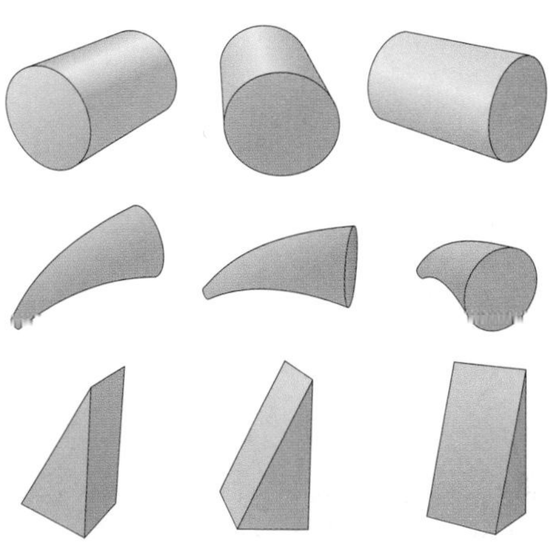

FIGURE 4.30 Three of the 36 or so geons in Biederman's "recognition by components" theory of object recognition. Each geon is shown in three orientations, illustrating the fact that they are easily recognizable from nearly any viewpoint.

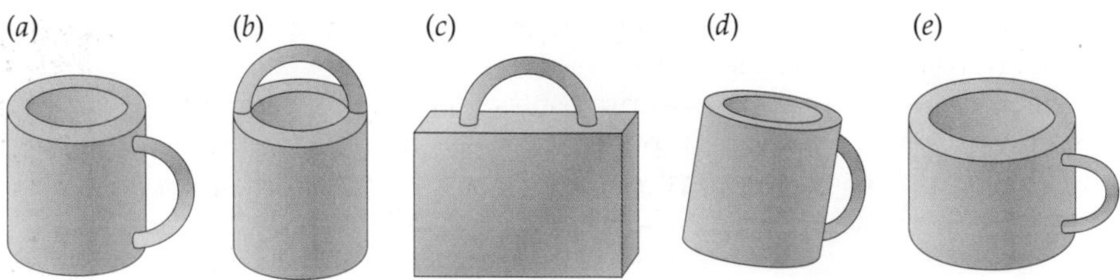

FIGURE 4.31 Combining geons can create a wide variety of object representations. (*a–c*) Three objects "spelled out" by different combinations of the cylinder, noodle, and brick geons. A different view of the coffee mug (*d*) and a different instance of this object class (*e*) would lead to the same structural description.

nonaccidental features (remember Figure 4.17?), so in theory, a visual system should be able to recognize a geon equally accurately and quickly, regardless of how the geon is oriented in space (as long as it's not an accidental view). Geons are featured in Biederman's **"recognition by components" model**, which we'll now describe in a bit more detail.

Just as the finite set of letters in the alphabet can be combined in various ways to produce an infinite number of words, the finite set of geons can be used to construct a very large number of object representations. Attaching a noodle to the side of a cylinder gives us a coffee mug (**Figure 4.31***a*). Moving the noodle to the top of the cylinder produces a pail (Figure 4.31*b*). Changing the cylinder to a brick gives us an attaché case (Figure 4.31*c*).

Because geons and relationships such as "A is beside B" are designed to be equally recognizable from many different vantage points, structural descriptions composed of these geons and relations should also be **viewpoint-invariant**. Minor shape variations also won't alter the structural descriptions of geons. As noted already, this is the great advantage of structural descriptions over templates: if we can recover the same structural description from any picture of the object (e.g., Figure 4.31*a*, *d*, and *e*), then we need to store only one representation of the object in memory.

Problems with Structural-Description Theories

We may have made too much progress. Viewpoint invariance is a good thing, but object recognition is not completely viewpoint-invariant. You were probably able to read that last sentence without turning your book upside down, but even Biederman would say that there is something quite clearly viewpoint-dependent about letter recognition and, more generally, object recognition. There are other problems with structural descriptions as well. For example, it is not clear that geons or any of the other "alphabets" proposed by structural-description models are adequate for the language of object recognition. Would the geon description of a cigar box differ from that of a book?

In response to these questions about structural-description models, researchers such as Michael Tarr, Heinrich Bülthoff, and others have returned to template-like representations that they call "views." Support for view-based representations generally comes from experiments that use novel, rather than familiar, objects. For example, Tarr and Pinker (1990) trained observers to recognize letterlike objects. During training, the objects were always shown in the upright orientation. Then, in a "surprise" phase of the experiment, the observers were asked to recognize rotated versions of the objects. The results revealed a linear relationship between orientation shift and the response time to recognize the object. The more the object was rotated, the longer the observers took to name it. This result suggests that the subjects may have stored a template-like representation of the object during the training phase, and then recognized the objects in the surprise phase by

"recognition by components" model Biederman's model of object recognition, which holds that objects are recognized by the identities and relationships of their component parts.

viewpoint invariance 1. A property of an object that does not change when observer viewpoint changes. 2. A class of theories of object recognition that proposes representations of objects that do not change when viewpoint changes.

mentally rotating the misoriented objects back to the upright views they had stored in memory.

Biederman and his colleagues protest that these types of stimuli aren't well described by geons, but even objects that can be identified on the basis of their "geons" show a dependence on viewpoint (Hayward and Williams, 2000). Gauthier et al. (1998) made novel objects that they named "greebles" out of geonlike parts (**Figure 4.32**). Recognition of these novel objects also appears to have a viewpoint-dependent component (**Web Activity 4.5: Viewpoint Effects** lets you test yourself in a short experiment using such objects). However, view-based models have their own problems, and the debate between structural-description and view-based theorists has been quite lively (Peterson and Rhodes, 2003).

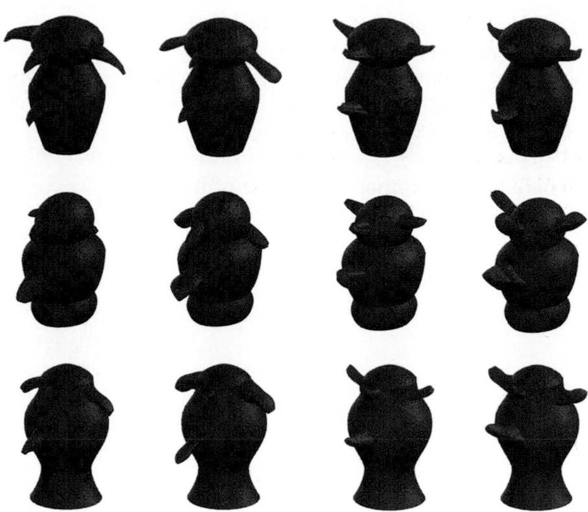

FIGURE 4.32 Recognizing these greebles does not seem to be entirely viewpoint-independent, even if they are made up of geonlike shapes. (From Gauthier et al., 1998.)

Multiple Recognition Committees?

If this chapter has had one theme, it is that no step on the road from image to recognition is taken by a single process acting alone. From the grouping of similar pieces of the image to the segregation of figure and ground, every step has been based on consensus—a committee decision. It seems likely that the act of recognition is similar. Indeed, recognition may not be a single act. We can recognize an object in multiple ways, perhaps simultaneously. As an example, **Figure 4.33***a* and *b* show two birds. In the termi-

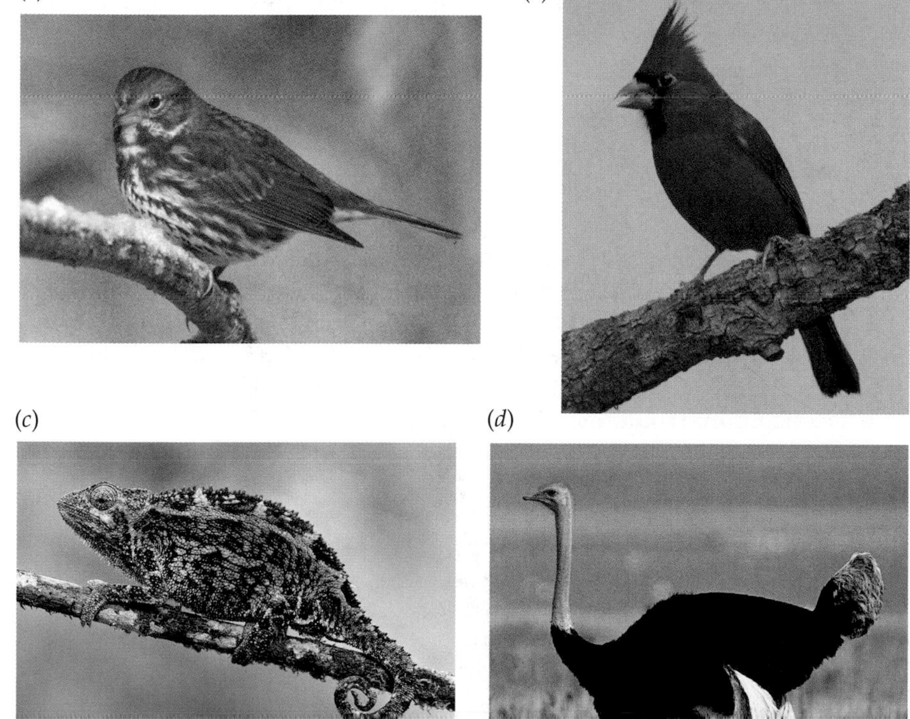

FIGURE 4.33 Two quite different birds (*a* and *b*), a yet more different animal (*c*), and a third "bird" (*d*).

entry-level category For an object, the label that comes to mind most quickly when we identify the object (e.g., *bird*). The object might be more specifically named; that's the "subordinate level" (e.g., *eagle*). The object might be more generally named; that's the "superordinate level" (e.g., *animal*).

nology of Pierre Jolicoeur and his colleagues (Jolicoeur, Gluck, and Kosslyn, 1984), "bird" is the **entry-level category** for these objects—the first word that comes to mind when we are asked to name them. But these objects are also quite clearly different. At a subordinate level—a more specific level beneath the entry level—Figure 4.33*a* shows a fox sparrow and Figure 4.33*b* shows a cardinal. At a superordinate level—a broader level above the entry level—these two objects, as well as the one in Figure 4.33*c*, are all animals.

We can imagine that each of these acts of recognition ("fox sparrow," "bird," "animal") might rely on different stored representations and different analyses of the visual stimulus. And we can imagine a geon account of "bird," but a geon description of "fox sparrow" would be harder to envision. Subordinate-level recognition seems better suited to a system in which the precise details of a particular view of the object are encoded. Recognizing Figure 4.33*a*, *b*, and *c* as animals seems like quite a different act.

Indeed, a number of studies have shown that it takes considerably longer to recognize objects at the subordinate or superordinate levels than at the entry level. Even more impressively, studies looking at brain recordings provide strong evidence that different parts of the brain are more active when people are engaged in subordinate-level recognition than when they are recognizing objects at the entry level (Palmeri and Gauthier, 2004). There are several more interesting twists. For example, when shown an atypical member of a category, such as the bird in Figure 4.33*d*, people are faster to name the object at a more subordinate level ("ostrich"). And when people become experts at recognizing a certain class of objects, subordinate-level recognition becomes as fast or faster than entry-level recognition (or, looked at another way, we might say that the entry level shifts down one level when one becomes an expert). (By the way, bird-watchers and dog show judges seem to be the most extensively studied such experts [Tanaka and Taylor, 1991].) All these results point to the conclusion that the visual system is employing several different object recognition committees, each working with their own sets of tools, at the same time.

Faces: An Illustrative Special Case

Faces are an interesting special case of object recognition. Take, for example, the images in **Figure 4.34**. You should have little difficulty recognizing these as faces, but you will probably have some difficulty quickly identifying the one that has been modified. If you turn the faces right side up, however, one of the pictures will look quite strikingly wrong (Thompson, 1980).

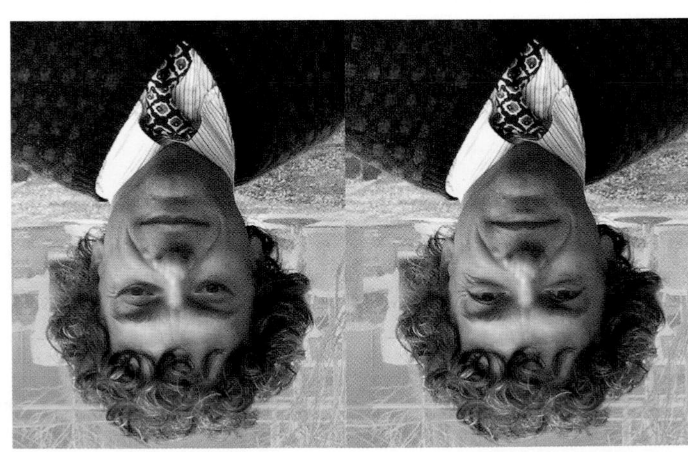

FIGURE 4.34 Which of these two photos has been altered? As you will see, both faces look fine upside down but one of them looks quite strikingly "wrong" when turned right way up. (After Thompson, 1980.)

This is another demonstration of the point made in the previous section—that different levels of categorization often seem to be subserved by different committees using different types of information. The processes that recognize a face as a face care little about inversion, and they don't seem to be disturbed by distortion of the face. The processes that recognize the face as belonging to a specific individual (in this case, one of the authors of this book) work poorly on inverted faces and are very concerned with the precise configuration of eyes, nose, and mouth. (See **Web Activity 4.6: The Face Inversion Effect**.)

Neuropsychology provides further evidence that the processes can be separated. Damage to specific areas in the temporal lobe of the brain can produce **prosopagnosia**, a disorder in which the patient can no longer identify faces. (See **Web Essay 4.3: Face Blindness**.) Though she may be able to recognize an object as a face, she will not know who the person might be. This is not to say that the two levels of face recognition are subserved by completely different systems (Gauthier, Behrmann, and Tarr, 1999). A neuropsychological mark of truly separate brain modules is **double dissociation**. Two functions, such as hearing and sight, are doubly dissociable if one can be damaged without harm to the other and vice versa. Thus, you can be blind and still hear or you can be deaf and still see. In face recognition, it is possible to lose the subordinate ability to recognize specific faces while retaining the ability to recognize an object as a face. It is not clear that the reverse even makes sense. How could you recognize a face as your mother without recognizing it as a face?

Further support for the notion that the two aspects of face recognition are linked comes from electrophysiological studies of the response properties of neurons in the temporal cortex of monkeys. Many of these cells have been shown to respond best to faces (Perrett, Rolls, and Caan, 1982; Perrett et al., 1984). Some seem more viewpoint-invariant than others (Perrett et al., 1992), and, most interestingly for the present point, evidence suggests that some of these neurons first signal that an object is a face (and not a hand or a house), and then later signal exactly whose face it is (Sugase et al., 1999).

Objects in the Brain

Cells that respond to faces? As you may have noticed, we've slipped back now from theoretical debates over how the visual system might go about recognizing objects to physiological studies of actual visual systems. Let's back up a bit and see how we get to these face cells.

Recall that cells in primary visual cortex (also called "striate cortex" because under a microscope it appears striped) are interested in the basic features of the visual image (see Chapter 3), responding to edges or lines of specific orientation, motion, size, and so forth. These neurons have relatively small and precise receptive fields. That is, a cell will respond to its preferred stimulus only if that stimulus is presented in a very specific location relative to the point where the observer (monkey, cat, human) is fixating gaze. Some of these striate cortex cells are involved in middle-vision processes such as grouping (Sugita, 1999) and texture segmentation (Nothdurft and Li, 1984). Other middle-vision tasks, such as the completion of illusory contours (Peterhans et al., 1986; von der Heydt, Peterhans, and Baumgartner, 1984), are handled in **extrastriate cortex**, a set of visual areas so called because they lie just outside the primary visual cortex.

From the extrastriate regions of the occipital lobe of the brain, visual information moves out along two main pathways (**Figure 4.35**). One pathway heads up into the parietal lobe. Visual areas in this pathway seem to be important in processing information relating to the location of objects in

prosopagnosia An inability to recognize faces.

double dissociation The phenomenon in which one of two functions, such as hearing and sight, can be damaged without harm to the other, and vice versa.

extrastriate cortex The region of cortex bordering the primary visual cortex and containing multiple areas involved in visual processing.

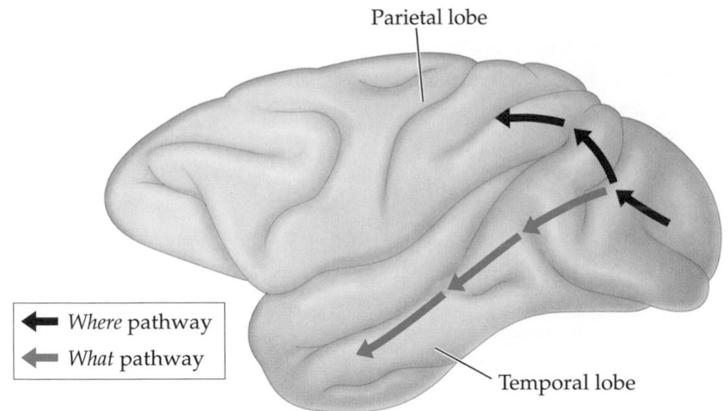

FIGURE 4.35 Visual cortical processing can be divided into two broad streams of processing. One, headed for the parietal lobe, can be thought of as being interested in *where* things are. The other, heading down into the temporal lobe, is concerned with *what* things are. This is a drawing of macaque monkey brain, but these pathways appear to exist in humans too.

space and the actions required to interact with them (moving the hands, the eyes, and so on). This pathway is sometimes known as the *where* pathway. As we will see in Chapter 8, it plays an important role in the deployment of attention. The other pathway, heading down into the temporal lobe, is known as the *what* pathway. This pathway appears to be the locus for the explicit acts of object recognition that we have been discussing in this chapter, though one should not become too addicted to this *what* and *where* distinction. Some basic object information is represented in both pathways (Konen and Kastner, 2008). Early evidence for a relationship between the temporal lobe and object recognition came from studies in which large sections of the temporal lobe were destroyed (**lesioned**) in monkeys. When Klüver and Bucy (1938, 1939) did this, they found that their monkeys behaved as though they did not know what they were seeing. This deficit, also seen in some human stroke victims, is known as **agnosia**, though Klüver and Bucy called it "psychic blindness."

Later work pointed to one part of the temporal lobe, the **inferotemporal (IT) cortex**, as particularly important in the visual problems of these monkeys. In the 1970s, Charlie Gross and his colleagues began to record the activity of single cells in this area. What they found was quite striking. Neurons in striate cortex are activated by simple stimuli and respond only if their preferred stimuli are presented in very restricted portions of the visual field (e.g., a cell might respond to a vertically oriented line between 3 and 4 degrees of visual angle northeast of the fovea). In contrast, cells in IT cortex were discovered to have receptive fields that could spread over half or more of the monkey's field of view. Even more striking were the sorts of stimuli that activated IT cells. The usual spots and lines didn't work well at all, but the silhouette of a monkey hand worked fantastically for some cells. Monkey faces excited other cells (**Figure 4.36**). There was even a cell with a distinct preference for a toilet brush shape (Gross, Rocha-Miranda, and Bender, 1972).

Findings like this led Horace Barlow (1972) and others to suggest a hierarchical model of visual perception (Pandemonium was a very early hierarchical model) in which the small receptive fields and simple features of visual cortex are combined with ever-greater complexity as one moves from striate cortex to IT cortex, eventually culminating in a cell that might fire when you see your grandmother or your *Sensation & Perception* textbook. Indeed, the term *grandmother cell*, coined by Jerry Lettvin, has entered the jargon of the field to stand for any cell that seems to be selectively responsive to one specific object (Barlow, 1995).

lesion In neuropsychology: 1. (n) A region of damaged brain. 2. (v) To destroy a section of the brain.

agnosia A failure to recognize objects in spite of the ability to see them. Agnosia is typically due to brain damage.

inferotemporal (IT) cortex Part of the cerebral cortex in the lower portion of the temporal lobe, important in object recognition.

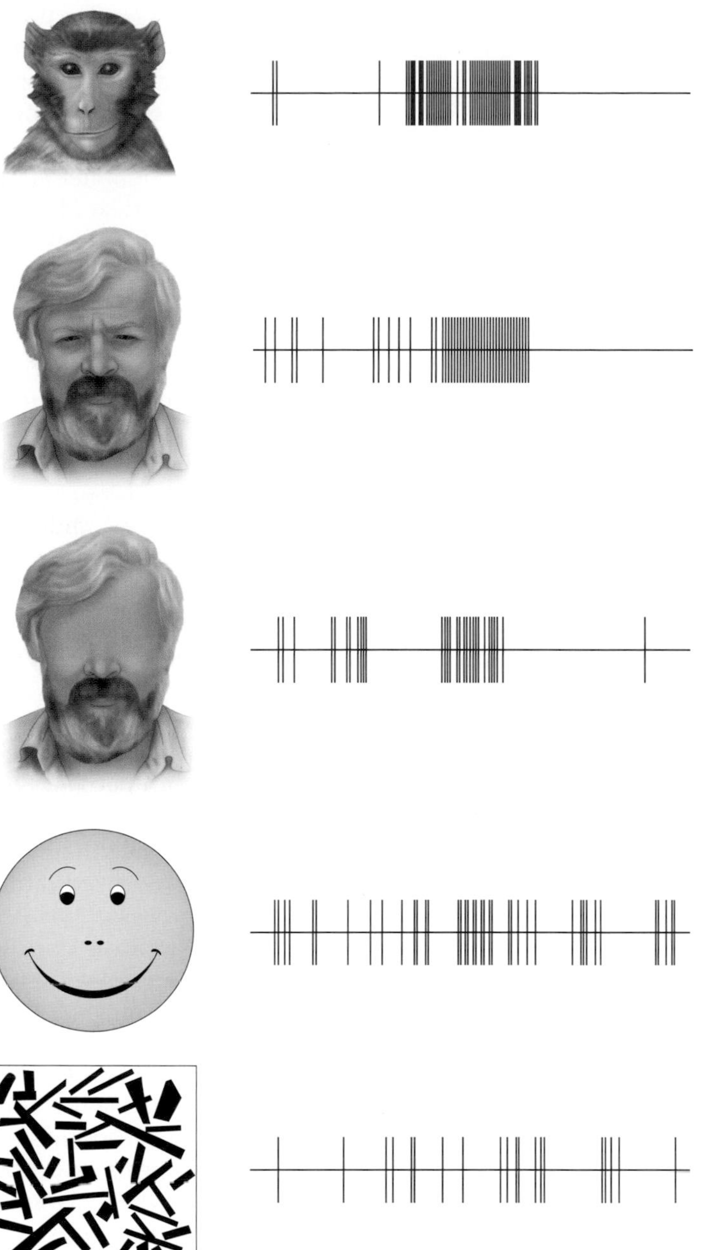

FIGURE 4.36 Cells in the inferotemporal cortex of macaque monkeys are interested in very specific stimuli. In this case, the cell responds vigorously to a monkey face and to some other stimuli that seem related. (After Gross, Rocha-Miranda, and Bender, 1972.)

We do not know what brain activity actually corresponds to your recognition of your grandmother. It is probably a bit extreme to imagine that this is the work of a single neuron in the IT cortex, and later work has cast doubt on the idea that IT cells respond to an object independent of its position in the visual field (DiCarlo and Maunsell, 2003). Nevertheless, it does seem clear that cells in that neighborhood are critically involved in object recognition. The IT cortex maintains close connections with parts of the brain involved with memory formation (notably the hippocampus). This is important because those IT cells need to *learn* their receptive-field properties. The receptive-field properties of primary visual cortex could be written into the genetic code in some manner, but neurons that respond to grandmothers clearly cannot be hardwired, since everyone's grandmother is different. Nikos Logothetis and his coworkers demonstrated that cells in IT cortex have precisely this type of plasticity (Logothetis, Pauls, and Poggio, 1995). After training monkeys to recognize novel objects, these researchers found IT neurons that responded with high firing rates to these objects, but only when the objects were seen from viewpoints similar to those from which they had been learned.

This brings us back to the Quiroga et al. (2005) discovery of Jennifer Aniston and Sydney Opera House responses in human visual cortex. Human cortex has areas that appear to be the equivalent of monkey IT cortex (the anatomy of human and macaque monkey brains is not identical, so we talk about **homologous regions**). However, we do not have a lot of systematic data on the responses of single cells in the human visual system. What we do have is evidence from brain lesions caused by strokes or other accidents. Like Klüver and Bucy's monkeys, humans with lesions in the temporal lobe often show symptoms of agnosia, the ability to see without the ability to know what we're seeing. Sometimes these agnosias can be quite specific. Prosopagnosia, the aforementioned inability to recognize faces, is one example. There are other interesting subdivisions of agnosia, such as the ability to recognize animate objects (e.g., animals) but not inanimate objects (e.g., tools) (Newcombe and de Haan, 1994). Studies using noninvasive imaging methods like functional magnetic resonance imaging (fMRI) also appear to support the idea of areas in the human brain that are more important for processing things like faces (Kanwisher, McDermott, and Chun, 1997) and places (Epstein and Kanwisher, 1998).

Should all this be taken as clear evidence for something like a grandmother cell model, with one piece of brain holding the "face cells" and others, perhaps, holding "tool cells"? It may not be that simple. Martha Farah (1992), for example, argues that effects appearing to be caused by differences between types of stimuli may reflect *how* an object is being recognized rather than *what* specific object it is. For example, faces must be processed holistically; that is, the precise relationship of eyes to nose to mouth is critical. Other objects may be quite successfully recognized by their collection of parts (e.g., keyboard + mouse + screen + box = computer, regardless of whether the mouse is 2 inches to the left or 10 inches to the right of the keyboard). It might also be unwise to think of specific cells in this part of the brain as being the neural substrate that recognizes grandma. Those cells might be more of a link between visual processes and stored memories (Quiroga et al., 2008). In our present state of understanding, it seems safe to say that our ability to recognize objects is critically dependent on brain structures in the temporal lobe. Exactly what those structures are doing remains a topic of active research.

Whatever those cells are doing, they are doing it very fast. Electrical activity from the brain can be recorded from electrodes placed on the scalp. If we flash a picture to an observer and ask if it contains an animal, we can record a signal in the observer that reliably differentiates animal from nonanimal scenes within 150 milliseconds from the onset of the stimulus (Thorpe, Fize, and Marlot, 1996). That is fast enough to mean that there cannot be a lot of feedback from higher visual or memory processes, suggesting that it must be possible to do some rough object recognition on the basis of the first wave of activity as it moves from retina to striate cortex to extrastriate cortex and beyond. That **feed-forward process** must be able to generate an "animal" signal from a wide range of animals in different positions, sizes, and so on.

Recently, computational neuroscientists used rules learned from studies of the properties of single cells to build models of the visual system that can perform a version of this task (DiCarlo and Cox, 2007; Serre, Oliva, and Poggio, 2007). Jack Gallant and his colleagues took similar ideas and used

homologous regions Brain regions that appear to have the same function in different species.

feed-forward process A process that carries out a computation (e.g., object recognition) one neural step after another, without need for feedback from a later stage to an earlier stage.

them to analyze human brain activity as recorded by fMRI. First, they showed the observer 1750 scenes and used the resulting fMRI output to train their model. In effect, they told the model, "This is what a house looks like, this is what a beach looks like," and so forth. Then they showed the observers 120 new scenes and asked the model to figure out which brain signal matched which new image. The model wasn't perfect but it did very well (72–92% correct) (Kay et al., 2008). We always knew there had to be a signal in the brain that corresponded to what was being seen. What is exciting about this new work is that we're getting to the point where we can read that signal.

Before we leave this topic, it is worth mentioning one very large part of the story that we've omitted up to now. There is good evidence that *attention* to an object is critical in recognition of that object. For example, a specialized piece of brain might be responsible for our ability to recognize a specific face. If so, that piece of brain probably requires a single face as its input—two eyes, a nose, and a mouth. If we're looking at a family photo, selective attention processes must come into play, lest we deliver a collection of a brother's eyes, sister's nose, and uncle's mouth to the face processor. Many of the brain structures critical for the deployment of attention seem to lie in the other main path coming out of the primary visual cortex, the one that goes toward the parietal lobe. This pathway, and the general topic of attention, is taken up in Chapter 8.

Summarizing Object Recognition

Object recognition remains an interesting puzzle for vision scientists, for much the same reason that a sporting match is interesting to watch. In a sport, we may know all the rules and we may be familiar with the capabilities of all of the players, but the actual game is an interaction of those rules and those players. The interaction is sufficiently complex and there are a sufficient number of unknown variables (e.g., did the pitcher sleep well last night?) that the result is not predictable. Similarly, we understand a good number of the basic principles in object recognition. We know what problems need to be solved. We also have experimental and physiological evidence for the existence of a number of "players" working on these problems. And we know the rules for simple situations in which, for example, the only relevant information is occlusion. However, the game is very complex. We want to understand how all these cues and clues interact to give rise to what appears to be a remarkably stable, coherent view of the world.

Summary

1. After early visual processes have extracted basic features from the visual input, it is the job of middle vision to organize these features into the regions, surfaces, and objects that can, in turn, serve as input to object recognition and scene-understanding processes.
2. Perceptual "committees" serve as an important metaphor in this chapter. The idea is that many semi-independent processes are working on the input at the same time. Different processes may come to different conclusions about the presence of an edge or the relationship between two elements in the input. Under most circumstances, we see the single conclusion that the committees settle on.
3. Multiple processes seek to carve the input into regions and to define the edges of those regions, and many rules are involved in this parsing of the image. For example, image elements are likely to group together if they are similar in color or shape, if they are near each other, or if they are connected

Refer to the
Sensation and Perception
website
(www.sinauer.com/wolfe2e)
for activities, essays, study questions, and other study aids

to each other. Many of these grouping principles were first articulated by members of the Gestalt school.

4. Other, related processes seek to determine if a region is part of a foreground figure (like this black *O*) or part of the background (like the white area around the *O*). These rules of grouping and figure–ground assignment are driven by an implicit understanding of the physics of the world. Thus, events that are very unlikely to happen by chance (e.g., two contours parallel to each other) are taken to have meaning. (Those parallel contours are likely to be part of the same figure.)
5. The processes that divide visual input into objects and background have to deal with many complexities. Among these are occlusion—the fact that parts of objects may be hidden behind other objects, and the fact that objects themselves have a structure. Is your nose an object or a part of a larger whole? What about glasses or hair or a wig?
6. Template models of object recognition hold that an object in the world is recognized when its image fits a particular representation in the brain in the way that a key fits a lock. It has always been hard to see how naïve template models could work, because of the astronomical number of templates required: we might need one "lock" for every object in every orientation in every position in the visual field.
7. Structural models propose that objects are recognized by the relationship of parts. Thus, an *H* could be defined as two parallel lines with a perpendicular line joining them between their centers. A cat would be more difficult, but similar in principle. In their pure form, such models are viewpoint-independent. The orientation of the *H* doesn't matter. Object recognition, however, is often viewpoint-dependent, suggesting that the correct model lies between the extremes of naïve template matching and pure structural description.
8. Faces are an interesting special case in which viewpoint is very important. Upright faces are much easier to recognize than inverted faces. Moreover, some regions of the brain seem to be specifically interested in faces. They lie near other regions in the temporal lobes that are important for recognition of other sorts of objects.
9. Recent physiological work showed very specific responses to very specific objects (e.g., the actress Jennifer Aniston) in the human temporal lobe. Other work showed that the first, rough acts of object recognition take place so fast that they must be accomplished by the first, feed-forward sweep of activity from the retina to the higher processing centers of the visual system.

CHAPTER 5

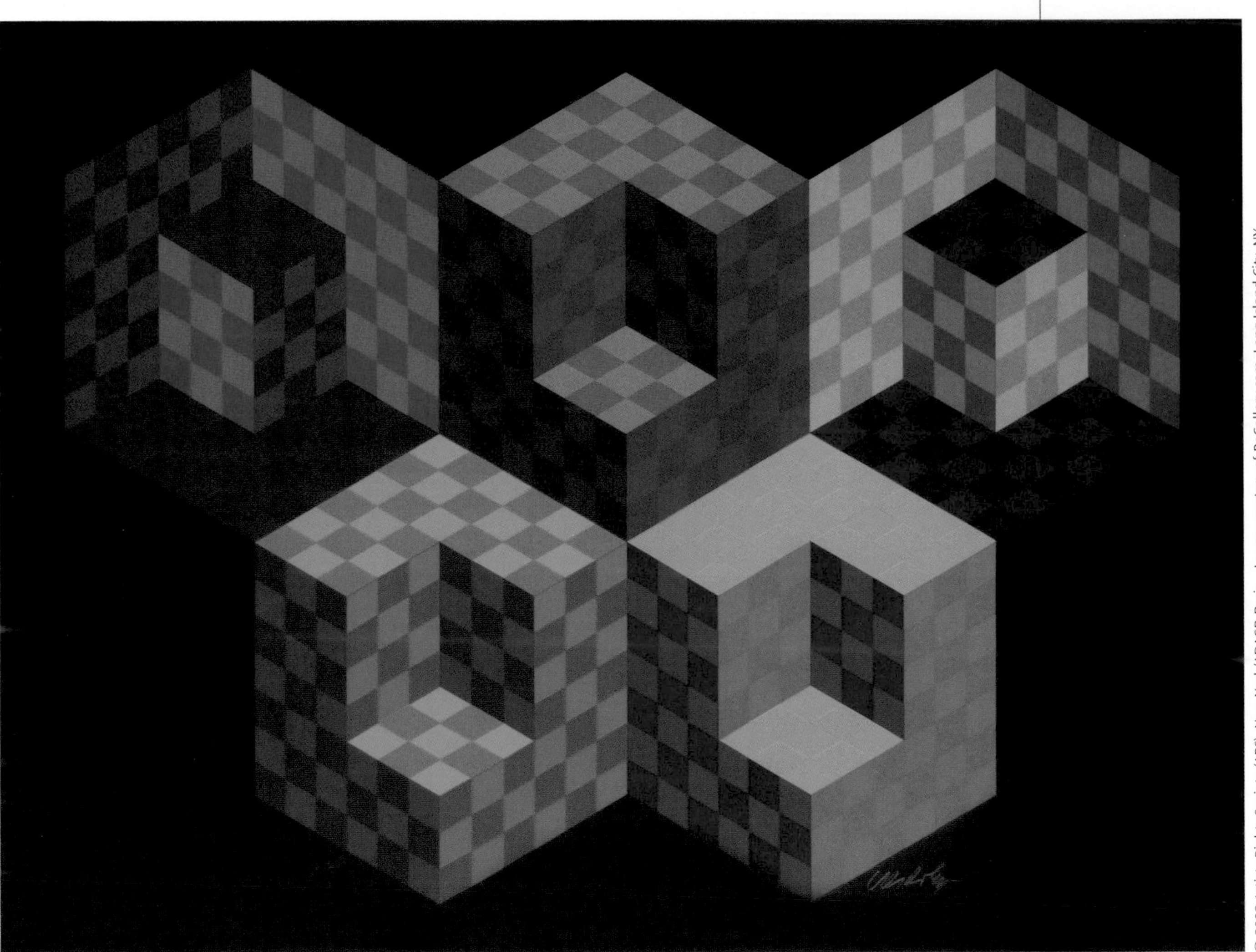

Victor Vasarely, *Hexa 5*, 1988

The Perception of Color

As you may recall from high school English class, there is a lot of blood in Shakespeare's *Macbeth*. If you didn't read *Macbeth*, take our word for it. The first words out of the lips of King Duncan of Scotland are, "What bloody man is that." Not long after, he is murdered offstage by Macbeth. When Macbeth reenters, he is so covered in blood that he concludes he would stain the ocean red if he tried to wash it off—an exaggeration, of course, but it makes sense because we know and we can see onstage that blood is red. As we will learn in this chapter, however, blood is *not* red. As strange as it may seem, color is not a physical property of things in the world; rather, it is a creation of the mind. Blood looks red because we look at it with our particular visual systems.

Basic Principles of Color Perception

Although color itself is not a physical property of things in the world, it is related to a physical property. As discussed in Chapter 2, humans see a narrow range of the electromagnetic spectrum between the wavelengths of about 400 and 700 nanometers (nm). The apparent color of a bit of the world is correlated with the wavelengths of the light rays reaching the eye from that bit of the world.

Most of the light that we see is reflected light. Typical light sources, like the sun or a lightbulb, emit a broad spectrum of wavelengths that hit surfaces in the world around us. Some wavelengths are absorbed by the surfaces they hit. The more light that is absorbed, the darker the surface will appear. Other wavelengths are reflected, and some of that reflected light reaches the eyes. The color of a surface depends on the mix of wavelengths that reach the eye from the surface (and, as we will see later, from the other surfaces and lights that are present). In the case of blood, more of the longer-wavelength light (>600 nm) is reflected into the eyes of the observer. Even though (almost) all humans would declare this collection of wavelengths to appear red, it would be a big mistake to think of specific wavelengths of light as being specific colors. As Steven Shevell (2003) puts it, "There is no red in a 700 nm light, just as there is no pain in the hooves of a kicking horse." Like pain, color is the result of the interaction of a physical stimulus with a particular nervous system.

The Problem of Univariance

To understand the interaction between the physics of the external world and the properties of the nervous system, let's examine the response of a single photoreceptor to a single wavelength of light. **Figure 5.1** shows how one kind of human photoreceptor responds to light of a specific wavelength

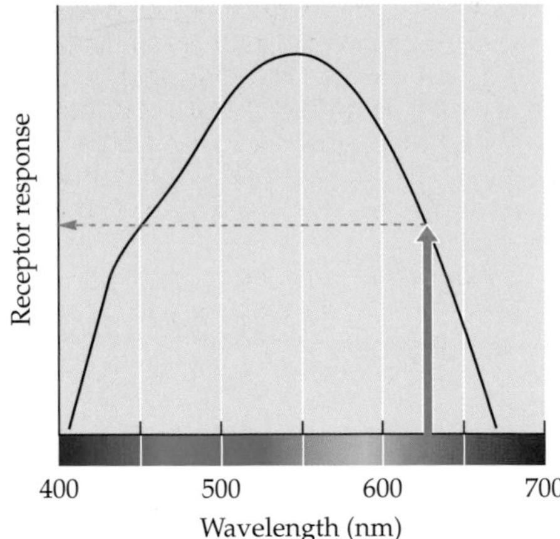

FIGURE 5.1 A single photoreceptor shows different responses to lights of different wavelengths but the same intensity. A 625-nm light of this intensity, indicated by the arrow, produces a response midway between the maximum and minimum responses.

while the intensity of the light is held constant. Because of the properties of the photopigment in the photoreceptor cell, 400-nm light produces only a small response in each cell of this type, 500-nm light produces a greater response, and 550-nm light even more. However, 600-nm light produces less than the maximal response, and 650-nm light produces a minimal response. Light of 625 nm produces a response of moderate strength.

So far, so good. We know that different wavelengths of light give rise to different experiences of color, and the varying responses of this photoreceptor to different wavelengths could provide a basis for color vision. But there is a problem, as illustrated in **Figure 5.2**. Suppose we change the wavelength to 450 nm. Figure 5.2 shows that an equal amount of 450-nm light will produce the same response from this photoreceptor that 625-nm light does. If we were looking at the output of the photoreceptor, we would have no way of distinguishing between the two lights. But when we look with a normal human color vision system, the 625-nm light looks orange and the 450-nm light looks violet.

Actually, the problem is even worse. Remember that Figures 5.1 and 5.2 represent the photoreceptor's response rate when all wavelengths are presented at the same intensity. Under these conditions, the graphs indicate that light at either 450 or 625 nm produces a response lower than the peak response obtained at about 535 nm. If we had a 535-nm light, we could reduce its intensity until it produced exactly the same level of response from our photoreceptor. Indeed, we could take a "white light" or any mix of wavelengths and, by properly adjusting the intensity, get exactly the same response out of the photoreceptor.

Thus, when it comes to seeing color, the output of a single photoreceptor is completely ambiguous. An infinite set of different wavelength–intensity combinations can elicit exactly the same response, so the output of a single photoreceptor cannot by itself tell us anything about the wavelengths stimulating it. This constraint is known as the **problem of univariance** (Rushton, 1972). (See **Web Activity 5.1: The Problem of Univariance.**) Obviously the human visual system has solved the problem, but not under all circumstances. Univariance explains the lack of color in dimly lit scenes, as we will see next.

problem of univariance The fact that an infinite set of different wavelength–intensity combinations can elicit exactly the same response from a single type of photoreceptor. One photoreceptor type cannot make color discriminations based on wavelength.

scotopic Light intensities that are bright enough to stimulate the rod receptors but too dim to stimulate the cone receptors. Compare *scotopic* and *mesopic*.

Trichromacy

Rods and Cones

As we learned in Chapter 2, the human retina contains two kinds of photoreceptors: rods and cones. Rods are sensitive to low (**scotopic**) light levels. All rods contain the same type of photopigment molecule: rhodopsin. Thus, they all have the same sensitivity to wavelength. As a consequence, although it is possible to tell light from dark under scotopic conditions, the problem of uni-

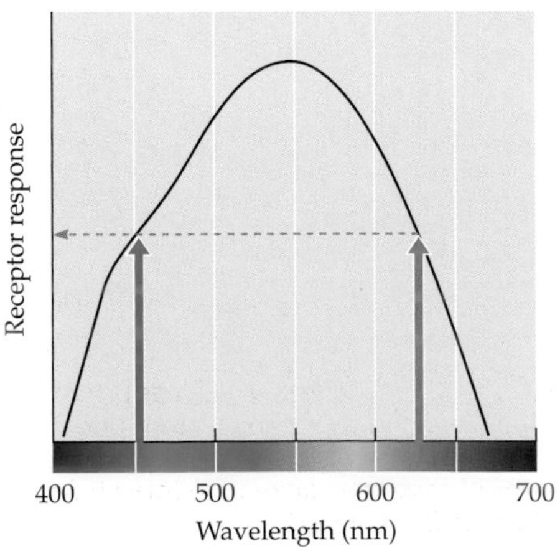

FIGURE 5.2 Lights of 450 and 625 nm each elicit the same response from the photoreceptor whose responses are shown here and in Figure 5.1. This is an illustration of the problem of univariance.

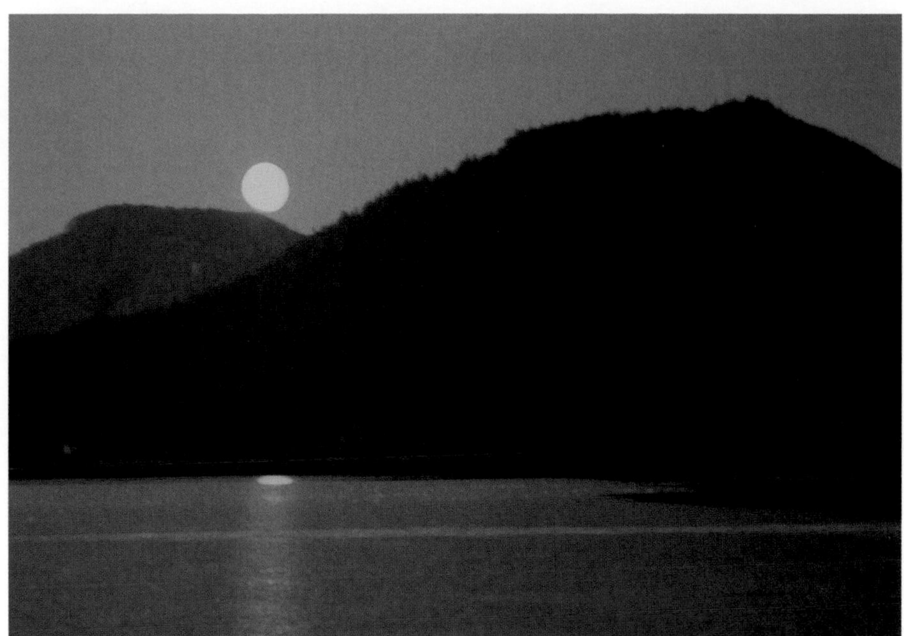

FIGURE 5.3 The moonlit world appears to be drained of color because we have only one type of rod photoreceptor transducing light under these scotopic conditions. With just one type of photoreceptor, we cannot make discriminations based on wavelength, so we cannot see color.

variance makes it impossible to discriminate colors. This is one hint that color is psychophysical and not physical. The world seen under a bright moon (**Figure 5.3**) has not been physically drained of color. The same mix of wavelengths that produces color perception during the day remains present on that moonlit night, but we fail to see colors under dim illuminants like moonlight because dim light stimulates only the rods, and the output of that single variety of photoreceptor does not permit color vision.

Cone photoreceptors are sensitive to higher, daylight light levels (**photopic**). Cones come in three varieties, each containing a slightly different photopigment. These different pigments give each type of cone a distinctive wavelength sensitivity, as shown in **Figure 5.4**.

The three cone types are named for where the peak of their sensitivity lies on the spectrum. Thus, the cones that have a peak at about 440 nm are known as short-wavelength cones (or **S-cones** for short). The middle-wavelength cones (**M-cones**) peak at about 535 nm, and long-wavelength cones

photopic Light intensities that are bright enough to stimulate the cone receptors and bright enough to "saturate" the rod receptors (i.e., drive them to their maximum responses). Compare *scotopic* and *mesopic*.

S-cone A cone that is preferentially sensitive to short wavelengths; colloquially (but not entirely accurately) known as a "blue cone."

M-cone A cone that is preferentially sensitive to middle wavelengths; colloquially (but not entirely accurately) known as a "green cone."

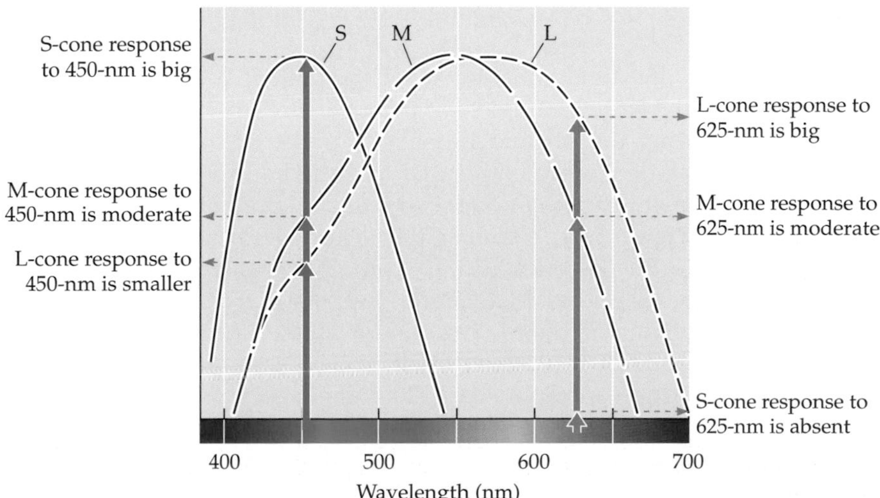

FIGURE 5.4 The two wavelengths that produce the same response from one type of cone (M), produce different patterns of responses across the three types of cones (S, M, and L).

(**L-cones**) peak at about 565 nm. You may be tempted to rename these "blue," "green," and "red" cones, but what you've learned so far should warn you that this is a bad idea. We do perceive long-wavelength light to be red. But if you had only L-cones, you would not see the world in shades of red. Rather, the problem of univariance would ensure that you would see a colorless (gray) world like the world that you see under moonlight, when just your rod photoreceptors are active. The L-cones are simply more sensitive to long wavelengths than the other cones are. So, it's *S-*, *M-*, and *L-*cones—not *blue*, *green*, and *red* cones.

The crucial message of Figure 5.4 is that, with three cone types, we can tell the difference between lights of different wavelengths. Look at the responses to the two wavelengths that produced the same response from the single cone in Figure 5.2. The two wavelengths of light—450 and 625 nm—still produce the same response from that type of cone, now revealed to be the M-cone. However, these two wavelengths produce different outputs from the L-cones and S-cones. In fact, as you will see if you try **Web Activity 5.2: Trichromacy**, any wavelength from about 420 to 660 nm produces a unique set of three responses from the three cone types. This combined signal can be used as the basis for color vision. (We can see from about 400 to 700 nm, but the very long and very short wavelengths stimulate only one type of cone.)

In our discussion of the univariance problem, we noted that we can make any wavelength look like any other by adjusting the intensity of the light. That doesn't happen in the three-cone world of human color vision. A specific light produces a specific set of responses from the three cone types. Suppose that the light produces twice as much M response as S response and twice as much S response as L response. If we increase the intensity of the light, the response sizes will change but the relationships will not. There will still be twice as much M response as S response, and twice as much S response as L response, and those relationships will define the color. The idea that the color of any light is defined in our visual system by the relationships among three numbers is the heart of **trichromacy** or, more elaborately, the **trichromatic theory of color vision**.

Metamers

The examples presented thus far involve the responses of the visual system to single wavelengths. Most of the time, however, we do not see pure wavelengths. As **Figure 5.5** shows, we usually see mixtures (here, reflected from a hamburger). How do our cones respond to such combinations of light wavelengths?

To answer this question, consider what happens if we mix two wavelengths. For the sake of the example, we will oversimplify by ignoring the S-cones and redrawing the M- and L-cones to make the numbers simpler. Imagine that we shine a wavelength that looks red and a wavelength that looks green onto a white piece of paper so that a mixture of both is reflected back to the eyes (**Figure 5.6*a***). Suppose the "green" light alone produces 80 units of activity in the M-cones and 40 in the L-cones (remember, we are ignoring the S-cones for now). In addition, suppose that the "red" light produces 40 units of activity in the M-cones and 80 in the L-cones. If we assume that we can add the cone responses together, then summing the "red" and "green" lights produces a response of 120 units in each cone. The absolute value is not important, because it could change if the intensity of the light changes. What is important is that this red plus this green produce a mixture that excites the L- and M-cones equally.

L-cone A cone that is preferentially sensitive to long wavelengths; colloquially (but not entirely accurately) known as a "red cone."

trichromatic theory of color vision (or trichromacy) The theory that the color of any light is defined in our visual system by the relationships of three numbers, the outputs of three receptor types now known to be the three cones. Also known as the *Young–Helmholtz theory*.

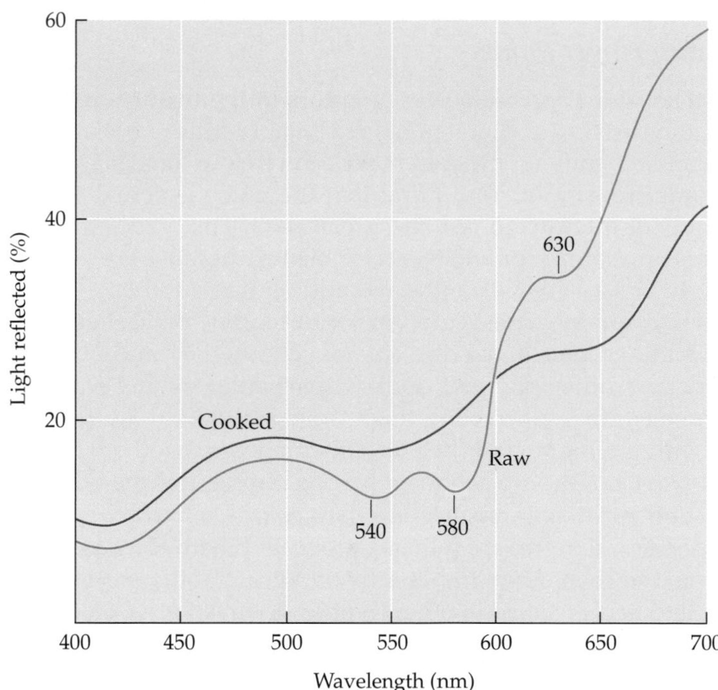

FIGURE 5.5 Objects in the real world reflect light across the spectrum in different amounts. This graph plots the reflectances of raw and cooked hamburger meat. Which one looks redder? Which one reflects more of the long wavelengths?

The key point is that the rest of the nervous system knows *only* what the cones tell it. If the mixture of "red" plus "green" lights produces the same cone output as the single wavelength of "yellow" light (Figure 5.6*b*), then the mixture and the single wavelength *must look identical*. Mixtures of different wavelengths that look identical are called **metamers**. The single wavelength that produces equal M- and L-cone activity will look yellow, and the "red" and "green" lights will mix to produce "yellow."

metamers Different mixtures of wavelengths that look identical. More generally, any pair of stimuli that are perceived as identical in spite of physical differences.

Two quick warnings:

1. Mixing wavelengths does *not* change the physical wavelengths. If we mix 500- and 600-nm lights, the physical stimulus contains 500 and 600 nm. It does not contain the average (550 nm). It does not contain the sum (1100 nm) (which we would not be able see anyway). Color mixture is a mental event, not a change in the physics of light.
2. For the mixture of a "red" light and a "green" light to look *perfectly* yellow, we would have to have just the right red and just the right green. Other mixes might look a bit reddish or a bit greenish.

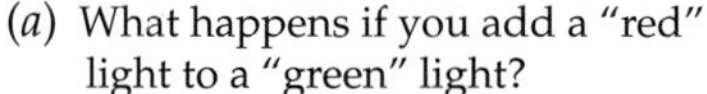
(*a*) What happens if you add a "red" light to a "green" light?

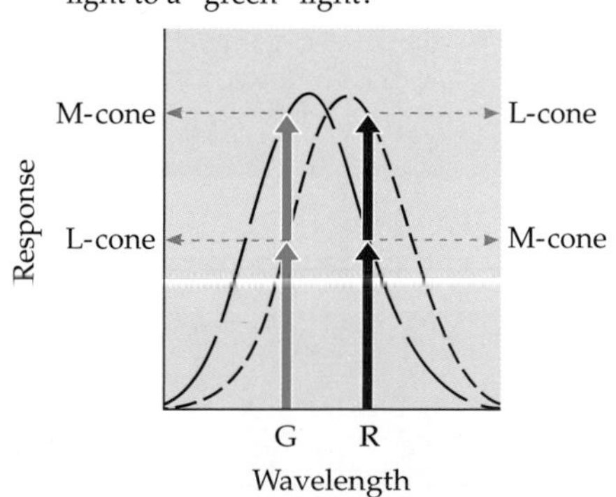

(*b*) "Yellow" produces equal L- and M-cone responses.

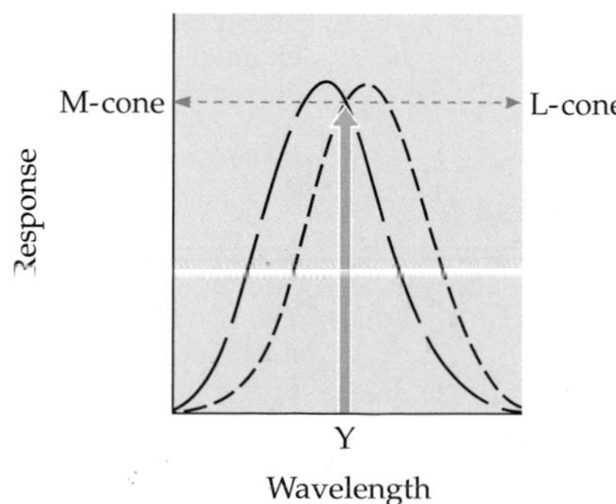

FIGURE 5.6 The long-wavelength ("red") and shorter-wavelength ("green") lights in part (*a*), if mixed together, produce the same response from the cones as the medium-wavelength ("yellow") light in part (*b*). If two sets of lights produce the same responses, they are metamers and must look identical.

Lights, Filters, and Finger Paints

The ubiquity of televisions and computer monitors in the twenty-first century may make color mixing and metamers reasonably intuitive. If you've never done so, find a magnifying glass and take a very close look at a yellow patch on your computer screen. You'll find that the patch is actually composed of thousands of intermixed red and green dots. The "red + green = yellow" formula is an example of **additive color mixture** because we are taking one wavelength or set of wavelengths and adding it to another.

For most of us, color mixture begins in kindergarten or earlier, with paints. In that world, red plus green don't make yellow; they make brown. A finger paint, or any other pigment, looks a particular color because it absorbs some wavelengths, subtracting them from white light falling on a surface covered with the pigment. When a toddler smears together red and green, almost all wavelengths are absorbed by one pigment or the other, so we perceive the **subtractive color mixture** as a dark color like brown.

Actually, finger paint mixtures are rather complicated, with some pigment particles sitting next to each other and effectively adding, others occluding each other, and still others engaged in other complex interactions. Colored filters, such as those you might put over stage lights, are a cleaner example of subtractive color mixture. As **Figure 5.7** shows, a subtractive mixture of blue and yellow produces green because the only wavelengths passing through both our "yellow" and "blue" filters fall into a middling range that appears green. All the other wavelengths have been subtracted out of the original white light. An additive mixture of blue and yellow lights looks white (**Figure 5.8**) because it includes a mix of wavelengths that stimulate the three cones roughly equally. (See **Web Activity 5.3: Color Mixing.**)

additive color mixture A mixture of lights. If light A and light B are both reflected from a surface to the eye, in the perception of color the effects of those two lights add together.

subtractive color mixture A mixture of pigments. If pigments A and B mix, some of the light shining on the surface will be subtracted by A, and some by B. Only the remainder contributes to the perception of color.

1. Take "white" light that contains a broad mixture of wavelengths.
2. Pass it through a filter that absorbs shorter wavelengths. The result will look yellowish.
3. Pass that through a bluish filter that absorbs all but a middle range of wavelengths.
4. The wavelengths that make it through both filters will be a mix that looks greenish.

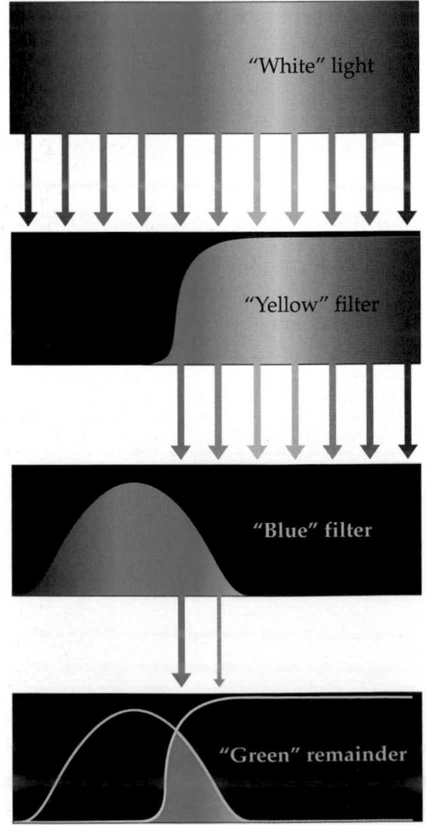

FIGURE 5.7 In this example of subtractive color mixture, "white"—broadband—light is passed through two filters. The first one absorbs shorter wavelengths, passing on a mix of wavelengths that looks yellow. The second absorbs longer wavelengths and the shortest wavelengths, passing on a mix that looks blue. The wavelengths that can pass through both filters without being subtracted are a middle range of wavelengths that appear green.

Additive color mixture with paints is possible. Georges Seurat (1859–1891) and other Postimpressionist artists of the late nineteenth century experimented with Pointillism, a style of painting that involved creating many hues by placing small spots of just a few colors in different textures (**Figure 5.9**). Viewing the painting in Figure 5.9 up close, we see each individual dot of color. Like the red, green, and blue phosphor dots on a computer monitor, the dots in the painting combine additively to produce a wide range of colors. Thus, from a distance, the man's face is appropriately skin colored even if, up close, it is composed of spots of color that would not be found on any normal face.

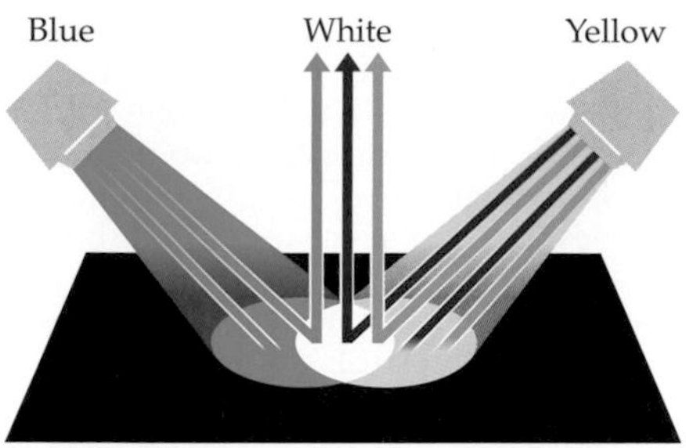

FIGURE 5.8 If we shine "blue" and "yellow" lights on the same patch of paper, the wavelengths will add, producing an additive color mixture. Remember that "yellow" is equivalent to a mix of a long wavelength and a medium wavelength, so blue plus yellow results in a mix of short, medium, and long wavelengths. The mixture looks white (or gray, if it is not the brightest patch in view).

Three Numbers, Many Colors

To summarize briefly, color vision is based on the output of three types of cone photoreceptors. Rods make a small, important contribution, but only in fairly dim light (Stabell and Stabell, 2002). Because we have exactly three different types of cone photoreceptors, the light reaching any part of the retina will be translated into three responses, one for each local population of cones. After that translation, the rest of the nervous system cannot glean anything more about the physical wavelengths of the light. If the light rays reflecting off two surfaces produce the same set of cone responses, the two surfaces must and will appear to be exactly the same color. They will be metamers, even if their physical characteristics are quite different. Thus, it is possible to produce blood-red color on the page without mimicking the physical properties of blood.

Three doesn't sound like very many, but it has been estimated that, with this system, we can discriminate more than 10 million different colors (Judd and Kelly, 1939). (We don't have this many distinctive color *names*, but we may be able to tell two colors apart even if we call them both "pea green.") Where do all these colors come from? Certainly there do not seem to be millions of discriminable colors on the spectrum from blue through green and yellow to red.

We can describe each of the colors in a rainbow with just a single number (the light wavelength), so the visible light spectrum defines a single color

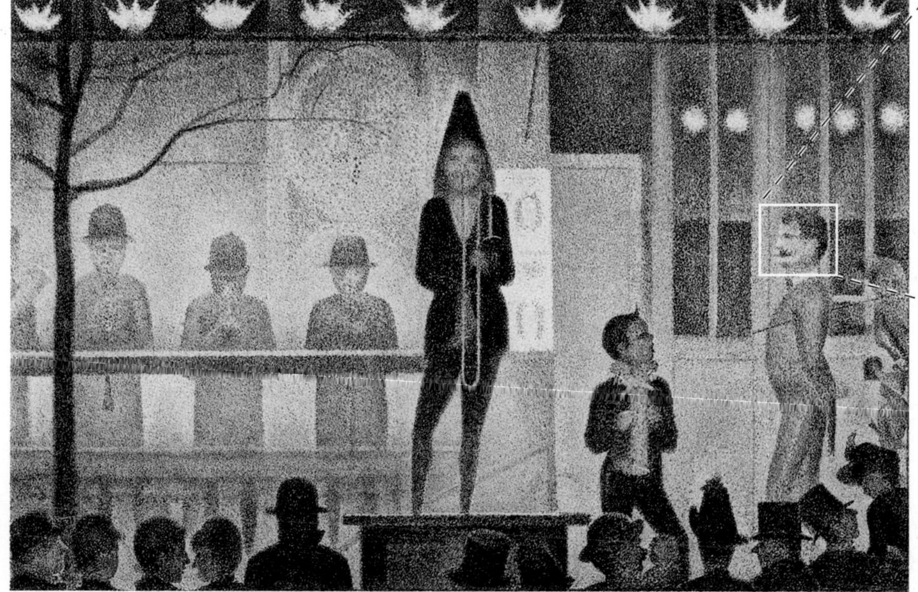

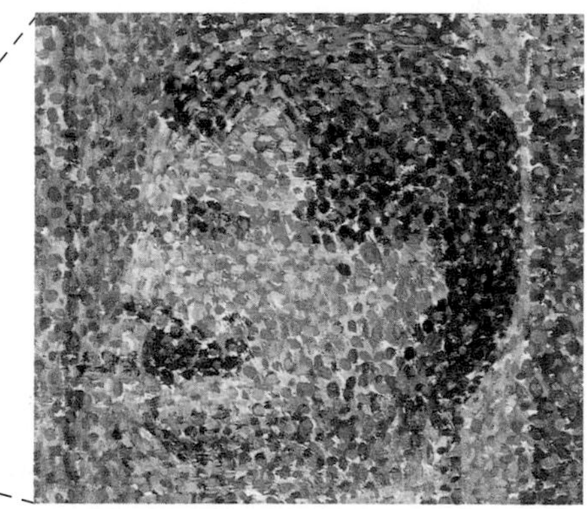

FIGURE 5.9 Georges Seurat's painting *La Parade* (1887–1888) illustrates the effect of additive color mixture with paints. Seurat used additive color mixture in the manner of a modern computer monitor. Small spots of color blend at a distance to give rise to other colors.

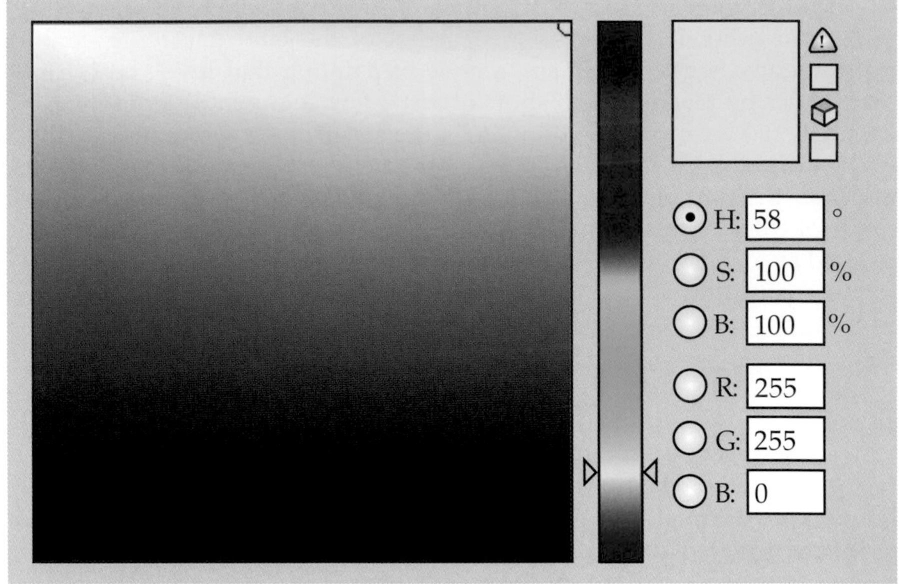

FIGURE 5.10 A color picker may offer several ways to specify a color in a three-dimensional color space. This one, found in Adobe Photoshop, offers two options on the far right. The first (upper) option defines the color space in terms of hue (H), saturation (S), and brightness (B). The second (lower) option uses the parameters red (R), green (G), and blue (B). See the text for details.

dimension. But with the three numbers we have available to us (the outputs of the three cone types), we should be able to define three dimensions; think of the height, length, and width of a cube. The range of our experience of color can be described by reference to a three-dimensional **color space**. It is worth exploring this space a little.

We can't talk about height, length, and width in color space; we need other terms. There are lots of possibilities. For example, take a look at the color picker in your favorite computer graphics program. The one shown in **Figure 5.10** offers two different ways to define colors in three dimensions. The controls in the lower part of the panel define color space in terms of red, green, and blue dimensions, corresponding to the relative intensities of the glowing red, green, and blue phosphors in a computer monitor. The "yellow" in the upper right-hand corner of the large square in Figure 5.10 is produced when red and green are set to the maximum (255 in this system) and blue is set to 0. (Yet again, "red" plus "green" looks yellow.)

More useful terms for describing the perceived attributes of a color are *hue*, *saturation*, and *brightness*, the terms that define the second mode of color definition illustrated in Figure 5.10. These dimensions are very different concepts from red, green, and blue, but notice that again the system is three-dimensional. **Hue** is the chromatic aspect of a light. For example, each point on the spectrum defines a different hue. The **saturation** dimension corresponds to the amount of hue present in a light. A pure white light has zero saturation; blood red is a saturated red. **Brightness** is the perceptual consequence of the physical intensity of a light. The physically intense light of the sun looks brighter than the less intense moon.

Hue is represented by the colorful vertical strip in Figure 5.10, and the large square region on the left represents a two-dimensional slice through the three-dimensional color space, with hue held constant. Brightness increases from the bottom to the top of the square, and saturation increases from left to right. In the upper left-hand corner of the square we see white, which is completely desaturated and has a brightness level of 100%. Along the bottom of the square, where brightness is at 0%, all the "colors" are black. In the upper right we see a "pure" yellow color: the point in the color space defined by 58° hue, 100% saturation, and 100% brightness.

color space The three-dimensional space, established because color perception is based on the outputs of three cone types, that describes the set of all colors.

hue The chromatic (colorful) aspect of color (red, blue, green, yellow, and so on).

saturation The chromatic strength of a hue. White has zero saturation, pink is more saturated, and red is fully saturated.

brightness The distance from black (zero brightness) in color space.

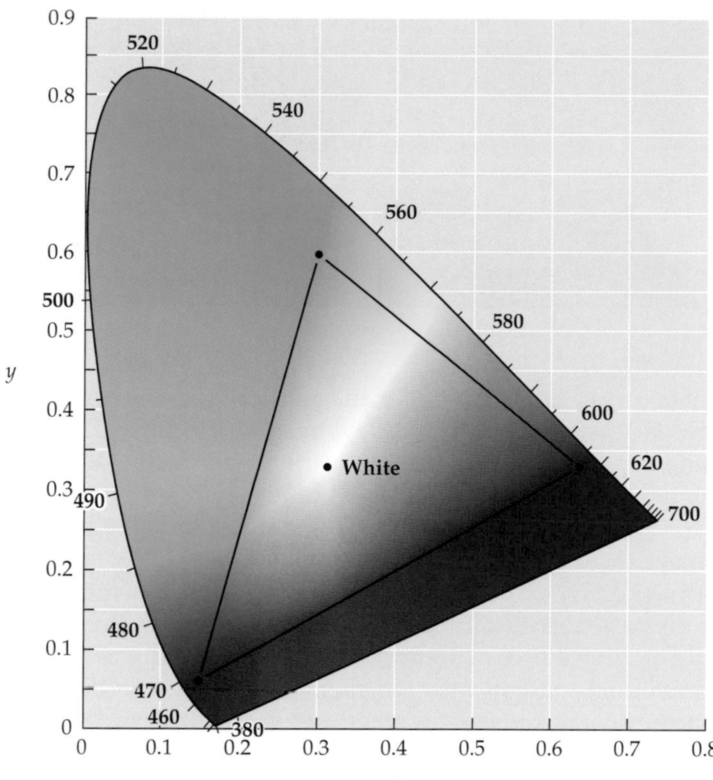

FIGURE 5.11 The curvaceous triangle shown here represents all the colors that can be seen (at one brightness level) by the human visual system. The smaller triangle contains all the colors that can be reproduced by a typical color monitor. Given this limitation, it is amazing that natural scenes on a monitor look as good as they do.

Now compare the hue strip in Figure 5.10 to the light spectrum at the bottom of Figure 5.4. Notice that some colors—for example, the purplish magentas between red and blue near the top of the hue strip—are not present in the spectrum. These colors are called, logically enough, "nonspectral hues," and they can result only from light mixtures. For example, suppose we combined a pure 420-nm light with a pure 680-nm light. As Figure 5.4 shows, this combination would strongly stimulate the L- and S-cones and produce minimal stimulation in the M-cones—a pattern that cannot be produced by any single light wavelength.

Another color space, illustrated in **Figure 5.11**, has dimensions that are somewhat opaquely labeled x, y, and Y. Again, the color space is three-dimensional, as it must be. This picture shows only the x and y dimensions (roughly, but not exactly, red and green). Capital Y is the luminance dimension of this space, so the figure shows all of the colors that we can see at one brightness level. The interesting feature is the smaller triangle. It contains all the colors that can be produced on a standard computer monitor or TV. Notice that many colors cannot be accurately produced on a monitor. It is a testimony to the flexible powers of the human visual system that a natural scene still looks quite natural when presented in this limited "gamut" of colors.

History of Trichromatic Theory

As mentioned already, the theory that color vision can be explained by the responses of three mechanisms with different sensitivities to the wavelengths of light is known as the "trichromatic theory of color vision." From what you've read so far in this book, you would be forgiven for supposing that clever anatomists and physiologists identified the three cone types and built a theory from there. Indeed, there have been beautiful experiments of

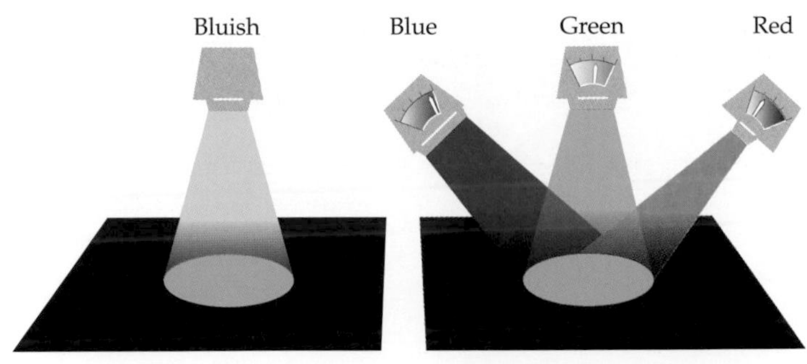

FIGURE 5.12 In a modern version of Maxwell's color-matching experiment, a color is presented on the left. On the right, the observer adjusts a mixture of the three lights to match the color on the left.

this sort. For instance, Julie Schnapf et al. managed to record the activity of single photoreceptors (Schnapf, Kraft, and Baylor, 1987). Jeremy Nathans et al. found the genes that code for the different photopigments (Nathans, Thomas, and Hogness, 1986). David Williams and his students even developed a method for photographing and identifying different cone types in the living human eye (see Figure 2.11).

Such research has cemented our understanding of the physical basis of trichromacy, but the basic theory was established by psychophysical experimentation, and theorizing started with Isaac Newton's great discovery that a prism would break up sunlight into the spectrum of hues and another prism would put the spectrum back together into white. In 1666, Newton understood that "the rays to speak properly are not coloured. In them is nothing else than a certain Power and Disposition to stir up a Sensation of this or that Colour" (from *Opticks*, published originally in 1704). Newton knew that color is a mental event.

The three-dimensional nature of the experience of color was worked out in the nineteenth century by Thomas Young (1773–1829), and subsequently by Hermann von Helmholtz (1821–1894). In their honor, trichromatic theory is often called the "Young–Helmholtz theory." James Clerk Maxwell (1831–1879) developed a color-matching technique that was central to Helmholtz's work on this topic. (Somehow Maxwell missed having his name attached, or we would have the Young–Maxwell–Helmholtz theory.) Maxwell's color-matching technique is illustrated in **Figure 5.12**. The observer in a modern version of such experiments would try to use different amounts of "primary" colored lights (e.g., the red, green, and blue lights on the right side of the figure) to exactly match another reference color (e.g., the cyan or bluish light on the left side).

The central observation from these experiments was that only three mixing lights are needed to match any reference light. Two primaries are not enough. Four are more than are needed. Long before physiology could prove it, these results led Young and Helmholtz to deduce that three different color mechanisms must govern the human experience of color.

Opponent Processes

Repackaging the Information

As discussed in earlier chapters, a lot of information is contained in the image of the world formed on the retina. Because the optic nerve that transports that information from eye to brain is of finite size, it is important to code the information efficiently. What should we do with the information from our three types of cones? We could send separate L, M, and S signals to the brain, but that approach would be less useful than one might think.

For example, the L- and M-cones have very similar sensitivities (see Figure 5.4), so most of the time they are in close agreement: L says, "Lots of light coming from location X." "Yes, lots of light coming from location X," M agrees.

Looking at the differences between cone responses turns out to be much more useful. The difference between L and M responses contains considerable information about color (possibly information that is particularly well suited to appreciating the differences between different amounts of blood in skin; think about blushing) (Changizi et al., 2006). Other information comes from the differences between L and M responses, and the S-cone responses. We could create (L – S) and (M – S) signals, but because L and M are so similar, a single comparison between S and (L + M) can capture almost the same information that would be found in (L – S) and (M – S) signals. Finally, combining L and M signals is a pretty good measure of the intensity of the light (S cones make a rather small contribution to our perception of brightness). Thus, on theoretical grounds it might be wise to convert the three cone signals into three new signals—(L – M), ([L + M] – S), and (L + M) (Buchsbaum and Gottschalk, 1983; Zaidi, 1997)—and the visual system does something reasonably close to this.

Opponent Cells in the Lateral Geniculate Nucleus

The earliest work on the combination of cone signals was done with fish (Svaetichin and Macnichol, 1959). By the 1960s, Russell De Valois and others had begun to show that these sorts of signals actually exist in the **lateral geniculate nucleus** (**LGN**) of macaque monkeys (De Valois, Abramov, and Jacobs, 1966). As described in Chapter 3, many ganglion cells in the retina and the LGN of the thalamus are maximally stimulated by spots of light. These cells have receptive fields with a characteristic center–surround organization. For example, some cells are excited when a light turns on in the central part of their receptive fields and inhibited when a light turns on in the surround (see Figure 2.13).

A similar antagonistic relationship characterizes color. Some of these retinal and LGN ganglion cells are excited by the L-cone onset in their center and inhibited by M-cone onsets in their surround. These (L – M) cells are one type of **color-opponent cell**, so named because different sources of chromatic information are pitted against each other. There are also (M – L), ([M + L] – S), and (S – [M + L]) cells—just the sorts of cells we would like to have to support a three-process opponent color system. The cells that were excited by light onset could be thought of as (L + M) cells. Thus, we have the three signals that we wanted on theoretical grounds.

Psychophysical Roots of Opponent Color Theory

Like trichromacy, **opponent color theory** has deep roots in the psychophysics of color vision. In the nineteenth century, Ewald Hering (1834–1918) described a curious feature of color vision: some combinations of colors are illegal. We can have a bluish green, a reddish yellow (which we would call "orange"), or a bluish red (which we would call "purple"), but reddish green and bluish yellow have never been seen, because they don't exist. Red and green are, in some fashion, opposed to each other, as are blue and yellow (Hering, 1878). Helmholtz was describing a trichromatic theory with three basic colors (red, green, and blue); Hering's theory had four basic colors in two opponent pairs: red versus green, and blue versus yellow. A black-versus-white component formed a third opponent pair, but this

lateral geniculate nucleus (LGN) A structure in the thalamus, part of the midbrain, that receives input from the retinal ganglion cells and has input and output connections to the visual cortex.

color-opponent cell A neuron whose output is based on a difference between sets of cones.

opponent color theory The theory that perception of color is based on the output of three mechanisms, each of them based on an opponency between two colors: red–green, blue–yellow, and black–white.

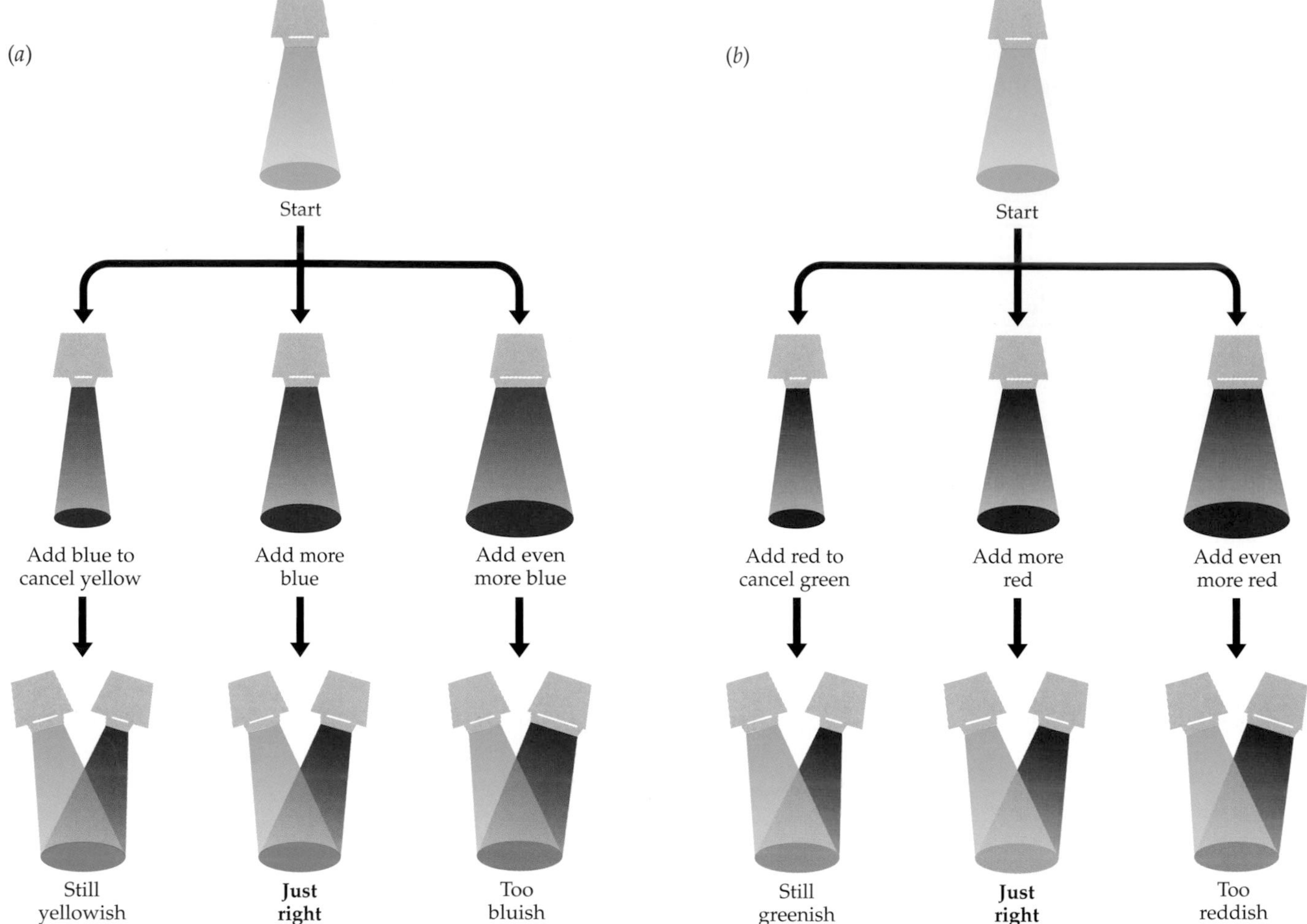

FIGURE 5.13 Hue cancellation experiments start with a color (here, yellowish green) and attempt to determine how much of the opponent color of one of the starting color's components must be added to eliminate any hint of that component from the starting color. In this example, the investigator might ask, (*a*) "How much blue must I add to eliminate any hint of yellow?" and (*b*) "How much red must I add to eliminate any hint of green?" For a reddish starting color, green would be added; for a bluish starting color, yellow would be added.

"opponency" is a bit different: although you can't have a reddish green, gray can be described as a blackish white.

Leo Hurvich and Dorothea Jameson (1957) revived Hering's ideas and developed one way to demonstrate this opponency. The method, called "hue cancellation," is shown in **Figure 5.13**. In this example, we start with a light that appears to be a yellowish green. We can cancel the yellowness by adding its opponent color, blue. We measure the amount of blue light needed to just remove all traces of yellow. We can do the same for the red–green opponency, adding just the right amount of red to make the patch of color lose all greenness. "But wait," the careful reader protests, "Earlier you said that red plus green makes yellow. Now it is making a gray or white. What's up?" Here we must plead that color language is a bit crude. Light from the "red" phosphor on a monitor, when added to light from the green phosphor, will look yellow, but that's because the "red" phosphor is actually orangish red. To make a pure red, we would need to add a bit of blue to the mix. That red mixed with the right green light will appear white.

Hue cancellation can be used for lights across the spectrum, as demonstrated in **Figure 5.14** (these are Dorothea Jameson's data; everyone has slightly different results). If we start at about 400 nm, the lights look reddish blue (or violet) and we need to add some green and some yellow to cancel them. But look what happens at about 470 nm. Here is a light that has no red or green to cancel; it looks perfectly blue. This location on the spectrum is known as **unique blue**. Continuing to scan along the spectrum in the figure reveals the locations of the other **unique hues**—hues that can be described

unique blue A blue that has no red or green tint.

unique hue Any of four colors that can be described with only a single color term: red, yellow, green, blue. Other colors (e.g., purple or orange) can be described as compounds (reddish blue, reddish yellow).

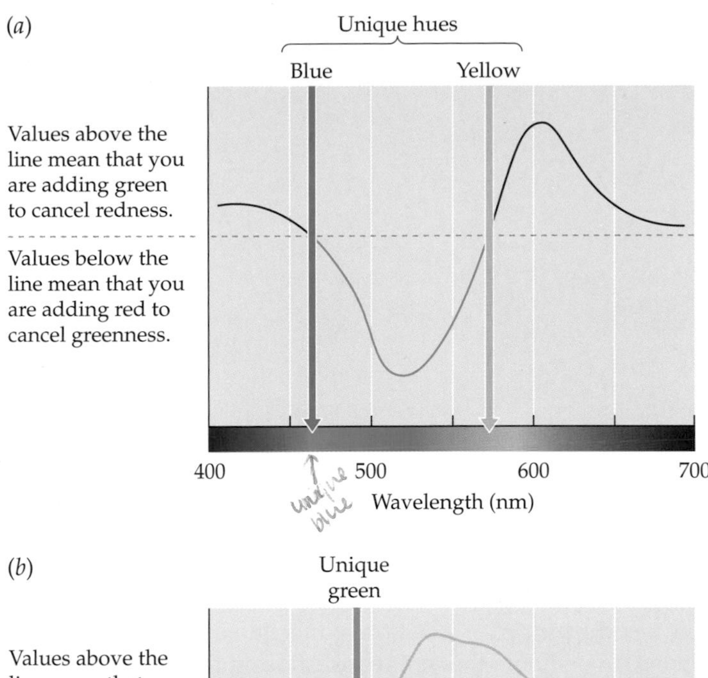

(b)
Unique green
Values above the line mean that you are adding blue to cancel yellowness.
Values below the line mean that you are adding yellow to cancel blueness.
400
500
600
700
Wavelength (nm)

FIGURE 5.14 These results from a hue cancellation experiment identify the locations where the hue cancellations cross the neutral midpoint as the locations of the unique blue, green, and yellow hues. "Unique red" is not defined by just one spectral locus. (After Hurvich and Jameson, 1957.)

with only a single color term. Only four hues can be described in this way. As you might guess, they are red, green, yellow, and blue. Only three of them have unique loci on the spectrum. All the very long wavelengths look red (with, maybe, a touch of residual yellow). The two crossings of the red–green function provide the loci of unique blue and unique yellow (Figure 5.14*a*). The point where the blue–yellow function crosses from positive to negative is the locus of "unique green," the green that has no blue or yellow in it (and, of course, no red) (Figure 5.14*b*). There are excellent exemplars of other colors, such as orange or purple, but they are not unique in the same way. Orange, no matter how pure, can still be described as a reddish yellow.

Afterimages

Another way to see opponent colors in action is to look at negative **afterimages**. If you look at one color for a few seconds, a subsequently viewed achromatic region will appear to take on a color opposite to the original color. The first colored stimulus is called the **adapting stimulus**. The illusory color that is seen afterward is the **negative afterimage**. (See **Web Activity 5.4: Afterimages.**)

Consider what would happen if you exposed your visual system to the red dot at the top of **Figure 5.15***b*. According to opponent color theory, a red

afterimage A visual image seen after the stimulus has been removed.

adapting stimulus A stimulus whose removal produces a change in visual perception or sensitivity.

negative afterimage An afterimage whose polarity is the opposite of the original stimulus. Light stimuli produce dark negative afterimages. Colors are complementary; for example, red produces green; yellow produces blue.

FIGURE 5.15 To understand what negative afterimages are, look at the image in part (*a*) and convince yourself that all the circles are gray. Now stare at the black dot in part (*b*). After 10 seconds or so, shift your fixation to the black dot in part (*a*). The circles should now look colored. This is a negative afterimage. Why does it happen? (If it didn't happen, try fixating more rigorously. Really look at the black dot.)

(*a*)

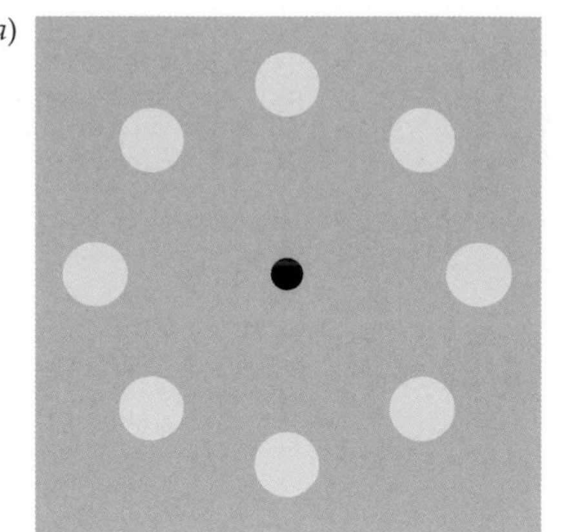

(*b*)

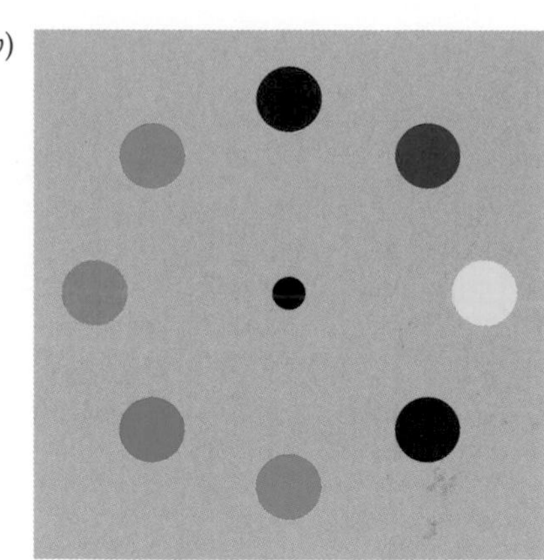

neutral point The point at which an opponent color mechanism is generating no signal. If red–green and blue–yellow mechanisms are at their neutral points, a stimulus will appear achromatic. (The black–white process has no neutral point.)

signal will be generated when the red–green opponent mechanism is pushed in the red direction. When you move your eyes to fixate the gray image (Figure 5.15*a*), the red is withdrawn from that area of the visual field, and like a released pendulum, the red–green mechanism swings back toward the **neutral point**, overshoots this point and slides into the green side. As a consequence, you see green until the opponent mechanism settles back to the neutral point. If you look at the green dot at the bottom of Figure 5.15*b* and then look back at the gray image (Figure 5.15*a*), you will see the result of pushing the red–green mechanism in the other direction. Other colors will produce other results, which you should now be able to predict.

Color in the Visual Cortex

This opponent-process story sounds as though it should go the way of the trichromacy story. Psychophysicists found three basic color processes: red–green, blue–yellow, and black–white opponency. And physiologists found three types of LGN cells using each of three different combinations of cone outputs: (L – M), ([L + M] – S), and (L + M) cells. It sounds perfect, and indeed those cells are sometimes described as red–green, blue–yellow, and black–white (De Valois, Abramov, and Jacobs, 1966). But there's a problem. If this were the case, an ([L + M] – S) cell should be a yellow–blue cell, maximally excited by unique yellow and maximally inhibited by unique blue; but a more detailed look reveals that adding and subtracting cone sensitivities produces cells that respond maximally along an axis extending from a purplish hue to a yellowish greenish hue.

The (L – M) cells aren't in quite the right place either. The L-cone end of the axis is near perceptual red, but the M-cone end is a bluish green (Eskew, 2008). Krauskopf, Williams, and Heeley (1982) call these endpoints the "cardinal directions" in color space. In **Figure 5.16**, these axes are superimposed on a slice of three-dimensional color space that shows hue and saturation but not brightness. The loci of perceptual red, yellow, green, and blue are also shown (Derrington, Krauskopf, and Lennie, 1984).

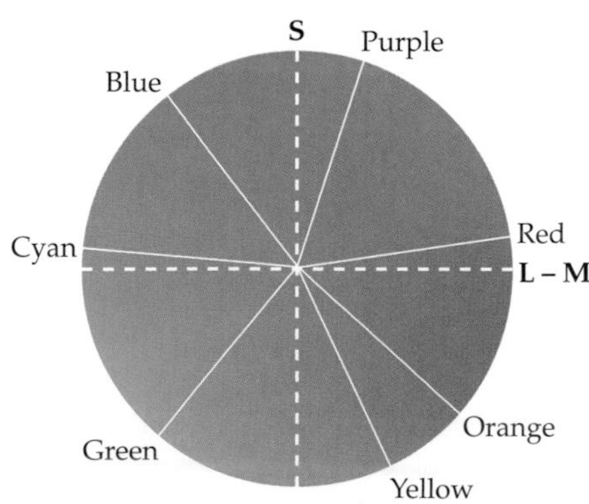

FIGURE 5.16 The colors that drive opponent cells most strongly are shown as the primary axes of this color space. They are not the same as the unique hues of perceptual experience. (After Gegenfurtner, 2003.)

This mismatch between color perception and the responses of LGN cells doesn't mean that someone is wrong. It means that the LGN is not the end of color processing. From the LGN, axons go to the visual cortex. Here matters are complex, and it is not clear how the physiology gives rise to perception (Gegenfurtner, 2003). The biggest controversy concerns the possibility of an area (or areas) in the brains of monkeys and humans specialized for color vision. There may be such an area in the pathway from the primary visual cortex (V1) into the temporal lobe (areas V2, V4, and V8) (Grill-Spector and Malach, 2004; Zeki, 1978). Indeed, certain cases of **achromatopsia**, a loss of color vision after brain damage, suggest that some pieces of cortex are vital for our perception of color (Zeki, 1990). This much seems clear: the LGN contains cells whose opponency is based on adding and subtracting the outputs of cones. The visual cortex takes that information and transforms it into a perceptually opponent experience of color that has red–green and blue–yellow axes. (See **Web Essay 5.1: Why Use Opponent Processes?**)

Does Everyone See Colors the Same Way?

Thus far, with a little caution, we have been talking about color as if we all see colors the same way, but do we? This is one of those questions that everyone asks at one point or another, often as a child. The answer will be "yes," "no," "maybe," or "we just don't know," depending on which version of the question is being asked.

Does Everyone See Colors the Same Way?—Yes

If you declare two lights to be metamerically matched, those around you will generally agree, but there will be some variation between individuals. For example, among different people unique green can vary from at least 495 to 530 nm (Nerger, Volbrecht, and Ayde, 1995). Some of these differences will be due to factors like age, which turns the lens of the eye yellow (J. S. Werner, Peterzell, and Scheetz, 1990). To a first approximation, however, your performance on standard measures of color vision will be the same as others'.

Does Everyone See Colors the Same Way?—No

There is a significant exception to the "yes" answer. Some 8% of the male population and 0.5% of the female population have a form of color vision deficiency commonly known as "color blindness," in which there is a malfunction in one or more of the genes coding the three cone photopigments. It's a "guy thing," because the genes that code for the M- and L-cone photopigments are on the X chromosome (Nathans, 1986). Males have only one copy of the X chromosome, so if one is defective, the male in question will have a problem. Females have two copies and can have normal color vision even if one copy is abnormal (actually, such women can end up with four different cone pigments) (Nagy, 1981). The S-cone photopigment is coded elsewhere, so everyone has two copies, and therefore S-cone color deficiencies are rare (Alpern, Kitahara, and Krantz, 1983). (See **Web Essay 5.2: Experiencing Color Blindness.**)

There are a number of different types of color blindness. One determining factor is the type of cone affected. A second factor is the type of defect; either the photopigment for that cone type is "anomalous"—that is, different from the norm—or the cone type is missing altogether. Although we call people who are missing one cone type "color-blind," it is a mistake to think that this means they cannot see colors at all. If you have two cone types rather than three, the normally three-dimensional color space becomes a two-dimensional space. If you have all three cones, you need three primary colors to make a metameric match with an arbitrary patch of color. The world will still be seen in color, but you will have a "flatter" color experience, different from that of people with normal color vision.

Because M- and L-cone defects are the most common, most color-blind individuals have difficulty discriminating lights in the middle- to long-

achromatopsia An inability to perceive colors that is caused by damage to the central nervous system.

deuteranope An individual who suffers from color blindness that is due to the absence of M-cones.

protanope An individual who suffers from color blindness that is due to the absence of L-cones.

tritanope An individual who suffers from color blindness that is due to the absence of S-cones.

color-anomalous A better term for what is usually called "color-blind." Most "color-blind" individuals can still make discriminations based on wavelength. Those discriminations are different from the normal—that is, *anomalous*.

cone monochromat An individual with only one cone type. Cone monochromats are truly color-blind.

rod monochromat An individual with no cones of any type. In addition to being truly color-blind, rod monochromats are badly visually impaired in bright light.

agnosia A failure to recognize objects in spite of the ability to see them. Agnosia is typically due to brain damage.

anomia An inability to name objects in spite of the ability to see and recognize them (as shown by usage). Anomia is typically due to brain damage.

wavelength range. For example, consider the wavelengths 560 and 610 nm. Neither of these lights activates S-cones very much, and the L-cones fire at about the same rate for both. But most of us can distinguish the lights on the basis of the M-cone outputs they elicit, which will be higher for the 560-nm light than for the 610-nm light (you can confirm these assertions by consulting Figure 5.4). English-speaking trichromats would label the colors of these two lights as "green" and "reddish orange," respectively.

Now consider a **deuteranope**, someone who has no M-cones. His photoreceptor output to these two lights will be identical. Following our maxim that the rest of the visual system knows only what the photoreceptors tell it, 560- and 610-nm lights must and will be classified as the same color by our deuteranopic individual.

A **protanope**—someone who has no L-cones—will have a different set of color matches based on the outputs of his two cone types (M and S). And a **tritanope**—with no S-cones—will be different again. Genetic factors can also make people **color-anomalous**. Color-anomalous individuals typically have three cone photopigments, but two of them are so similar that these individuals experience the world in much the same way as individuals with only two cone types.

We actually have some notion of exactly what the world looks like to color-deficient individuals, because there are a few, very rare cases of individuals who are color-blind in only one eye. They can compare what they see with the color-blind eye to what they see with the normal eye, so we can reconstruct the appearance of the color-blind world (MacLeod and Lennie, 1976).

True color blindness comes in a few, rare forms. It is possible to be a **cone monochromat**, with only one type of cone in the retina. Cone monochromats (who also have rods) live in a one-dimensional color space, seeing the world only in shades of gray. Even more visually crippled is the **rod monochromat**, who is missing cones altogether. Because the rods work well only in dim light and are generally absent in the fovea, these individuals have very poor acuity and serious difficulties seeing under normal daylight conditions, in addition to lacking the ability to discriminate colors.

We already mentioned one other very interesting class of color blindness, coming not from photoreceptor problems but from damage to the visual cortex. Lesions of specific parts of the visual cortex beyond primary visual cortex can cause achromatopsia. An achromatopsic individual sees the world as drained of color, even while showing evidence that wavelength information is processed at earlier stages in the visual pathway. Brain lesions can also produce various forms of color agnosia or anomia (Oxbury, Oxbury, and Humphrey, 1969). In an **agnosia**, the patient can *see* something but fails to know what it is. **Anomia** is an inability to name—in this case, an inability to name colors. A patient with anomia might be able to pick the banana that "looks right" but unable to report that the banana is or should be yellow.

Does Everyone See Colors the Same Way?—Maybe

With the exception of color-deficient individuals, all the readers of this book would agree about the "redness" of a good example of red or the "greenness" of a good green. There might be some disagreement about marginal colors (is that a reddish orange or an orangish red?) but there would be no substantive disagreement about the basics. Does this consensus grow from learned custom or from underlying physiological mechanisms? One way to examine this question is to analyze the color terms used in different languages to see whether most languages honor the same color categories. We are still not quite sure whether this is the case.

We do know that the number of "basic" color terms differs dramatically across cultures. What makes a color term basic? Berlin and Kay (1969) asserted that it must be common (like *red* and not like *beige*), not an object or substance name (excluding *bronze* and *lavender*), and not a compound word (no *blue-green*). This classification is a little subjective (is *beige* that uncommon?), but Berlin and Kay argued that, in English, these rules yield a list of 11 terms: *red, green, blue, yellow, black, white, gray, orange, purple, brown,* and *pink*. Other languages have different numbers of basic terms—some as few as 2 or 3.

cultural relativism In sensation and perception, the idea that basic perceptual experiences (e.g., color perception) may be determined in part by the cultural environment.

At one time it was thought that the differing numbers of basic color terms in different languages meant that color categorization was arbitrary. This notion was called **cultural relativism**, meaning that each group was free to create its own linguistic map of color space. Berlin and Kay's important discovery was that the various maps used in different cultures are actually rather similar (Lindsey and Brown, 2006). After surveying many languages, they found that the 11 basic color terms in English are about as many as any group possesses. Of course, the words themselves differ, but *red* is *rouge* (French) is *adom* (Hebrew). Moreover, languages do not select randomly among the possible color names. If a language has only two basic color terms, speakers of the language divide colors into *light* and *dark*. If a language has three color terms (one chromatic term beyond *light* and *dark*), what do you think the third usually is? If you guessed *red*, you are correct. Next enters *yellow*, then *green* and *blue*.

Of course, these findings raise another interesting question: if a language has only two basic color terms, do its speakers *see* colors differently than we do with our 11 basic terms? Eleanor Rosch (Heider, 1972) studied this question among the Dani of New Guinea, a tribe whose language has only two basic color terms: *mola* for light-warm colors and *mili* for dark-cool colors. Now, it is hard enough to ask your neighbor to define the experience of blue and then to ask if that is the same as your experience of blue. It is much more difficult to ask these questions across a great cultural divide. But there are tricks, as the experiment illustrated in **Figure 5.17** demonstrates.

Suppose you are shown a bluish color chip and asked to remember it. Then you are shown two test chips and asked to pick the color you saw before. Obviously, the less similar the two test colors are, the easier this task is. But more important, you will do better if the wrong choice is on the other side of a color categorical boundary. Color boundaries are sharper than you might think. If you show people a collection of colors and ask, "Which are

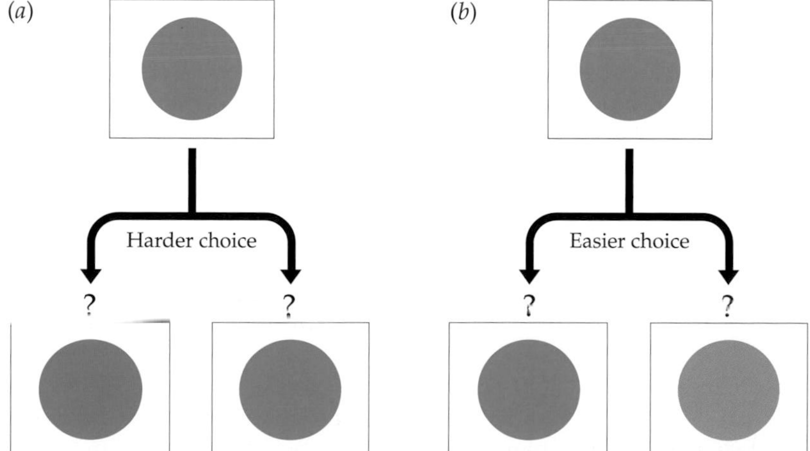

FIGURE 5.17 It is easier to remember which of two colors you have seen if the choices are categorically different. For example, suppose you had to remember the "blue" patch shown at the top of each part of the figure. Picking between two "blues," as in part (*a*), would be rather hard. The task would be easier if one of the choices were "blue" and the other "green," as in part (*b*), even if the distance in color space were the same in the two cases.

blue and which are green?" people do the task without much difficulty. If you have to remember a color, as in the task shown in Figure 5.17, you are likely to give it a label like "green" or "blue." If the next color has the same label, you are more likely to be confused than if it has a different label.

Rosch found that the Dani's performance on such tasks reflected the same color boundaries, even when their language did not recognize the distinction between the two colors (a Dani might call all the colors in Figure 5.17 *mili* but would still do better with the task on the right). This finding leads to the conclusion that color perception is not especially influenced by culture and language; blue and green are *seen* as categorically different, even if one's language does not employ color terms to express this difference.

In the late 1990s, Debi Roberson went up the Sepik River in New Guinea to study the Berinmo, whose language, like the Dani's, has a limited set of basic color terms. Unlike previously studied groups, the Berinmo have terms that form novel boundaries in color space. For example, their *nol/wor* distinction lies in the middle of colors we categorize as green, and may roughly distinguish live from dead or dying foliage. Moreover, when the Berinmo did the color memory task, they performed better across their *nol/wor* boundary than across the blue/green boundary. English speakers showed the opposite result (Davidoff, Davies, and Roberson, 1999). More recently, similar results have been found in a comparison of English and Russian subjects across the Russian categorical distinction between light blues (*goluboy*) and dark blues (*siniy*) (Winawer et al., 2007). So, can language or culture influence color perception? For many years, we thought the answer was "no." Now, thanks to Roberson's work, we are not so sure.

From the Color of Lights to a World of Color

Up to this point we have largely confined ourselves to discussing how the human visual system perceives colored lights in isolation. However, our eyeballs spend most of their time gathering reflected light that has bounced off the surfaces of a host of visible objects. Many new and complex issues arise when we turn our attention from the perception of isolated colors, or **unrelated colors** (Shevell, 2003), in the laboratory to the perception of multicolored objects in the real world. For example, nothing in all of the preceding discussion of color will explain "brown" or "gray," because there is no such thing as an unrelated light that appears brown or gray.

Brown, gray, and a host of other colors exist only as **related colors**, colors that can be seen only in the context of other colors. As we look around, the colors of objects are not determined exclusively by their own reflective properties. The color we see on one object depends in complex ways on the colors of other objects in the vicinity. For example, gray is an achromatic color that is seen when other nearby regions are lighter. Browns are really dark yellows or oranges (depending on the brown). They look brown only if accompanied by other lighter colors. Seen in isolation, an unrelated "gray" patch will look white and a "brown" patch will look yellow or orange.

We can distinguish something on the order of a few thousand unrelated colors. Allowing for context effects is what boosts the number of distinguishable colors to the millions (Shevell, 2003).

unrelated color A color that can be experienced in isolation.

related color A color, such as brown or gray, that is seen only in relation to other colors. A "gray" patch in complete darkness appears white.

illuminant The light that illuminates a surface.

Color Constancy

Another problem we face when studying real-world color perception concerns the nature of the **illuminant**, the light that illuminates a surface. The problem is that not all illuminants are the same, as **Figure 5.18** illustrates.

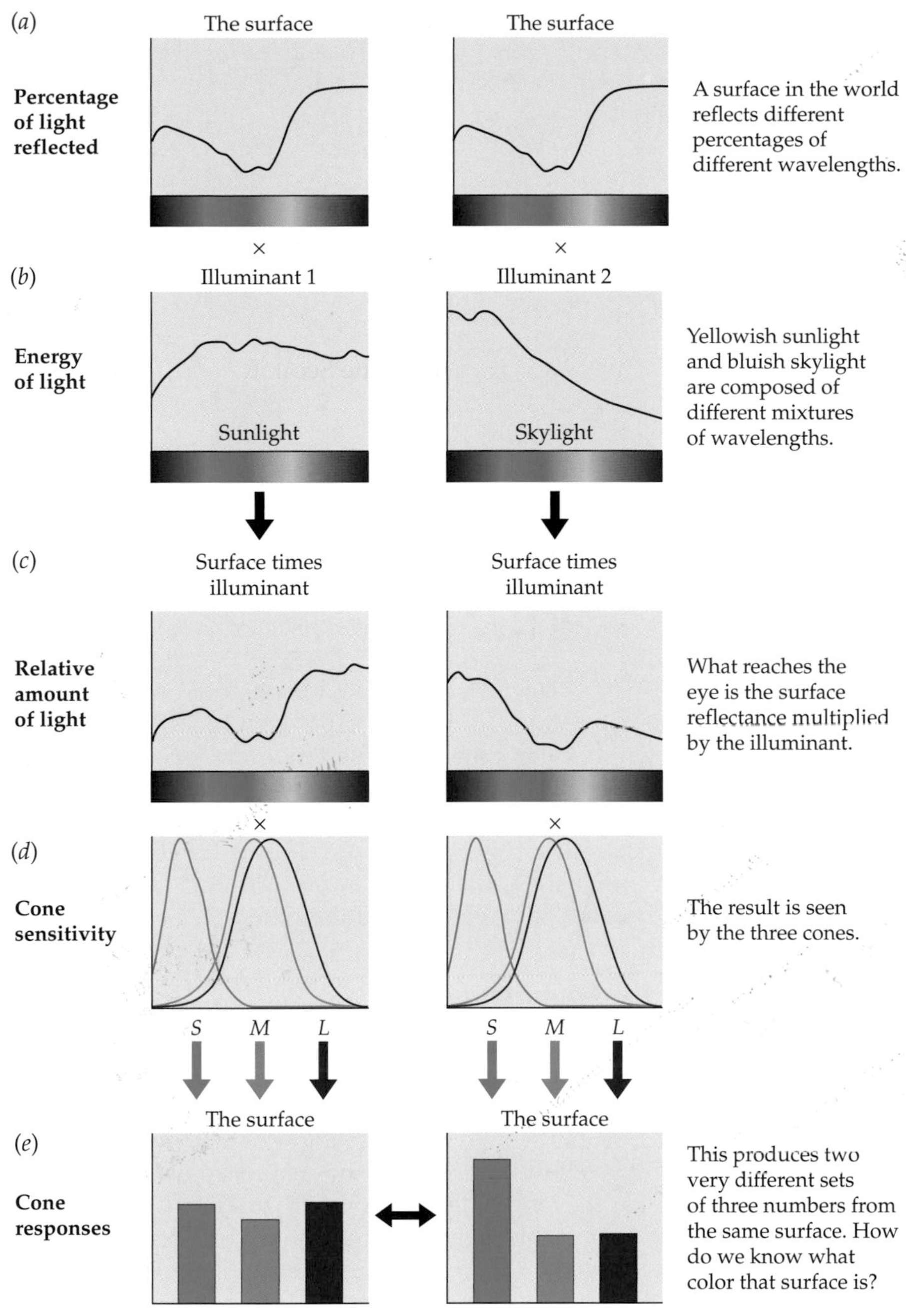

FIGURE 5.18 The same surface (*a*) illuminated by two different lights (*b*) will generate two different patterns of activity in the S-, M-, and L-cones (*c–e*). However, the surface will appear to be the same color under both illuminants. This phenomenon is known as color constancy. (After Smithson, 2005.)

Figure 5.18*a* shows the **spectral reflectance function** for a surface—the percentage of each wavelength that is reflected from the surface. With its preponderance of long and short wavelengths, it probably looks purplish. Let's call it "lilac." Figure 5.18*b* shows the **spectral power distribution**—the relative amount of light at different visible wavelengths—of two different types of "daylight": sunlight and skylight. Sunlight is a yellowish light, richer in middle and long wavelengths; skylight is more bluish. Figure 5.18*c* shows that the light reflected to our eyes is the product of the surface and the illumination. For example, a surface might reflect 90% of 650-nm light, but no 650-nm light would reach the eye unless there was some in the original illumination. Figure 15.18*d* shows that those two different products of surface

spectral reflectance function The function relating the wavelength of light to the percentage of that wavelength that is reflected from a surface.

spectral power distribution The physical energy in a light as a function of wavelength.

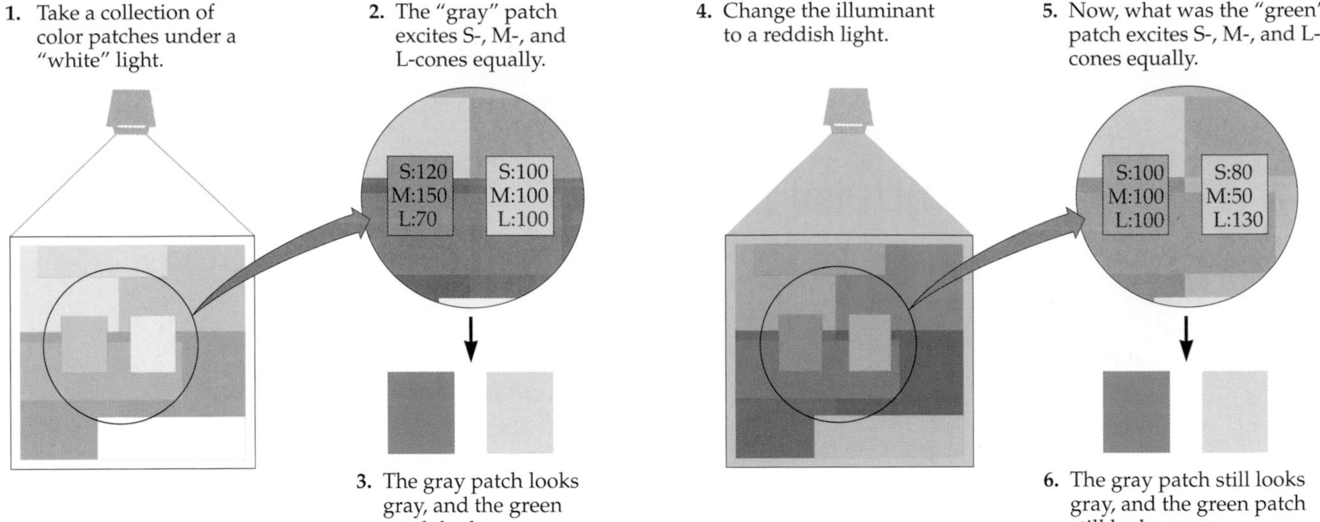

FIGURE 5.19 This color constancy experiment was conducted by McCann, McKee, and Taylor (1976). In a rich context, the perceived color of a patch is not determined only by the excitation of the S-, M-, and L-cone populations at the location of the patch. It is also strongly influenced by its environment.

and illumination are converted into two different sets of three numbers by the L-, M- and S-cones.

Here's the puzzle: That lilac surface will look lilac-colored under both illuminants. White paper will look white. A banana will look yellow. This phenomenon is known as **color constancy**, the tendency for the colors of objects to appear relatively unchanged in spite of substantial changes in the illuminant. Color constancy is good because we just want to know the color of the object. We are generally uninterested in the nature of the illuminant or its interactions with an object's surface. In more technical language, we would say that we "discount" the role of the illuminant.

The Problem with the Illuminant

Discounting the role of the illuminant is a fine goal, but it is not trivial to accomplish. Let's think about this as a math problem. In simple terms, we have an illuminant (call it I) and a surface (S). As shown in Figure 5.18*c*, what we can sense is $I \times S$, but what we want to know is S. It is as if we were given a number (say, 48), told that it is the product of two other numbers, and asked to guess what they might be. The answer could be 12 and 4. Or it could be 16 and 3. Or 6 and 8. Given just the number 48, we cannot solve the problem. Nevertheless, given $I \times S$, the visual system does a pretty good job of figuring out S.

McCann, McKee, and Taylor (1976) brought color constancy into the lab (**Figure 5.19**). They created a setup in which the left eye was looking at a set of color patches under one light source while the right eye looked at other patches under an independent light source in a different part of the visual world. With this setup they could ask observers to look at a patch shown only to the left eye and match it to the appearance of a patch shown to the right eye. These collections of patches are often called "Mondrians" in honor of Piet Mondrian, the twentieth-century artist whose abstract works look *a little* like these collections of rectangular patches (you decide; see **Figure 5.20**).

In panel 1 of Figure 5.19, the critical patches are the gray and green ones at the center. Under a "white" light, the gray patch reflected equal amounts of S-, M-, and L-wavelength light. The patches in the other eye were illuminated with white light of the same composition. Naturally enough, observers

color constancy The tendency of a surface to appear the same color under a fairly wide range of illuminants.

matched the gray patch in the left eye to the gray patch in the right, and they matched green to green.

In panel 4 of Figure 5.19, the illumination of the Mondrian has been changed; it has been made redder. In the illustration, you can see this. In the experiment, the change might not have been noticed, just as you might not notice a change from sunlight to skylight. Under the white light, the green patch produced 120 units of S-cone excitation, 150 units of M-cone, and 70 units of L-cone. If the illuminant were made a bit redder, the same green patch could now be made to produce 100 units each of S-, M-, and L-cone excitation, *exactly* the same as what the gray patch produced under the white light.

If seen in isolation, the "green" patch would now appear gray, because the three cone types would all be firing at approximately equal rates in response to the light reflecting off the patch. In the context of the Mondrian, however, the patches kept their original, "true" colors. Green looked green, and gray looked gray. The presence of the other colors allowed the colors of the test patches to remain constant over a fairly dramatic change in the nature of the illumination. How is this possible?

FIGURE 5.20 A real Mondrian: Piet Mondrian's *Composition in Gray, Red, Yellow, and Blue* (1920). (Courtesy of the Granger Collection.)

Physical Constraints Make Constancy Possible

Because there is always an infinite set of lights and surfaces that will produce any given image on the retina, the problem of color constancy cannot be solved if one tries to use just the three cone activation numbers that come from each spot in the image. More information is needed. Fortunately, more information is available. For instance, some intelligent guesses can be made about the illuminant. In Figure 5.19, it's possible that each patch has its own dedicated light source. Thus, the brown, L-shaped region in the lower left corner could really be a white surface, illuminated by a carefully shaped, dim yellow light source.

Although such situations can be concocted in the laboratory by devilishly clever perception researchers, they are very, very unlikely to occur in the real world. Sharp borders in an image are almost always the result of boundaries between surfaces, not boundaries between light sources. Shadow borders can be an exception to this rule (Adelson, 1993; Cavanagh and Leclerc, 1989). Shadow borders, however, change mainly the brightness and not the chromatic properties of a region. It is easy to see the image in **Figure 5.21***a* as three rectangles with a shadow lying across their middles. In Figure 5.21*b*, the top and bottom are brighter than the middle, but for that difference to be the result of a shadow we know that the shadow would have to be coinci-

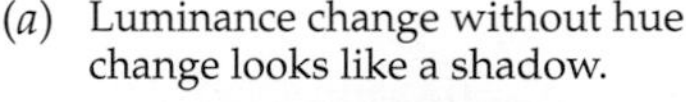
(*a*) Luminance change without hue change looks like a shadow.

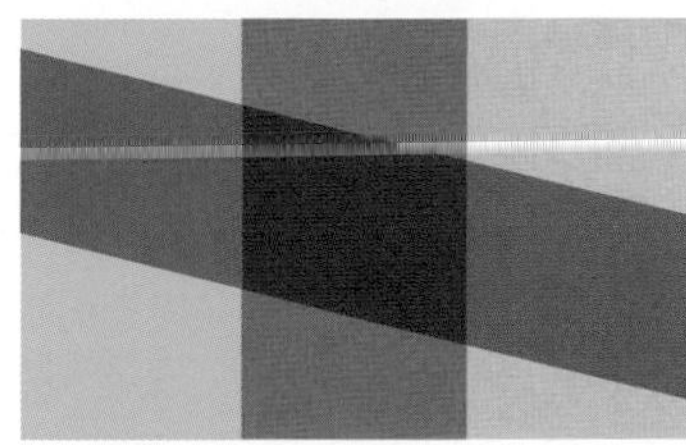

(*b*) Luminance change *with* hue change looks less like a shadow.

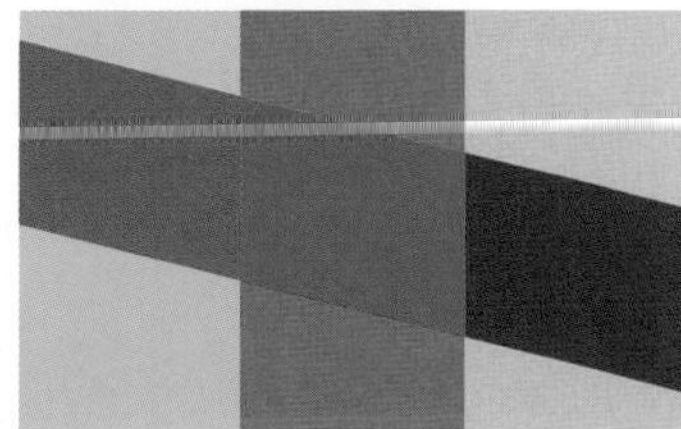

FIGURE 5.21 The visual system "knows" that brightness changes across a shadow boundary but hue does not. As a result, (*a*) looks like a shadow, but (*b*) does not.

reflectance The percentage of light hitting a surface that is reflected and not absorbed into the surface. Typically reflectance is given as a function of wavelength.

dently aligned with the hue change (Smithson, 2005). Our implicit knowledge of these sorts of constraints helps us sort out the visual world.

We aren't completely sure which assumptions are most important for color constancy, but let's review some of the known constraints on the distribution of wavelength information in the real world. Natural light sources (and most artificial ones, such as standard lightbulbs) are generally "broadband." That is, they contain many wavelengths, even if some wavelengths are not as intense as others. Furthermore, their spectral composition curves (see Figure 5.18) are usually smooth; spikes at particular wavelengths are uncommon, though this generalization is violated by some artificial light sources. Highly unnatural (e.g., monochromatic) light sources make the world look highly unnatural—a fact exploited in clubs the world over. Indeed, with a monochromatic source, color vision is impossible, though not much broadband light is needed to get color back.

Real surfaces also tend to be broadband in their **reflectances** (recall the hamburger distributions of Figure 5.5). It would be very unlikely, for example, to find a surface that reflected 100% of 535-nm light, 0% of 538-nm light, and 100% again of 540-nm light. Even surfaces that are nearly metameric with single wavelengths of light are actually reflecting a wide range of wavelengths. There are limits on the reflectivity of real surfaces. The whitest surface rarely reflects more than 95% of any wavelength, and the blackest rarely reflects less than 5%. The brightest thing in the visual field is likely to be white. A "specular reflection" (like the shiny spot on a billiard ball) has a wavelength composition very similar to that of the illuminant.

Cues like this, perhaps in clever combination, can be used to solve the otherwise unsolvable problem of color constancy (Smithson, 2005). Returning to the earlier math example, if you were told that two smaller integers multiplied to make 48 and that one of those integers had to be odd, you

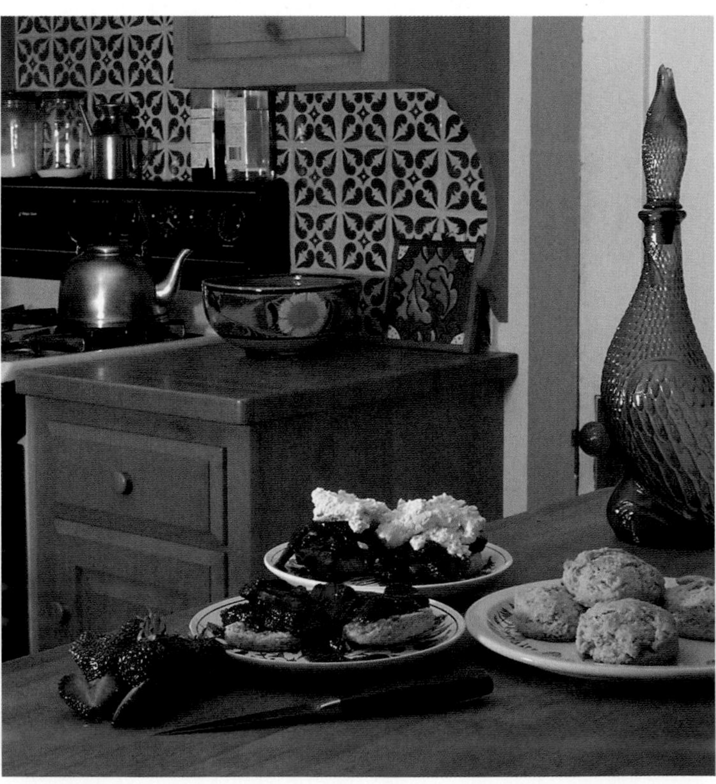

FIGURE 5.22 The strawberries in a complex scene will look red even if there is not much long-wavelength light in the illuminant.

could determine with certainty that the integers were 16 and 3. Something like this restriction of the possible solutions is going on in color vision, too.

How might the visual system use these assumptions to achieve color constancy? Suppose, for example, that you are standing in a kitchen illuminated by a light source composed primarily of short and middle wavelengths (**Figure 5.22**). None of the surfaces in your visual field will reflect much long-wavelength light, because there isn't much of this light to be reflected. But given the assumption that the illumination is evenly distributed around the room, you will still perceive the strawberries as red because they will be reflecting *more* long-wavelength light than any other surface does.

The subtlety of the visual system's understanding of the physics of light and reflection is evident in an elegant experiment by Bloj, Kersten, and Hurlbert (1999) (**Figure 5.23**). They took a card that was half red and half white (Figure 5.23, Step 1) and folded it so that the red region faced the white region (Step 2). As a result, some of the light reflected from the red side bounced off the white side and into an observer's eye (Step 3). Seen in isolation, that formerly white area would have looked mildly pink. However, the visual system seems to "know" about mutual reflection. Observers saw the white region as white because their visual systems had a way to explain the pinkness as being due to illumination (Step 4).

Now comes the clever part. Using an optical trick, Bloj et al., in effect, switched the left and right eyes, making the card look like a roof rather than a corner (Step 5). If it were a roof, the red and white areas would not be able to face each other, and consequently, the red area would not be able to reflect onto the white. Because this was a trick, however, all of the actual wavelengths were identical. But the visual system had lost its explanation for the long-wavelength light bouncing off the white region. As a result, the white region now looked quite pink (Step 6). If the pinkness could not be attributed to illumination, it had to be attributed to the actual color of the surface.

1. Start with a card half red, half white.

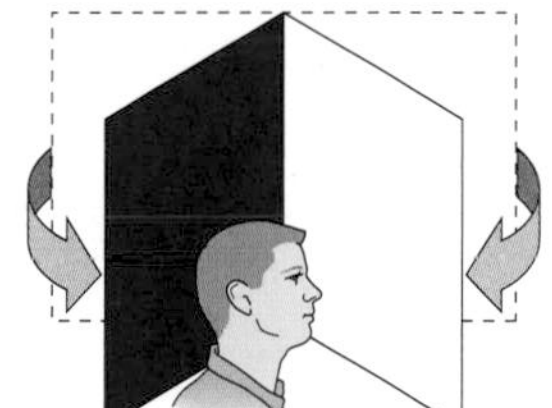

2. Fold it so that red faces white.

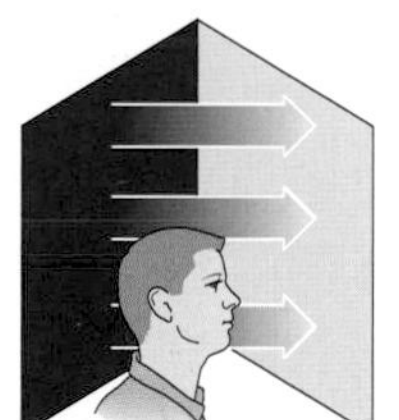

3. Light reflects from red onto white.

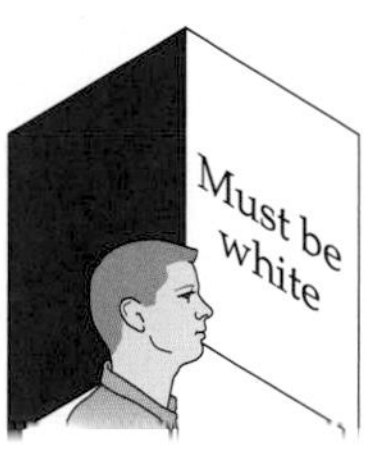

4. The visual system "knows" about the reflection and knows to discount it.

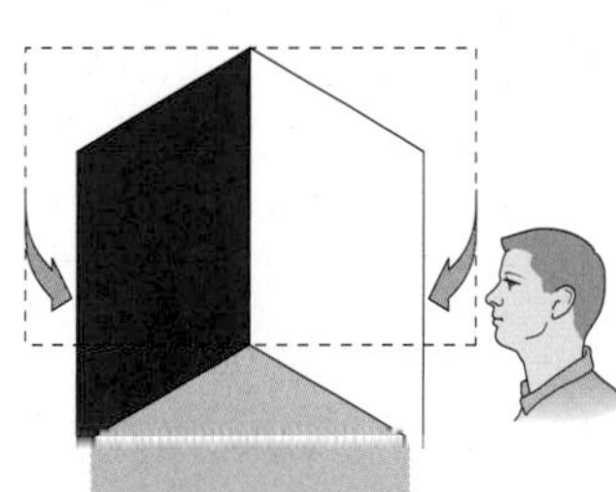

5. Now, fool the visual system into thinking the card is folded like a roof.

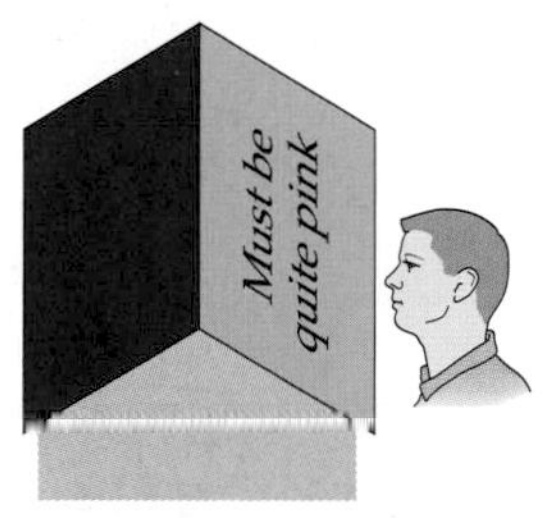

6. Without the reflection explanation, the white side now looks quite pink.

FIGURE 5.23 The experiment of Bloj, Kersten, and Hurlbert (1999) shows us how assumptions about the physics of the world influence the psychophysics of color perception.

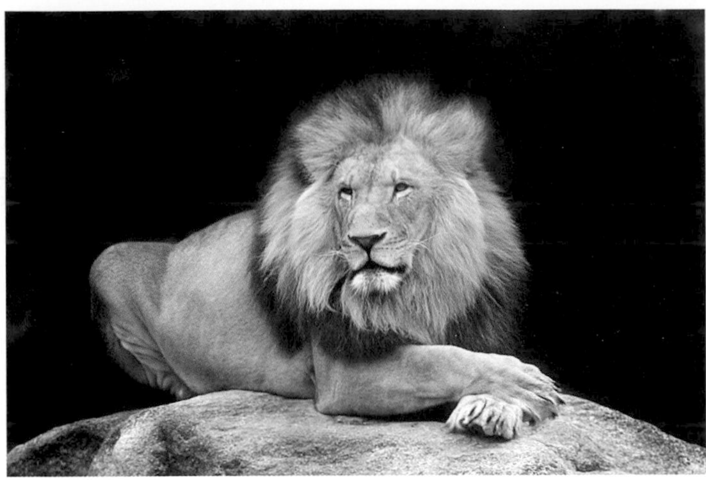

FIGURE 5.24 A black-and-white lion is still a lion.

We dwell on this experiment not because the perception of folded cards is vitally important, but because the experiment, like many others, neatly illustrates that vision is not just a simple translation of the world from photons to neurons. Vision is the nervous system's best guess about what is happening in the world. (See **Web Activity 5.5: Illusions of Lighting** for more on this point.)

Color Vision in Animals

The ability to use wavelength information has evolved several times in several ways during the course of evolution. Evolutionary theory tells us that, for this to be true, color vision must provide an advantage that makes it worth the trouble. An animal can certainly survive without color vision. If we cannot make wavelength discriminations, we can still identify a lion (**Figure 5.24**) and we can still find our way through the forest. Although color vision might make the lion stand out a bit better from the trees, we would be much more impaired if we lacked "orientation vision" or "motion vision." Across the animal kingdom, however, there seem to be at least two realms of behavior where color vision is especially useful: eating and sex.

Having color vision does seem to make it easier to forage for food. Would you rather pick ripe berries with (**Figure 5.25***a*) or without (Figure 5.25*b*) color vision? The colors of wildflowers did not develop to please the aesthetic sense of humans. They are advertisements to bees and other insects offering to trade food for sex (well, at least for pollination). In fact, many flowers have dramatic patterns that we cannot see because they are variations in the reflection of short-wavelength ("ultraviolet") light, which is outside our range. Bees can see these short wavelengths, and it is the bees that flowers are designed to attract (**Figure 5.26**).

Colorful displays—from the dramatic patterns on tropical fish (**Figure 5.27***a*) to the neck and beak of a toucan (Figure 5.27*b*) to the face of the baboon (Figure 5.27*c*)—are all sexual signals. What makes the toucan with the most colorful neck and beak the most desirable mate for a female toucan?

FIGURE 5.25 Picking a strawberry is easier if you have color vision.

(*a*)

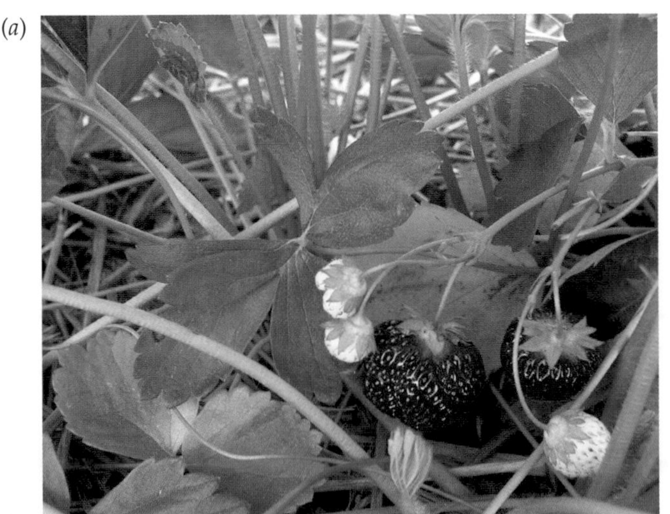

(*b*)

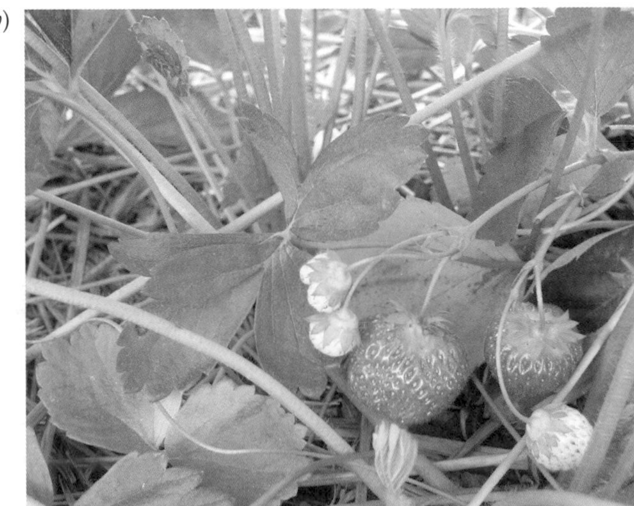

(*a*)

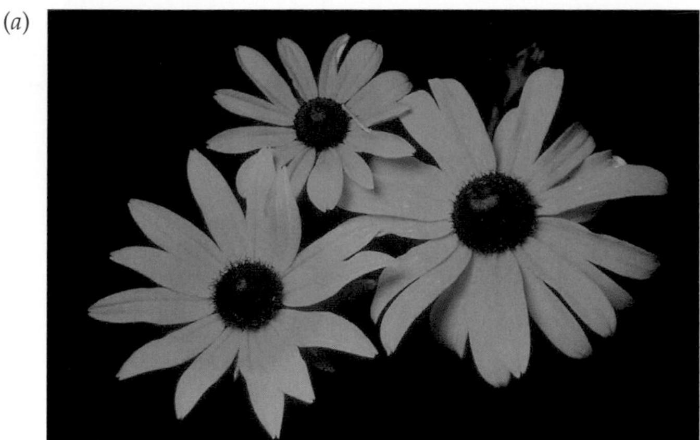

(*b*)

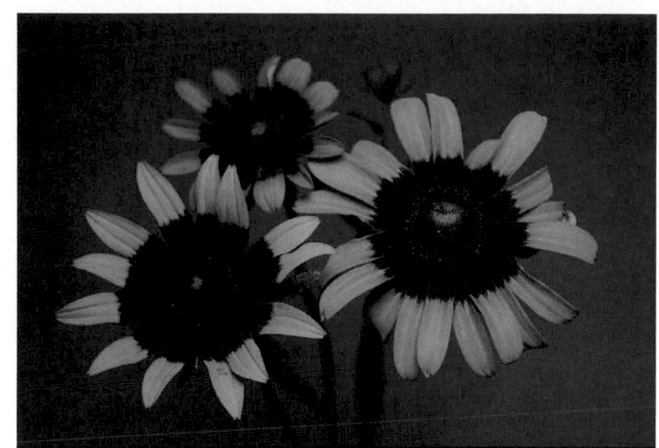

FIGURE 5.26 Color vision in different species. (*a*) These black-eyed Susans are shown as seen with human photoreceptors and color vision. (*b*) A honeybee can see UV light. In UV, the flower's "black eye" (or maybe the pupil of that eye) is much larger—a better target for the bee. (Courtesy of Tom Eisner.)

We can't ask her, of course, but a colorful neck and beak might somehow indicate that this toucan's genes are better than his competitors'. A female toucan that sees the world in black and white won't be able to perceive this information and will therefore be at an evolutionary disadvantage. As noted earlier, primate color vision may be particularly well suited to detect the amount of blood in a blushing or blanched cheek (Changizi et al., 2006).

Color vision is accomplished in different ways in different species. We are trichromats, with three different types of photoreceptors. Dogs appear to be dichromats, with two types of photoreceptors (Neitz, Geist, and Jacobs, 1989). Chickens, surprisingly enough, turn out to be tetrachromats, with four (Okano, Fukada, and Yoshizawa, 1995). There is not much gain in information if the number of photoreceptor types is increased beyond three or four (Maloney, 1986), which probably explains the lack of octachromats or dodecachromats—individuals with 8 or 12 types of cones, respectively.

Our S-, M-, and L-cones are different because they contain different photopigments (**Figure 5.28***a*). It is also possible to use a single photopigment to create more than one functional type of cone. The trick is to put a different filter in front of each type of cone so that some wavelengths are subtracted before light reaches the photoreceptor (Figure 5.28*b*). A cone with a reddish oil droplet in front of it will respond more vigorously to long-wavelength light than will a cone covered by a greenish droplet. Chicks and other birds have these droplets, as do a variety of reptiles (Govardovskii, 1983).

FIGURE 5.27 The colors of animals—from tropical fish (*a*) to toucans (*b*) to baboons (*c*)—are often an advertisement to potential mates.

(*a*)

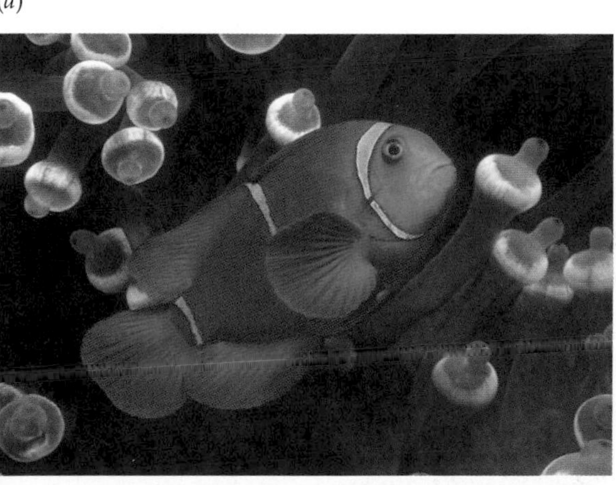

(*b*)

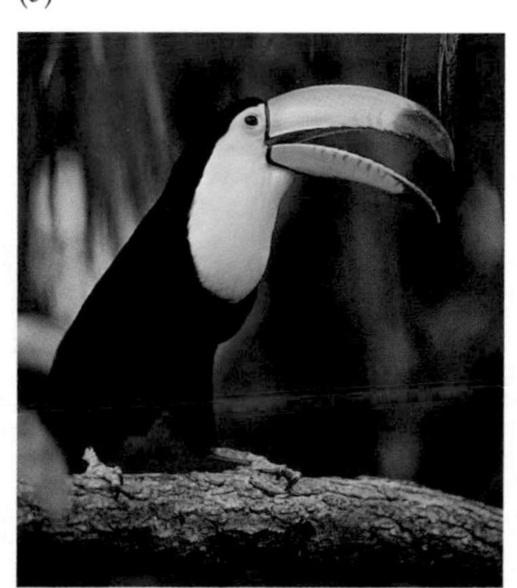

(*c*)

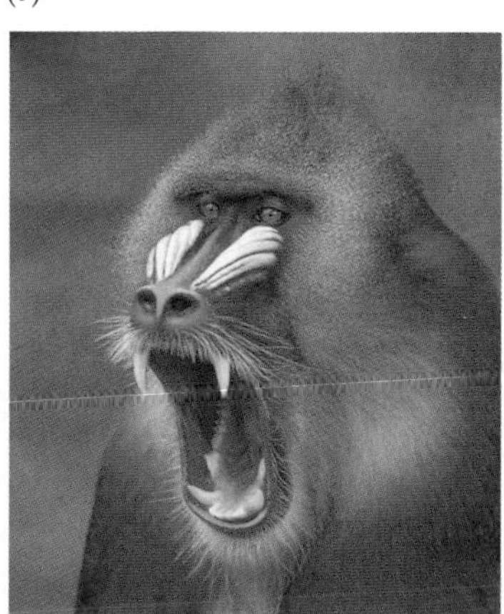

FIGURE 5.28 Two ways to make photoreceptors with different spectral sensitivities. (*a*) Our S-, M-, and L- cones are different because they contain different photopigments. (*b*) Some animals have only one type of photopigment. These animals can have color vision because colored oil droplets sitting on top of photoreceptors create groups of photoreceptors with different sensitivities to wavelength.

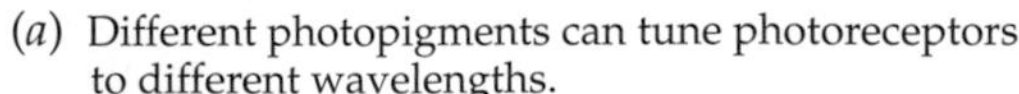

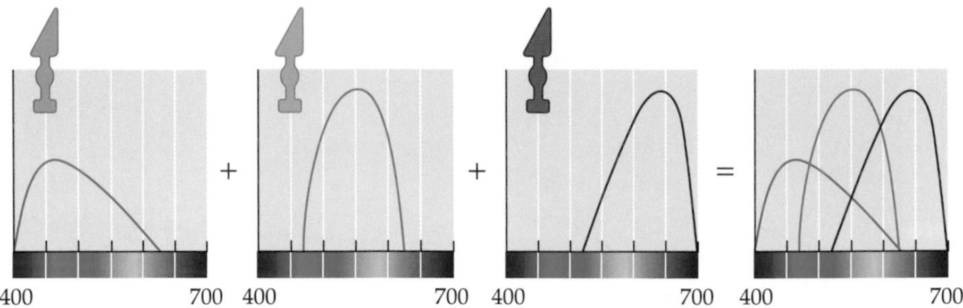

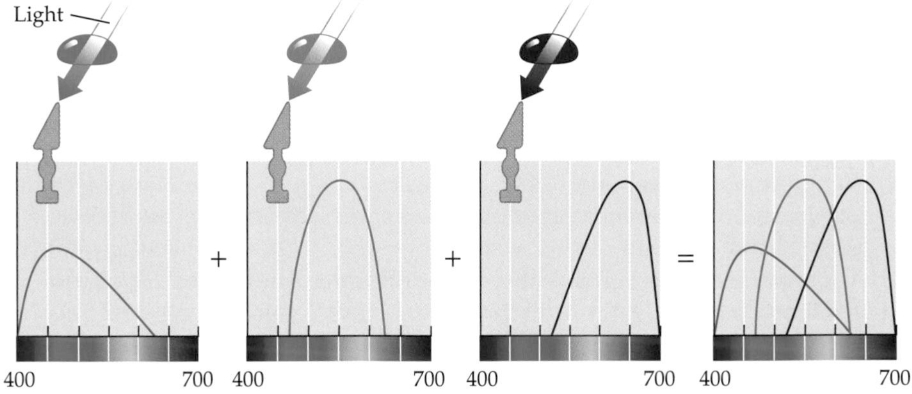

Even fireflies get into this act in a limited way. Fireflies signal each other with bioluminescence: they make their own light. Different species have different lights, and each species' visual system appears to be tuned to its particular wavelength signature. A combination of a photopigment and a colored filter makes signals of conspecifics (members of the same species) appear brighter than the flashes of other fireflies in the vicinity (Cronin et al., 2000). With this sort of visual system, the firefly will never appreciate the palette of colors in a sunset. But it will be able to locate an appropriate mate, and that, after all, was the pressure shaping the development of this limited sensitivity to wavelength.

Like humans, other animals are interested in the properties of surfaces, not the properties of illuminating lights. Therefore, color constancy is a goal of all animals with dichromatic, trichromatic, or tetrachromatic vision. Researchers have found that animals with quite different color vision systems do, in fact, show color constancy. Take the honeybee, for example. Annette Werner trained honeybees to land on a region of one color in order to get food and to ignore two other colors (A. Werner, Menzel, and Wehrhahn, 1988). She could then alter the illuminating light so that the light reflecting off a "bad" color had the same effect on the bee photoreceptors under the new light that the "good" color had had under the old light. Nevertheless, the bees still flew to the good color. (You should recognize this as the bee analog to the McCann, McKee, and Taylor experiment illustrated in Figure 5.19.) We cannot tell what the bees "saw," but they behaved as though the perceived colors stayed constant when the illumination changed. Much the same experiment has been done with goldfish, with much the same result (Dorr and Neumeyer, 1996; Ingle, 1985).

These studies of animals remind us of two important points about color perception. First, if we think about the oil droplets of fireflies, the tetrachromacy of chickens, and so forth, we are reminded that color is a mental experience and not a physical property. These animals can make discriminations according to the wavelength of light, but they live in a different color world than the one we perceive. Second, the experiments on color constancy illustrate that, even though different organisms have different color vision apparatus, all must solve the same basic problems. The physics of the world do not change for different species. If a human needs to ignore the color of the illuminant, so does a bee.

Summary

1. Probably the most important fact to know about color vision is that lights and surfaces look colored because a particular distribution of wavelengths of light is being analyzed by a particular visual system. Color is a mental phenomenon, not a physical phenomenon. Many animal species have some form of color vision. It seems to be important for identifying possible mates, possible rivals, and good things to eat. Color vision has evolved several times in several different ways in the animal kingdom.
2. Rod photoreceptors are sensitive to low (scotopic) light levels. There is only one type of rod photoreceptor. It yields one "number" for each location in the visual field. Rods can support only a one-dimensional representation of color from dark to light. Thus, scotopic vision is achromatic vision.
3. There are three types of cone photoreceptors with different sensitivities to the wavelength of light. Cones operate at brighter light levels, producing three "numbers" at each location; the pattern of activity over the different cone types defines the color.
4. If two regions of an image produce the same response in the three cone types, they will look identical; that is, they will be metamers. And they will look identical even if the physical wavelengths coming from the two regions are different.
5. In additive color mixture, two or more lights are mixed. Adding a light that looks blue to a light that looks yellow will produce a light that looks white (if we pick the right blue and yellow). In subtractive color mixture, filters, paints, or other pigments that absorb some wavelengths and reflect others are mixed. Mixing a typical blue paint and a typical yellow paint will subtract most long and short wavelengths from the light reflected by the mixture, and the result will look green.
6. Information from the three cones is combined to form three opponent processes. Cones sensitive to long wavelengths (L-cones) are pitted against medium-wavelength (M) cones to create an (L – M) process that is *roughly* sensitive to the redness or greenness of a region. (L + M) cones are pitted against short-wavelength (S) cones to create a process *roughly* sensitive to the blueness or yellowness of a region. The third process is sensitive to the overall brightness of a region.
7. Color blindness is typically caused by the congenital absence or abnormality of one cone type—usually the L- or M-cone, usually in males. Most color-blind individuals are not blind to differences in wavelength. Rather, their color perception is based on the outputs of two cone types instead of the normal three.
8. The goal of color vision is to describe the properties of surfaces in the world (e.g., a "red" strawberry) and to ignore the color of the light shining on the surface (e.g., sunset versus high noon). Mechanisms of color constancy use implicit knowledge about the world to correct for the influence of different illuminants and to keep the strawberry looking red under a wide range of conditions.

Refer to the
Sensation and Perception
website
(www.sinauer.com/wolfe2e)
for activities, essays, study questions, and other study aids.

CHAPTER 6

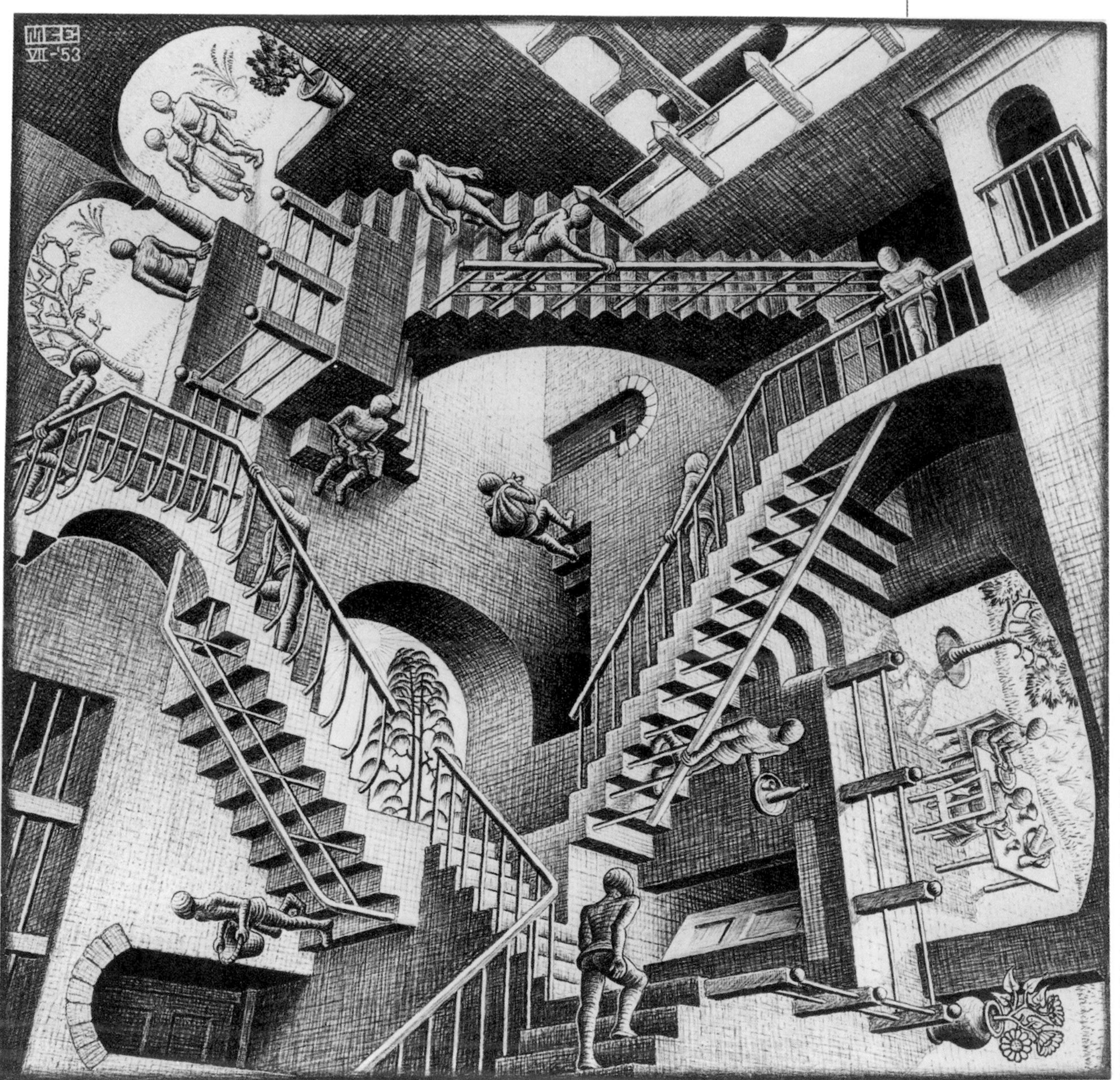

M. C. Escher, *Relativity*, 1953

Space Perception and Binocular Vision

Imagine that you're moving quietly through a meadow, trying to get close enough to a bear cub to get a good picture. Suddenly you discover that Mother Bear is not happy about your photo session. She charges, and you run—back across the field, through a thicket of trees. A quick leap across a stream brings you to a slope that leads down to the road where your partner is waiting in the jeep. You dive into the passenger side and roar off down the track to safety. As the bear lumbers off and your heartbeat returns to normal, your thoughts naturally turn to the acts of visual space perception that you have just performed. You picked a path through the three-dimensional world that brought you to safety. You behaved as though you knew where the trees were. You acted as though you understood how far it was across the stream. All in all, you demonstrated a sophisticated grasp of the layout of the physical world around you.

Humans share this sophistication with a large part of the animal kingdom. Faced with the same bear, a rabbit or deer would have shown a similar grasp of the relevant issues in space perception (without the jeep). The ability to perceive and interact with the structure of space is one of the fundamental goals of the visual system. It is also quite a formidable accomplishment, and in this chapter we'll explore how we do it.

As a starting place, let's assume that the external world exists. This is a philosophical position known as **realism**. It is not the only possibility. The **positivists** note that all you really have to go on is the evidence of your senses, so the world could be nothing more than an elaborate hallucination. For less philosophical elaborations of this viewpoint, we could consult the writings of Philip K. Dick and other science fiction authors; in this book, we'll just assume that there is a real world out there to perceive.

The geometry of that real world is **Euclidean** (named in honor of the ancient Greek geometer Euclid, of the third century BCE). This means that parallel lines remain parallel as they are extended in space, that objects maintain the same size and shape as they move around in the space, that the internal angles of a triangle always add to 180 degrees, and so forth. All that stuff you learned in high school math classes is true in the real world.

Euclidean geometry is not the only geometry. Although the real world is Euclidean, the geometry of retinal images of that world is decidedly *non*-Euclidean. The geometry becomes non-Euclidean when the three-dimensional world is projected onto the curved, two-dimensional surface of the retina. Parallel lines in the world do not necessarily remain parallel in the retinal image, as **Figure 6.1** illustrates. The angles of triangles don't always add up to 180 degrees. The retinal area occupied by an object gets smaller as the object moves farther away from the eyeball. What all this means is that if we want to appreciate the Euclidean world, we have to reconstruct it from non-Euclidean input.

realism A philosophical position arguing that there is a real world to sense.

positivism A philosophical position arguing that all we really have to go on is the evidence of the senses, so the world might be nothing more than an elaborate hallucination.

Euclidean Referring to the geometry of the world, so named in honor of Euclid, the ancient Greek geometer of the third century BCE. In Euclidean geometry, parallel lines remain parallel as they are extended in space, objects maintain the same size and shape as they move around in space, the internal angles of a triangle always add to 180 degrees, and so forth.

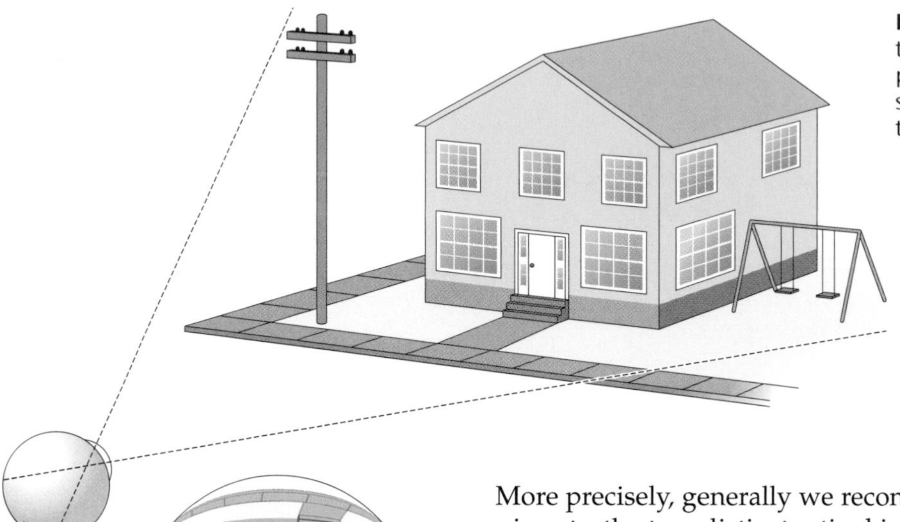

FIGURE 6.1 The Euclidean geometry of the three-dimensional world (where, for example, parallel lines don't converge) turns into something quite different on the curved, two-dimensional retina.

More precisely, generally we reconstruct the world from two non-Euclidean inputs: the two distinct retinal images. Close your left eye, stretch your left arm out in front of you, and hold up your left index finger. Then hold up your right index finger about 6 inches in front of your face, so that it appears to be positioned just to the left of the left index finger (see **Figure 6.2**). Now quickly open your left eye and close your right eye. If you positioned your fingers properly, your right finger will jump to the other side of your left finger. Although this demonstration is designed to exaggerate the different views of your two eyes, the point is a general one: the two retinal images always differ. They differ because the retinas are in slightly different places. Just as you and the person standing next to you see somewhat different views of the world, so do your two eyes. Much of this chapter will be devoted to explaining how the visual system goes to quite elaborate lengths both to exploit and to reconcile these differences.

Why have two eyes at all? Perhaps most fundamentally, having two eyes confers the same evolutionary advantage as having two lungs, two kidneys,

(*a*)

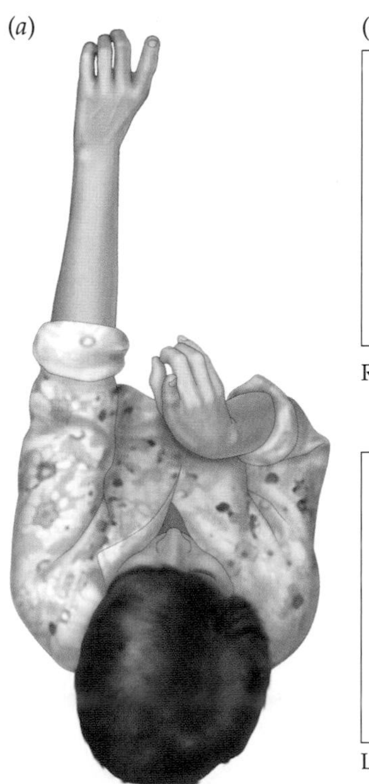

(*b*)

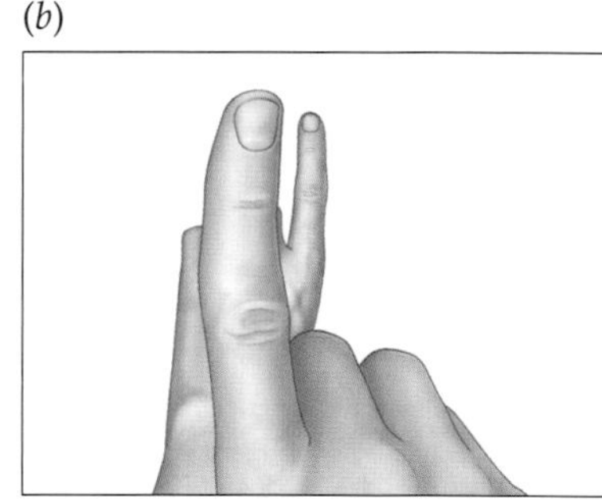

Right retinal image

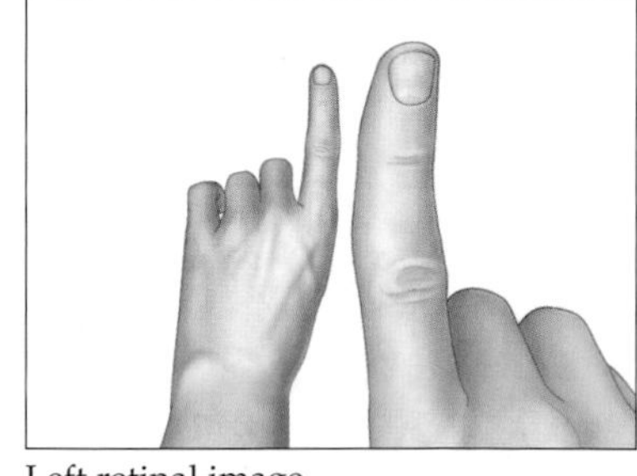

Left retinal image

FIGURE 6.2 The two retinal images of a three-dimensional world are not the same. See the text for details.

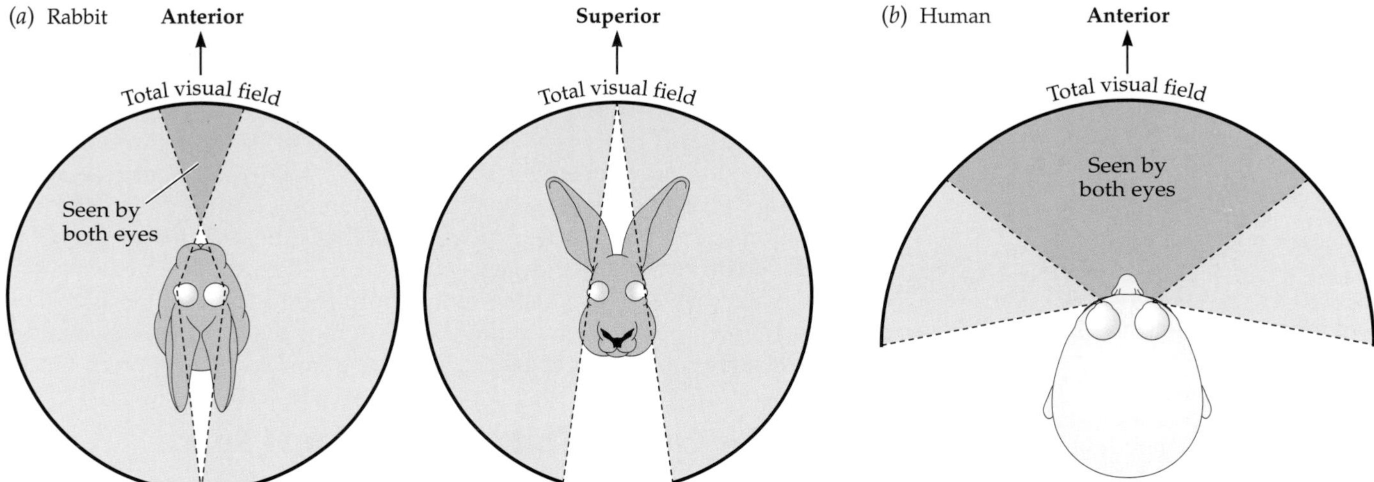

FIGURE 6.3 Visual fields vary, depending on the species. (*a*) A rabbit's visual field is like a planetarium dome (with ears). (*b*) A human visual field is more like a windshield covering a large region in front of the eyes.

and two brain hemispheres: you can lose one eye and still be able to see. A second advantage to doubling the number of eyes is that they enable you to see more of the world. This explains why it is so hard to sneak up on a rabbit. Its visual field actually extends a full 360 degrees (**Figure 6.3***a*), and it can also see straight up (Hughes, 1977).

Our visual field is limited to about 190 degrees from left to right, 110 degrees of which is covered by both eyes (Figure 6.3*b*). The field is more restricted vertically: about 60 degrees up from the center of gaze and 80 degrees down, as was shown in Figure 2.19—limited by the anatomy of cheeks and eyebrows. Overlapping, binocular visual fields give predator animals such as humans a better chance to spot small, fast-moving objects in front of them that might provide dinner (e.g., those rabbits, whose dome-shaped visual fields are adapted to avoid being caught). Having two eyes looking for dinner is rather like having two people looking. If each person had a 50% chance of finding the rabbit and the two people were independent, together they would have a 75% chance. In vision, this **binocular summation** principle may have provided the evolutionary pressure that first moved eyes to the front of some birds' and mammals' faces. Under most circumstances, we do not get such a large benefit from binocular summation. The 50% to 75% benefit assumes two completely independent observers, but the two eyes are still embedded in one person. Nevertheless, you will do better at many tasks with two eyes than you would do with just one (Jones and Lee, 1981).

Once the eyes moved to the front, though, evolution found an additional use for overlapping visual fields. Try this. Take the top off a pen and hold the top in one hand, the pen in the other, about a foot in front of your face. Now, close one eye and try to quickly put the cap on the pen. Repeat the same task with both eyes open. For most (but not all) people, this task is easier with two eyes than with one. This is a quick demonstration of the usefulness of **binocular disparity**—the differences between the two retinal images of the same world. Disparity is the basis for a vivid perception of the three-dimensionality of the world that is not available with purely **monocular** (one-eyed) vision. The technical term for this binocular perception of depth is **stereopsis**. The geometric and physiological bases for stereopsis are the topic of a large portion of this chapter.

When you decide you need a break from reading this chapter, take that break with one eye closed. You should be able to notice the loss of stereopsis (and of part of your visual field), but a period of one-eyed visual experience

binocular summation The combination (or "summation") of signals from each eye in ways that make performance on many tasks better with both eyes than with either eye alone.

binocular disparity The differences between the two retinal images of the same scene. Disparity is the basis for stereopsis, a vivid perception of the three-dimensionality of the world that is not available with monocular vision.

monocular With one eye.

stereopsis The ability to use binocular disparity as a cue to depth.

depth cues Information about the third dimension (depth) of visual space. Depth cues may be monocular or binocular.

monocular depth cue A depth cue that is available even when the world is viewed with one eye alone.

binocular depth cue A depth cue that relies on information from both eyes. Stereopsis is the primary example in humans, but convergence and the ability of two eyes to see more of an object than one eye sees are also binocular depth cues.

occlusion A cue to relative depth order in which, for example, one object obstructs the view of part of another object.

will also make it clear that stereopsis is not a necessary condition for depth perception or space perception. Rabbits do very well with very little binocular vision, and painters and movie directors manage to convey realistic impressions of depth on flat canvases and movie screens. On the other hand, stereopsis does add a richness to the perception of the three-dimensional world, as vividly described by Oliver Sacks (2006) in his article about "Stereo Sue," a neuroscientist who regained stereopsis at the age of 48.

Returning from your break, you will find that a description of the set of **monocular depth cues** to three-dimensional space is the first major topic of this chapter. After that, we turn to the more complicated topic of the **binocular depth cue** of stereopsis. Then, in the last section of the chapter, we consider how the various cues are combined to produce a unified perception of space.

Monocular Cues to Three-Dimensional Space

M. C. Escher (1898–1972) titled the picture at the start of this chapter *Relativity*. Escher was a master of the rules that govern our perception of space. Each bit of stairway, each landing, every person is drawn using cues that enable us to infer three dimensions from two. However, when we try to follow those stairs, we find that Escher's drawing cleverly fails to add up to a coherent representation of a place that could exist. Even when no one is trying to fool us, it is geometrically impossible (not to mention computationally infeasible) for the visual system to create a perfectly faithful reconstruction of Euclidean space, given the non-Euclidean input we receive through our eyes. The best we can do is to use depth cues to infer aspects of the three-dimensional world from our two-dimensional retinal images. On the basis of the retinal images and an implicit understanding of physics and geometry, each cue provides a hint about the likely structure of the space in front of us and the disposition of objects in that space.

Unless we are stuck in an extremely impoverished perceptual environment (say, the Sahara desert during a sandstorm), every view of the world provides multiple depth cues. Usually the cues reinforce each other, combining to produce a convincing and reliable representation of the three-dimensional world. Occasionally, however, the cues are contradictory. Escher could fool us by deliberately manipulating depth cues and other routine visual inferences. He arranges sensible local cues into a globally implausible story. What cues does the visual system use to infer depth relations, and how do we use those cues to create a representation of the three-dimensional world? (See Web Activity 6.1: Monocular Depth Cues.)

Occlusion

FIGURE 6.4 Occlusion makes it easy to infer relative position in depth.

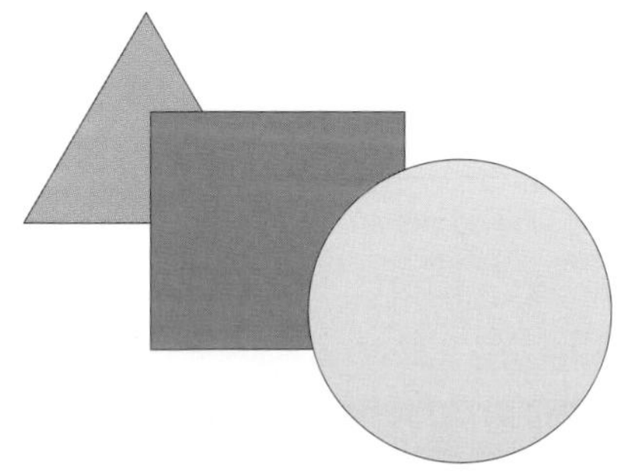

Some of the cues to the layout of the three-dimensional world were introduced earlier in this book, because hints to the layout of space can also be hints about the structure of objects in that space. **Occlusion** is an example (see the section titled "Finding Edges" in Chapter 4). In Chapter 4, occlusion was a cue to the presence of an otherwise invisible edge. As a depth cue, occlusion gives information about the relative position of objects. Thus, in **Figure 6.4** we are happy to infer a circle in front of a square in front of a triangle. Occlusion is present in almost every visual scene (we challenge you to find a situation in normal life where nothing blocks your view of anything else), and many researchers argue that it is the most reliable of all the depth cues. It is wrong only in the case of "accidental viewpoints" (remember those from Chapter 4?). That is, the retinal image shown in Figure 6.4 could be produced by a circle and two oddly shaped puzzle pieces, as shown in

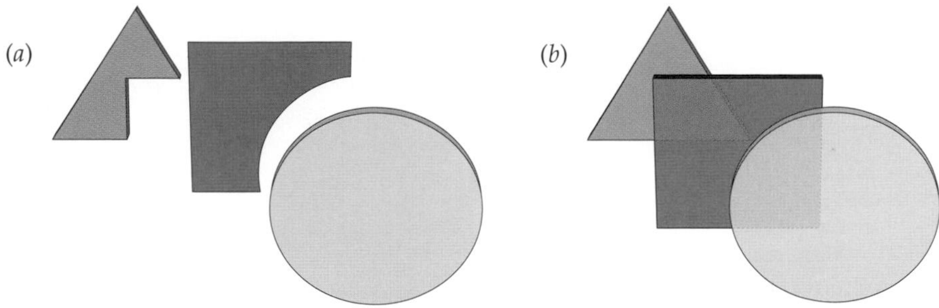

FIGURE 6.5 Figure 6.4 could be an "accidental" (unlikely) view of the pieces shown here in (*a*). It is much more likely, however, that it is a generic view of circle, square, and triangle, as shown in (*b*).

Figure 6.5*a*. That scenario would require careful placement of the objects and the viewer. It is much more likely that Figure 6.4 would arise from a more generic view of a circle occluding a square occluding a triangle (Figure 6.5*b*).

We do not know from the occlusion cue alone if the red square in Figure 6.4 is in front of a small green triangle, a larger but more distant triangle (maybe a green tree), or an even larger but even more distant green mountain. Occlusion is a **nonmetrical depth cue**; it just gives us the relative orderings of occluders and occludees. A **metrical depth cue** is one that does provide information about distance in the third dimension.

nonmetrical depth cue A depth cue that provides information about the depth order (relative depth) but not depth magnitude (e.g., his nose is in front of his face).

metrical depth cue A depth cue that provides quantitative information about distance in the third dimension.

projective geometry For purposes of studying perception of the three-dimensional world, the geometry that describes the transformations that occur when the three-dimensional world is *projected* onto a two dimensional surface. For example, parallel lines do not converge in the world, but they do in the two-dimensional projection.

relative size A comparison of size between items without knowing the absolute size of either one.

Size and Position Cues

The image on the retina formed by an object out in the world gets smaller as the object gets farther away. (See Web Activity 3.1: Visual Angle for a review.) Moreover, your visual system knew this fact of **projective geometry** implicitly before you ever picked up this book and learned it explicitly. Projective geometry describes how the world is *projected* onto a surface. For example, a shadow is a projection of an object onto a surface. An implicit understanding of the rules of projective geometry can be said to undergird many of the depth cues described here. In this case, the visual system knows that, all else being equal, smaller things are farther away. Hence, the plasticine balls in **Figure 6.6** may appear to lie in different depth planes. We can call this depth cue **relative size**.

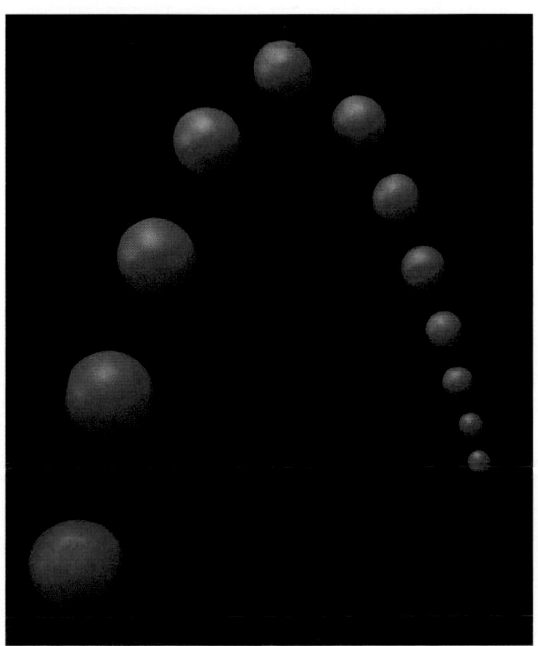

FIGURE 6.6 All of these plasticine balls are resting on the same surface; the small ones appear to be farther away. Some portion of the visual system assumes that all of these items are the same. If one ball projects a smaller image on the retina and if the balls really are the same size, then the smaller one must be farther away. This is the cue of relative size.

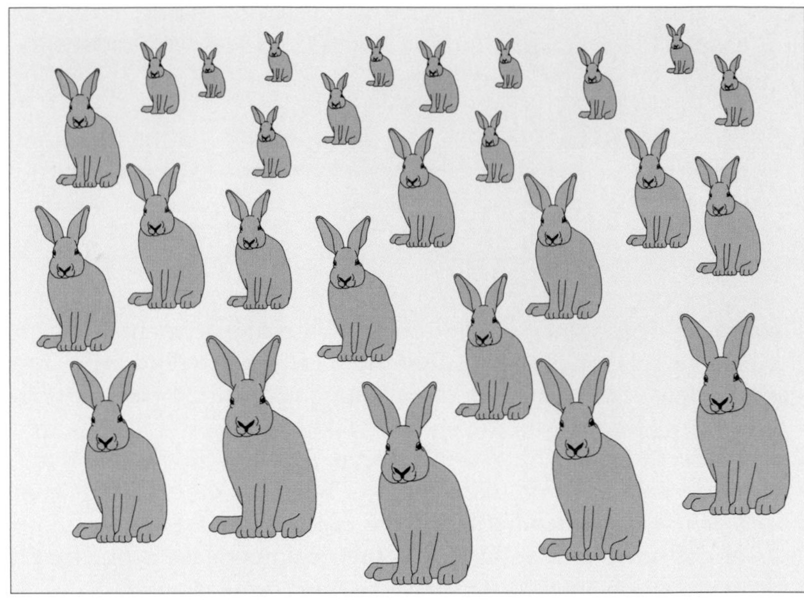

FIGURE 6.7 This rabbit texture gradient shows that the size cue is more effective when size changes systematically.

texture gradient A depth cue based on the geometric fact that items of the same size form smaller images when they are farther away. An array of items that change in size across the image will appear to form a surface in depth.

relative height As a depth cue, the observation that objects at different distances from the viewer on the ground plane will form images at different heights in the retinal image. Objects farther away will be seen as higher in the image.

The impression of three-dimensionality in **Figure 6.7** is more powerful than that in Figure 6.6 because we have added another cue. The critical difference is in the organization of the objects in the two figures. In Figure 6.7, the rabbits form an orderly **texture gradient**, with larger objects in one area and smaller objects in another. Because smaller is interpreted as farther away, this arrangement creates the perception of a ground plane receding into the distance.

In **Figure 6.8**, the rabbits are again arrayed in an orderly texture, but here we get less of a sense of depth. The difference between Figures 6.8 and 6.9 is that the former includes another depth cue that is not present in the latter: **relative height**. Imagine that that you're actually standing in a field of rabbits. Consider the rabbit at your feet (**Figure 6.9**). It will project its image in your lower visual field. The smaller image of a more distant rabbit will be

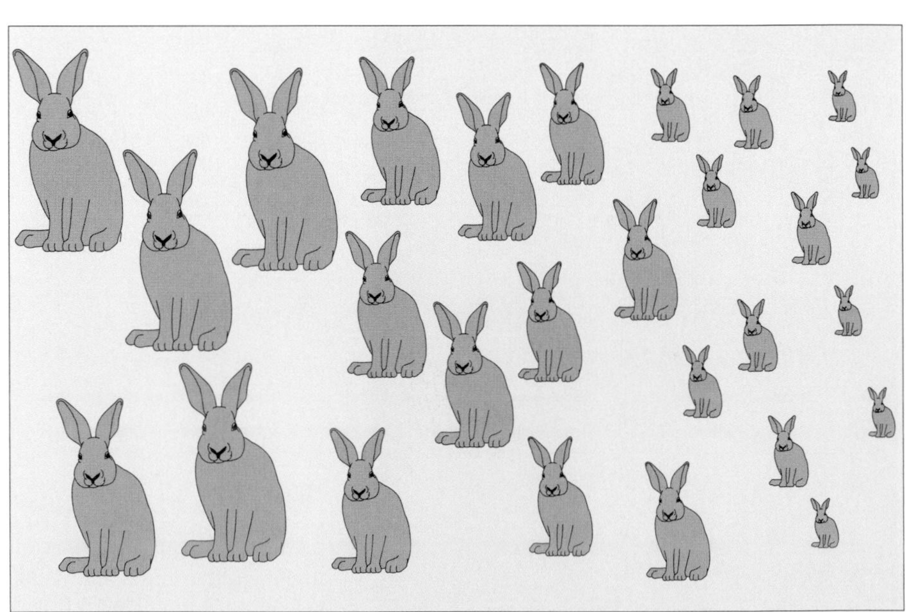

FIGURE 6.8 Organized differently, this illustration of the same rabbits as those shown in Figure 6.7 does not produce the same sense of depth. A size cue is most effective when it is consistent with an object arranged on the ground, not on a wall.

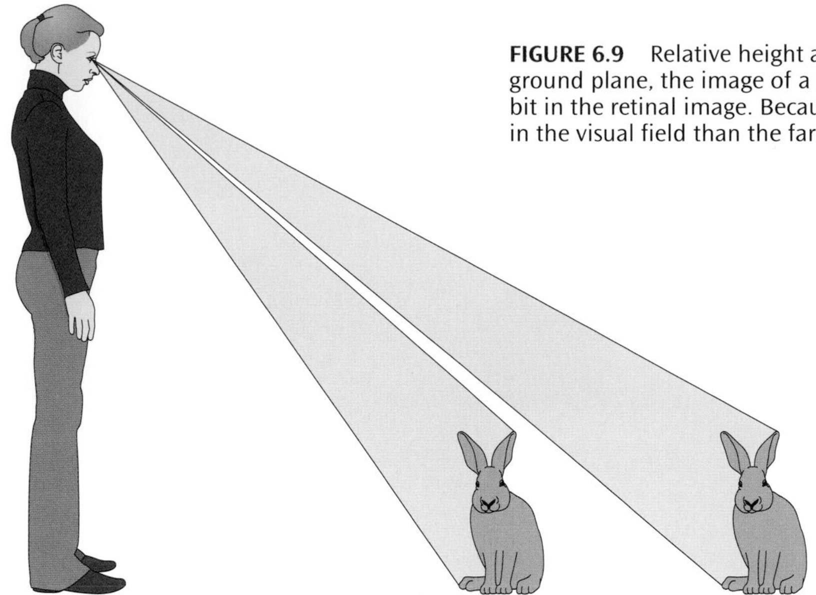

FIGURE 6.9 Relative height as a cue to depth. If we are looking down at the ground plane, the image of a closer rabbit will lie above the image of a farther rabbit in the retinal image. Because the image is inverted, the closer rabbit lies lower in the visual field than the farther rabbit.

projected higher in the visual field. Here, then, is another geometric regularity produced by projective geometry that the visual system can exploit: for objects on the ground plane, objects that are more distant are higher in the visual field.

Texture fields that provide an impression of three-dimensionality are really combinations of relative size and relative height cues. Like the metaphor of perceptual committees in Chapter 4, this is a case in which multiple cues interact to produce a final perception. **Figure 6.10** shows how this interaction can give rise to a size illusion. The little rabbits in the top center and lower right of the figure are actually the same physical size on the page, but the one at the bottom looks smaller to most of us than the one at the top. Why? We infer, on the basis of relative height, that the rabbit at the bottom must be closer. If it is closer and it forms an image of the same size as the little rabbit at the top, it follows that the little rabbit at the bottom must be really little.

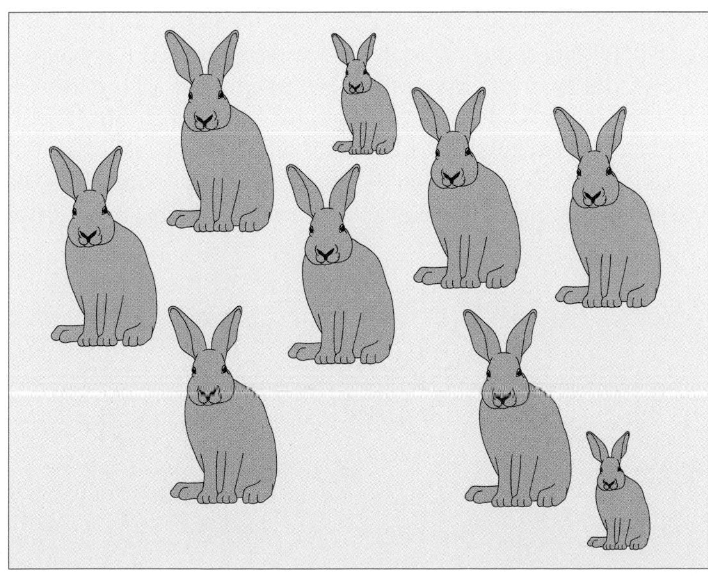

FIGURE 6.10 The two smaller rabbits in the image are the same size. Why don't they look the same size?

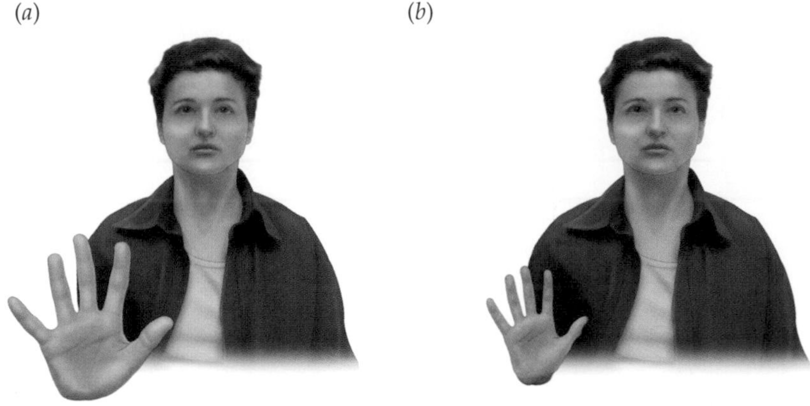

FIGURE 6.11 The cue of familiar size. The hand in (*a*) looks closer than the one in (*b*) because we know how big hands should be relative to heads.

familiar size A depth cue based on knowledge of the typical size of objects like humans or pennies.

relative metrical depth cue A depth cue that could specify, for example, that object A was twice as far away as object B without providing information about the absolute distance to either A or B.

absolute metrical depth cue A depth cue that provides absolute information about the distance in the third dimension (e.g., his nose sticks out 4 centimeters in front of his face).

If we know what size something *ought* to be, that knowledge can be a depth cue in its own right. We infer that the woman in **Figure 6.11***a* is holding her hand out at the end of an outstretched arm. Why do we make this guess? One alternative is that she is holding her hand near her shoulder, as in Figure 6.11*b*. But if that were the case in Figure 6.11*a*, the hand would need to be a *very* big hand. Here, our knowledge of the normal relationship of hand size to head size makes all the difference. This is the depth cue of **familiar size**.

Recall that occlusion is a nonmetrical cue, providing only depth *order*. The relative size and relative height cues, especially taken together, provide some metrical information. This is illustrated in **Figure 6.12**, where the three balls appear to lie at measurable distances from each other. The red and blue balls seem closer in depth than the blue and green, for example. Relative size and height do not tell us the *exact* distance to an object or between objects. These are **relative metrical depth cues**. Familiar size, however, could be an **absolute metrical depth cue**. If your visual system knew the actual size of an object and the visual angle of the object's projection on the retina, it could (at least in theory) calculate the exact distance from object to eye. In practice, however, even if you know that your friend is 5 feet 10 inches tall, the visual system does not seem to know that fact with a precision that would let you know he is standing exactly 12 feet away.

Aerial Perspective

In addition to its implicit knowledge of geometry and its learned knowledge of familiar size, the visual system "knows" about properties of the atmosphere. The triangles in **Figure 6.13***a* give only a faint sense of depth, if any. They are just an array of identical shapes. Adding some grayscale information, however, as in Figure 6.13*b*, provides the impression of something like a mountain range receding in the distance. More specifically, the fainter

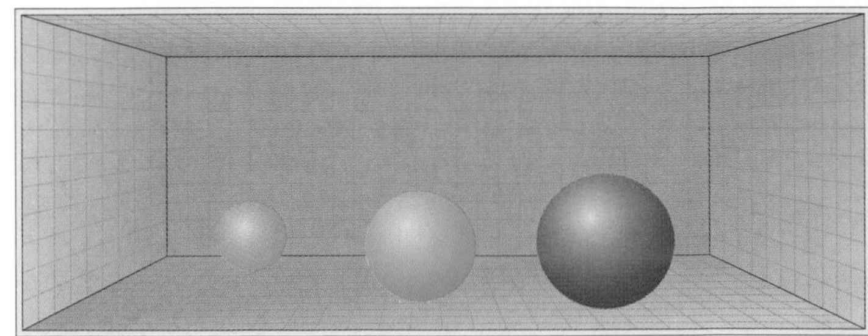

FIGURE 6.12 The metrical cues of relative size and height can tell the visual system more than a nonmetrical cue like occlusion can. Not only does the red sphere in this image appear to be closest and the green sphere farthest away, but also the blue sphere is seen to be closer to the red sphere than it is to the green sphere.

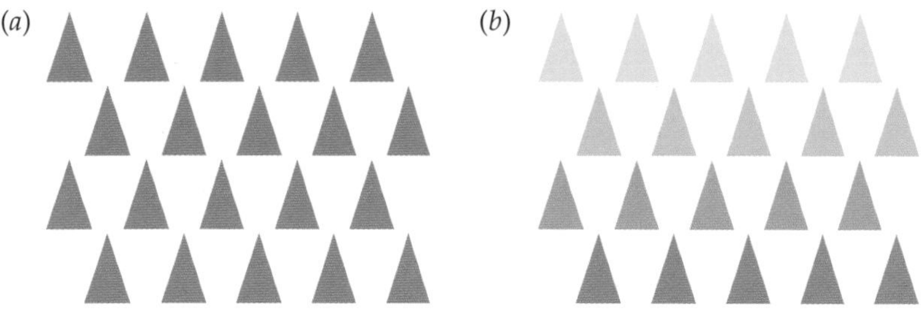

FIGURE 6.13 The triangles seem to recede into depth more in (*b*) than in (*a*). The depth cue here is called "haze" or "aerial perspective."

mountains (triangles) may appear to be farther away than the darker ones. The depth cue at work here relies on an implicit understanding that light is scattered by the atmosphere, and that more light is scattered when we look through more atmosphere. Thus, more distant objects are subject to more scatter and appear fainter and less distinct. This cue is known as **haze** or **aerial perspective**. **Figure 6.14** shows a real-world example. Short wavelengths (blue) are scattered more than medium and long wavelengths. This is why the sky looks blue and why more distant objects look not only hazy, but bluish. The real image gives a stronger sense of depth. By now, it should be clear that this effect results from the inclusion of other depth cues beyond the blue haze. Note the occlusion and the known size of trees and swans.

aerial perspective (or haze) A depth cue based on the implicit understanding that light is scattered by the atmosphere. More light is scattered when we look through more atmosphere. Thus, more distant objects are subject to more scatter and appear fainter, bluer, and less distinct.

linear perspective A depth cue based on the fact that lines that are parallel in the three-dimensional world will appear to converge in a two-dimensional image.

Linear Perspective

In the six lines shown in **Figure 6.15**, it is not difficult to see a simple representation of the view out the windshield of a car moving down a road in a flat landscape. The depth cue in this case, **linear perspective**, is based on the rules that determine how lines in three-dimensional space are projected onto a two-dimensional image. The core piece of projective geometry in this case

FIGURE 6.14 A real-world example of aerial perspective. Scattering of light by the atmosphere makes more distant features appear hazy and blue.

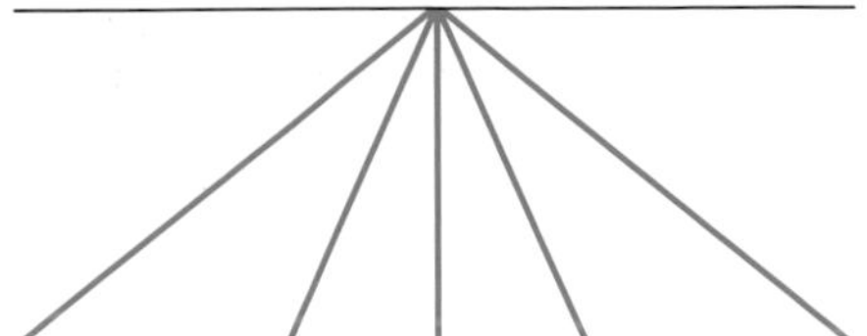

FIGURE 6.15 Linear perspective. If we titled this image "Driving across Kansas," you would understand because the converging lines give the impression of parallel lines receding toward the horizon.

is that lines that are parallel in the three-dimensional world will appear to converge in the two-dimensional image, except when the parallel lines lie in a plane that is parallel to the plane of the two-dimensional image. Thus, if we were standing in front of the closed door in **Figure 6.16***a*, the parallel sides of that door would remain parallel in the retinal image. If we opened the door onto a hallway, however, the parallel lines formed by the walls, floor, and ceiling would converge in the two-dimensional retinal image as they receded into the distance in the three-dimensional world (Figure 6.16*b*). Indeed, if the hall went back far enough, the walls, floor, and ceiling would seem to meet at a point called the **vanishing point**.

Like texture gradients, linear perspective can be seen as a special case of the relative size and height cues. Assuming that the five blue lines in Figure 6.15 are parallel in three dimensions is tantamount to assuming that the distance between the lines remains constant. But the retinal distance between the lines is larger at the bottom of the image and smaller at the top. Therefore, the lines must be farther away at the top of the image than at the bottom. Like the relative size and height cues, linear perspective provides relative, but not absolute, metrical depth information.

Pictorial Depth Cues and Pictures

As a group, the depth cues discussed so far are known as the **pictorial depth cues**. These are the cues produced by the projection of the three-dimensional world onto the two-dimensional surface of the retina. A realistic picture or photograph is the result of projecting the three-dimensional world onto the two-dimensional surface of film or canvas. When that image is viewed from the correct position, the retinal image (in one eye, at least) formed by the two-dimensional picture will be the same as the retinal image that would have been formed by the three-dimensional world, and hence we see depth in the picture. In theory, this means that a picture should look correct from only one, precise viewing position. In fact, pictures look reasonable over quite a range of views. Were this not so, there would be only one good seat in the movie theater.

To correctly interpret the shape of three-dimensional objects from two-dimensional pictures, people take the orientation of the flat surface of the image into account so that they can understand both that the picture is, in fact, a picture and not the real thing and, at the same time, calculate an accurate

vanishing point The apparent point at which parallel lines receding in depth converge.

pictorial depth cue A cue to distance or depth used by artists to depict three-dimensional depth in two-dimensional pictures.

(*a*)

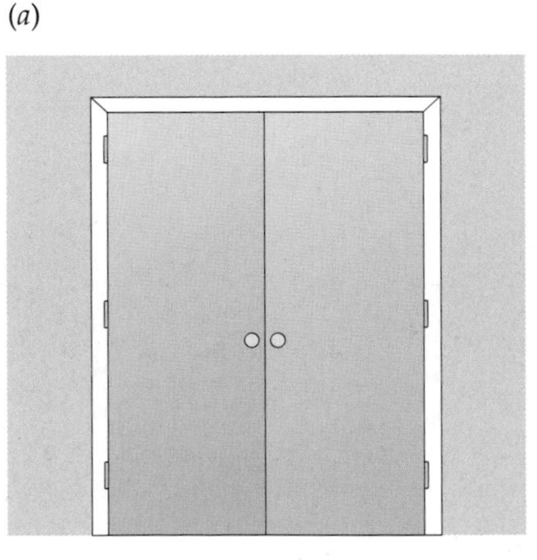

(*b*)

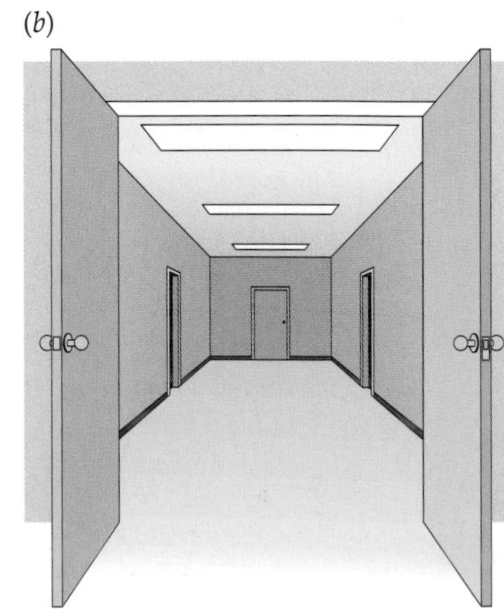

FIGURE 6.16 Parallel lines in the image plane, such as those defining the door in (*a*), remain parallel in the image. But parallel lines in other planes, such as the ground, ceiling, and side walls in the hall in (*b*), converge as they recede into the distance.

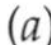

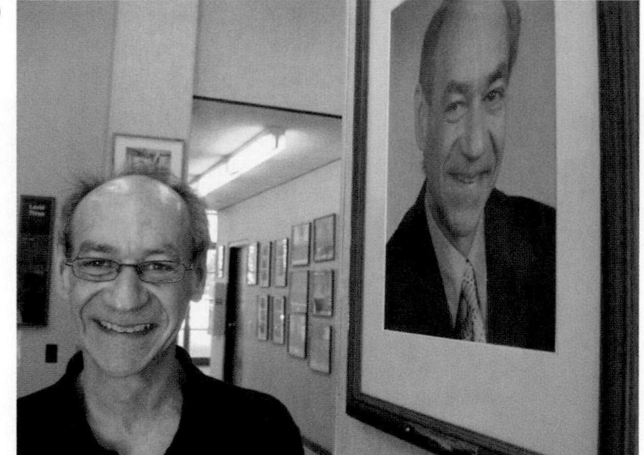

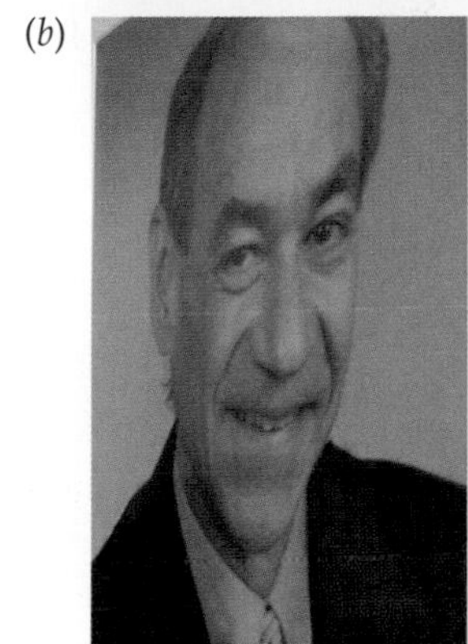

FIGURE 6.17 Picture in a picture. (*a*) One of the authors, Dennis Levi, is seen standing next to a photograph of himself. In this panel the "picture in the picture" appears reasonable. (*b*) The framed picture, isolated without the context. Does the picture appear distorted? (Courtesy of Martin S. Banks.)

impression of the thing that is portrayed (Vishwanath, Girshik, and Banks, 2005). To illustrate this point, Marty Banks snapped the photo of a guy standing alongside a picture of himself shown in **Figure 6.17***a*; here the "picture in the picture" appears reasonable. When isolated without the context, however, the framed picture appears distorted (Figure 6.17*b*), showing that our visual system compensates for the perceptual distortion in the first picture, where the context enables us to take the orientation of the surface into account.

Artists and photographers sometimes use a technique know as **anamorphosis** or **anamorphic projection**. In anamorphic projection, the rules of linear perspective are pushed to an extreme in which the projection of three dimensions into two creates a picture that is recognizable only from an unusual vantage point (or sometimes with a curved mirror). The results are known as "anamorphic art." In Hans Holbein's sixteenth-century painting *The Ambassadors* (**Figure 6.18***a*), the odd

anamorphosis (or anamorphic projection) Use of the rules of linear perspective to create a two-dimensional image so distorted that it looks correct only when viewed from a special angle or with a mirror that counters the distortion.

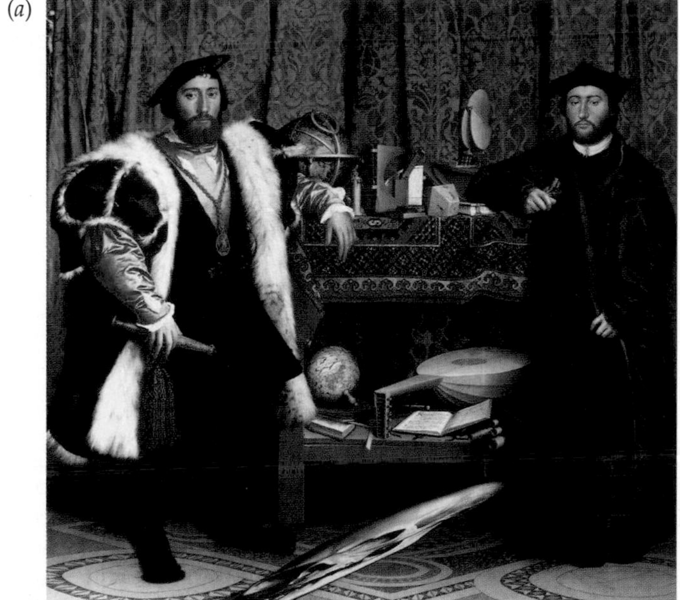

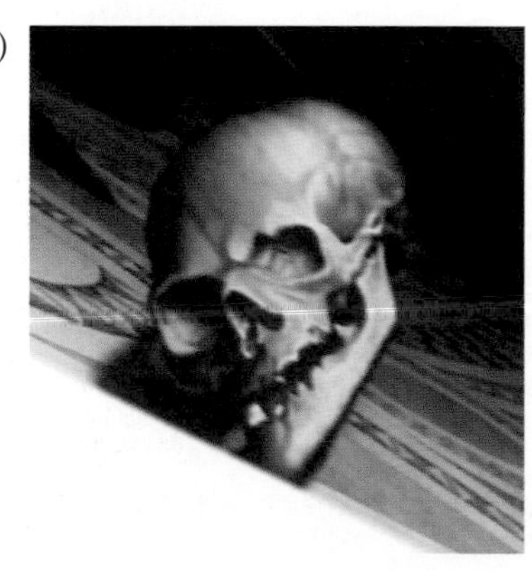

FIGURE 6.18 In 1533, Hans Holbein painted the double portrait in (*a*) with an odd object at the feet of the two men. Viewed from the correct position (*b*), the object proves to be a skull, making it an example of anamorphic art. No one is sure why Holbein put the anamorphic skull in the picture. Maybe it is intended as a reminder that we all must die, or maybe he included it just to show off his abilities.

(a)

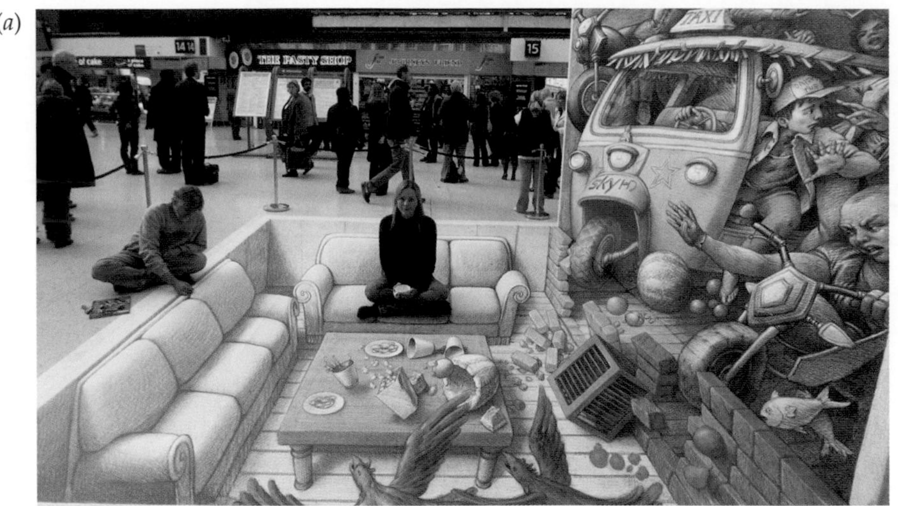

(b)

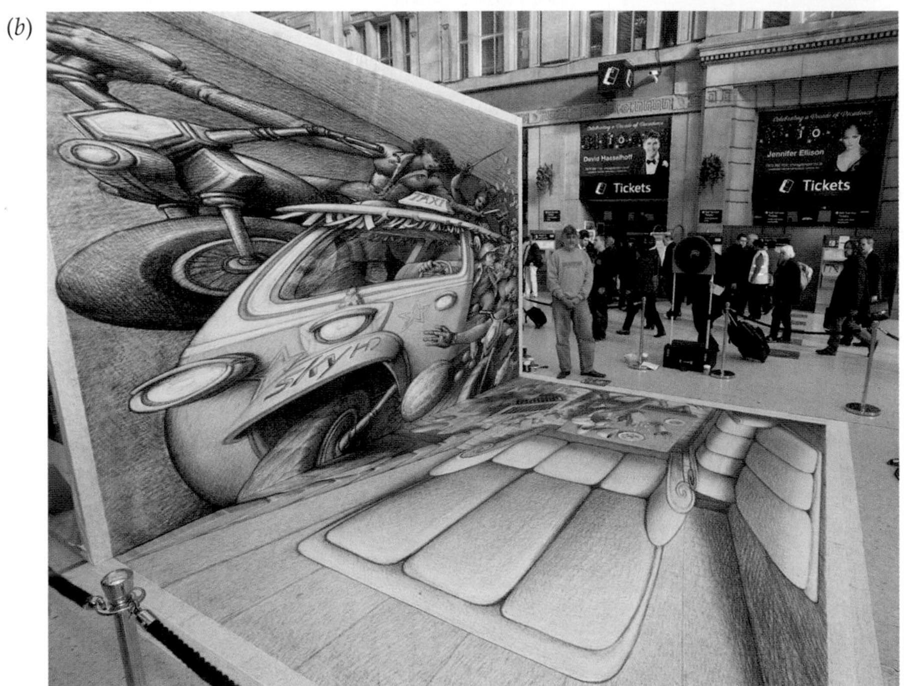

FIGURE 6.19 Modern-day anamorphic art. (*a*) In this photograph, it looks like a young woman is sitting in a pit on the sidewalk. But, as shown in (*b*), this is just a clever bit of anamorphic art by street artist Kurt Wenner. It is just a flat image that looks three-dimensional when viewed from the correct position.

diagonal smear at lower center proves to be a skull when correctly viewed (Figure 6.18*b*). In our own day, the sidewalk chalk artist Kurt Wenner creates amazing anamorphic images that look spectacularly real from the right vantage point and spectacularly distorted from elsewhere (**Figure 6.19**). More on the role of pictorial depth cues in art can be found in **Web Essay 6.1: Making the Implicit Explicit**.

Motion Cues

motion parallax An important depth cue that is based on head movement. The geometric information obtained from an eye in two different positions at two different times is similar to the information from two eyes in different positions in the head at the same time.

Beyond the pictorial depth cues, a number of additional sources of information are available to our visual system when we view real-world scenes that cannot be reproduced in a static two-dimensional picture. The first nonpictorial depth cue we will discuss is **motion parallax**. To appreciate its power (and to understand why photographs of the forest often don't come out

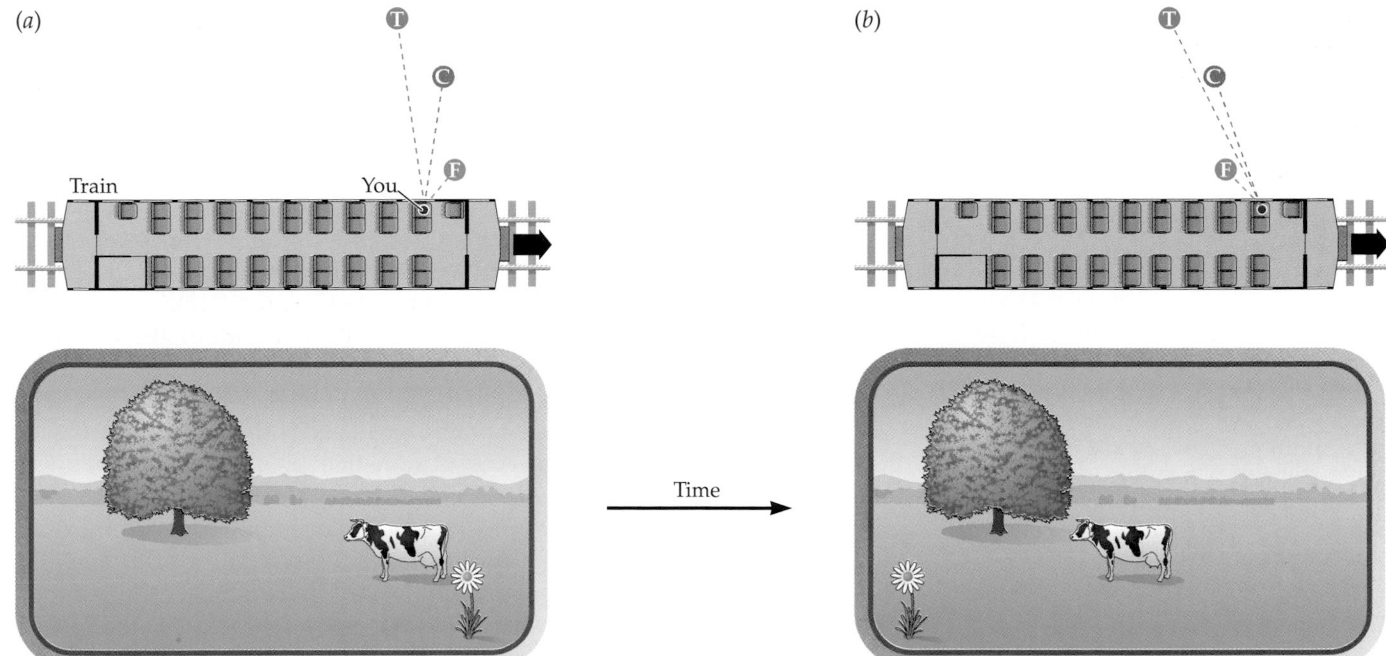

FIGURE 6.20 Motion parallax. As you look out the window of a moving train, objects closer to you (the flower in this illustration) shift position more quickly than objects farther away (the tree) from one moment (*a*) to the next (*b*). This regularity can be exploited as a depth cue.

well), the best thing to do is to go outside and lie under a tree. Gaze up into the branches and leaves with one eye covered and your head stationary. You will notice that leaves and branches form a relatively flat texture. You can see all the details, but you may have trouble deciding if one little branch lies in front of or behind another. If you open the other eye, stereopsis (introduced earlier and discussed in detail later in the chapter) will allow the branches and leaves to fill out a three-dimensional volume that was lacking before. Close the eye and the volume collapses again. Now, move your head from side to side, and motion parallax will restore the sense of depth.

How does motion provide a cue for depth? Suppose you're sitting on a train, looking out the window at the countryside. At one instant you see the scene sketched in **Figure 6.20***a*. A moment later, the scene has changed to the one in Figure 6.20*b*. Notice that, as your train moved from left to right in the figure, all the objects shifted from right to left. But note that some things shifted more than others. The flower moved almost all the way across your retinal image, the cow moved a much shorter distance, and the tree hardly changed positions at all. The term *parallax* refers to the geometric relationship revealed here: when your eyes move, objects closer to you shift position more than objects farther away when you change your viewpoint. Of course, you don't need to be on a train; just moving your head will do. The geometric information obtained from an eye in two different positions at two different times (motion parallax) is similar to the information by two eyes in different positions in the head at the same time (stereopsis) (Durgin et al., 1995; Rogers and Collett, 1989).

Motion parallax provides relative metrical information about how far away objects are; and as the experiment with the tree branches proves, it can provide a compelling sense of depth in some situations in which other cues are not very effective. The downside of motion parallax is that it works only if the head moves (just moving the eyes back and forth won't do, as you can easily prove to yourself). Now you know why a cat might bob her head back and forth as she plans a spectacular leap from the sofa to the table.

accommodation The process by which the eye changes its focus (in which the lens gets fatter as gaze is directed toward nearer objects).

convergence The ability of the two eyes to turn inward, often used in order to place the two images of a feature in the world on corresponding locations in the two retinal images (typically on the fovea of each eye). Convergence reduces the disparity of that feature to zero (or nearly zero).

divergence The ability of the two eyes to turn outward, often used in order to place the two images of a feature in the world on corresponding locations in the two retinal images (typically on the fovea of each eye). Divergence reduces the disparity of that feature to zero (or nearly zero).

Accommodation and Convergence

Like a camera, the eyes need to be focused to see objects at different distances clearly. As we learned in Chapter 2, the human eye focuses via a process called **accommodation**, in which the lens gets fatter as we direct our gaze toward nearer objects. We also have to point our eyes differently to focus on objects at different distances. As the disembodied eyeballs in **Figure 6.21** move from the red dot to the blue dot, they rotate inward—a process called **convergence** (Figure 6.21*a*); refocusing on the red dot would require rotation outward, which is known as **divergence** (Figure 6.21*b*).

If we could monitor our state of accommodation and/or the extent to which our eyes were converged, we could use this information as a cue to the depth of the object we were trying to bring into focus: the more we have to converge and the more the lens has to bulge in order to focus on the object, the closer it is. When we focus on objects more than about 2 to 3 meters away, the lens is as thin as it can get and the eyes are diverged about as much as possible, so neither cue provides much useful information. But careful studies have shown that the visual system takes advantage of both cues for objects closer than this limit. Convergence is used more than accommodation (Fisher and Ciuffreda, 1988; Owens, 1987). Moreover, these cues are the only ones besides familiar size that can tell us the *exact* distance to an object. Chameleons, for example, use the absolute metrical depth information from convergence to catch prey insects with their sticky tongues (Harkness, 1977).

Binocular Vision and Stereopsis

As defined earlier, the term *binocular disparity* refers to differences between the images falling on our two retinas, and *stereopsis* refers to the impression of three-dimensionality—of objects "popping out in depth"—that most humans get when they view real-world objects with both eyes. Like the accounts of other depth cues, the story of the route from binocular disparity to stereopsis is a story of the visual system exploiting the regularities of projective geometry to recover the three-dimensional world from its projections, this time, onto two two-dimensional surfaces. We will illustrate the transla-

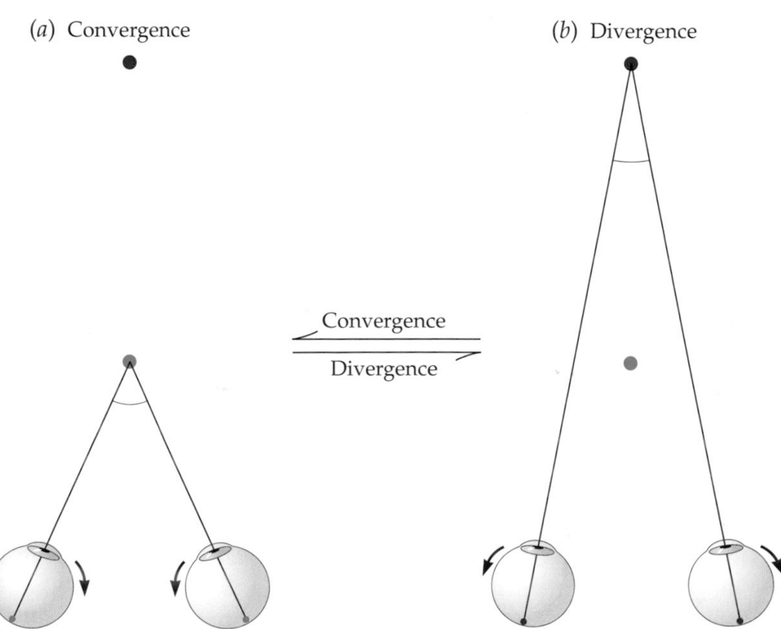

FIGURE 6.21 Vergence. (*a*) As we shift focus from a far to a near point, our eyes converge. (*b*) As we go from near to far, the eyes diverge.

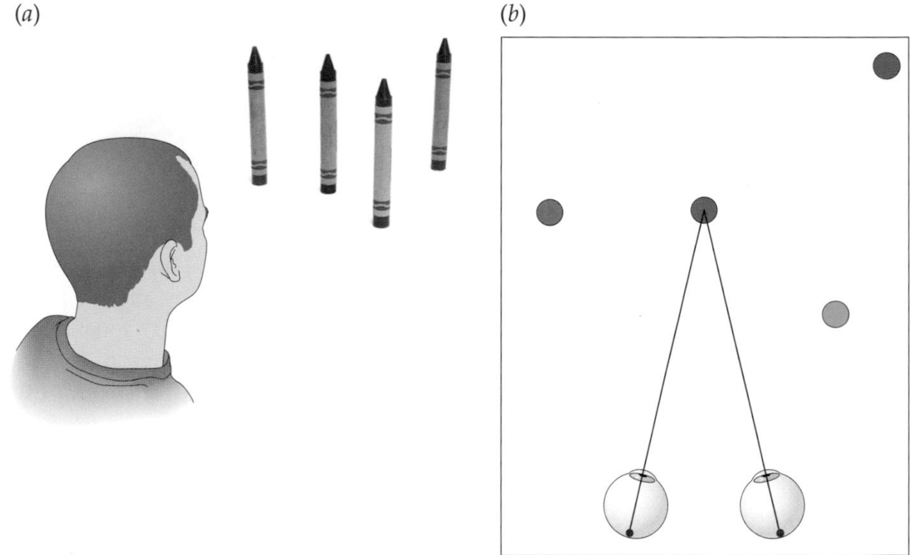

FIGURE 6.22 This simple visual scene illustrates how geometric regularities are exploited by the visual system to achieve stereopsis from binocular disparity. (*a*) The viewer, Bob, is assumed to be fixating his gaze on the red crayon. (*b*) This top view traces the rays of light bouncing off the red crayon onto Bob's retinas.

tion from disparity to stereopsis using the situation shown in **Figure 6.22***a*, in which the viewer (call him Bob) is facing a scene that includes four colored crayons at different depths. Suppose that Bob is focusing his gaze on the red crayon, as shown in Figure 6.22*b*. The two lines in this figure trace the paths of the light rays that reflect off the red crayon and onto Bob's two retinas. (Bob's experiences with crayon scenes are also demonstrated in Web Activity 6.2: Binocular Disparity.)

corresponding retinal points A geometric concept stating that points on the retina of each eye where the monocular retinal images of a single object are formed are at the same distance from the fovea in each eye. The two foveas are also corresponding points.

Because the visual system is designed so that the object of our gaze *always* falls on the fovea, the rays from the red crayon fall on the fovea in each of Bob's eyes. **Figure 6.23** shows the retinal images for the crayons in each eye. The red crayon is in the center of both images. We've added a narrow vertical line behind this crayon in each image to emphasize the fact that this is the location of the fovea.

Now consider the retinal images of the blue crayon. Because the optics of the eye reverse the retinal image, the blue crayon on the right side of the scene falls on the left side of the two retinal images. In our imaginary scene, the blue crayon is placed so that the monocular retinal images of that crayon are formed at the same distance from the fovea in each eye. We say that this crayon's images fall on **corresponding retinal points**. The same can be said of the images of the red crayon, which fall on the two foveas.

In fact, any object lying on the imaginary circle that runs through the two eyeballs and the object on which Bob is fixated should project to correspon-

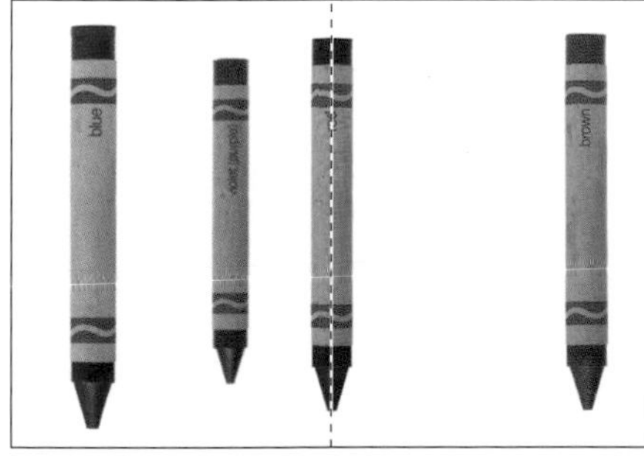

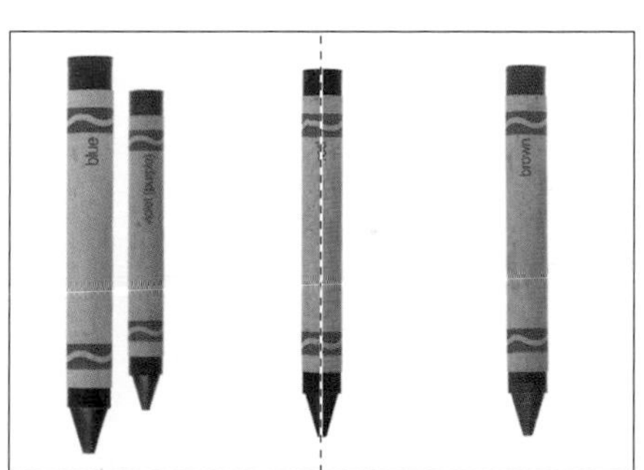

FIGURE 6.23 The overlapping portions of the images falling on Bob's left and right retinas. Because the retinal image is reversed, the blue and purple crayons on the right side of the scene project to the left side of each retina, whereas the brown crayon on the left side of the scene projects to the right side of each retina. The size differences between the retinal images of the crayons in the two retinas are exaggerated in this figure compared to the differences we would observe if we saw this scene in the real world.

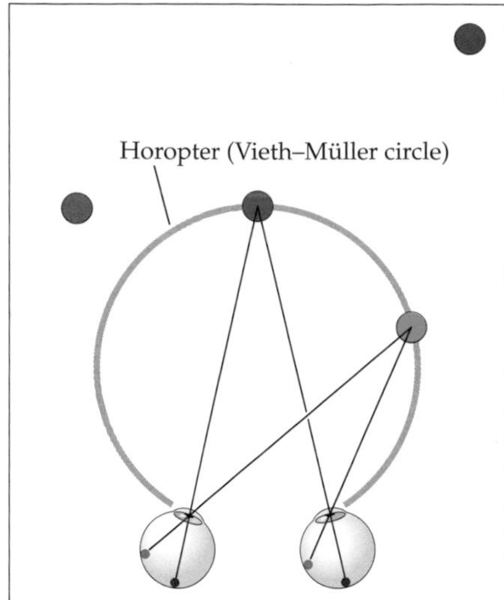

FIGURE 6.24 Bob is still gazing at the red crayon. This view from above traces the light rays reflecting from the red and blue crayons onto Bob's retinas. The blue crayon projects to corresponding retinal points—positions that are equidistant from and on the same side of the fovea. The same would be true of any object falling on the gray line shown in the figure. (The horopter and Vieth–Müller circle are not exactly the same, but they would be very similar in this case.)

ding retinal points. This imaginary circle, called the **Vieth–Müller circle**, is drawn in gray in **Figure 6.24**. Objects that fall on corresponding retinal locations are said to have zero binocular disparity. If the two eyes are looking at one spot (such as the red crayon), then there will be a surface of zero disparity running through that spot. That surface is known as the **horopter**. Any object placed on that imaginary surface in the world will form images on corresponding retinal locations. As it happens, the horopter and the Vieth–Müller circle are not quite the same. If you are *extremely* fond of rather complicated geometry, you may want to pursue this topic (Howard and Rogers, 1995, 2001; Tyler, 1991). Otherwise, the important point is that there is a surface of zero disparity whose position in the world depends on the current state of convergence of the eyes.

Vieth–Müller circle The location of objects whose images fall on geometrically corresponding points in the two retinas. If life were simple, this circle would be the horopter, but life is not simple.

horopter The location of objects whose images lie on corresponding points. The surface of zero disparity.

diplopia Double vision. If visible in both eyes, stimuli falling outside of Panum's fusional area will appear diplopic.

Panum's fusional area The region of space, in front of and behind the horopter, within which binocular single vision is possible.

Objects that lie on the horopter are seen as single objects when viewed with both eyes. Objects significantly closer to or farther away from the surface of zero disparity form images on decidedly noncorresponding points in the two eyes, and we see two of each of those objects. This double vision is known as **diplopia**. Objects that are close to the horopter but not quite on it can still be seen as single objects. This region of space in front of and behind the horopter, within which binocular single vision is possible, is known as **Panum's fusional area** (Panum, 1940).

Armed with this terminology, let's return to Bob and his crayons. Consider the retinal images of the brown crayon, lying just off the horopter. As Figure 6.23 and the view from above in **Figure 6.25***a* show, rays of light bouncing off this crayon do *not* fall on corresponding retinal points: the crayon's image is farther away from the fovea on the left retina than on the right retina. Rela-

(*a*)

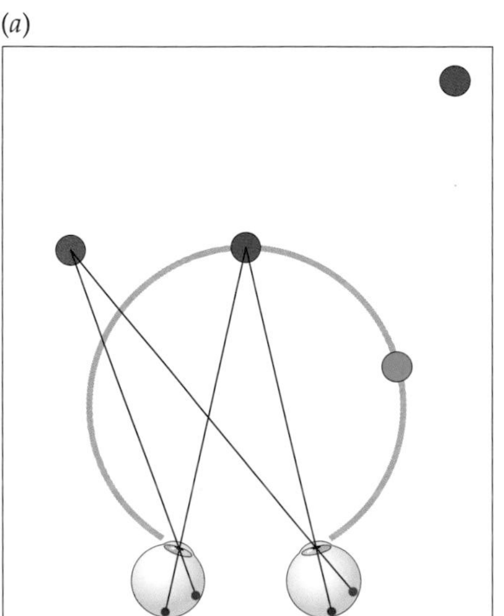

(*b*)

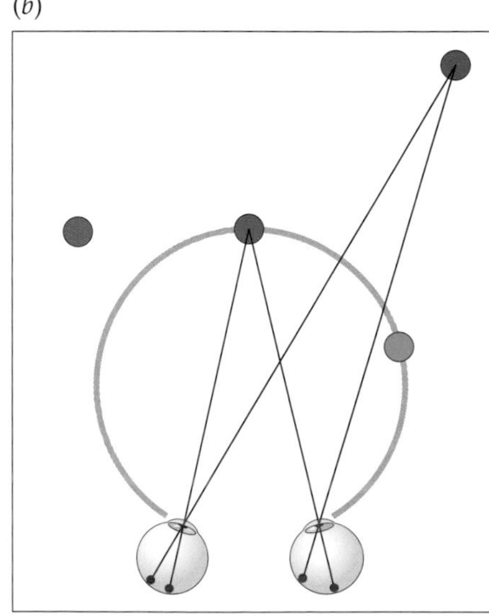

FIGURE 6.25 Light rays projecting from the brown (*a*) and purple (*b*) crayons onto Bob's retinas as he continues to gaze at the red crayon.

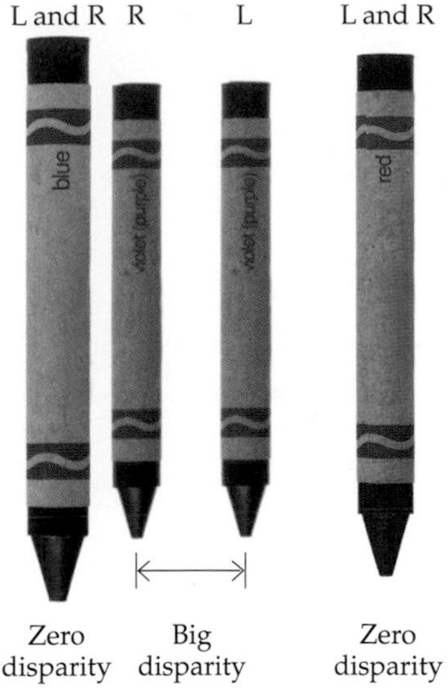

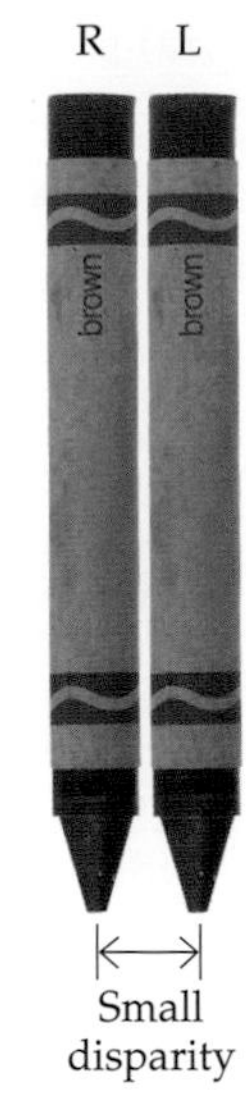

FIGURE 6.26 Superposition of Bob's left (L) and right (R) retinal images of the crayons in Figure 6.23, showing the relative disparity for each crayon. Size differences are ignored here. The red and blue crayons sit on the horopter and have zero disparity. They form retinal images in corresponding locations. The brown crayon forms images with a small binocular disparity. The purple crayon, farther from the horopter, has larger binocular disparity.

tive to the horopter, this crayon forms a retinal image with a nonzero binocular disparity. The purple crayon is even farther off the horopter (Figure 6.25*b*); it forms retinal images that are even more disparate (**Figure 6.26**).

The geometric regularity that the visual system uses to extract metrical depth information from binocular disparity should now be growing clear. The larger the disparity, the greater the distance in depth of the object from the horopter.

The direction in depth is given by the *sign* of the disparity, as illustrated in **Figure 6.27**. Suppose that Bob is looking at a red crayon with his eyes converged so that the red crayon falls on the fovea in each eye. A closer, blue crayon will form images on noncorresponding, disparate points. On the left retina, blue will lie to the left of red. Because the image is reversed, this means that, viewed from the left eye, blue is to the right of red. Viewed from the right eye, blue is to the left. Right in left, and left in right; that is **crossed disparity** (Figure 6.27*a*), and crossed disparity always means "in front of the horopter." In Figure 6.27*b*, Bob is looking at the blue crayon, and the red is seen to the left with the left eye and to the right with the right; that is **uncrossed disparity**, and uncrossed disparity always means "behind the horopter."

crossed disparity The sign of disparity created by objects in front of the plane of fixation (the horopter). The term *crossed* is used because images of objects located in front of the horopter appear to be displaced to the left in the right eye, and to the right in the left eye.

uncrossed disparity The sign of disparity created by objects behind the plane of fixation (the horopter). The term *uncrossed* is used because images of objects located behind the horopter will appear to be displaced to the right in the right eye, and to the left in the left eye.

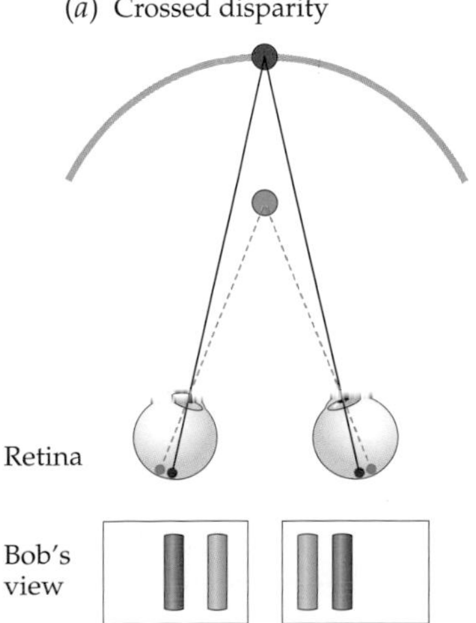

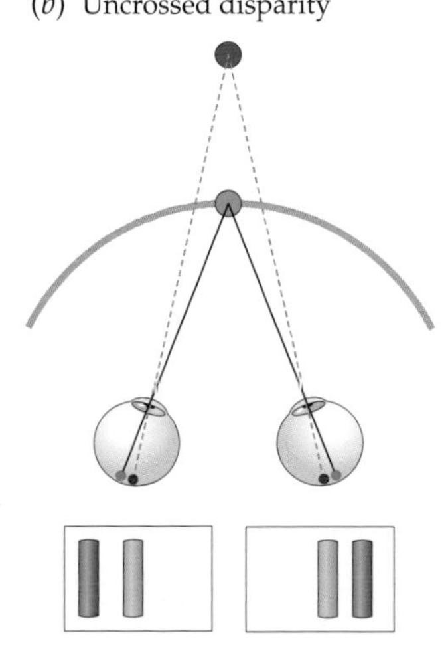

FIGURE 6.27 Crossed and uncrossed disparity. (*a*) Here Bob is foveating the red crayon. In the Bob's-eye views, the closer, blue object is seen to the right in the left eye and to the left in the right eye. This situation is crossed disparity. (*b*) Here Bob has shifted his gaze and his horopter to the blue crayon. In the Bob's-eye views, the farther, red object is seen to the left in the left eye and to the right in the right eye. This situation is uncrossed disparity.

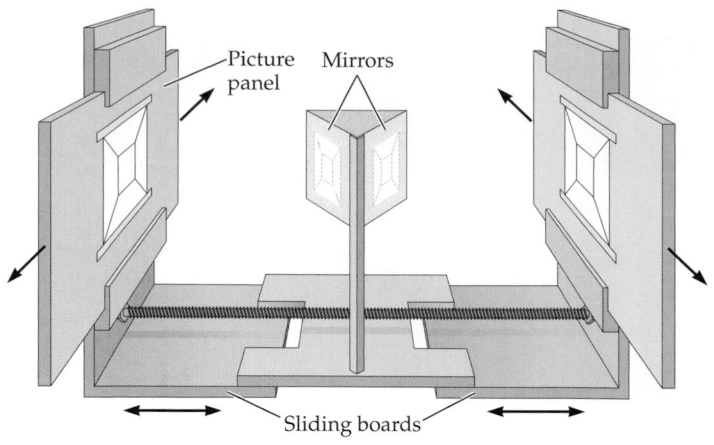

FIGURE 6.28 Wheatstone's stereoscope. The viewer would bring her nose up the vertical rod at the center of the apparatus so that each eye was looking at the image reflected in one of the two mirrors. (From Howard and Rogers, 1995.)

Stereoscopes and Stereograms

stereoscope A device for presenting one image to one eye and another image to the other eye. Stereoscopes can be used to present dichoptic stimuli for stereopsis and binocular rivalry.

Interestingly, although scientists had studied the geometry of binocular vision for millennia (the geometer Euclid was at it in the third century BCE), not until the nineteenth century was binocular disparity properly recognized as a depth cue. In the 1830s, Sir Charles Wheatstone invented a device called the **stereoscope** (**Figure 6.28**) that presented one image to one eye and a different image to the other eye. The stereoscope proved that the visual system treats binocular disparity as a depth cue, regardless of whether the disparity is produced by actual or simulated images of a scene.

For the average citizen the stereoscope was not science; it was home entertainment. The Wheatstone stereoscope had two different images in two different places. In the 1850s, however, David Brewster and Oliver Wendell Holmes invented viewers (**Figure 6.29***a*) that held a card with a double image like that shown in Figure 6.29*b*. The double images were captured by cameras with two lenses separated by about 2 inches, the distance between the average human's eyes. This arrangement allows stereo cameras to take a pair of pictures that mimic the images produced by the projective geometry of human binocular vision. Photographers traveled the world with these stereo cameras, capturing far-off scenes in a way that enabled a London schoolchild to see, for example, the British Army in Cape Town, South Africa, in a vivid three dimensions. (For a guide to more of these historical images, as well as many other stereograms, see **Web Essay 6.2: Stereo Images on the Web**.)

FIGURE 6.29 Stereopsis for the masses. (*a*) This Holmes stereoscope—among others—brought stereo photos into the homes of many mid-nineteenth-century homes. (*b*) A stereo photo of South African Light Horse, a scouting regiment of the British Army, on Adderly Street, in Cape Town, South Africa, 1900. If you can "free-fuse" (see the next section) you will be able to see this scene jump out in depth.

(*a*)

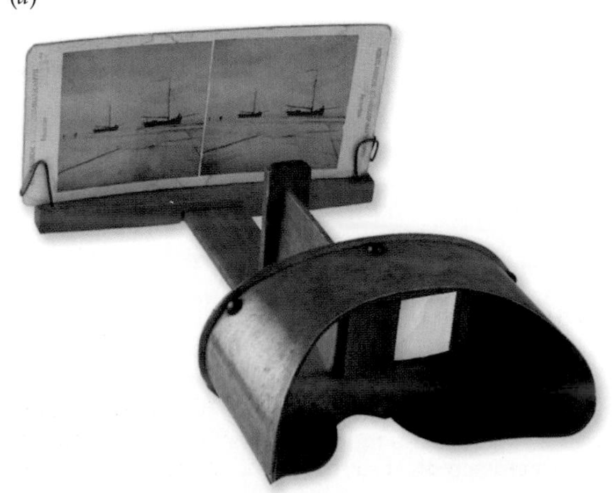

(*b*)

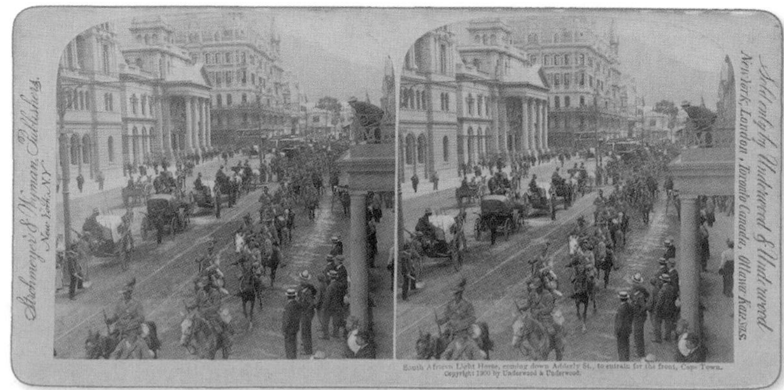

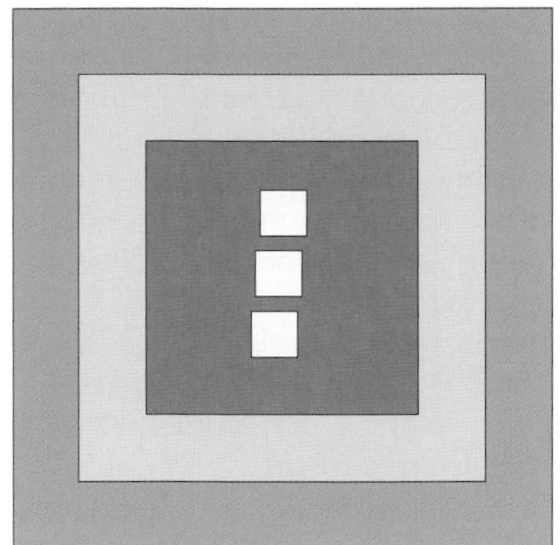
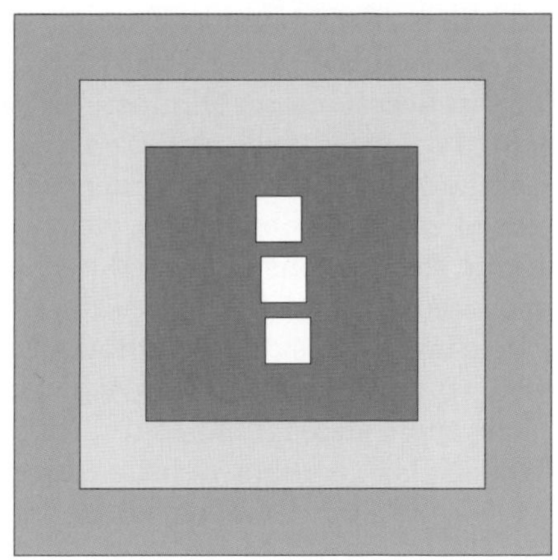

FIGURE 6.30 Try to converge (cross) or diverge (uncross) your eyes so that you see three (rather than two or four) sets of squares here. If you succeed, you will probably be able to see that the three white squares lie at different depths in the central image.

A stereoscope is very helpful, but you don't actually need it to experience stereopsis. You can teach yourself a technique known as **free fusion**, which John Frisby (1980) called "the poor man's stereoscope." **Figure 6.30** contains two copies of almost identical pictures. If you cross your eyes hard, you should see four sets of squares. This is the phenomenon of double vision (diplopia), described in the previous section. Two of those sets are seen with the left eye and two with the right. The trick is to relax just a bit until you see just three sets of squares. The far left set is seen only in the left eye; the far right, only in the right, but the middle set is the fusion of a set seen by the left eye and another set, seen by the right eye. This fusion of the separate images seen by the two eyes makes stereopsis possible. It is also possible to get there by diverging the eyes, relaxing them until you see three sets of squares.

Achieving the perception of three, instead of four or two, sets of squares in Figure 6.30 is the first step toward free fusion. The second step is to bring the middle set into focus. As noted earlier, convergence and accommodation normally work in lockstep, so crossing your eyes automatically leads your ciliary muscles to make your lenses more spherical. Similar problems (in the opposite direction) will occur if you diverge your eyes. To see the middle set of squares clearly, you have to decouple accommodation and convergence. If you can manage it, then the image will come into focus and the three white squares will appear to lie at different depths in the middle of the three sets of squares that you're seeing. When viewed normally, notice that the white squares in the left and right panels look misaligned in opposite directions. Those are the monocular views. When you free-fuse, the opposite misalignments become the binocular disparity and your visual system converts that disparity into a perception of depth.

The depth that you see depends on whether you converged or diverged your eyes. We described crossing, or converging, the eyes. It is also possible to free-fuse the images in Figure 6.30 by *diverging* your eyes. Divergence requires focusing on a point beyond the plane of the page, so that the image of the left-hand set of squares falls on the left fovea and the image of the right-hand set falls on the right fovea. Because the images falling on the two retinas in the divergence method are reversed compared to the convergence situations, the disparities are reversed and the perceived depth will be reversed. If you converge, the top square will be the farthest back. If you diverge, it will appear closest to you. Either converging or diverging will produce a clear stereoscopic effect, so give it a try.

Before we go on, we should note that approximately 3% to 5% of the population lacks stereoscopic depth perception—a condition known as **stereo-**

free fusion The technique of converging (crossing) or diverging the eyes in order to view a stereogram without a stereoscope.

stereoblindness An inability to make use of binocular disparity as a depth cue. This term is typically used to describe individuals with vision in both eyes. Someone who has lost one (or both) eyes is not typically described as "stereoblind."

random dot stereogram (RDS) A stereogram made of a large number (often in the thousands) of randomly placed dots. Random dot stereograms contain no monocular cues to depth. Stimuli visible stereoscopically in random dot stereograms are cyclopean stimuli.

cyclopean Referring to stimuli that are defined by binocular disparity alone. Named after the one-eyed Cyclops of Homer's *Odyssey*.

blindness. Stereoblind individuals might be able to achieve the perception of three sets of squares in Figure 6.30, but the little white squares will not pop out in depth. Stereoblindness is usually a secondary effect of childhood visual disorders such as strabismus, in which the two eyes are misaligned. If you had such a visual disorder during childhood and/or you've been diagnosed with stereoblindness, we apologize but you just won't perceive depth in the stereograms presented here and on the website. That said, most people who try and fail to see depth in stereograms have "normal" vision (wearing glasses doesn't count as abnormal). Those people just need practice, so don't give up. Web Activity 6.3: Stereoscopes and Stereograms provides more stereograms for practice, and Web Essay 6.2: Stereo Images on the Web leads to another website with more tips for free-fusing.

Random Dot Stereograms

For 100 years or so after the invention of the stereoscope, it was generally supposed that stereopsis occurred relatively late in the processing of visual stimuli. The idea was that the first step in free-fusing images such as those in **Figure 6.31**, would be to analyze the input as a face. We would then use the slight disparities between the left-eye and right-eye images of the nose, eyes, chin, and other objects and parts to enrich the sense that the nose sticks out in front of the face, that the eyes are slightly sunken, and so on.

Bela Julesz, a Hungarian radar engineer who spent most of his career at Bell Labs in New Jersey, thought the conventional wisdom might be backward. He theorized that stereopsis might be used to *discover* objects and surfaces in the world. Why would this be useful? Julesz thought that stereopsis might help reveal camouflaged objects. A mouse might be the same color as its background, but out in the open it would be in front of the background. A cat that could use stereopsis to break the mouse's camouflage would be a more successful hunter. (Cats do have stereopsis, by the way [Blake, 1988; R. Fox and Blake, 1971].) To prove his point, Julesz (1964, 1971) made use of **random dot stereograms** (**RDSs**), an example of which is shown in **Figure 6.32**. If you can free-fuse these images, you will see a pair of squares, one sticking out like a bump, the other looking like a hole in the texture (which one is the bump and which is the hole depends, again, on whether you converge or diverge your eyes).

The important point about RDSs is that we cannot see the squares in either of the component images. We cannot see the squares using any monocular depth cues. These are shapes that are defined by binocular disparity alone. Julesz called such stimuli **cyclopean**, after the one-eyed Cyclops of Homer's *Odyssey*. Wheatstone showed with his stereoscope that binocular disparity is a necessary condition for stereopsis. Julesz demonstrated with the RDS that disparity is *sufficient* for stereopsis. To understand how random dot stereograms are made, visit Web Activity 6.3: Stereoscopes and Stereograms,

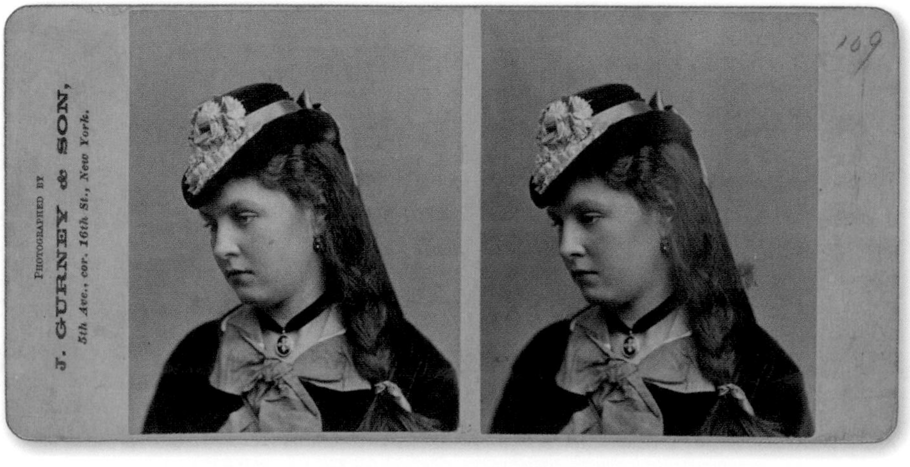

FIGURE 6.31 A stereo photograph of a woman's face.

FIGURE 6.32 If you can free-fuse this random dot stereogram, you will see two rectangular regions: one in front of the plane of the page, the other behind the page. Which is which depends on whether you converge or diverge in order to fuse the two squares.

FIGURE 6.33 Is this a simple picture or a complicated computational problem?

which also explains "magic eye" or "wallpaper" stereograms, known more technically as "autostereograms."

Stereoscopic Correspondence

If you successfully free-fused the random dot patterns in Figure 6.32, you solved a truly daunting problem. Even if you didn't, if you have normal binocular vision you are solving the **correspondence problem** all the time. The correspondence problem is the problem of figuring out which bit of the image in the left eye should be matched with which bit in the right eye. **Figure 6.33** uses an extremely simple situation to illustrate why correspondence is so tricky. There are, of course, just three dots in Figure 6.33. **Figure 6.34*a*** traces the paths of rays of light from the printed circles on the page to the images on your retinas. The retinal images of the circles are labeled to make it clear which image on the left retina corresponds to which image on the right retina, but your visual system has no such labels. All it knows about is the retinal images, as shown in Figure 6.34*b*. Figure 6.34*c* shows another possible

correspondence problem (binocular vision) The problem of figuring out which bit of the image in the left eye should be matched with which bit in the right eye. The problem is particularly vexing when the images consist of thousands of similar features like dots in random dot stereograms.

FIGURE 6.34 Interpreting the visual information from the three circles in Figure 6.33.

(*a*) The actual situation

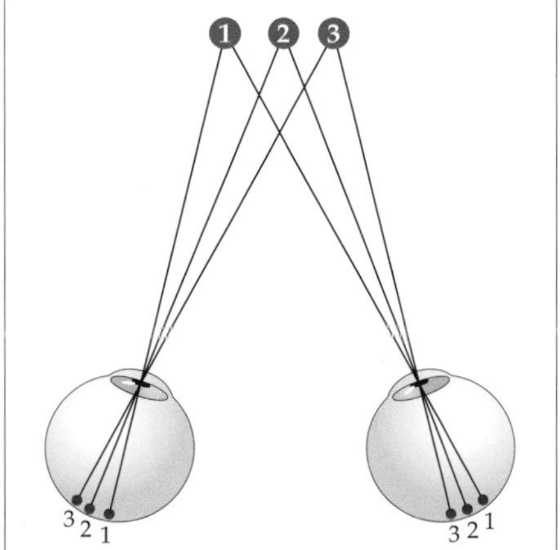

(*b*) What the visual system knows

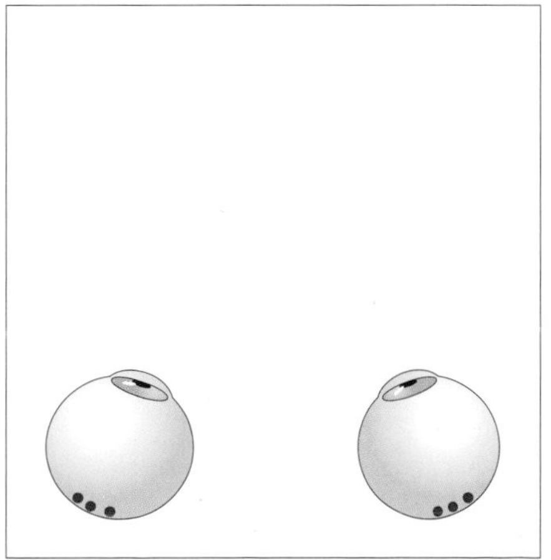

(*c*) Another plausible interpretation

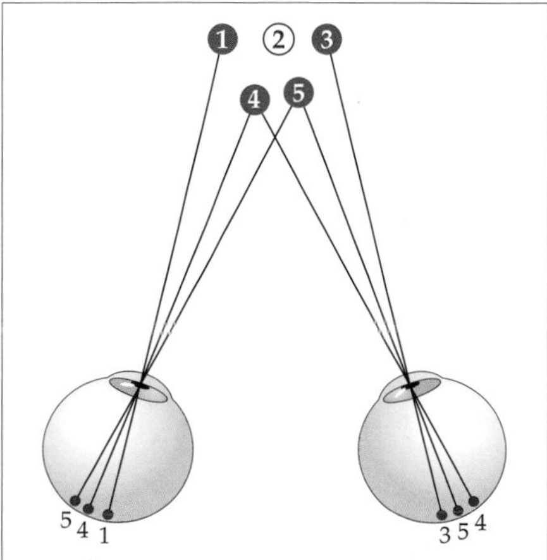

uniqueness constraint In stereopsis, the observation that a feature in the world is represented exactly once in each retinal image. This constraint simplifies the correspondence problem.

continuity constraint In stereopsis, the observation that, except at the edges of objects, neighboring points in the world lie at similar distances from the viewer. This is one of several constraints that have been proposed to help solve the correspondence problem.

geometric interpretation of the situation: if the left retinal image of circle 2 is matched to the right retinal image of circle 1, and the left retinal image of circle 3 is matched to the right retinal image of circle 2, you will perceive *four* circles, with the inner pair of circles perceived as floating in front of the outer pair. (In fact, you may be able to see this if you can cross your eyes correctly.)

With only three elements in the visual scene, it isn't hard to imagine how the visual system might achieve the proper correspondence: first match the two circles whose images fall on the foveas; then match the two images to the left of the foveas with each other; then match the two images to the right of the foveas. Before random dot stereograms, a similar logic seemed reasonable for more complex scenes too. Go back to the face in Figure 6.31. Our visual systems could solve the correspondence problem by first finding the parts of the faces and then matching nose to nose, mouth to mouth, and so forth. The random dot stereogram in Figure 6.32, however, contains thousands of identical black and white dots falling on each retina. How can we be sure that the dot in the center of the fovea in one eye corresponds to the dot in the center in the other eye? Even if we knew that, could we really match each dot in the right eye with just one dot in the left eye? If there were a little dirt on the page, would the whole process collapse? How in the world does our visual system succeed in making the proper matches?

Matching thousands of left-eye dots to thousands of right-eye dots in Figure 6.32 would require a lot of work for any computational system. However, the problem is simpler if we look at a blurred version of the stereogram. Blurring leaves only the low-spatial-frequency information. **Figure 6.35** shows the low spatial frequencies of the stereogram from Figure 6.32. Now, rather than thousands of dots, we have just a few large blobs. If you free-fuse the images in Figure 6.35, you won't see the rectangles clearly. You may not see them at all; but, as David Marr and Tomaso Poggio (1979) realized, if you match the low-spatial-frequency blobs, you have a good approximation to the answer of what goes with what. You can work from there to determine how to match up the high-frequency dots, edges, and so forth.

Marr and Poggio also suggested two additional heuristics for achieving correspondence: the uniqueness and continuity constraints. The **uniqueness constraint** is the reality that a feature in the world is represented exactly once in each retinal image. Working in the opposite direction, the visual system knows that each monocular image feature (e.g., a nose or a dot) should be paired with exactly one feature in the other image. The **continuity constraint** holds that, except at the edges of objects, neighboring points in the world lie at similar distances from the viewer. Accordingly, disparity should change

FIGURE 6.35 A low spatial frequency–filtered version of the stereogram in Figure 6.32. Correspondence is much easier to achieve here. If you free-fuse these two images, you will be able to tell roughly where the rectangles lie. The high-frequency information in Figure 6.32, however, gave more precise information.

smoothly at most places in the image. (These constraints are difficult to illustrate on a static page, but **Web Activity 6.4: Stereoscopic Correspondence** provides dynamic explanations of them.)

The Physiological Basis of Stereopsis

Now that we know something about the theoretical basis of stereopsis, we can ask how it is implemented by the human brain. The most fundamental requirement is that input from the two eyes must converge onto the same cell. As noted in Chapter 3, this convergence does not happen until striate cortex, where most neurons are binocular (Hubel and Wiesel, 1962). A binocular neuron has two receptive fields, one in each eye. In binocular striate cortex neurons, these two receptive fields are generally very similar in the two eyes, sharing nearly identical orientation and spatial frequency tuning, as well as the same preferred speed and direction of motion (Hubel and Wiesel, 1973). Thus, these cells are well suited to the task of matching images in the two eyes.

Many binocular neurons respond best when the retinal images are on corresponding points in the two retinas, thereby providing a neural basis for the horopter. However, many other binocular neurons respond best when similar images occupy slightly *different* positions on the retinas of the two eyes (Barlow, Blakemore, and Pettigrew, 1967; Pettigrew, Nikara, and Bishop, 1968). In other words, these neurons are tuned to a particular binocular disparity.

Figure 6.36*a* illustrates the binocular receptive fields of two disparity-sensitive cells of this sort. These cells would be in striate cortex (the figure omits synapses in retina and LGN). The neurons' receptive fields overlap on the right retina, but on the left retina the blue neuron has a receptive field on one side of the fovea, while the red neuron has its receptive field on the

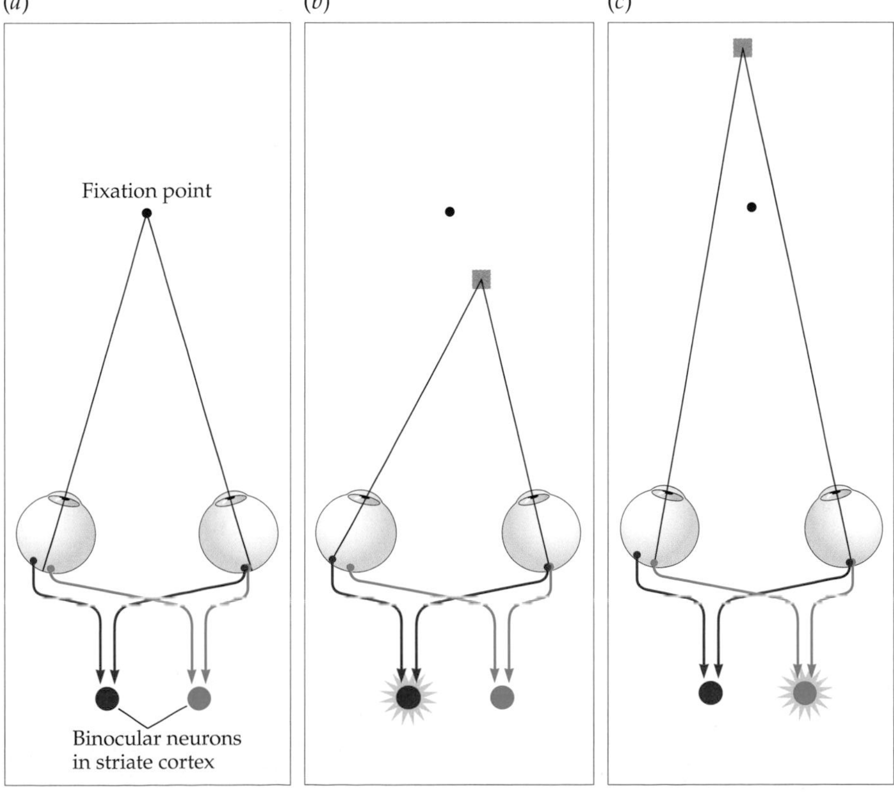

FIGURE 6.36 In these simplified diagrams of receptive fields for two binocular disparity–tuned neurons in striate cortex, the red neuron "sees" stimuli falling on the red receptive fields, and the blue neuron responds to stimuli falling on the blue receptive fields (these receptive fields overlap on the right retina). (*a*) The overall picture, showing the fixation point in relation to the two retinas. (*b*) The red neuron responds best to a stimulus closer to and slightly to the right of the fixation point. (*c*) The blue neuron responds best if its preferred stimulus is behind and slightly to the left of fixation.

other side. The red neuron will respond maximally to a stimulus closer than the point of fixation (Figure 6.36*b*), and the blue neuron will respond optimally to a stimulus lying beyond fixation (Figure 6.36*c*). Imagine covering Panum's fusional area with neurons whose receptive fields occupied different parts of that three-dimensional space.

Cells with similar but binocularly disparate receptive fields are, at best, just the beginning of the neural substrate of stereopsis. Gian Poggio and his colleagues (Poggio and Talbot, 1981) found that more than half of the neurons in V1 are tuned to disparity, and that the percentage of disparity-tuned neurons increases in V2 and higher areas. Some neurons responded positively to disparities near zero—that is, to images falling on corresponding retinal points—but some were inhibited by these stimuli. Other neurons, rather than being tuned to a specific spot in depth, were broadly tuned to a range of crossed (near) or uncrossed (far) disparities. Ohzawa and Freeman (1986a, 1986b) described how disparity could be coded by neurons that had quite different receptive fields in each eye. Then, once information about disparity is extracted from the image, the correspondence problem must be solved and little local signals about depth must be combined into surfaces and objects in a three-dimensional world.

The brain can make use of two different types of disparity information: absolute and relative. Consider Figure 6.24. Both of Bob's eyes are fixating on the red crayon. The image of the red crayon falls on the fovea of each eye. The image of the blue crayon lands at different positions on the left and right retinas. If Bob decides to fixate the blue crayon directly, he will need to rotate his eyes by different angles. The difference of angles is called the **absolute disparity** (which corresponds to the difference in visual direction from the two eye's views) and is used to control convergence. When we fixate a target, convergence places the images of the object on the fovea of each eye and reduces the disparity to zero (or nearly zero).

Suppose Bob needs to estimate the relative depths or distances of the red and blue crayons (that is, how far in front of the red crayon is the blue one?). To make an accurate estimate, the visual system uses **relative disparity** (which is the difference in absolute disparities of objects or parts of an object). We are very much more sensitive to relative than to absolute disparity, and evidence shows that absolute and relative disparity are probably processed in different areas of the brain (Cumming and Parker, 1999; Thomas, Cumming, and Parker, 2002; see Parker, 2007, for a detailed discussion).

Combining Depth Cues

If the chapters of this book were novels, this chapter could be said to have the same plot as the discussion of object recognition in Chapter 4 but with different characters. In Chapter 4 we described a set of cues that enabled us to group local features together into possible objects and then to recognize those objects. We described the process as a sort of committee effort in which different sources of information each contributed their opinions. In this chapter we have covered multiple sources of depth information and they, too, need to be combined. Any or all of these cues might be available to the visual system when we're viewing any visual scene. None of the cues are foolproof, and none work in every possible situation. For example, relative height produces inconsistent or misleading information if we can't see the point at which an object touches the ground. All we really have is a collection of guesses about possible depth relations between different objects in our visual field.

By carefully combining and weighting these guesses, the visual system generally arrives at a coherent, and more or less accurate, representation of

absolute disparity A difference in the actual retinal coordinates in the left and right eyes of the image of a feature in a visual scene.

relative disparity The difference in absolute disparities of two elements in a visual scene.

three-dimensional space. Helmholtz, writing in the nineteenth century (and translated into English in the twentieth), called this automatic cue combination process "unconscious inference" (Helmholtz, 1924). In recent years, a number of vision researchers have been attempting to put this sort of argument on a more rigorous mathematical footing by using what is called a **Bayesian approach**, named after the Bayes' theorem in statistics, which, in turn, is named after the Reverend Thomas Bayes (1702–1761) (Yuille and Kersten, 2006).

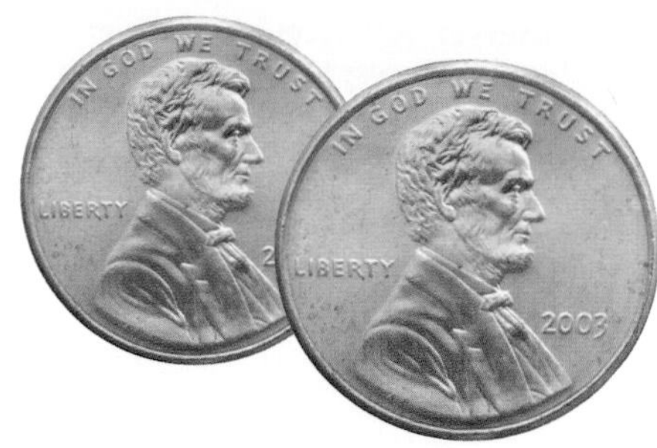

FIGURE 6.37 Retinal image of a simple visual scene.

The Bayesian Approach

The basic insight of Reverend Bayes, described in a paper that was not published until after his death, was that prior knowledge could influence estimates of the probability of a current event. In the present context, the "event" is the particular visual scene we are currently viewing, and Bayes' theorem states that $P(S_X \mid I)$ (the probability of a scene X, given the visual input we're currently receiving) is proportional to $P(S_X)$ (the overall probability of the scene), multiplied by $P(I \mid S_X)$ (the probability of *this* input, given *this* scene):

$$P(S_X \mid I) \approx P(S_X) \times P(I \mid S_X)$$

Enough math. Let's unpack Bayes' observations with a concrete example. Suppose our visual system is confronted with the retinal image shown in **Figure 6.37**. There are an infinite number of possible ways to produce this retinal image. Three of these are shown in **Figure 6.38**. Maybe the two pennies are the same size, but the one on the left is slightly farther away than the one on the right (Figure 6.38*a*). Maybe the penny on the right is much smaller, but also much closer, than the penny on the left (Figure 6.38*b*). Maybe the two pennies are equidistant, but the penny on the left is smaller and has had a bite taken out of it (Figure 6.38*c*). If you don't think the set of possibilities is

Bayesian approach A statistical model based on Reverend Thomas Bayes' insight that prior knowledge could influence our estimates of the probability of a current event.

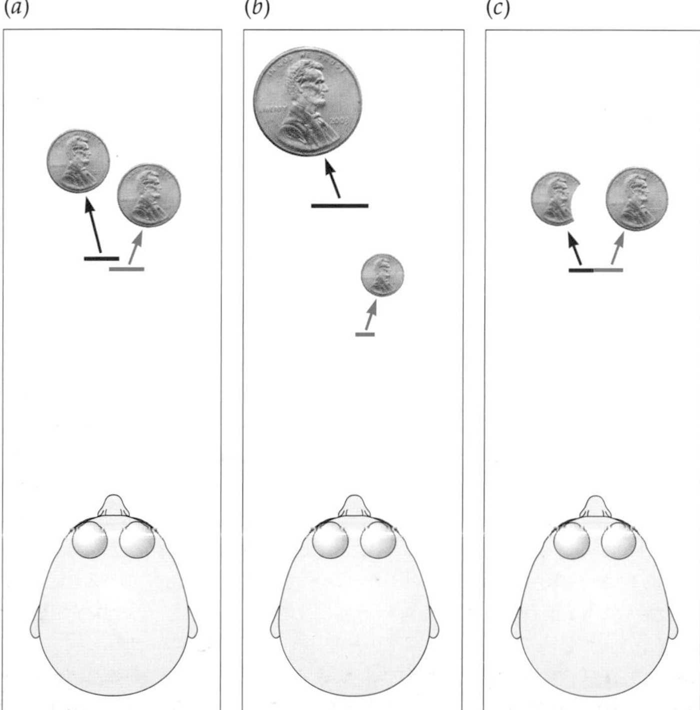

FIGURE 6.38 Three of the infinite number of scenes that could generate the retinal image in Figure 6.37.

ideal observer A theoretical observer with complete access to the best available information and the ability to combine different sources of information in the optimal manner. It can be useful to compare human performance to that of an ideal observer.

infinite, remember that if the size can vary, the distances can vary forever. One penny could be on the moon (it would have to be a really big penny).

How does the visual system decide what we're actually seeing? Which interpretation seems more likely? That is the core of the Bayesian approach (except that it's all automatic; our conscious selves do not get to make the decision). In our experience, all pennies are the same size. This familiar size cue is one source of prior knowledge in this case. It makes $P(S_A)$, the *a priori* probability of scene A, higher than $P(S_B)$ or $P(S_C)$. Furthermore, for the scene in Figure 6.38*c* to produce the retinal image in Figure 6.37, we would have to be seeing the scene from one of those unusual and unlikely "accidental viewpoints." It is much more likely that the points of contact between penny 1 and penny 2 reflect occlusion. Thus, $P(S_C \mid I)$, the probability that scene C is the origin of the image is very low. If we were to plug all these probabilities into Bayes' equation, we would find that $P(S_A \mid I)$ is highest. Given the image in Figure 6.37, the most likely answer is the scene depicted in Figure 6.38*a*.

How precisely do we actually know the size of a penny? Are they all absolutely identical or do they vary? If we measured them, there would be some error in the measurement. We simply could not be perfect. That imperfection is a feature of any of the cues we have discussed here. How precisely can we calculate binocular disparity, for instance? That error puts a limit on reliability of the cue. As an analogy, this is why you were taught about "significant figures" in high school science. It makes no sense to give your weight as 175.489673969 pounds, because the scale just is not that precise. If we know the quality of each source of information, we can determine the best possible performance of someone using that information. This is known as **ideal observer** analysis (W. S. Geisler, 1989; Hillis et al., 2004).

For the two pennies of Figure 6.37, it is interesting that we and our committees are so willing to come to the quick conclusion that a closer penny is occluding a farther penny. After all, the real answer is that the stimulus is an image on a flat page. There are no pennies and no depth. Moreover, other depth cues, such as stereopsis and convergence, are telling the visual system that the two objects in the scene are equidistant. The unconscious decisions we make involve a complex set of cue combination rules that are only beginning to be worked out. It is not a matter of one cue, one vote. Here, for example, stereopsis information does not contribute to our interpretation of the depth relationships in Figure 6.37. Nevertheless, it probably does provide one of the cues that tell us that this is a flat book illustration.

Illusions and the Construction of Space

If visual perception of the world is a best guess about the causes of visual input, then interesting things should happen when a guess is wrong. In some sense, as with the pennies we just discussed, a guess is wrong whenever we look at a two-dimensional picture and see it as three-dimensional. As noted, however, we are not really fooled into thinking that the picture actually is three-dimensional. It would be more accurate to say that we make a plausible guess about the three-dimensional world that is being represented in the two-dimensional picture.

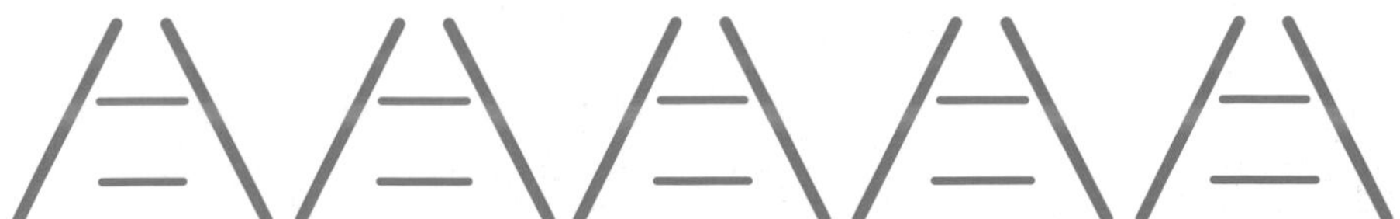

FIGURE 6.39 In which image are the two horizontal lines the same length?

What about a situation like that shown in **Figure 6.39**? In one of the five pairs of horizontal lines, the two lines are the same length. Can you pick the correct pair? In fact, it is the second from the left. Odds are you picked the third or fourth pair, even though the bottom line in both of those images is physically longer than the top line. This is known as the Ponzo illusion, named after Mario Ponzo, who described the effect in 1913. What causes this illusion? For many years, a popular family of theories has held that the illusion is a guess gone wrong—a situation in which we overinterpret the depth cues in a two-dimensional image. The basic idea is shown in **Figure 6.40**. Maybe the two tilted lines that induce the illusion in each image of Figure 6.39 are being interpreted by the visual system as linear perspective cues like the train tracks in Figure 6.40. If so, then objects that were the same size in the two-dimensional image would represent objects of different sizes in the three-dimensional world.

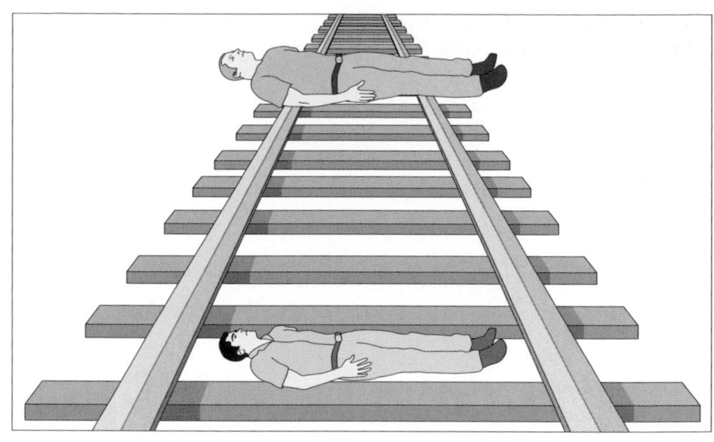

FIGURE 6.40 The two figures lying across these train tracks are the same size in the image. You can verify this by measuring them. However, if they were really in the three-dimensional world shown in the image, then the more distant person would need to be much larger to have this appearance.

Such accounts are very compelling and exist for a wide range of visual illusions (Gillam, 1980). (See **Web Essay 6.3: The Moon Illusion**.) They are consistent with the view that the job of the visual system is to use the available cues to make an intelligent guess about the world (Gregory, 1966, 1970). Just because an answer is plausible, however, doesn't mean it's right. In **Figure 6.41**, line B looks longer than line A. That makes sense if we see the context lines lying at different distances on the wall of the colonnade. As in the Ponzo illusion, if line B is farther away than A, then the same image size implies a larger size in the real world. But what about lines C and D? Surely D would be interpreted as farther away than C. Does it look convincingly larger?

(*a*)

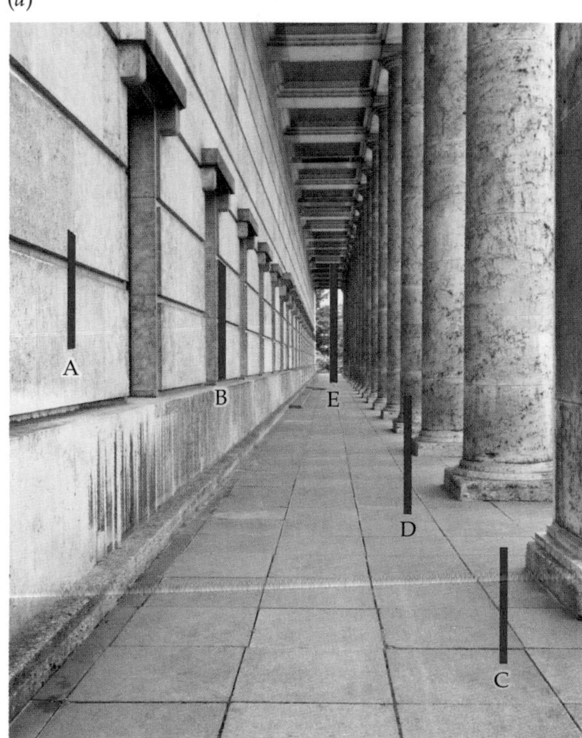

(*b*)

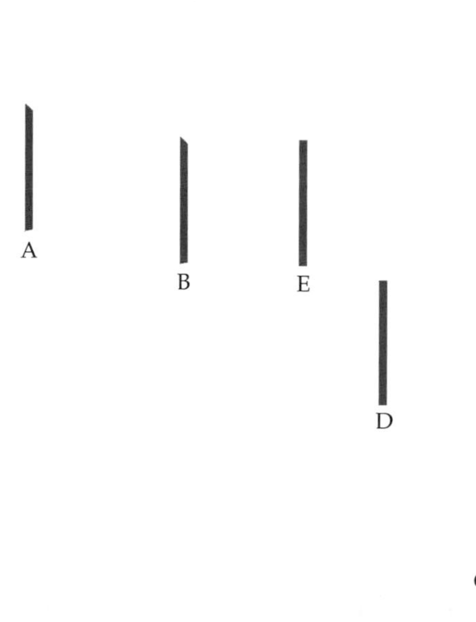

FIGURE 6.41 All of the red lines in this illustration are the same length. Does B look bigger than A? Does D look bigger than C? In each case, which line is farther away if this is a colonnade?

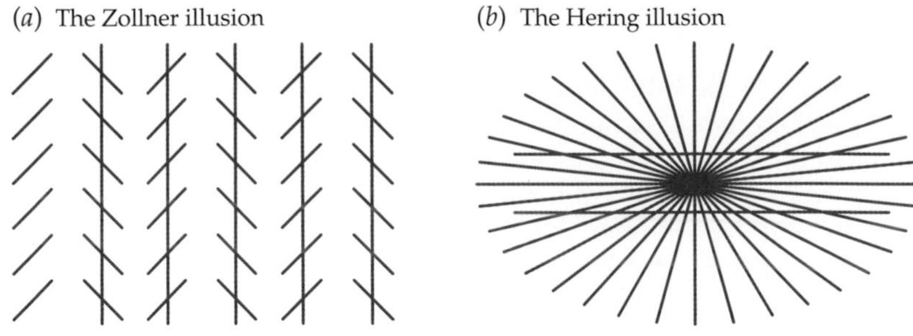

FIGURE 6.42 The vertical lines are parallel in (*a*), as are the horizontal lines in (*b*).

Prinzmetal, Shimamura, and Mikolinski (2001) use a demonstration like this as part of their argument that the Ponzo illusion is not a by-product of depth cues at all. They argued that it reflects a more general aspect of the visual system's response to tilted lines, and is related to illusions like the Zollner and Hering illusions illustrated in **Figure 6.42** (which we will *not* try to explain) (see Prinzmetal and Beck, 2001). The point is debatable. After all, line E looks very big down there at the apparent end of the colonnade. Who is right? This note of caution reminds us that even the best theory must always face the next experiment. It will be interesting to see how many of the convincing ideas in this book still seem credible in a generation.

Binocular Rivalry and Suppression

The preceding sections demonstrated that objects in the world often project images on our two retinas that do not overlap (that is, the images fall on noncorresponding retinal points), and that the visual system is physiologically prepared to deal with these discrepancies via disparity-tuned neurons in striate cortex and beyond. But what happens when completely different stimuli are presented to the two eyes? You can answer this question for yourself by fixating on a small object across the room, such as a clock, and moving your hand up so that your fingers occlude the object in the right eye (making sure the left eye still has an unobstructed view). It would seem a bad idea to fuse the fingers and the clock into a single perception of something that does not exist in the world. Accordingly, the visual system chooses instead to *suppress* one image and perceive the other. In the present situation, you probably see the clock as though you were looking through a hole in your hand. (For an even more compelling perception of a hole in your hand, try the demonstration of suppression in Web Activity 6.2: Binocular Disparity.)

How does the visual system "decide" what to see? The more interesting of the two stimuli is likely to be dominant. *Interesting* in this case (*salient* might be a better word) means interesting to the early stages of cortical visual processing. High contrast is more interesting than low contrast, bright is better than dim, moving objects are more interesting than stationary ones, and so forth (Fahle, 1982). The meaning of the stimulus may have an effect, but if so, it is a very small effect (Yu and Blake, 1992).

binocular rivalry The competition between the two eyes for control of visual perception, which is evident when completely different stimuli are presented to the two eyes.

The competition between the two eyes for control of visual perception, known as **binocular rivalry**, is never completely won by either eye (Alais and Blake, 2005; Wheatstone, 1852) or either stimulus (Blake and Logothetis, 2002). If you stare at the combination of the clock and hand long enough, your fingers will eventually conquer the visual territory, only to surrender it back to the clock a moment later. The battle is easier to see if the two combatants are more closely matched. If you free-fuse the two panels of **Figure**

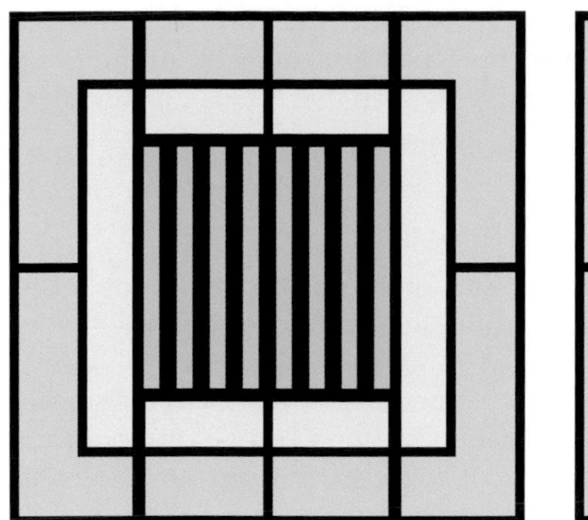
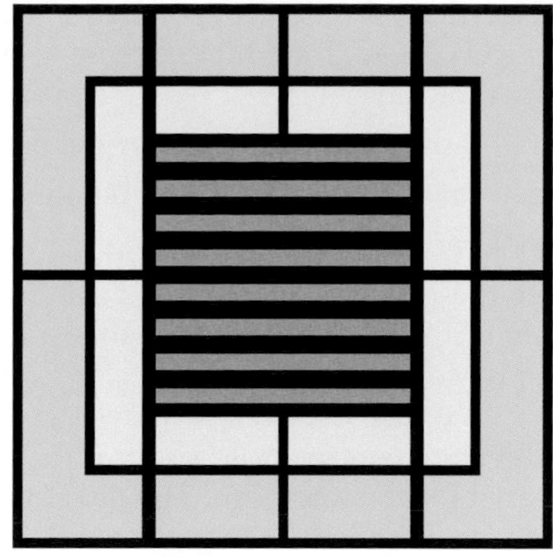

FIGURE 6.43 Binocular rivalry. If you free-fuse these two images, you will be able to watch the blue verticals and orange horizontals engage in the perceptual battle known as binocular rivalry.

6.43, your visual system will not actually combine the perpendicular stripes. Instead, you will see a battle between the vertically and horizontally striped patches, with regions of dominance growing and shrinking over time as illustrated in **Figure 6.44**.

Binocular rivalry might seem an odd situation that would arise only in a vision lab or a perception course, but a moment's reflection should convince you that the stimuli for rivalry are actually very common. Recall that Panum's fusional area is the region of space surrounding the horopter within which images on the two retinas can be fused. As noted earlier, objects located too far off the horopter—outside Panum's area—are subject to diplopia. In fact, the proportion of the three-dimensional visual world that falls *inside* Panum's area is actually fairly small. Think about two pairs of corresponding points: A_L and A_R, and B_L and B_R (the *L* and *R* stand for "left" and "right," respectively). Now imagine that one object falls on two noncorresponding retinal points: A_L and B_R. It follows that *something else* must be forming an image on A_R. There will be noncorresponding images on the corresponding points A_L and A_R (and, similarly, on B_L and B_R). Those are the conditions for rivalry.

The fact that the two eyes are seeing different images brings us to an ancient problem: the problem of binocular single vision. Why, when we see one elephant in one eye and one elephant in the other eye, don't we perceive two elephants? Given what we've learned in this chapter, we're now in a position to answer this question. If the elephant is within Panum's area, we fuse its two images into a single stereoscopic perception. If it is outside Panum's area, we normally suppress one of the copies. Why don't we see the rivalry? In part, because we aren't looking. Our attention and eyes are typically directed toward the foveated object or toward objects falling on roughly corresponding points in each eye. Moreover, acuity is so bad in the periphery of the visual fields that, even when objects are vying for binocular precedence, the rivalry is quite indistinct.

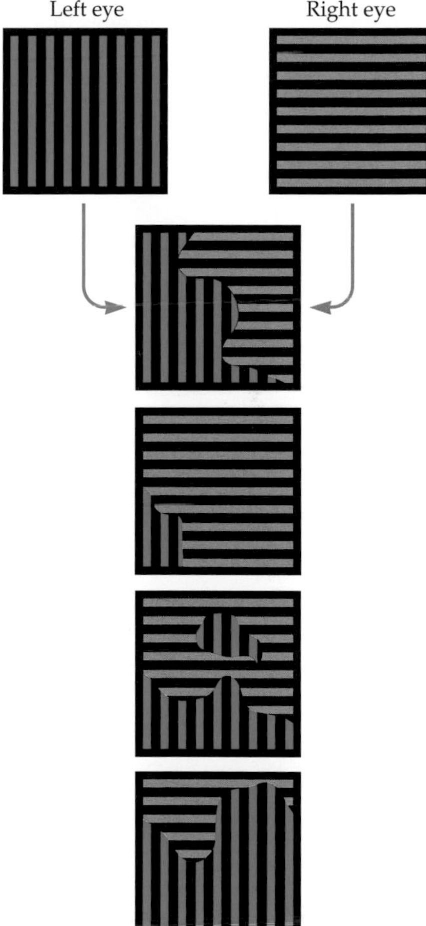

FIGURE 6.44 If blue vertical bars are shown to one eye while orange horizontal bars are shown to the other, the two stimuli will battle for dominance, with different stimuli dominating at different times in different parts of the visual field.

Development of Binocular Vision and Stereopsis

What is binocular vision like in infants? Babies are born with two eyes, but are they born with stereopsis? If not, how does binocular function develop? In a wonderful conversation about visual development, Davida Teller and

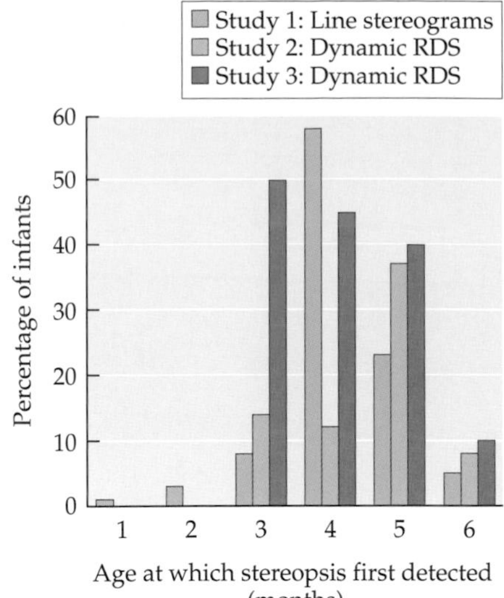

FIGURE 6.45 The onset of stereopsis. This figure shows the percentage of infants demonstrating stereopsis for the first time as a functon of their age. In three separate studies (the three different colors) almost all infants showed stereopsis for the first time between 3 and 5 months. (After Birch, 1993.)

stereoacuity A measure of the smallest binocular disparity that can generate a sensation of depth.

Tony Movshon (1986) recalled a lecture by a disillusioned developmental psychologist, John McKee, who argued that the field could be summed up by three laws:

1. As children get older, they get better at things.
2. Whatever it is, girls do it before boys.
3. Everything develops along with everything else.

To these "laws" Teller added a summary statement: "Things start out badly, then they get better; then, after a long time, they get worse again" (Teller and Movshon, 1986).

As it turns out, research over the last 25 years or so has shown that visual development provides support for the first and second "laws," but not for a strict form of the third. The development of binocular vision and stereopsis provides one of the strongest violations of that third law.

Most visual functions indeed start off badly (but not as badly as we used to think) and then improve steadily until they reach adult levels; however, the development of stereopsis is surprising, in that infants are essentially blind to disparity until about 4 months of age. At that point stereopsis appears quite suddenly—almost out of the blue. Of course, measuring stereopsis (or anything else) in infants is no easy task, but developmental psychologists have been very inventive in designing methods for assessing development.

Remarkably, despite differences in techniques and procedures, most investigators agree about the onset of stereopsis. **Figure 6.45** summarizes the results of several studies, showing the age at which stereopsis can first be detected. These studies (and others like them) looked for evidence that infants could reliably detect a large binocular disparity (typically on the order of 30 to 60 arc minutes). The agreement among the studies is remarkable. Infants are essentially stereoblind before 3 months, with most infants showing a sudden onset of stereopsis between 3 and 5 months.

Stereopsis is not an all-or-none phenomenon. Just as an individual's acuity is a measure of his ability to resolve spatial detail, **stereoacuity** is a measure of the smallest binocular disparity that can generate a sensation of depth. Once an infant develops stereopsis, stereoacuity increases rapidly to near adult levels (**Figure 6.46**). Birch and Petrig (1996) found that stereoacuity rose from essentially nothing before 4 months to near adult levels by 6 months! This time course is very different from the time course of development of simple acuity. Though coarsely present at birth, basic acuity takes years to reach adult levels. The same difference between basic acuity and stereoacuity is seen in monkeys (O'Dell and Boothe, 1997), but the overall rate of development is faster. Interestingly, not only stereoacuity but several other visual functions develop at a rate approximately four times faster than in humans, as if one monkey week were the equivalent of one human month. In keeping with this rule of one human month being equal to one monkey week, stereopsis can be detected in monkeys within the first 3 to 5 weeks of life compared to the 3- to 5-month window of onset observed in humans.

How, then, do we explain the sudden emergence of stereopsis in humans at about 4 months? Although newborn infants make convergence eye movements to track a target as it approaches their nose, accurate and consistent convergence probably does not occur until they are 3 to 4 months old. But we can't conclude that inaccurate convergence prevents stereopsis from developing earlier than 4 months, because convergence need not be very accurate in order to detect large disparities. Moreover, several studies used repeating gratings (like striped wallpaper), which would be fused at some disparity even if convergence were inaccurate. Before 4 months, babies don't respond to these stereoscopic stimuli either.

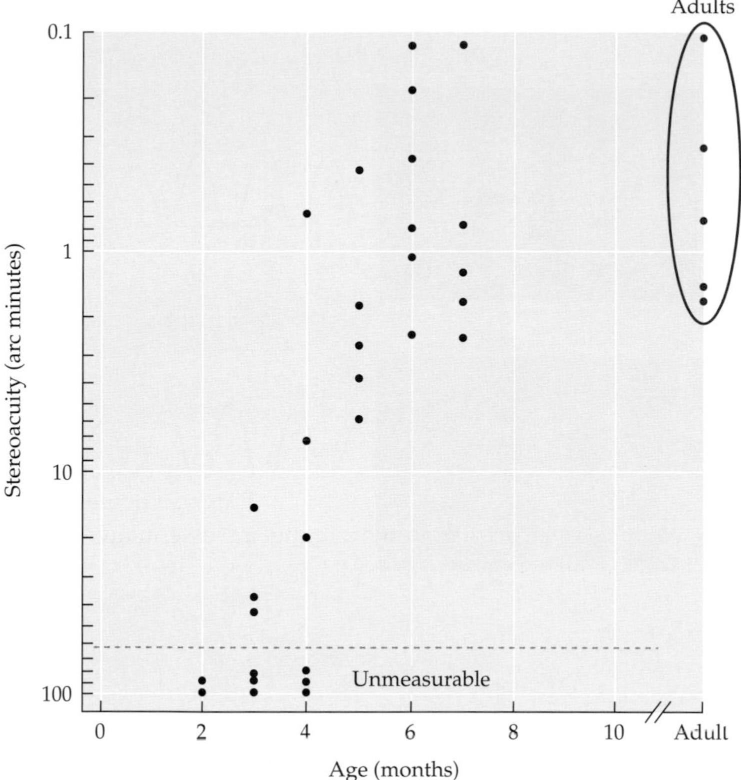

FIGURE 6.46 The development of stereoacuity. Stereoacuity develops to adult levels within the first 6–7 months of life. (After Birch and Petrig, 1996.)

An alternative view is that the failure of stereopsis to develop prior to 4 months might mean that some part of the visual system is immature. Disparity-sensitive neurons in V1 are one plausible candidate for that immature part, but recent anatomical and physiological data suggest that we need to look beyond V1 for an explanation of why infants do not exhibit stereopsis.

Yuzo Chino and his colleagues made the most detailed quantitative study of the binocular responses of V1 neurons of infant monkeys (Chino et al., 1997). They presented a pair of drifting sine wave gratings **dichoptically** (one to each eye). The sine waves were identical in spatial frequency, orientation, contrast, and velocity, and these values were chosen to maximize the cell's response. A phase difference between the two monocular gratings creates binocular disparity. When the relative spatial phase of the two drifting sine waves was varied, the response of a binocular neuron waxed and waned. For the cell whose responses are illustrated in **Figure 6.47**, note that the binocular response was considerably higher than the response through either eye alone (dashed horizontal lines) for some interocular phase differences. At other interocular phase differences, the binocular response was lower than the response through either eye alone. This sinusoidal binocular phase tuning is the hallmark of binocular neurons in the visual cortex. Using this sensitive method, Chino et al. (1997) found that within the first week of life—well before the onset of stereopsis—infant monkeys had practically the same proportion of phase disparity–sensitive neurons as did adults in primary visual cortex.

In addition, the ocular dominance properties (see Chapter 3) of these infant monkeys were essentially identical to those of adults. Others have also found that ocular dominance columns in the input layers of V1 are essentially adultlike at birth (Horton and Hocking, 1996).

dichoptic Referring to the presentation of two stimuli, one to each eye. Different from *binocular* presentation, which could involve both eyes looking at a single stimulus.

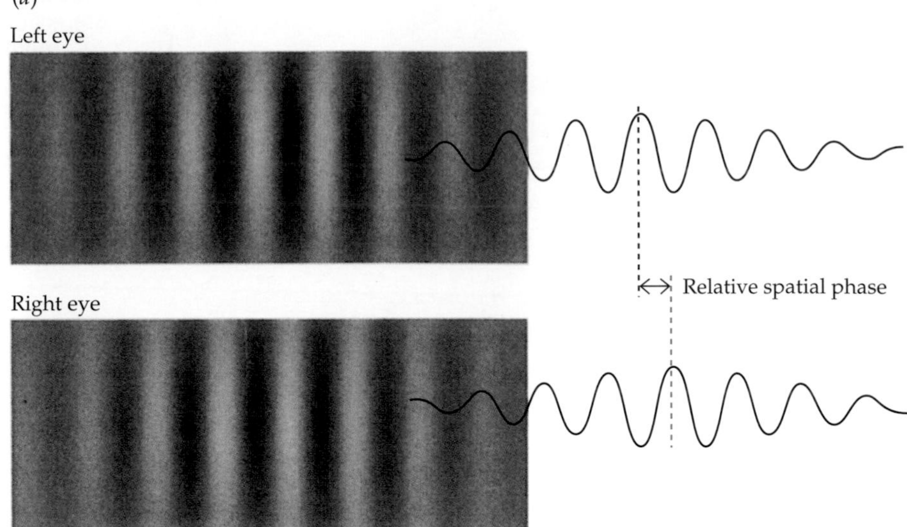

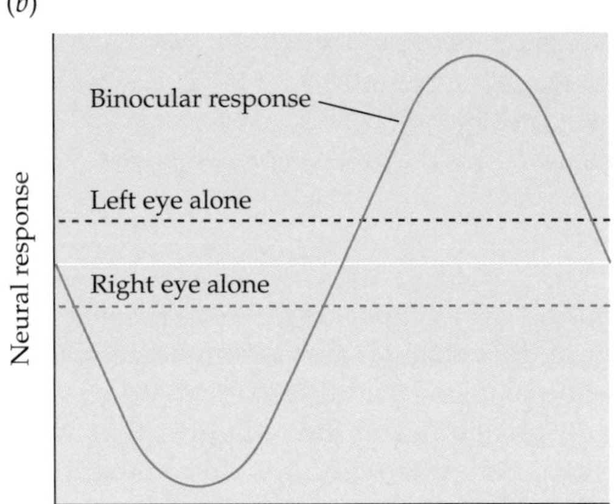

FIGURE 6.47 Interocular phase difference gratings are used to study disparity tuning. (*a*) Two sinusoidal gratings drift differently in each eye, producing a sinusoidal change in spatial phase disparity. (*b*) The response of a binocular neuron. Notice that the binocular response varies with phase, and the monocular responses do not. (After Chino et al., 1997.)

What do these studies tell us about the development of stereopsis? The results suggest that the neural apparatus in V1 of newborns is capable of combining signals from the two eyes and that it is sensitive to interocular disparities. So why are newborns blind to disparity? One possibility is that the extraction of relative disparity, which is needed for stereoacuity, takes place beyond V1, possibly in V2. At this time, we do not know much about the responses of V2 neurons to disparity in newborns, but emerging evidence suggests that other receptive-field properties mature later in V2 than in V1 (Zhang et al., 2005; Zheng et al., 2007).

On the other hand, maybe the problem is in V1. Although V1 cells of newborn monkeys are adultlike in their response to interocular phase disparity, these neurons remain immature in several important ways. They do not have adult sensitivity to monocular spatial frequency or direction of motion. Moreover, they are much less responsive overall than adult neurons (that is, their peak firing rates are considerably lower). In addition, these neurons display more interocular suppression than adult neurons do. Thus, it is also possible that because of the immaturity in V1 neurons, the signals they send to the next stage of processing are too weak or confused to support stereopsis.

Abnormal Visual Experience Can Disrupt Binocular Vision

The presence of all this binocular hardware, even if it is immature, strongly suggests that extensive binocular visual experience is not necessary for binocular connections to form in V1. These connections are present at birth or very shortly thereafter, so we don't need to "learn" or develop binocular vision. The development of adult binocular vision and stereopsis, however, does require visual experience. In Chapter 3 we learned about Hubel and Wiesel's work on the **critical period**, the period during early visual development when normal binocular visual stimulation is required for normal cortical development. During this period, the visual cortex is highly susceptible to any disorder that alters normal binocular visual experience. In cats and monkeys this critical period is approximately the first 3 to 4 months of life.

How can we estimate the critical period in humans during which we cannot look at the details of the organization of visual cortex? Some humans are born with two eyes that do not point at the same spot in the world. This not uncommon disorder is known as **strabismus**, as we learned in Chapter 3. The incidence is about 3%. In **esotropia**, one eye is pointed too far toward the nose ("cross-eyed"). In **exotropia**, the deviating eye is pointed too far to the side. There a various ways to treat strabismus. For example, it is possible to surgically correct the position of the eyes. For the present discussion, however, the important point is that it is possible to test adults who had misaligned eyes at different points and for different durations during childhood.

Recall from Chapter 3 that exposure to lines tilted to one side of vertical will make vertical lines appear tilted to the other side. This is known as the tilt aftereffect. One characteristic of the tilt aftereffect is that it shows interocular transfer (transfer of the effect from one eye to the other). If we show the adapting lines to one eye, we can measure an aftereffect through the other eye. This result is generally taken to show that the cells responsible for the effect are binocular; they receive input from both eyes (for some details, see Wolfe and Held, 1981). Individuals who exhibited strabismus during the first 18 months of life do not show normal interocular transfer (Banks et al., 1975; Hohmann and Creutzfeldt, 1975). This result provides an indirect estimate of the period during which binocular connections in humans are susceptible to abnormal input.

Let's examine in a bit more detail why strabismus disrupts binocular vision. We will use left esotropia as an example. In left esotropia (**Figure 6.48**), the left eye is turned in. As a consequence, although the object of fixation (the yellow brick in this case) lands on the fovea of the right eye, it lands on a region in the "nasal" retina of the left eye. (The nasal retina is the half of the retina closest to the nose.) This means that the images of the yellow brick are in noncorresponding points in the two eyes. What will the patient see? If an adult becomes esotropic (perhaps because of an injury), she will experience diplopia (double vision), seeing two bricks instead of one. However, children who exhibit strabismus early in life often experience no such problem. Why? Notice that *something* is present at the fovea of the left eye. In Figure 6.48, this something is a purple pentagon. Thus, in strabismus, normally corresponding points in the two eyes receive conflicting information (this situation is known—not unreasonably—as confusion). To eliminate diplopia and confusion, the brain **suppresses** one of the two images. It is simply not consciously perceived. In esotropia, the most common pattern is suppression of the input from the eye that is turned in. So, in the example in Figure 6.48, the patient would most likely suppress visual input from the left eye.

critical period In the study of development, a period of time when the organism is particularly susceptible to developmental change. There are critical periods in the development of binocular vision, human language, and so on.

strabismus A misalignment of the two eyes such that a single object in space is imaged on the fovea of one eye, and on a nonfoveal area of the other (turned) eye.

esotropia Strabismus in which one eye deviates inward.

exotropia Strabismus in which one eye deviates outward.

suppression In vision, the inhibition of an unwanted image. Suppression occurs frequently in persons with strabismus.

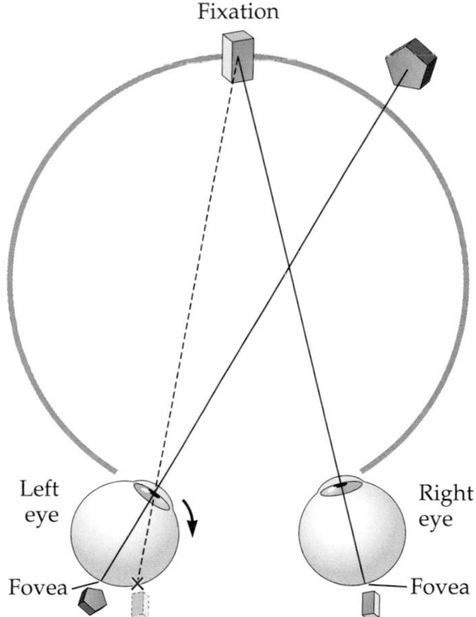

FIGURE 6.48 Left esotropia. The patient wants to fixate on the yellow brick, but the left eye is turned too far toward the nose and, as a result, the left fovea is pointing at a different location (here the purple pentagon) while the image of the yellow brick falls to the right of the left fovea.

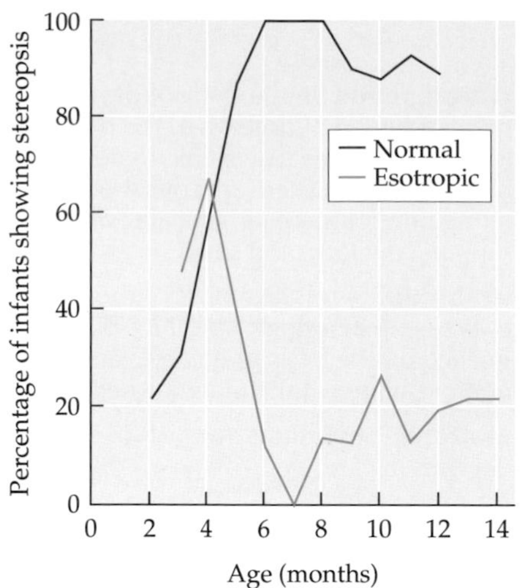

FIGURE 6.49 Development of stereopsis in normal infants (red line) and in esotropes. Beyond 4 months, very few esotropic infants demonstrated stereopsis. (After Stager and Birch, 1986.)

Binocular rivalry is a form of suppression, so some suppression is an important part of normal visual experience. Unfortunately, early-onset strabismus can have other, more serious effects on the developing visual nervous system, and on visual performance. For example, strabismus greatly reduces the number of binocular neurons in the visual cortex (Wiesel, 1982)). Cells that would normally be driven by both eyes are dominated by only one. You would be correct if you suspected that this situation would disrupt stereopsis. Birch and her colleagues (e.g., Stager and Birch, 1986) followed the development of stereopsis in normal and esotropic infants. **Figure 6.49** illustrates the percentage of infants who showed a measurable ability to perceive stereoscopic depth. The red line shows that by about 6 months of age, almost all normal infants demonstrate stereopsis. In contrast, the esotropes (all of whom were diagnosed with esotropia by 6 months) initially demonstrated a normal pattern of stereopsis development. After 4 months, however, very few esotropic infants demonstrated stereopsis.

This result has an interesting parallel in cortical physiology. Chino and his colleagues (Kumagami et al., 2000) made otherwise normal monkeys strabismic. They found that a brief period of experimental strabismus shortly after the age of onset of stereopsis produced a greater loss of disparity sensitivity and more binocular suppression in V1 neurons than did an earlier episode of strabismus. These physiological and perceptual deficits appear to be permanent and have important implications for the surgical treatment of infantile esotropia. Almost all surgeons agree that treatment should be early, but there has been a lot of debate about just how early. These results suggest that the treatment should take place before the age at which stereopsis normally develops, in order to minimize the damage done by esotropia.

Refer to the **Sensation and Perception** website **(www.sinauer.com/wolfe2e)** for activities, essays, study questions, and other study aids.

Summary

1. Reconstructing a three-dimensional world from two, non-Euclidean, curved, two-dimensional retinal images is one basic problem faced by the brain.
2. Having two eyes is an advantage for a number of reasons, some of which have to do with depth perception. It is important to remember, however, that it is possible to reconstruct the three-dimensional world from a single two-dimensional image. Two eyes have other advantages over just one: expanding the visual field, permitting binocular summation, and providing redundancy if one eye is damaged.
3. A number of monocular cues provide information about three-dimensional space. These include occlusion, various size and position cues, aerial perspective, linear perspective, motion cues, accommodation, and convergence.
4. Having two laterally separated eyes connected to a single brain also provides us with important information about depth through the geometry of the small differences between the images in each eye. These differences, known as binocular disparities, give rise to stereoscopic depth perception.
5. Random dot stereograms show that we don't need to know what we're seeing before we see it in stereoscopic depth. Binocular disparity alone can support shape perception.
6. The difficulty of matching an image element in one eye with the correct element in the other eye is known as the correspondence problem. The brain uses several "tricks" to solve the problem. For example, it reduces the initial complexity of the problem by matching large "blobs" in the low-spatial-frequency information before trying to match every high-frequency detail.
7. Single neurons in primary visual cortex and beyond have receptive fields that cover a region in three-dimensional space, not just the two-dimensional image plane. Some neurons respond to a wide range of depths (e.g., stimuli beyond the current distance of fixation). Others have more precise receptive fields.

8. When the stimuli on corresponding loci in the two eyes are different, we experience a continuous perceptual competition between the two eyes known as binocular rivalry.
9. All of the various monocular and binocular depth cues are combined (unconsciously) according to what prior knowledge tells us about the probability of the current event. Making the wrong guess about the cause of visual input can lead to illusions.
10. Stereopsis emerges suddenly at about 4 months of age in humans, and it can be disrupted through abnormal visual experience during a critical period early in life.

CHAPTER 7

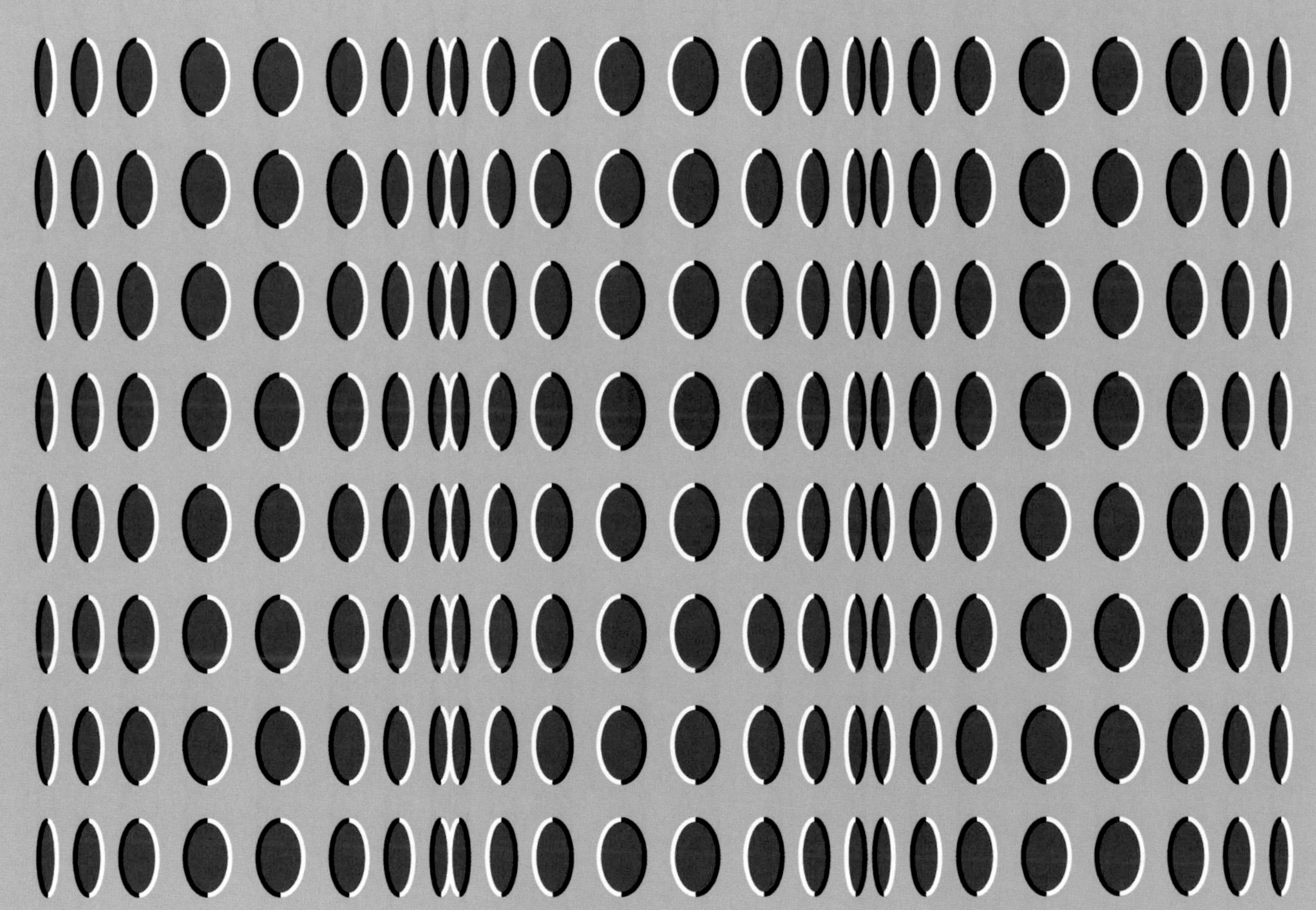

Akiyoshi Kitaoka, *Rollers*, 2004

Motion Perception

Take a look at the insect in **Figure 7.1**. Like any self-respecting ladybug, it flits around from leaf to leaf. At time 1 it is on the lowermost leaf; at time 2 it has moved to the middle leaf. Our visual system distinguishes the bug by a number of features, such as its shape, its location in space, and its color. Previous chapters have established these features as fundamental perceptual dimensions: characteristics of visual stimuli that are directly encoded by neurons fairly early in the visual system.

Is the ladybug's motion also a fundamental perceptual dimension? At first glance, we might think not. After all, motion is really just a change in an object's location over time. If we already have neural mechanisms set up to determine position, why go to the extra expense of adding more low-level machinery to process motion?

Though the added investment might seem unnecessary, consider this question from the position of the primordial vertebrates that "invented" the visual system we eventually inherited. Many bugs move pretty quickly, so if we depend on catching them for our supper, fast detection of their direction of motion will be important to our survival. Similarly, if other animals are trying to catch us for their supper, we need to be adept at detecting the motion of these predators too. In Chapter 6, we saw that motion parallax is an important cue for depth perception. And from a more modern perspective, it would be hard to believe that hockey goalies, baseball batters facing knuckleball pitchers, and boxers trying to avoid being pummeled by their opponents could do their jobs without having a mechanism for very quickly determining the movements of pucks, balls, and fists.

In fact, we've already seen some strong indications that motion is a low-level perceptual phenomenon—in Chapter 3, where we learned that many cells in primary visual cortex selectively respond to motion in one particular direction. A phenomenon called the "waterfall illusion" provides another piece of evidence that there is something special about motion. Here's how Robert Addams (1834) described this illusion after a visit to the waterfall of Foyers (**Figure 7.2**):

> Having steadfastly looked for a few seconds at a particular part of the cascade, admiring the confluence and decussation of the currents forming the liquid drapery of waters, and then suddenly directed my eyes to the left, to observe the face of the sombre age-worn rocks immediately contiguous to the water-fall, I saw the rocky surface as if in motion upwards, and with an apparent velocity equal to that of the descending water, which the moment before had prepared my eyes to behold that singular deception.

The "deception" that Addams described—which had also been noted by Aristotle (384–322 BCE)—has more recently been dubbed the **motion aftereffect (MAE)**. After viewing motion in a constant direction for a sustained

motion aftereffect (MAE) The illusion of motion of a stationary object that occurs after prolonged exposure to a moving object.

period of time (at least 15 seconds or so), we see any stationary objects that we view subsequently (like the rocks around the waterfall) as moving in the opposite direction. This phenomenon may seem a lot like the color aftereffects we studied in Chapter 5, and that's no coincidence. Just as color aftereffects are caused by opponent processes for color vision, the MAE is caused by opponent processes for motion detection. We'll discuss these processes in detail later in the chapter. Let's back up first and take a broader look at how the visual system might go about detecting motion.

The waterfall illusion is just one of many motion illusions. Akiyoshi Kitaoka's *Rollers* at the beginning of this chapter shows another powerful illusion of motion. (See **Web Essay 7.1: Perceiving Motion in Static Images.**) The picture is stationary on the page, but it can produce a strong illusion of motion if you allow your eyes to drift across it. How does this work? We don't yet have a consensus, but recent work suggests that patterns like the rollers and equally compelling rotating snakes elicit directional responses

Time 1

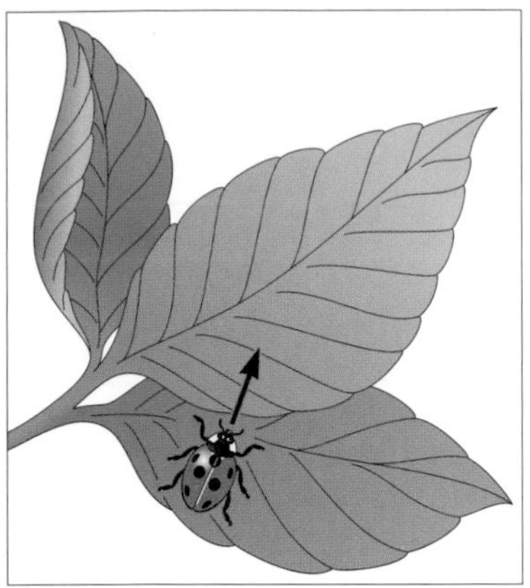

Time 2

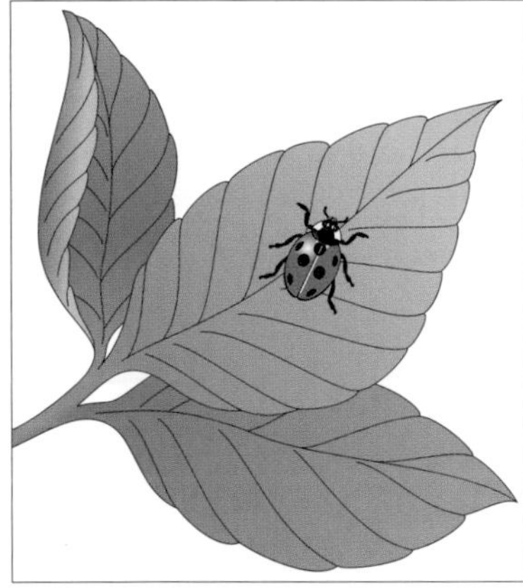

FIGURE 7.1 Motion is a change in position over time, as the movements of this ladybug demonstrate.

FYERS, UPPER FALL.
Dim seen through rising Mists and ceaseless show'rs —
The hoary cavern, wide-surrounding, low'rs.
Still thro' the gap the struggling river toils,
And still below, the horrid cauldron boils.

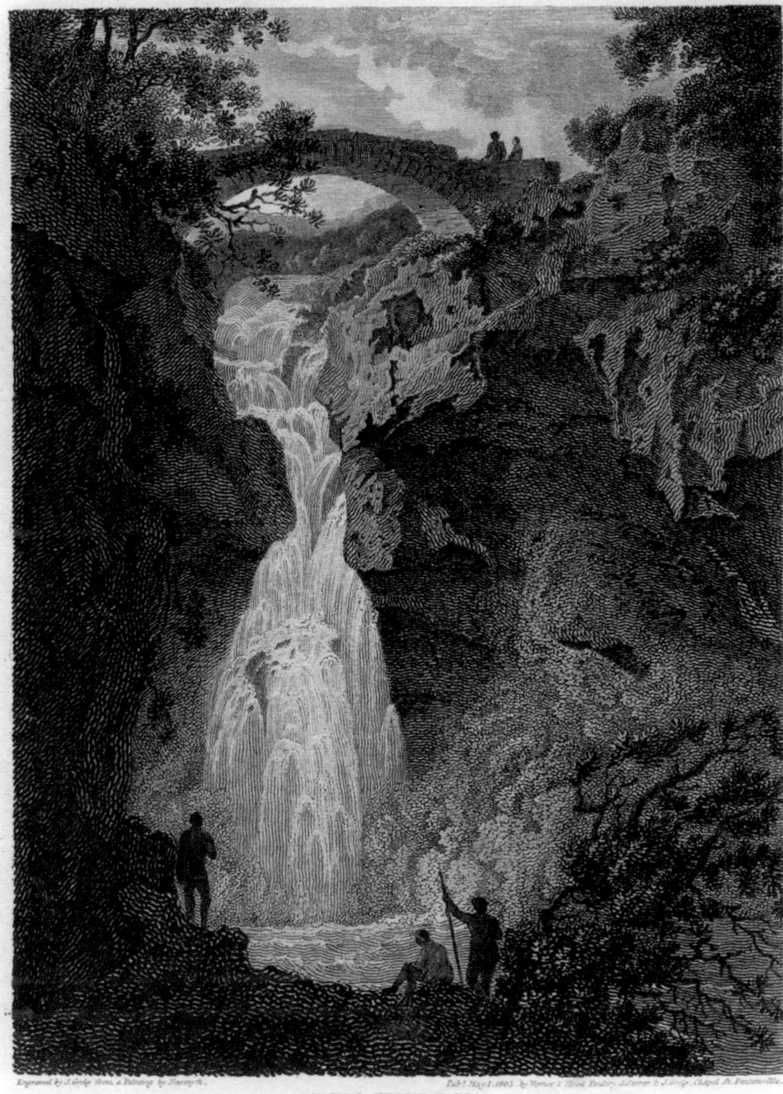

FIGURE 7.2 A print from the lower falls of Foyers (hand-colored by Grieg, 1803, after a painting by Nasmyth), with the last four lines of the poem that Robert Burns (1759–1796) wrote while visiting the falls. (From Peter Thompson's website: www.hip.atr.co.jp/departments/Dept5/MAEWWW/MAE-history/History.html; courtesy of Frans A. J. Verstraten.)

from neurons in monkey cortex that correspond closely to the directions perceived by humans (Conway et al., 2005).

Computation of Visual Motion

How would you build a motion detector? Because motion involves a change in position over time, a logical place to start is with two adjacent receptors (call them neurons A and B) separated by a fixed distance. A bug (or a spot of light) moving from left to right would first pass through neuron A's receptive field, then a short time later would enter receptor B's receptive field (**Figure 7.3***a*). In theory, a third cell that "listens" to neurons A and B should be able to detect this movement.

However, our motion detection cell (M) cannot simply add up excitatory inputs from A and B. Given such a neural circuit, M would fire in response to the moving bug, but it would also respond to a large, stationary bug that covered both receptive fields (Figure 7.3*b*). To solve this problem, we need two additional components in our neural circuit, as shown in Figure 7.3*c*. The first new cell, labeled "D" in the figure, receives input from A and delays transmission of this input for a short period of time. Cell D also has a fast adaptation rate. That is, it fires when cell A initially detects light, but quickly stops firing if the light remains shining on A's receptive field. Cells B and D are then connected to neuron X, a multiplication cell. This multiplication cell will fire only when both cells B and D are active. By delaying receptor A's response (D) and then multiplying it by receptor B's response (X), we can create a mechanism that is sensitive to motion.

This mechanism would be direction-selective: it would respond well to motion from left to right, but not from right to left. The mechanism would also be tuned to velocity because when the bug is moving at just the right speed, the delayed response from receptor A and the direct response from receptor B occur at the same time and therefore reinforce each other. This simple "bug" motion detector is based on a model developed by Werner Reichardt in the 1950s to explain how flies detect motion (Reichardt, 1986). Almost all models of human motion detection are, at their core, an elaboration of Werner Reichardt's model adapted to the spatial-frequency filtering properties of the human visual system (see Chapter 3).

One elaboration, developed by Barlow and Levick (1965), uses what electrical engineers would call an "AND gate." Cell X fires if and only if *both* its inputs (B and D) are firing simultaneously, and it passes this message on to

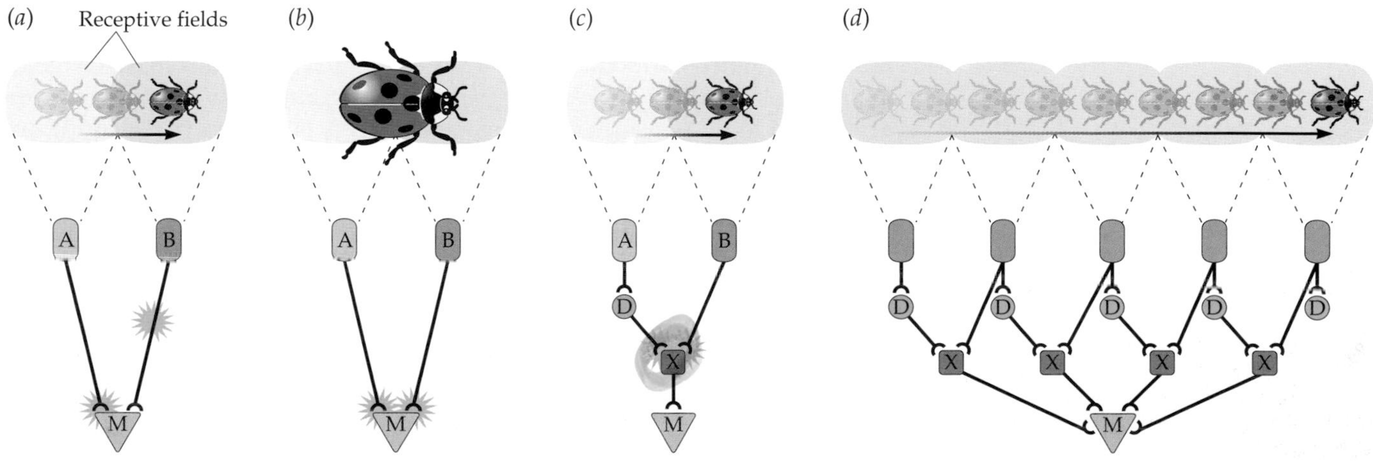

FIGURE 7.3 Constructing a neural circuit for the detection of rightward motion. See the text for details.

the motion detection cell M. The AND concept is almost certainly not correct, and a more elaborate version—which was developed by Adelson and Bergen (1985) and is based on linear filters that delay, sum, and then are followed by nonlinearities—seems closer to the "truth." In **Web Activity 7.2: Motion Detection Circuit**, which presents a more elaborate version of this neural circuit, you can interactively move spots of light around and see how it works.

Now that we've constructed our neural circuit, consider what happens when our bug moves into cell A's receptive field and then into cell B's receptive field. Cell A will activate cell D, which, after a short delay, will communicate its response to cell X. If the bug is flying at just the right speed, it will move into cell B's receptive field just as cell D begins to fire. The signals from B and D will be multiplied by X, and X will drive cell M, the motion detector, to fire. Note that M will not respond to our large sedentary bug, because of the fast adaptation of the D cell. Furthermore, M will respond to motion in only one particular direction (left to right in Figure 7.3). A bug moving from cell B's receptive field into cell A's receptive field would cause B and D to fire in the wrong order, so X would not receive its two inputs simultaneously, and M would not fire. Our motion detector is also velocity-sensitive: if the bug moves too fast or too slow, the outputs from B and D will again be out of sync. A more realistic circuit would include additional receptors to detect longer-range motion, as shown in Figure 7.3*d*. Here, the M cell fires continuously as the bug moves across the fields of the five receptors at the top of the circuit.

Apparent Motion

One possible objection to this neural circuit is that it does not, in fact, require continuous motion in order to fire. An image of a bug that appears in A's receptive field, then disappears, and then reappears in B's receptive field a short time later will drive M to respond just as strongly as if the image had moved smoothly across the two receptive fields. Although it raises a valid concern, this observation turns out to be a virtue rather than a liability for the Reichardt model, because it provides an excellent explanation for a visual illusion that modern humans experience on a daily basis.

Called **apparent motion**, this illusion was first demonstrated by Sigmund Exner in 1875. Exner set up a contraption that would generate electrical sparks separated from each other by a very short distance in space and a very short period of time. Even though there were two separate sparks—two different perceptual objects—observers swore that they saw a single spark moving from one position to another. (Apparent motion is demonstrated in **Web Activity 7.1: Types of Motion**.)

We in the twenty-first century experience apparent motion every time we watch television, go to a movie, or use a computer. You are probably aware that an animated cartoon is really a series of still drawings. Objects such as Daffy Duck (**Figure 7.4**) change positions each frame, and when the frames are shown to us at a sufficiently fast speed (e.g., 60 frames per second), we perceive these position changes over time as motion. **Web Activity 7.1: Types of Motion** shows the two frames in Figure 7.1, from which you will have little difficulty inferring motion. Live-action movies and television programs work exactly the same way, except that the frames are still photographs rather than drawings.

apparent motion The (illusory) impression of smooth motion resulting from the rapid alternation of objects that appear in different locations in rapid succession.

The Correspondence and Aperture Problems

Although apparent motion turns out to be a win for our motion detection circuit, two more of the classic perceptual "problems" that we've discussed over

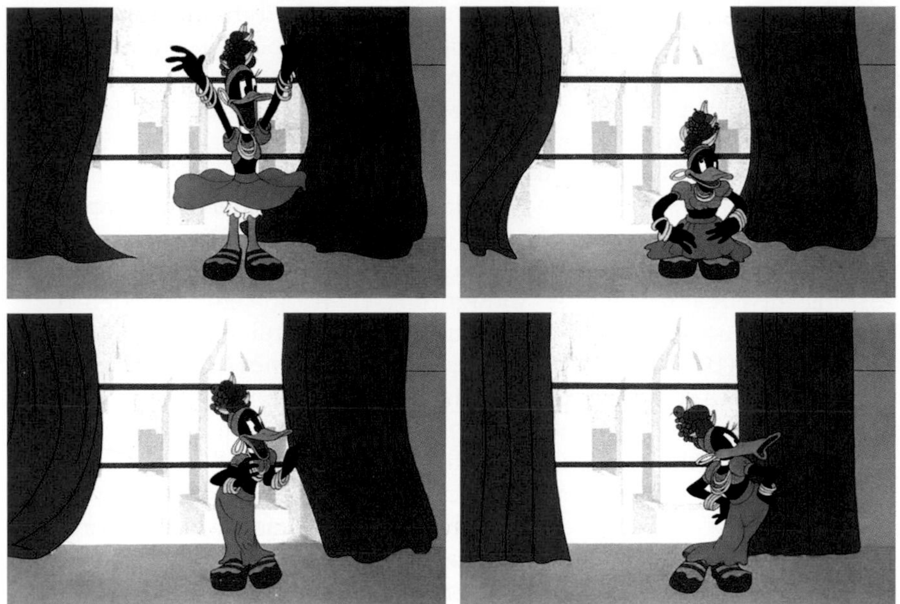

FIGURE 7.4 Daffy Duck impersonates Carmen Miranda in these four stills from the Looney Tunes animation *Yankee Doodle Daffy*.

and over in this book remain issues for the Reichardt model. We can illustrate these problems with the movies diagrammed in **Figure 7.5**. Each movie has two frames that alternate back and forth. The only difference between the two frames is that the only object in the movie, the red square studded with small circles, has been shifted diagonally by a short distance. (These movies are animated in **Web Activity 7.1: Types of Motion**. Viewing the animations as you read this section will make the following discussion much clearer.)

aperture An opening that allows only a partial view of the object.

If you view the first version of the movie (depicted in Figure 7.5*a*) on the website (click on "The Aperture Problem" and select "Movie 1"), you will clearly detect diagonal motion. This scenario appears to present no problem to our motion detector: the square moves down and to the right, and then back up and to the left, and detectors sensitive to these directions pick up and signal this movement. Now consider Movie 2 (depicted in Figure 7.5*b*), where we cover most of the square with a black "mask," leaving three of the circles viewable through a small **aperture** (in Figure 7.5*b*, the mask is illustrated as transparent so that you can see what's behind it, but in the movie the mask is opaque). Beneath the mask, the square moves exactly as before, but if you view the movie, you will quite clearly perceive up-and-down, *not* diagonal, motion! (You really have to see the animation to appreciate the difference in the motion perceived in the two movies.)

FIGURE 7.5 Movies illustrating the aperture and correspondence problems. See **Web Activity 7.1: Types of Motion** for animated versions.

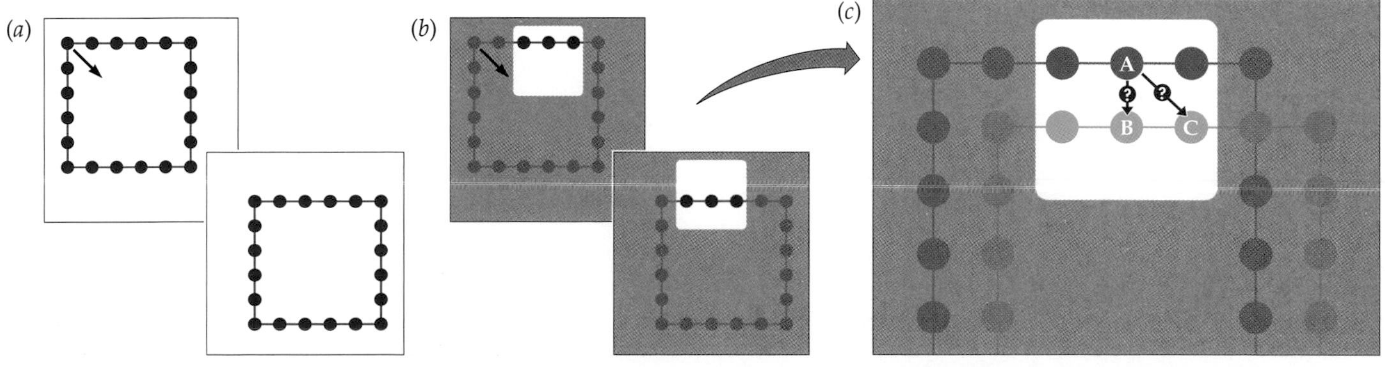

correspondence problem (motion) The problem faced by the motion detection system of knowing which feature in frame 2 corresponds to a particular feature in frame 1.

aperture problem The fact that when a moving object is viewed through an aperture (or a receptive field), the direction of motion of a local feature or part of the object may be ambiguous.

The larger issue that these movies bring up is called the **correspondence problem** for motion detection. It is similar to the correspondence problem we encountered in Chapter 6 for stereoscopic depth perception. Consider the close-up view of the situation in Figure 7.5*b*, shown in Figure 7.5*c*. Here we superimposed the two frames, coloring the square and circles blue in their frame 1 positions and green in their frame 2 positions. The difficulty for our motion detection system is this: how does it know which circles in frame 2 correspond to which circles in frame 1? Because we have motion detectors for all directions, one detector will sense the diagonal motion implied by matching the circle labeled "A" in Figure 7.5*c* with the circle labeled "C." But another detector will sense the vertical motion implied by matching circle A with circle B. These detectors compete to determine our overall perception. (You can see some other demonstrations of the correspondence problem in **Web Activity 7.3: Motion Correspondence**.)

The **aperture problem** gets its name from the fact that a different detector may win this competition when an object is viewed through an aperture than would win if we could see the whole object, as is the case in our demonstration here. Without the mask, the diagonal-motion detector clearly determines which direction we perceive the square to be moving. But when we view the square through the aperture, the system appears to impose some kind of shortest-distance constraint, and thus the vertical-motion detector wins.

At this point you may be thinking it's rather silly to claim that an artificial situation such as the one we've set up here poses a broad challenge to the visual system. After all, how often is our view of a moving object limited to a small window as in the movies here? To understand the broader implications of the correspondence and aperture problems, consider the fact that every neuron in V1 (the primary visual cortex) has a limited receptive field. In other words, *every V1 cell sees the world through a small aperture*. Therefore, as illustrated in **Figure 7.6**, none of the V1 cells (which are represented in the

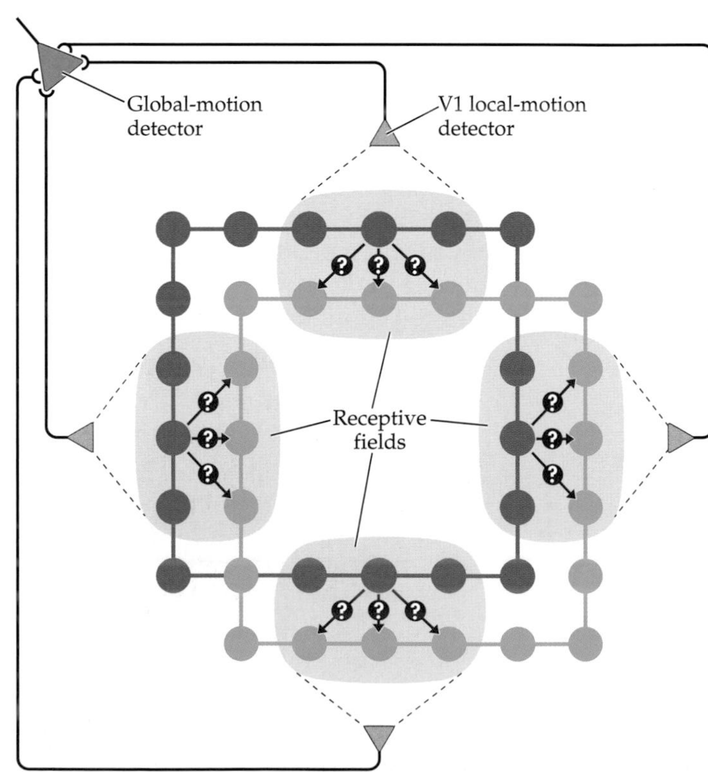

FIGURE 7.6 Building a global-motion detector. See the text for details.

figure as gray triangles) can tell with certainty which visual elements correspond to one another when an object moves, even when no mask is present.

The solution to this problem is to have another set of neurons listen to the V1 neurons and integrate the potentially conflicting signals. As Figure 7.6 shows, only one direction—down and to the right—is consistent with what all four V1 cells are seeing here, and this is the direction we perceive when we see the object as a whole. If the neuron represented by the orange triangle in Figure 7.6 has access to all the V1 cells detecting local-motion directions, it will be in a position to compare their outputs and find this common denominator. Of course, we haven't specified *how* this global-motion detector performs this comparison, but that question would lead us beyond the scope of this book.

middle temporal lobe (MT) An area of the brain thought to be important in the perception of motion.

Detection of Global Motion in Area MT

Though a discussion of how global-motion detectors work would be too broad for this text, we can say something about *where* the global-motion detectors are. We saw in Chapter 3 that lesions to the magnocellular layers of the LGN (lateral geniculate nucleus) impair the perception of large, rapidly moving objects. Information from magnocellular neurons feeds into V1 and is then passed on to (among other places) the **middle temporal lobe** of the cortex, an area commonly referred to as **MT** (**Figure** 7.7). The vast majority of neurons in MT are selective for motion in one particular direction, but they show little selectivity for form or color. But do these MT cells correspond to the orange neuron in Figure 7.6, which responds to large-scale motion of whole objects, or are they the low-level motion detectors represented by the gray triangles in Figure 7.6?

To find out, Newsome and Pare (1988) trained a group of monkeys to respond to correlated dot motion displays, illustrated in **Figure 7.8**. (Note that, in the actual stimuli, all dots are the same color and no arrows are present. You can get a much better feel for what Newsome and Pare's monkeys were experiencing by visiting the "Correlated Dot Motion" section of **Web Activity 7.1: Types of Motion**). In Figure 7.8*a*, all the dots (100%) are moving to the right. In Figure 7.8*b*, 50% of the dots have correlated motion (that is, they are moving in the same direction), while the motion of the rest of the dots is uncorrelated (these dots are moving in random directions). In Figure

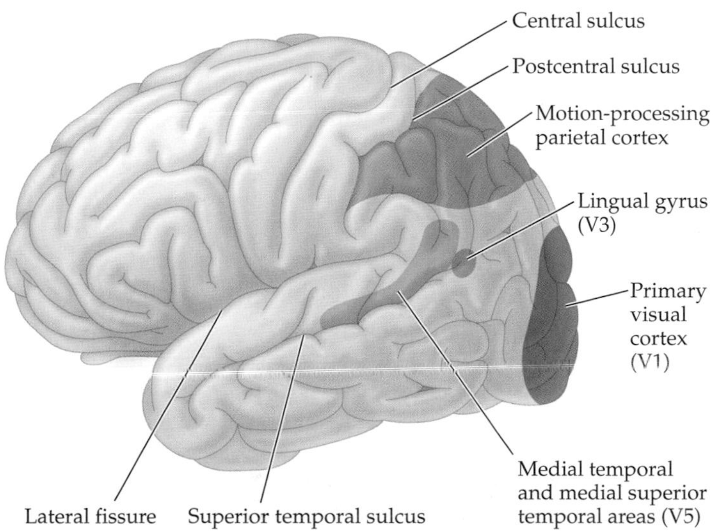

FIGURE 7.7 The middle temporal lobe and other regions of the cortex involved in motion perception.

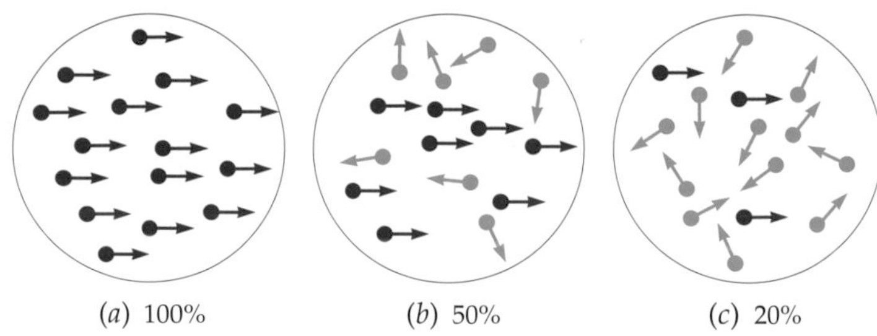

FIGURE 7.8 The Newsome and Pare paradigm. The observer's task is to identify the direction of motion of the correlated dots, shown in purple here. (In the actual stimuli, the dots are not colored and there are no arrows.)

7.8*c*, only 20% of the dots are in correlated motion. Just as in the aperture problem demonstration, no single dot in these displays is sufficient to determine the overall direction of correlated motion. So, to detect the correlated direction, a neuron must integrate information from many local-motion detectors.

Once they were fully trained, the monkeys in Newsome and Pare's study could recognize the correlated motion direction when only 2% to 3% of the dots were moving in this direction. The researchers then lesioned the monkeys' MT areas. Following the surgery, the monkeys needed about ten times as many correlated dots in order to correctly identify the direction of motion. However, the monkeys' ability to discriminate the orientation of stationary patterns was generally unimpaired. Interestingly, the monkeys' performance in the correlated dot motion task improved markedly during the weeks following the lesion, presumably because they learned to use other brain areas to discriminate motion.

Lesion studies have been central to our understanding of the specificity of brain areas. However, such studies are often less than completely compelling, because lesions (even nice "clean" chemical lesions, like those used by Newsome and Pare) may be incomplete or may influence other structures. To test the involvement of MT neurons in global-motion perception more directly, Newsome et al. (Salzman, Britten, and Newsome, 1990) trained a new group of monkeys to discriminate correlated motion directions, then poked around in the monkeys' MT areas to find groups of neurons that responded to one particular direction. Once they had found a group of neurons that responded, for example, to rightward motion, they showed the monkey a new set of stimuli and electrically stimulated the identified MT neurons. Remarkably, the monkeys showed a strong tendency to report motion in the stimulated neurons' preferred direction, even when the dots they were seeing were actually moving in the opposite direction! These results make a very strong case that MT is the site of global-motion detection neurons in the visual system.

Motion Aftereffects Revisited

We know that the monkey brain is very similar to the human brain, but it is always nice to establish converging evidence suggesting that results from monkey labs apply to human vision as well. In the case of motion perception, researchers have looked for this evidence using the MAE (motion aftereffect). As we noted earlier, the existence of the MAE implies an opponent-process system much like the one that plays a role in color vision (discussed in Chapter 5). When we view a stationary object, the responses of neurons tuned to different directions of motion are normally balanced. That is, neurons sensitive to upward motion fire at the same rate as neurons sensitive to downward motion, so the signals cancel out and no motion is perceived. But when we look at a waterfall for a prolonged period, the detectors sensitive to downward motion become fatigued. When we then switch our gaze to a stationary object, the neurons sensitive to upward motion fire faster than the tuckered-out downward-sensitive neurons, and we therefore perceive the rocks as drifting up.

You might wonder why *any* motion detectors would fire in response to a stationary rock, but as we will see in a bit, our eyes are constantly drifting around, so there is always a small amount of retinal motion to stimulate motion detectors at least slightly. You might also wonder what happens when we adapt to downward motion and then see something moving horizontally. Make a prediction and then test your hypothesis using **Web Activity 7.4: Motion Aftereffects**.

Here's another experiment to try with this activity: adapt for 15 seconds or so to rightward motion with your right eye open but your left eye closed, then quickly switch eyes, closing your right eye and opening your left. You should experience an aftereffect that is only slightly reduced in magnitude compared to the aftereffect you get with both eyes open the whole time. What does this **interocular transfer** tell us about the locus of the MAE in the visual system? Could motion aftereffects be subserved by neurons in the retinas? What about neurons in the LGN?

The fact that a strong MAE is obtained when one eye is adapted and the other tested means that the effect must be reflecting the activities of neurons in a part of the visual system where information collected from the two eyes is combined (e.g., Raymond, 1993). As we learned in Chapter 3, input from both eyes is not combined until cortical area V1, where neurons show a preference for input from one eye or another but respond to some extent to stimuli in both eyes. Recent advances in functional imaging techniques may make it possible to locate the site of motion aftereffects even more precisely. The emerging evidence suggests that the MAE in humans is caused by the same brain region shown to be responsible for global-motion detection in monkeys: cortical area MT. For example, David Heeger and his colleagues (Huk, Ress, and Heeger, 2001), after controlling for the important effects of attention, demonstrated that the direction-selective adaptation produced a selective imbalance in the fMRI signal in human MT, providing evidence that MAE is due to a population imbalance in area MT.

Up to this point, our discussion has focused on **first-order motion**—that is, about **luminance-defined objects** that change position over time; in the next section, however, we describe another interesting motion phenomenon: **second-order motion**, in which **texture- or contrast-defined objects** change position over time.

Second-Order Motion

Second-order motion, illustrated in **Figure 7.9**, is an interesting phenomenon. The three frames in the figure look like collections of random black and white dots, which is what they are. But if you go to the website and look at the sequence of frames played as a movie, you will clearly perceive a set of leftward-moving stripes. (**Web Activity 7.1: Types of Motion** includes some additional frames that will lead to the perception of an infinite loop in which the stripes move leftward off the edge of the movie and reappear on the right side.)

This movie is constructed from a combination of two patterns: a random collection of small white and black dots, and a series of wide white and black stripes. The patterns are overlaid and combined in such a way that dots covered by white bars are inverted (black dots turn white and vice

interocular transfer The transfer of an effect (such as adaptation) from one eye to the other.

first-order motion The motion of an object that is defined by changes in luminance.

luminance-defined object An object that is delineated by changes in reflected light.

second-order motion The motion of an object that is defined by changes in contrast or texture, but not by luminance.

texture-defined (contrast-defined) object An object that is defined by changes in contrast or texture, but not by luminance.

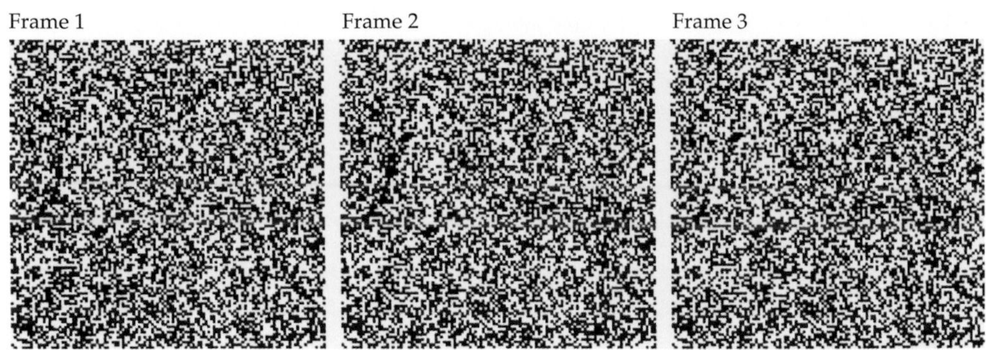

FIGURE 7.9 Three frames from a movie demonstrating second-order motion. See **Web Activity 7.1: Types of Motion**, in which you will quite clearly see stripes moving from right to left across the field of dots.

versa), and dots covered by black bars are left alone. The frames of the movie are made by the process of shifting the bars to the left while the dots remain stationary. The resulting perception of movement is called "second-order motion."

As in first-order apparent motion displays, nothing actually moves in second-order motion. Even more incredibly, there is nothing *to* move in second-order motion. As **Figure 7.10** shows, the only thing that changes in our second-order motion movie is that strips of dots are inverted from one frame to another: from frame 1 to frame 2 the dots in the orange strip are inverted; then from frame 2 to frame 3 the dots in the blue strip are inverted. Just as random dot stereograms prove that matching discrete objects across the two eyes is not necessary for stereoscopic depth perception, second-order motion proves that matching discrete objects across movie frames is not necessary for motion perception.

Several lines of evidence suggest that the visual system includes specialized mechanisms for second-order motion. For example, Lucia Vaina et al. (Vaina and Cowey, 1996; Vaina et al., 1998) described one neurological patient who suffered brain damage that caused impaired perception of first-order motion but not of second-order motion. A second patient showed the opposite pattern: impaired second-order but spared first-order motion perception. These two patients had lesions in different brain areas, and together they demonstrate a "double dissociation" of function, which would not be possible if there were a single motion mechanism. Tim Ledgeway demonstrated a motion aftereffect for second-order motion and found that the second-order MAE transfers even more completely between eyes than does the first-order MAE (Ledgeway, 1994; Ledgeway and Smith, 1994).

Why did we evolve a motion detection system for something as esoteric as second-order motion? It turns out that second order–like motion does

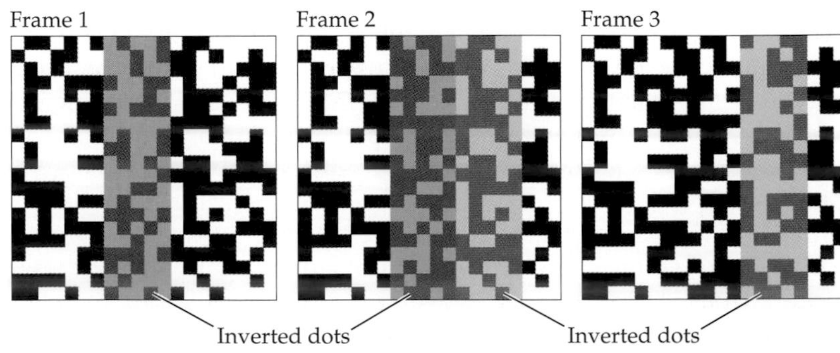

FIGURE 7.10 Close-ups of one section of the frames in Figure 7.9, illustrating the changes from frame to frame.

occur in the real world, especially when an object is effectively camouflaged. This chapter's home page on the website shows a situation in which something like second-order motion makes an otherwise invisible object spring to life. (See **Web Essay 7.2: Beyond Second-Order Motion**.)

optic array The collection of light rays that interact with objects in the world in front of a viewer. Term coined by J. J. Gibson.

optic flow The changing angular positions of points in a perspective image that we experience as we move through the world.

focus of expansion The point in the center of the horizon from which, when we are in motion (e.g., driving on the highway), all points in the perspective image seem to emanate. The focus of expansion is one aspect of optic flow.

Using Motion Information

Now that we know something about how the motion perception system works under the hood, let's consider some ways we might use motion information to interpret the world around us.

Going with the Flow: Using Motion Information to Navigate

For sighted people, getting around is easy. Our vision effortlessly guides our motion through space, whether we are walking or driving, so that we usually reach a destination quite safely and efficiently. Indeed, safe navigation is one of the primary functions of the visual system. What information does the visual system use to help us navigate our way across a busy intersection? Or consider the challenge that confronts a pilot landing an airplane at high speed. In an attempt to improve World War II pilots' performance in such situations, J. J. Gibson (1957), who was working for the US Army at the time, developed an influential theory about the **optic array**—the collection of light rays that interact with objects in the world in front of a viewer. Some of these rays strike our retinas, enabling us to see. Gibson argued that, when we move through our environment, we experience patterns of **optic flow** that our visual systems use to determine where we're going.

Consider a pilot coming in to land her plane. As the plane approaches the ground, the optic array will expand outward, in a pattern known as "radial expansion" (**Figure 7.11**). The pilot's heading—the specific point at which she is aiming her plane—will always be the center, or **focus of expansion**, of the optic array. As indicated in Figure 7.11, the focus of expansion is the one place in the visual field that will be stationary, so if the pilot's visual system can locate this stationary point, it can determine the heading. (For a relevant demonstration, see **Web Activity 7.1: Types of Motion**.)

Gibson was able to derive a number of optic flow heuristics that the visual system might use to navigate around the world. At the most basic level, the mere presence of optic flow indicates locomotion, and a lack of flow is a signal that you are stationary. If you have ever left your car in neutral with the brake off at the top of a hill, you may have experienced a situation in which optic flow alone tells you that you are in (unintentional) motion. Outflow (flow toward the periphery, as depicted in Figure 7.11) indicates that you are approaching a particular destination; inflow indicates retreat (assuming that your head is facing forward; you will also experience outflow when you look over your shoulder as you walk forward). And as mentioned already, the focus of expansion, or "focus of constriction" if you're driving in reverse, tells you where you are going to or coming from.

Are humans actually able to make use of optic flow information? Laboratories like Bill Warren's have used elaborate computer-generated displays of moving dots and lines to simulate optic flow information, and they have made a good deal of progress in understanding both the utility and complexity of optic flow information. For example, Warren et al. (W. H. Warren, Morris, and Kalish, 1988) demonstrated that humans could estimate their direction of heading to within about 1 or 2 degrees solely on the basis of the pattern of optic flow simulated by the moving dots, even when the display contained only a very small number of dots.

FIGURE 7.11 This schematic illustrates the optic flow field produced by movement forward in space. FOE = focus of expansion. (After W. H. Warren and Saunders, 1995.)

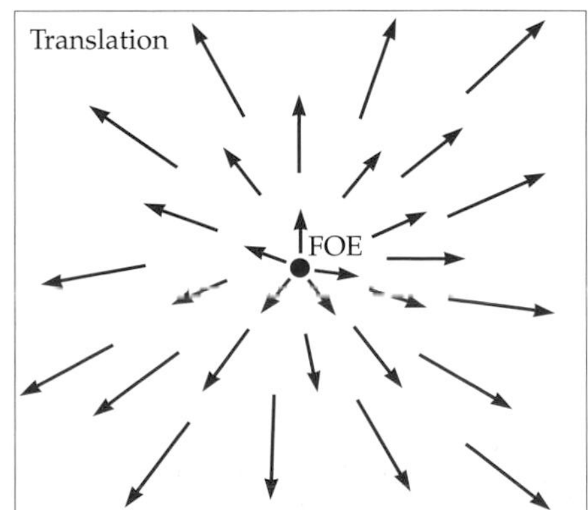

biological motion The pattern of movement of living beings (humans and animals).

Of course, the nice clean optic flow pattern diagrammed in Figure 7.11 occurs only if the head and eyes remain fixed and pointed straight ahead. As soon as gaze is shifted to one side, a new "radial" component is introduced to the optic flow. However, W. H. Warren and Hannon (1990) showed that observers were able to discount these radial components, both when the observers moved their own eyes and when the computer-generated display mimicked the radial flow caused by an eye movement. If the radial shift is relatively slow, observers can compensate for simulated eye movements just as readily as they do for real eye movements; but with faster simulated eye movement speeds, performance breaks down (Royden, Banks, and Crowell, 1992). This result implies that the visual system can make use of the copies of eye muscle signals sent to the comparator when it is processing optic flow information.

Something in the Way You Move: Using Motion Information to Identify Objects

The fact that we use motion information to guide us as we move through our environment is not all that surprising. What may be less obvious is that motion can also help inform us about the nature of objects. Some 30 years ago, Gunnar Johansson (1975) recognized that there might be something special about the motion of animals and people—**biological motion**—that helps us identify both the moving object and its actions.

Consider the tennis player in the top panel of **Figure 7.12***a*. It's clear from the contours of his body that he's in the act of moving to smash an innocent little tennis ball in the direction of his opponent. Figure 7.12*b* shows the same tennis player in the dark. All we can see are the little lights attached to his ankles, knees, hips, elbows, wrists, and shoulders. There's not very much in the static pattern of the lights to inform us that the contour is a human (let alone a man), or that he/it is engaged in athletic activity. What Johansson

(*a*)

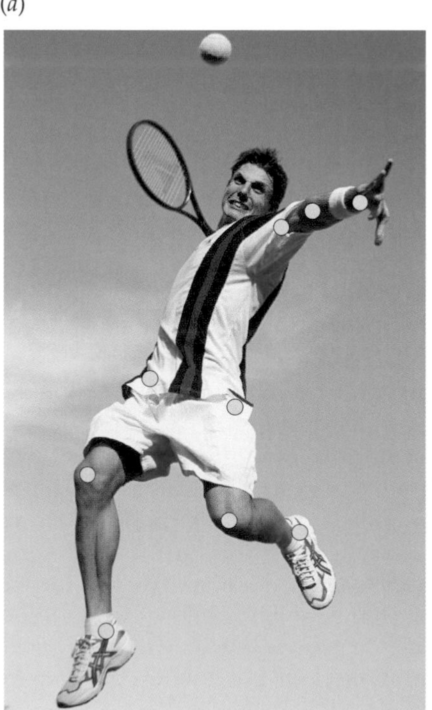

(*b*)

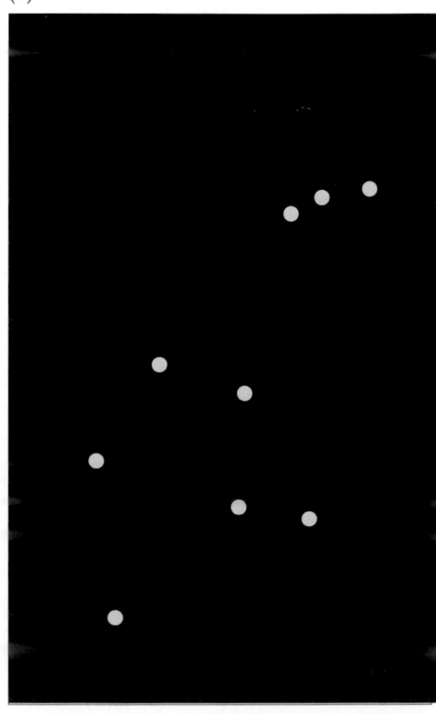

FIGURE 7.12 Biological motion can be seen compellingly when lights attached to a moving human are viewed in total darkness.

discovered, though, is that when the lights move, their motion gives the viewer an immediate and very compelling impression of a live human being in action. Once again, you really need to see this to appreciate it, so watch the classic "dot walker" movie in **Web Activity 7.1: Types of Motion**.

There is even evidence that observers can use biological motion to identify whether a set of moving lights is attached to a male or female walker. How do they do that? As we walk, when the right leg is in front of the left leg, the right shoulder is behind, and vice versa. If we draw one line connecting the left shoulder with the right hip and another connecting the right shoulder with the left hip, the intersection of the two lines is the center of the walker's motion. Because males typically have broader shoulders and narrower hips than females, the average male's center of motion is higher than that of females. James Cutting et al. (Barclay, Cutting, and Kozlowski, 1978) have suggested that observers use estimates of the center of motion as a cue to the walker's gender. Other studies (e.g., Mather and Murdoch, 1994) suggest that, in certain views, the amount of body sway might provide an even more salient gender cue; and recent work (Neri, Morrone, and Burr, 1998) shows that the mechanisms that analyze biological motion obey different rules for integrating motion over space and time than do mechanisms for other forms of complex motion.

Biological motion appears to play an important role in how we understand human actions. Recent studies of biological motion with two "actors" either dancing or fighting show that we are much more efficient in discriminating biological motion of a human when two humans are acting in synchrony (e.g., fighting or dancing) than when they are out of sync. This finding suggests that when we watch two people interacting, knowing what one is doing helps us understand the actions of the other. We can think of this phenomenon as proof of the old adage that "it takes two to tango" (Neri, Luu, and Levi, 2006).

time to collision (TTC) The time required for a moving object (such as a cricket ball) to hit a stationary object (such as a batsman's head). TTC = distance/rate.

tau (τ) Information in the optic flow that could signal TTC (time to collision) without the necessity of estimating either absolute distances or rates. The ratio of the retinal image size at any moment to the rate at which the image is expanding is tau, and TTC is proportional to tau.

Avoiding Imminent Collision: The Tao of Tau

In cricket, as in so much of life, the object is to keep your eye on the ball and to stay out of trouble. Indeed, much of our visual apparatus may be designed to do just that. The batsman shown in **Figure 7.13** evidently did not keep his eye on the ball. Luckily, accidents like this are not too common, because cricketers are extremely good at judging precisely when a tiny ball, hurtling toward them at speeds approaching 100 miles per hour, is about to collide with their head (Regan, 1991). What visual information do we use to avoid imminent collisions, or to achieve collision when catching or batting a ball? To rephrase somewhat more precisely, how do we estimate the **time to collision** (**TTC**) of an approaching object?

Consider a small, red cricket ball, thrown by a large, rather angry-looking man (on the other team), that bounces off the ground about 10 feet way from you. At this distance, if the ball hurtles toward the bridge of your nose at a constant rate of 50 feet per second, it will collide with your face in 0.20 second (TTC = distance/rate = 10/50). The most direct way to estimate TTC would therefore be to estimate the distance and speed of the ball. However, determining absolute distances in depth is a tricky proposition, as we saw in Chapter 6, and humans are far better at judging TTC than would be predicted on the basis of their distance judgment abilities.

In an attempt to reconcile this apparent discrepancy, D. N. Lee (1976) and others have pointed out that there is an alternative source of information in the optic flow that could signal TTC without absolute distances or rates having to be estimated. Lee called this information source **tau** (τ). Here's how tau works. As it approaches your nose, the image of the ball on your retina

FIGURE 7.13 This batsman has just been hit by a very hard cricket ball.

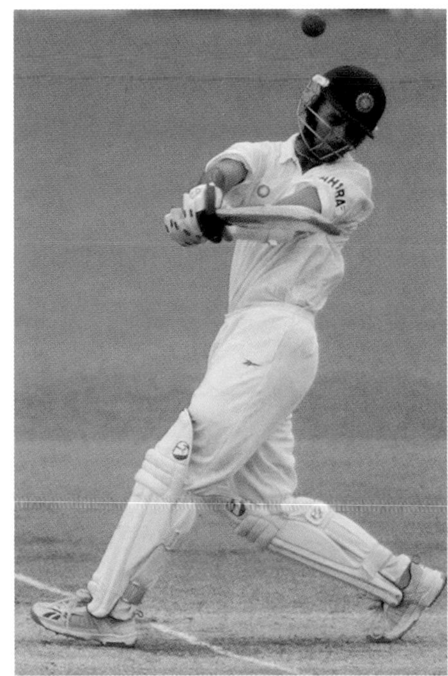

smooth pursuit A type of eye movement in which the eyes move smoothly to follow a moving object.

will grow larger (if you don't believe this, have someone throw a ball—preferably a soft one—at your face and see for yourself). The ratio of the retinal image size at any moment to the rate at which the image is expanding is tau, and TTC is proportional to tau. The great advantage of using tau to estimate TTC is that it relies solely on information available directly from the retinal image; all you need to do is to track the visual angle subtended by the cricket ball as it approaches your eye.

Do we actually make use of tau? The jury is still out. It is clear that estimating the time to imminent collision is critically important to animals and humans, and almost every species tested will attempt to avoid a simulated collision. There is also evidence that certain neurons in the visual systems of pigeons and locusts respond to objects on a collision course with them and can signal a particular time to collision (e.g., Rind and Simmons, 1999; Wang and Frost, 1992). However, Tresilian (1999) recently concluded that tau is just one of a number of different sources of visual information that can be used to judge the time to collision.

Eye Movements

Place a blank piece of paper on the desk in front of you and draw a small black dot right in the center of the paper. Close your left eye and focus your right eye's gaze on the dot; then position a pencil so that it is near the bottom right corner of the paper. Keeping your eye trained on the dot, move the pencil slowly across the sheet to the left side, as shown in **Figure 7.14***a*. What did you perceive? The image of the pencil just swept across your retina from right to left, so assuming that your rightward-motion detectors are functioning correctly, you should have perceived movement in this direction. (You may have thought that the word *rightward* in the previous sentence was a typo, but technically the image sweeps across the retina in the opposite direction from the actual movement, since the right side of the world projects to the left side of the retina and vice versa. To avoid confusion, we'll ignore this inconvenient bit of physics for now and pretend that images move on the retina in the same direction that the objects in the world are moving. **Web Activity 7.5: Eye Movements** provides illustrations of these phenomena that honor physics.)

Now try a slightly different demonstration. Start with the pencil near the bottom left corner of the paper, fixate on the eraser, and track it with your eye as you move it back across the sheet of paper to the right corner (Figure 7.14*b*). Congratulations! You have just executed a type of eye movement called **smooth pursuit**, which kept the image of the pencil stationary on the

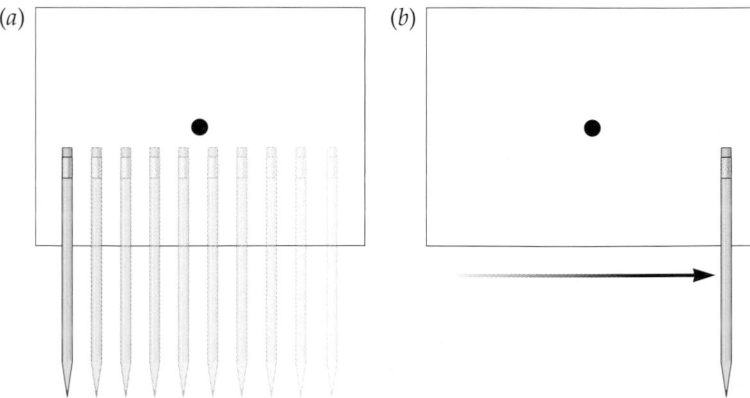

FIGURE 7.14 Studying eye movements. (*a*) Keeping our gaze fixated on the dot while the pencil moves to the left causes the pencil to generate motion across the retina, and we perceive the pencil to be moving in this direction. (*b*) Keeping our gaze fixated on the pencil while it moves to the right causes the dot to generate motion in the same direction across the retina, but we do not perceive the dot to move.

retina while it was in motion. But think about what happened to the image of the dot just above your finger. When the pencil was on the left side of the page, the dot was to the right of your fixation point. As you tracked the pencil, the dot shifted to the center of your retina, then slid to the left of fixation once the pencil reached the right side of the paper. However, you should *not* have perceived the dot to be moving in this case, even though the image of the dot made essentially the same journey across your retina as the image of the pencil did in Figure 7.14*a*.

We hope you have convinced yourself that the retinal image movement of the pencil when you keep your gaze centered on the dot (see Figure 7.14*a*) is essentially the same as the retinal image movement of the dot when you keep your gaze centered on the pencil (see Figure 7.14*b*). The question is, Why do we perceive the pencil to be in motion in the first case, but perceive the dot to be stationary in the second case? The reason is that in one case there's an eye movement. Think about how the visual system might accomplish this balancing act while we back up and describe eye movements in a bit more detail.

Physiology and Types of Eye Movements

As **Figure 7.15** shows, six muscles are attached to each eye, arranged in three pairs. These muscles are controlled by an extensive network of structures in the brain. One way to get some inkling of the role of these brain structures is to stimulate them with small electrical signals and observe the movements of the eyes. For example, if a cell in the midbrain (**superior colliculus**) of a monkey is stimulated, the monkey's eyes will move by a specific amount in a specific direction. Every time that cell is stimulated, the same eye movement will result. Stimulating a neighboring cell will produce a different eye movement (Stryker and Schiller, 1975). (The superior colliculus also gets some input directly from retinal ganglion cells; this input presumably helps with the planning of eye movements.) By contrast, in response to stimulation of some of the cells in the frontal eye fields (and, indeed, certain superior colliculus cells too), the monkey will move its eyes to fixate a specific spot in space. Depending on where the eyes start, this adjustment may require an eye movement up, down, left, or right. In this case, it is

superior colliculus A structure in the midbrain that is important in initiating and guiding eye movements.

(*a*)

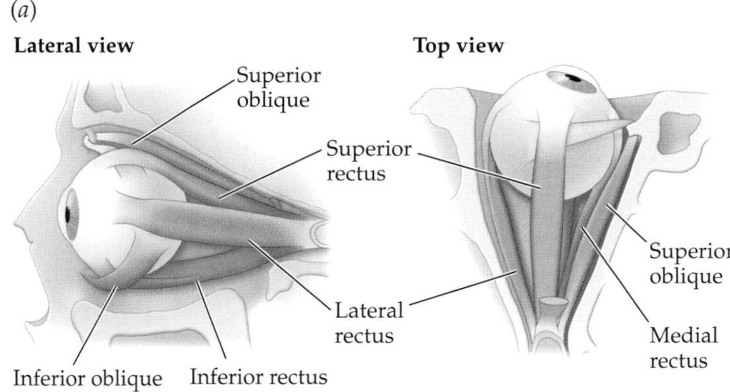

(*b*)

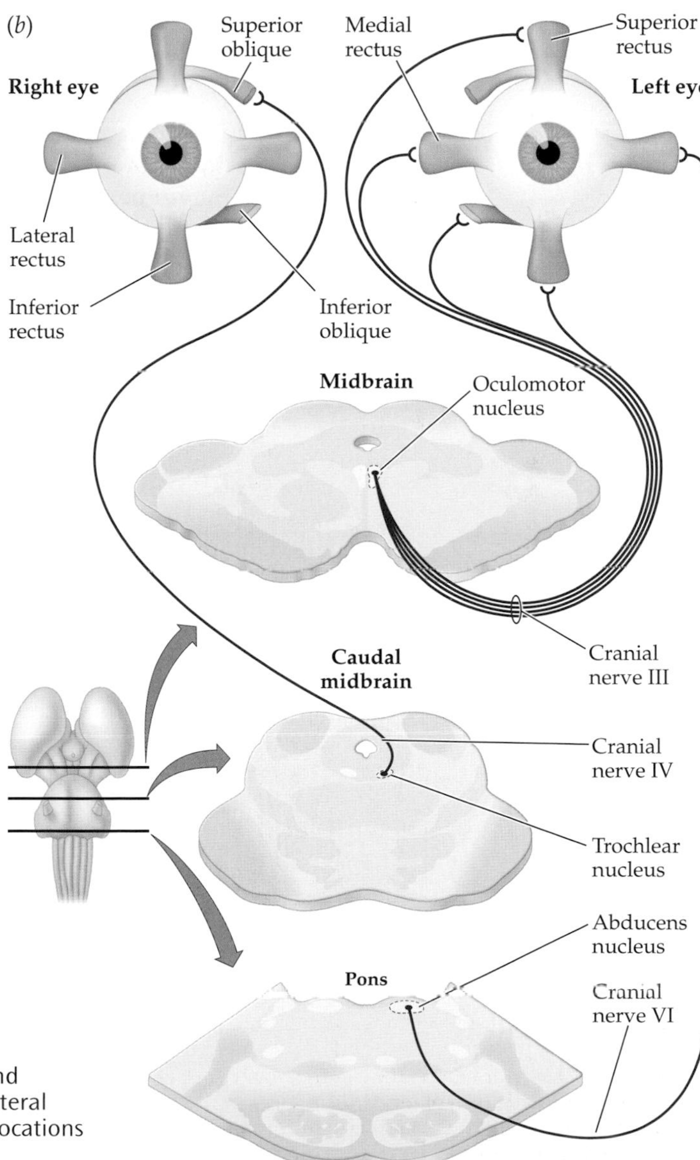

FIGURE 7.15 Six muscles—arranged in three pairs (superior and inferior oblique, superior and inferior rectus, and medial and lateral rectus)—are attached to each eye. Part (*b*) shows the midbrain locations of the cranial nerves that innervate the six muscles.

vergence A type of eye movement in which the two eyes move in opposite directions—for example, both eyes turn toward the nose (convergence) or away from the nose (divergence).

saccade A rapid movement of the eyes that changes fixation from one object or location to another.

reflexive eye movement A movement of the eye that is automatic and involuntary.

the destination and not the movement that is coded (Mays and Sparks, 1980; Schiller and Sandell, 1983).

This description merely scratches the surface of a motor system that is not only very complex, but very active. For example, even when we try to hold our eyes completely stationary, they continue to execute small but important movements. These involuntary eye drifts and small jerks keep the retinal image "fresh"; if the eye muscles are temporarily paralyzed—say, as a result of taking curare (it's amazing what some people will subject themselves to in the name of science!) (Matin et al., 1982)—the entire visual world gradually fades from view.

In addition to involuntary eye movements, there are three types of voluntary eye movements. Most obvious, perhaps, are the previously discussed smooth-pursuit movements that we make when tracking a moving object. **Vergence** eye movements occur when we rotate our eyes inward (converging the eyes) or outward (diverging the eyes) to focus on a near or far object. The third type of voluntary movements are **saccades**: fast jumps (up to 1000 degrees per second) (Bahill and Stark, 1979) of the eye that shift our fixation point from one spot to another. We can decide to make a saccade deliberately, but whether we are thinking about it or not, we will make three or four saccades every second of every minute of every waking hour of the day. That's something like 3 saccades × 60 seconds × 60 minutes × 16 hours = 172,800 saccades per day—before we count the saccades that we make during our dreams in rapid-eye-movement (REM) sleep (Maquet et al., 1996).

When we view a scene, our saccades are not random. We tend to fixate the "interesting" places in the image. Thus, the eyes are more likely to make saccades in response to contours than to broad featureless areas of an image (**Figure 7.16**). Interest also has a richer semantic meaning: We make eye movements that are based on the content of a scene and on our specific interests in that scene (Yarbus, 1967). Our pattern of eye movements as we enter the cafeteria will be different if we're looking for lunch than if we're looking for love.

There are also **reflexive eye movements**—for example, when the eyes move to compensate for head and body movement while maintaining fixation on a particular target. These are known as vestibular eye movements and operate via the vestibulo-ocular reflex (VOR) (see Chapter 15). Optokinetic nystagmus (OKN) is another reflexive eye movement, in which the eyes will involuntarily track a continuously moving object. OKN is characterized by

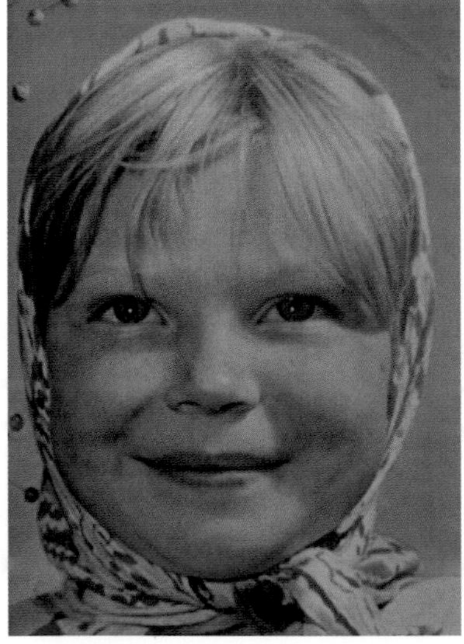
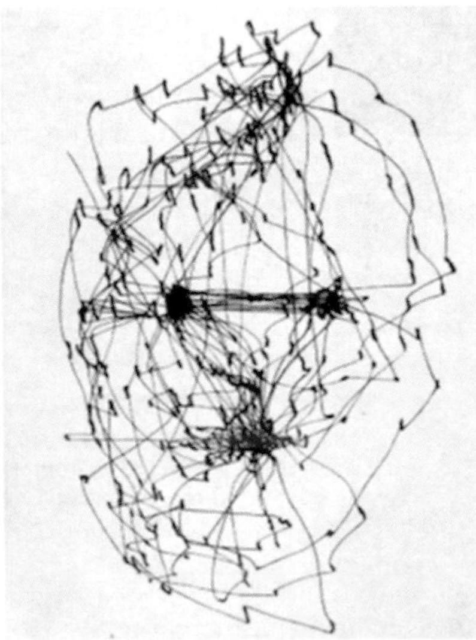

FIGURE 7.16 A classic scan path (right) showing the pattern of eye movements during inspection of the picture of the girl (left). (From Yarbus, 1967.)

the eyes moving smoothly to (say) the right in pursuit of an object moving to the right, and then snapping back. The presence of OKN in response to moving stripes has often been used as a measure of visual acuity in infants.

Eye Movements and Reading

If you are reading this chapter, then your eyes are doing a lot of moving! Reading English involves fixating for roughly a quarter of a second, and then making a saccade of about 7 to 9 letter spaces. We make saccades in order to bring the text into our fovea, because print that's too far from our fixation cannot be read, in part because of crowding (see Chapter 3 and Levi, 2008). Interestingly, readers of English are able to gain information from up to 15 characters to the right of fixation, but only 3 to 4 characters to the left. Thus, the perceptual span is asymmetrical. Readers of Hebrew (which is read from left to right) have the reverse asymmetry. Readers of both Hebrew and English can switch this asymmetry depending on which language they are reading (reviewed by Rayner, 1978), so the asymmetry is attentional, not a product of limitations imposed by the visual system.

As discussed next, there is no information processing during saccades, so while we are reading, all of the information processing must take place during the fixations. Interestingly, such processing occurs during a small fraction of the fixation. "Disappearing text" experiments (in which the words actually disappear off of the computer screen while participants are reading) reveal that if a word remains on the screen for only 50 milliseconds after first fixated, reading proceeds normally (Rayner et al., 2003). There are many other interesting aspects of eye movements in scene perception and in visual search and attention (see Chapter 8).

Saccadic Suppression and the Comparator

Now we'll return to the tricky problem of discriminating motion across the retina that is due to eye movements versus object movements. Let's do one more demonstration using that white piece of paper with the dot in the middle. Close your left eye again and gaze just to the left of the dot; then execute some saccades, shifting your eyes back and forth to the right and then to the left of the dot. The dot will be moving across your retina, but you should not experience any perception of movement. Now, with your left eye still closed, fixate on the dot, place your right index finger on the right side of your right eye socket, and gently "jiggle" your eyeball. *Now* the dot (as well as the paper and the desk the paper is sitting on) *should* appear to move back and forth! What's going on here?

Part of the answer is **saccadic suppression**. When we make a saccade, the visual system pretty much shuts down for the duration of the eye movement (visual activity is suspended in a similar way when we blink). To be a bit more precise, the visual system does not shut down altogether. Saccadic suppression acts mainly to suppress information carried by the magnocellular pathway.

To observe saccadic suppression, you need to find a mirror. As you look at yourself in the mirror, fixate first on one eye and then on the other. You will notice that you do not see the saccadic eye movements that you must be making. If you are concerned that the saccades might be too small to see, find a friend to help you. Have this person stand in front of you and move his or her fixation from one of your eyes to the other. You will have no trouble seeing your friend's saccades even though you are quite blind to your own.

Although saccadic suppression eliminates the smear of the moving world during a saccade, it seems as if we should still be disturbed by the sudden

saccadic suppression The reduction of visual sensitivity that occurs when we make saccadic eye movements. Saccadic suppression eliminates the smear from retinal image motion during an eye movement.

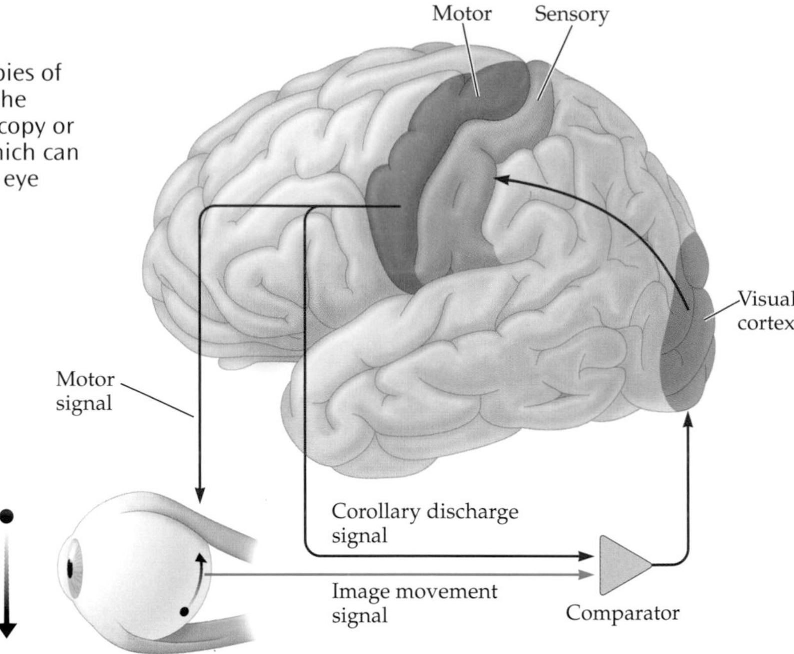

FIGURE 7.17 The comparator. The brain sends two copies of each order to move the eyes. One copy goes directly to the extraocular muscles; the other (known as the efference copy or "corollary discharge signal"), goes to the comparator, which can in turn compensate for image changes produced by the eye movement.

displacement of the objects in front of us. In any case, no suppression takes place when we execute smooth-pursuit eye movements, as in the earlier exercise with the pencil.

By sending out two copies of each order to move the eyes, the motor system solves the "problem" of why an object in motion may appear stationary. One copy goes to the eye muscles; another (often referred to as the "efference copy") goes to an area of the visual system that has been dubbed the **comparator** (**Figure 7.17**). The comparator can then compensate for the image changes caused by the eye movement, inhibiting any attempts by other parts of the visual system to interpret the changes as object motion. When we jiggle the eyeball with a finger, no signal is sent from the eye muscles to the comparator (the eye muscles are not what move the eye), so the visual input is interpreted as our world being rocked. (For interactive demonstrations of the similarities and differences between eye movements and object movements, see **Web Activity 7.5: Eye Movements**.)

Development of Motion Perception

Sensitivity to visual motion does not develop all at once. Some aspects of motion perception are already evident at birth. For example, reflexive eye movements to moving targets (OKN) are present in newborns (as long as the targets are sufficiently large), and physiological studies show that neurons in V1 have adultlike sensitivity to visual direction. On the other hand, sensitivity to global motion, which is thought to reflect processing in MT, appears to develop more slowly, reaching maturity at about 3 to 4 years of age, while sensitivity to motion-defined form and biological motion takes even longer (Freire et al., 2006; Parrish et al., 2005).

comparator An area of the visual system that receives one copy of the order issued by the motor system when the eyes move (the other copy goes to the eye muscles). The comparator can compensate for the image changes caused by the eye movement.

The Man Who Couldn't See Motion

Recall what it's like to experience a motion aftereffect. You stare at a waterfall and then shift your gaze to the cliff next to the falls. You know that the rocks are not moving, and you can see that they aren't actually going anywhere, yet you still experience an otherworldly sense of "disembodied" motion. (Review the phenomenon in **Web Activity 7.4: Motion Aftereffects**, if you haven't tried it for a while.)

Now imagine the opposite experience: objects change position, and you are fully aware of these location shifts but you experience *no* perception of motion. As bizarre as it seems, this is exactly what happens in a rare neuropsychological disorder known as **akinetopsia**, described in the following case report (Horton and Trobe, 1999):

akinetopsia A rare neuropsychological disorder in which the affected individual has no perception of motion.

> A 47-year-old man reported seeing streams of multiple, frozen images trailing in the wake of moving objects. As soon as motion ceased, the images collapsed into each other. He compared his vision to a scene lit by a flashing strobe, except that stationary elements were perceived normally. In fact, if nothing was in motion and he held perfectly still, his vision was entirely normal. The moment anything moved, however, it left a stream of static copies in its path. For example, while out for an evening stroll, he saw a pack of identical dogs lined up behind his West Highland terrier. Driving was impossible because he was confused by multiple snapshots of cars, streets, and signs. Moving lights were followed by a long comet trail.

Another patient reported that when she watched her own arm moving, "passage of the limb would be reduplicated by multiple, fuzzy images, the way a cartoonist might draw motion."

Not surprisingly, akinetopsia appears to be caused by disruptions to cortical area MT. For the two patients described here, the disruptions were side effects of a prescription antidepressant drug, and their motion perception problems disappeared once they were taken off the drug. In other cases, akinetopsia is brought on by direct trauma to area MT due to stroke or elective brain surgery (e.g., surgery to alleviate epileptic seizures). Patients in the latter category sometimes regain normal motion perception abilities several weeks after surgery, indicating that, as in Newsome's monkeys, the human brain can sometimes rearrange its connections so that different areas take over MT's motion-processing functions.

Summary

1. Like color or orientation, motion is a primary perceptual dimension, which is coded at various levels in the brain. Motion information is used to determine where objects are going and when they are likely to get there, and to help us move through our environment without being hit in the head by flying objects.
2. We can build a simple motion-detecting circuit by using linear filters that delay and sum information (and are followed by nonlinearities).
3. V1 neurons view the world through a small window, leading to the well-known "aperture problem" (that is, a V1 neuron is unable to tell which elements correspond with one another when an object moves through its receptive field).
4. There is strong physiological and behavioral evidence that the middle temporal area (MT) is involved in the perception of global motion.
5. Aftereffects for motion, like those for orientation or color, can provide important insights into the underlying mechanisms in humans.
6. There appear to be separate systems for analyzing luminance-defined (first-order) motion and contrast- or texture-defined (second-order) motion.
7. The brain has to figure out which retinal motion arises in the world, and which arises because of eye movements. Moreover, the brain must suppress the motion signals generated by our eye movements, or the world will be pretty "smeared."
8. Motion information is critically important to us for navigating around our world, avoiding imminent collision, and recognizing the movement of animals and people.

Refer to the
Sensation and Perception
website
(www.sinauer.com/wolfe2e)
for activities, essays, study questions, and other study aids.

CHAPTER 8

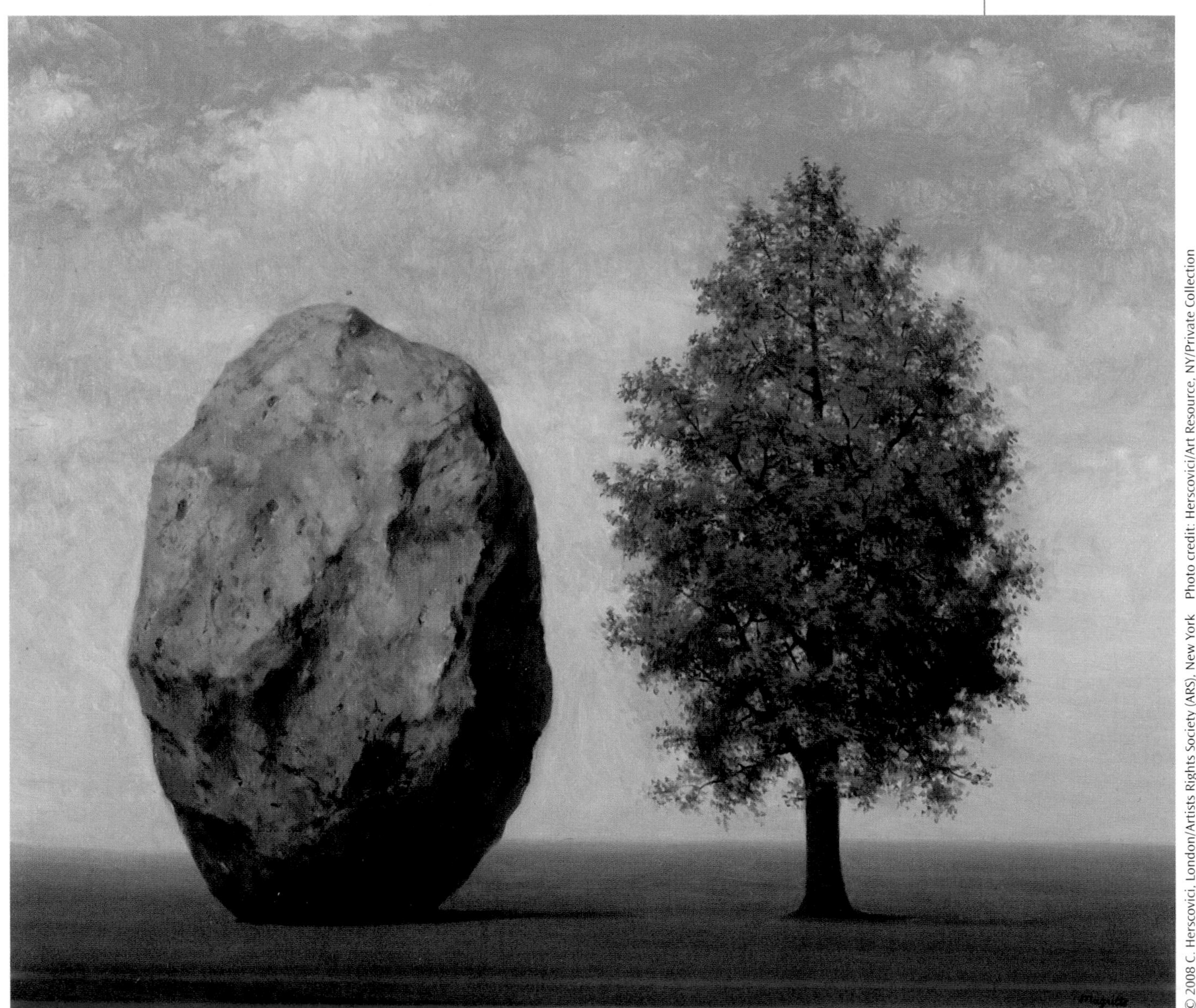
René Magritte, *La Leçon de Politesse* (*The Etiquette Lesson*)

Attention and Scene Perception

If you're reading this, you are probably a student. If you are a student, you are probably taking more than one course and are therefore very busy. Here's an idea: Why not read two books at the same time? One reason this doesn't work is that peripheral visual acuity is limited, as you may recall from Chapter 2: if you're looking at the words on this page, you won't be able to make out the print in another book. This problem can be overcome if the size of the print is increased, as in **Figure 8.1**, but try simultaneously looking at the column of Xs in the figure and reading the two sentences. It should be quite clear that, even with nice large letters, we still cannot read two messages at the same time. Note that we *can* read the words on one side or the other of the Xs while looking at the Xs. We just can't read both sides simultaneously.

This is a specific example of a more general problem. The retinal array contains far more information than we can process. **Figure 8.2** shows another example. We cannot possibly recognize all the objects in this picture at once. That's why "Where's Waldo?" and "I Spy" games are a challenge.

Why can't we process everything at once? Quite literally, we don't have the brains for it. Remember from Chapter 4 that recognizing a single object like an elephant requires a sizable chunk of the brain and its processing power, especially when the elephant could be seen in many different orientations, under different lighting conditions, at different retinal sizes, and so on. Moreover, in order to understand Figure 8.2, we also need to process the relationships between objects—like the fact that the elephant is dousing the yellow car with its trunk. If we do the math for even a fairly small subset of all possible visual stimuli, it turns out that processing everything, everywhere, all at once requires a brain that will not fit in the human head (Tsotsos, 1990).

If it is not possible to process everything all at once, what should be processed? This can't be left to chance. If we're crossing a road, we need to determine that no car will hit us. Devoting our visual processes exclusively to the doughnut shop on the other side of the street could be dangerous. To deal with this problem, we "pay attention" to some stimuli and not to others. As we will see in this chapter, **attention** is not a single *thing*, and it does not have a single locus in the nervous system. Rather, *attention* is the name we give to a family of mechanisms that restrict processing in various ways.

Here are some of the distinctions we can make when considering varieties of attention. Attention can be overt or covert. *Overt attention* usually refers to directing a sense organ at a stimulus—fixating the eyes on a single word, for example. If you point your eyes at this page while directing attention to a person of interest off to the left, you are engaging in *covert attention*. Reading this text while continuing to be aware of music playing in the room is an example of *divided attention*. Watching the pot to note the moment the water begins to boil is *sustained attention*. In this chapter we will be most concerned with **selective attention**, the ability to pick one (or a few) out of many stimuli.

attention Any of the very large set of selective processes in the brain. To deal with the impossibility of handling all inputs at once, the nervous system has evolved mechanisms that are able to restrict processing to a subset of things, places, ideas, or moments in time.

selective attention The form of attention involved when processing is restricted to a subset of the possible stimuli.

These	x	Is
letters	x	it
are	x	time
big	x	for
and	x	a
easy	x	quick
to	x	snack
read.	x	yet?

FIGURE 8.1 Even though the letters are big enough to resolve while looking at the *X*s, we simply cannot read the left-hand and right-hand sentences at the same time.

These are not mutually exclusive terms. Staring straight ahead while attending only to an interesting person to the exclusion of all else might be described as an act of sustained, covert, selective attention.

Although we will focus on visual attention, it is important to remember that attentional mechanisms operate in all of the senses. Getting a shot in the doctor's office may hurt more than an equivalent injury on the playing field because of the different amounts of attention we give to each event. We can also use attentional mechanisms to give priority to one sense over others. Right now, you are probably selecting visual stimuli over auditory, even if you have music on in the background. And you didn't even notice the pressure of your posterior on the seat until we mentioned it (sorry for disrupting your attention).

In this chapter, first we discuss evidence that we attend to only one (or perhaps a few) objects at any single moment. We consider attentional selection in space (I am attending to this object and not that object) and selection in time (I was attending to that object, but now I have selected this object). Next we examine the changes that occur in the brain when we attend to

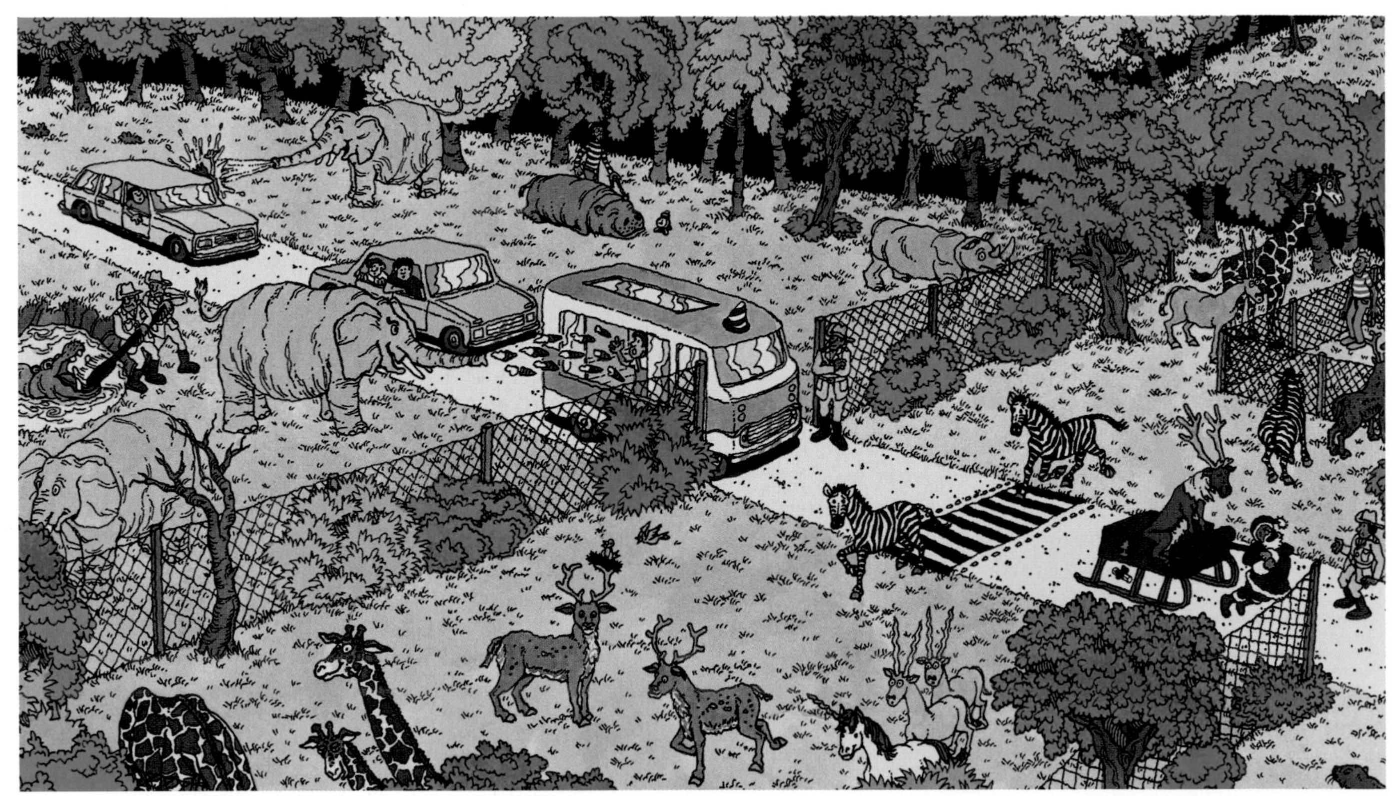

FIGURE 8.2 Search for the raised hand (straight up in the air) in this piece of a "Where's Waldo?" picture. (From *Where's Waldo?* © Martin Handford 2005.)

one object rather than another, and we will see what happens when the neural substrate of attention is damaged. Having convinced you, we hope, that we can recognize only one object at a time, we will turn to scenes. If we are attending to one object, what does it mean to say that we see a whole scene?

reaction time (RT) A measure of the time from the onset of a stimulus to a response.

cue A stimulus that might indicate where (or what) a subsequent stimulus will be. Cues can be valid (correct information), invalid (incorrect), or neutral (uninformative).

Selection in Space

To begin, let's consider what it means to "pay attention." A good place to start is with a cueing experiment of the sort pioneered by Michael Posner (1980). Start with the situation shown in **Figure 8.3***a*. The subject in the experiment fixates on a central point (*). After a variable delay, a test probe appears in one of the two boxes. All the subject needs to do is hit a response key as fast as possible when the probe appears. The measure of interest is the average **reaction time (RT)**—the amount of time that elapses between the point when the probe appears and the point when the subject hits the response key.

Suppose now that the situation is slightly changed: during the waiting period, the subject is given a **cue**, a stimulus that provides a hint about where the target might appear. In Figure 8.3*b*, the cue is a change in the outline color of one of the two boxes (call this a "peripheral cue"). Because the test probe appears in the cued location, this peripheral cue is said to be a "valid" cue. Given a valid cue, Posner found that RT decreases. Compared to the no-cue control, the subject generally responds faster to the probe, because she is "paying attention" to the correct location. In Figure 8.3*c*, we have a different kind of cue. The arrow is a "symbolic" cue but it can also direct attention. In this case, however, the cue would be misleading, or "invalid," because the cued location is on the left but the probe appears on the right. RTs are slower here than in the control condition because the subject has been fooled into attending to the wrong location. We could have valid or invalid instances of either peripheral or symbolic cues. Of course, the experimenter doesn't tell the subject whether a cue will be valid. In a typical experiment, the cue might be valid on 80% of the trials and invalid on the remaining 20%. That would make it in the subject's interest to attend to the cue and would still let the experimenter measure the RTs for plenty of invalid trials.

How long does it take for a cue to redirect our attention? It depends on the nature of the cue. At the beginning of a trial in a Posner cueing experiment, the subject is attending to the fixation point (time 1

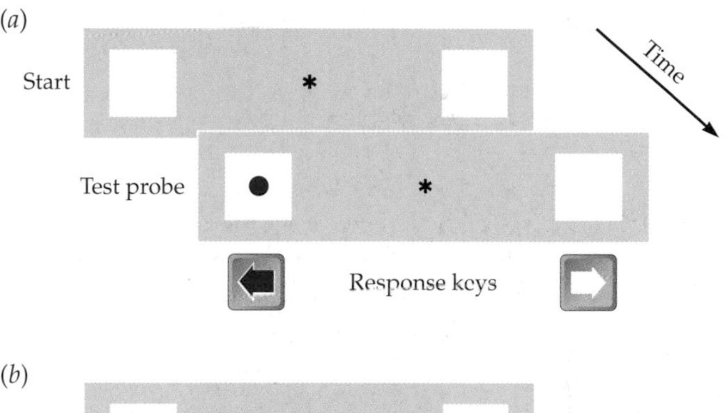

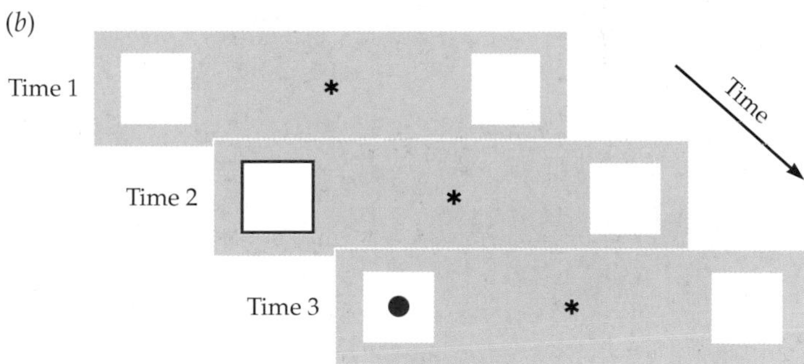

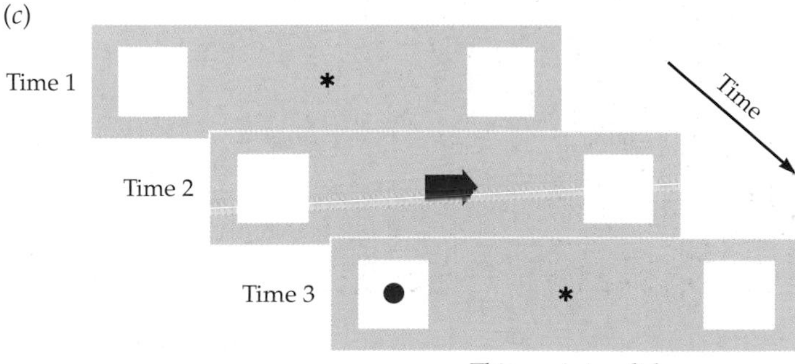

FIGURE 8.3 The Posner cueing paradigm. (*a*) This simple probe detection experiment has two possible probe locations. Here all you have to do is hit one key if the probe appears on the left and another if it appears on the right. (*b*) A valid cue. Here a cue indicates where the target will be. This time the cue is valid; we are telling the truth. (*c*) An invalid cue. This cue points to the wrong side. (This is also a different kind of cue—a symbolic cue. Symbolic cues direct attention more slowly.)

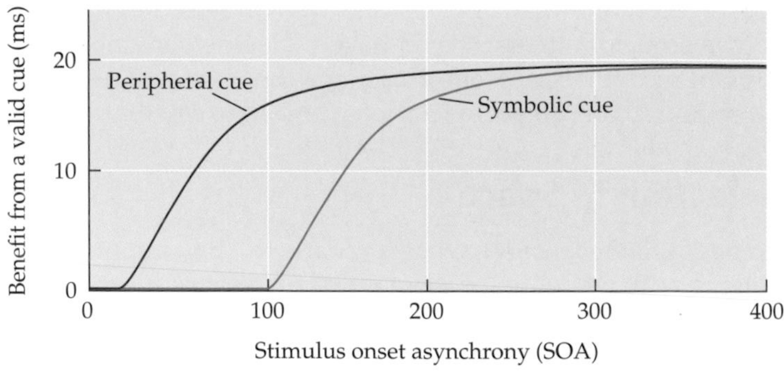

FIGURE 8.4 The effect of a cue develops over time. A peripheral cue (like that in Figure 8.3*b*) becomes fully effective 100 to 150 milliseconds after it appears. A symbolic cue (see Figure 8.3*c*) takes longer to get started and to rise to full effect.

stimulus onset asynchrony (SOA) The time between the onset of one stimulus and the onset of another.

in Figure 8.3*b* or *c*). The cue appears at time 2 and the probe appears at time 3. We can measure the timing of the attention shift by varying the interval between time 2 and time 3. This is called the **stimulus onset asynchrony**, a psychophysical variable that typically goes by its acronym, **SOA**. If the SOA is 0 milliseconds (ms), the cue and probe appear simultaneously. There is no time for it to be used to direct attention, and there is no difference between the effects of a valid or invalid cue. As the SOA increases to about 150 ms, the magnitude of the cueing effect from a valid peripheral cue increases, as shown by the red line in **Figure 8.4**. After that, the effect of the cue levels off or declines a bit.

Symbolic cues take longer to work presumably because we need to do some work to interpret the arrow (blue line, Figure 8.4). Interestingly, some rather symbolic cues behave like fast, peripheral cues. For example, we are very quick to deploy our attention in response to a pair of eyes looking one direction or the other (**Figure 8.5**), as if we were built to get information from the gaze of others (Friesen, Ristic, and Kingstone, 2004). You can try the cueing experiment in some of its important variations in Web Activity 8.1: Attentional Cueing.

The "Spotlight" of Attention

In a cueing experiment, attention starts at the fixation point and somehow ends up at the cued location. But does it actually *move* from one point to the next? Attention could be deployed from spot to spot in a number of ways. It might move in a manner analogous to the movements of our eyes. When we shift our gaze, our point of fixation sweeps across the intervening space (although, as we saw in Chapter 7, saccadic suppression keeps us from noticing, and being disturbed by, this movement). Attention might sweep across space in a similar manner, like a spotlight beam (Posner, 1980).

The spotlight metaphor makes good sense and has become, perhaps, the most common way for cognitive psychologists to talk about attention. But there are other possibilities. For example, attention might expand from fixation, growing to fill the whole region from the fixation spot to the cued location, and then shrink to include just the cued location. This would be a version of a zoom lens model of attention (Eriksen and Yeh, 1985). Or, when attention is withdrawn from the fixation spot, it might not move at all. It might simply melt away at that location and then reappear at the cued location (Sperling and Weichselgartner, 1995). It is hard to say for sure which metaphor is "correct," because we have no direct way to measure the location and extent of attention. However, the best evidence suggests that attention is not *moving* from point to point the way a physical spotlight would move (Cave and Bichot, 1999).

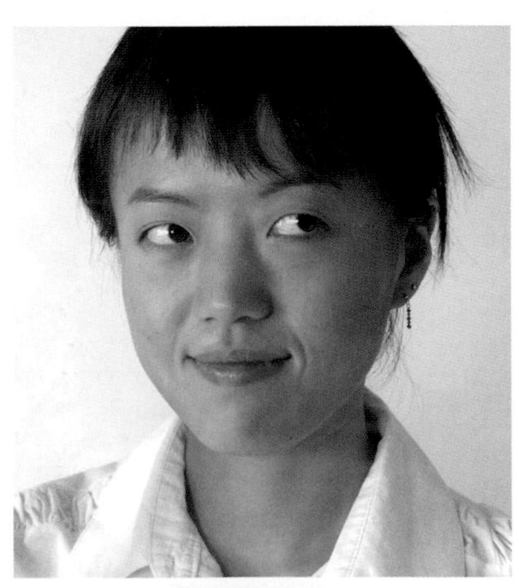

FIGURE 8.5 Which way does your attention shift when you look at this picture?

Visual Search

Cueing experiments provide important insight into the deployment of attention. But the situation is rather artificial, in that all of the experiments involve telling the observer exactly when and where to attend. **Visual search** experiments provide a closer approximation of the actions of attention in the real world. In a typical visual search experiment, the observer looks for a **target** item among **distractor** items. Visual searches are ubiquitous in the real world: we look for faces in a crowd, mugs in a cupboard, books on a shelf, and so forth. Some searches are so easy that we hardly think of them as searches (e.g., finding the cold-water tap on a sink). Others, like looking for one raised hand in the "Where's Waldo?" puzzle of Figure 8.2, are much more demanding.

visual search Looking for a target in a display containing distracting elements.

target The goal of a visual search.

distractor In visual search, any stimulus other than the *target*.

The quest to understand what makes some search tasks easy and others hard has proven to be one of the most productive and interesting lines of cognitive psychology research in the past quarter century. **Figure 8.6** shows examples of the simplified visual search tasks performed in the lab. In Figure 8.6*a* and *b*, the target is a red vertical bar. In Figure 8.6*c*, the target is the

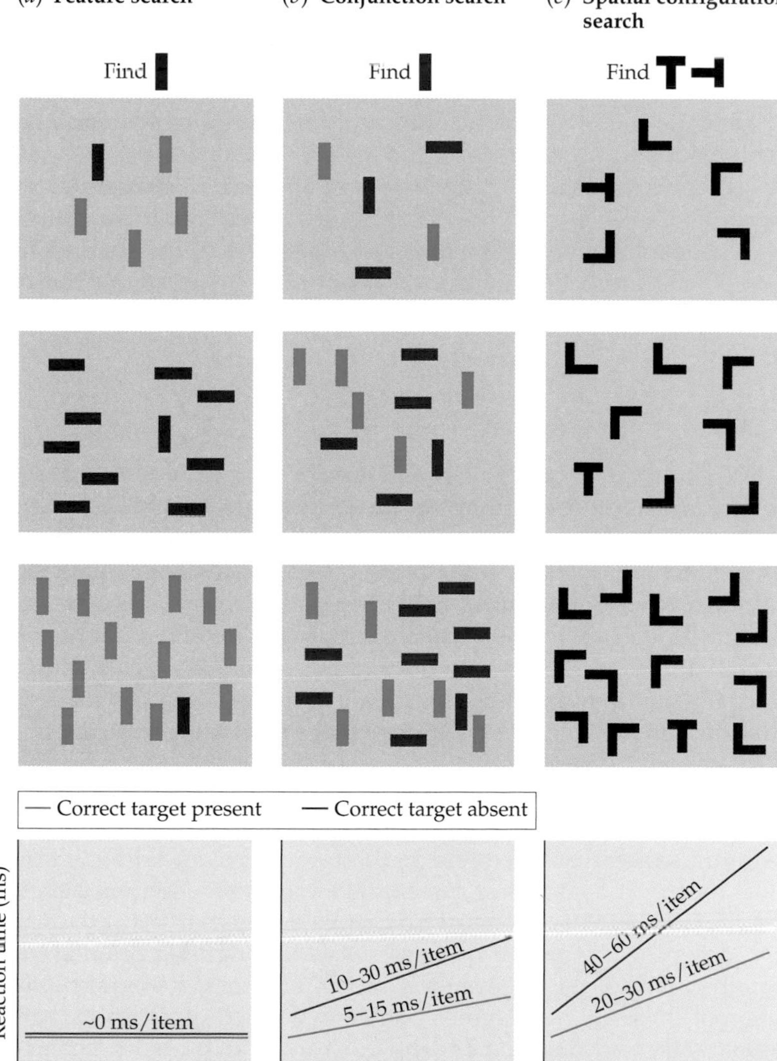

FIGURE 8.6 Laboratory visual search tasks. Each part of the figure shows a different search task, with difficulty increasing from (*a*) to (*c*). Each row shows a different number of items (the set size), with difficulty increasing as set size increases. Here we show only examples with the target present. In a typical experiment, a target might be absent in half of the trials. The graphs at the bottom depict typical patterns of results for each type of task. The red line in each graph represents average reaction times for different set sizes on target-absent trials; the blue line shows results for target-present trials.

letter *T* (in any of four possible rotations). Two factors are being varied in this figure: First, the tasks increase in difficulty from (*a*) to (*c*). Second, each row of the display shows a different **set size**, the number of items in the display. As a general (and unsurprising) rule, it is harder to find a target as the number of items increases.

One of the standard measures of the ease of search is to ask how much time is added (on average) for each item added to the display. Observers perform the same type of search over and over while the experimenter measures the RT required for the subject to say "yes" if the target is present or "no" if there is no target in the display. As the task becomes harder, the slope relating RT to set size grows steeper. These slopes are plotted at the bottom of Figure 8.6. Saying "yes" the target is present (blue) is faster than saying "no" (red) because, even in the hardest task, if the subject is lucky she might stumble on the presence of the target with her first deployment of attention, but it is not possible to stumble on the *absence* of the target in the same way.

Although all the displays in Figure 8.6 include a target, in a typical experiment the target is present in 50% of the trials and absent in the other 50%. At the end of the experiment, the researcher averages the RTs of all the trials from all the experimental subjects for each set size, for target-present trials and target-absent trials. Typical results for each task are shown at the bottom of Figure 8.6. In each graph, the lower line represents RTs for target-present trials, and the upper line represents RTs for target-absent trials. You can try a number of different visual search tasks in **Web Activity 8.2: Visual Search**. It's much easier to get a feel for the difficulty of these tasks when you do them yourself.

One way to compare search tasks is to talk about the "efficiency" with which we can work our way through the display. If we can direct attention to the target as soon as the display appears, regardless of the set size, then we have an efficient search. If we must examine each item in turn until we find the target, then we have an inefficient search. Different types of search tasks differ in their efficiency.

Feature Searches Are Efficient

The task in Figure 8.6*a* is called a simple **feature search**. Here the target is defined by the presence of a single feature. Each example contains an item with a unique color or orientation. If the unique item is sufficiently **salient** (that is, if it stands out visually from its neighbors), it really doesn't matter how many distractors there are. The target seems to "pop out" of the display. Apparently, we can process the color or orientation of all the items at once (in **parallel**). When we measure the RT, it does not change with the set size. The results will approximate the flat lines plotted at the bottom of Figure 8.6*a*; more technically, the slope of the function relating RT to set size is about 0 ms per item.

Between one dozen and two dozen basic attributes seem to be able to support parallel visual search (Wolfe and Horowitz, 2004). These include obvious stimulus properties like color, size, orientation, and motion (Treisman, 1986a, 1986b), and some less obvious attributes, like lighting direction (Enns and Rensink, 1990). In **Figure 8.7***a*, look for the bar that is oriented differently in depth. This task is quite easy, even though the orientation of all items in the plane of the page is the same. In Figure 8.7*b*, we take a similar collection of three-colored regions but we make two-dimensional rather than apparently three-dimensional items. Now it is much harder to find the odd item.

set size The number of items in a visual display.

feature search Search for a target defined by a single attribute, such as a salient color or orientation.

salience The vividness of a stimulus relative to its neighbors.

parallel In visual attention, referring to the processing of multiple stimuli at the same time.

(*a*)

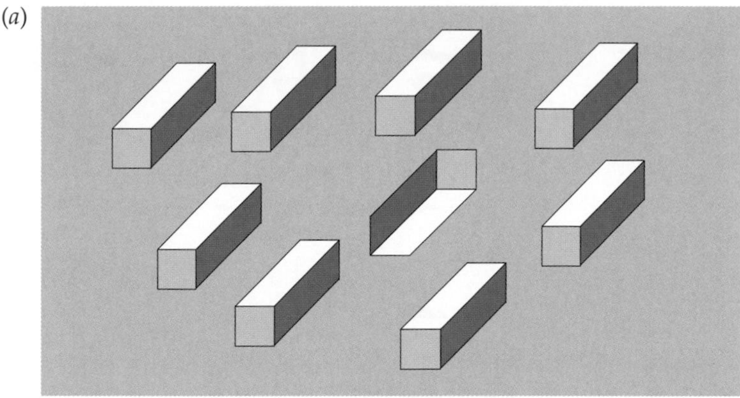

(*b*)

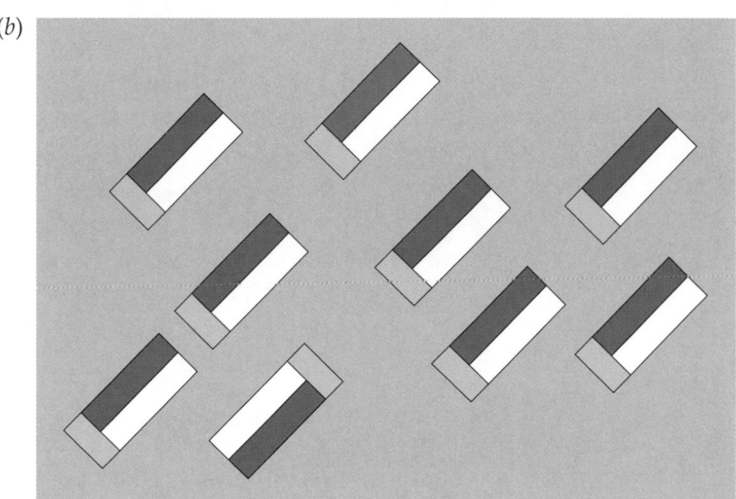

FIGURE 8.7 Three-dimensional orientation is a basic feature used in the guidance of search. (*a*) The oddly oriented bar in this image is easy to find, even though all bars have the same orientation in the two-dimensional image plane. (*b*) To show that the ease of the task in (*a*) had to do with the three-dimensional effects and not just with the relative positions of different regions, the experiment was repeated with apparently two-dimensional items composed of similar parts in similar positions. Now it is harder to find the odd item. (After Enns and Rensink, 1990.)

Many Searches Are Inefficient

When the target and distractors in a visual search task contain the same basic features, as in Figure 8.6*c*, search is inefficient. Here, we are looking for *T*s among *L*s where both targets and distractors are composed of a vertical and a horizontal bar. It is not hard to distinguish a *T* from an *L*, but we need to attend to each item until we stumble on the target. Even if, as in Figure 8.1, the letters are big enough that we don't have to move our eyes to distinguish *T* from *L*, each additional distractor adds about 20 to 30 ms to a successful search for a target and about twice that amount of time (40–60 ms) to a search that ends without finding a target. Given the terms of this discussion, that is an inefficient search.

Why do we get this particular pattern of results? One straightforward proposal is that these tasks involve a **serial self-terminating search**, in which items are examined one after another (serially) either until the target is found or until all items have been checked. Consider the case in which a target is present. Sometimes the observer will get lucky and find the target on the first deployment of attention. Sometimes she will be unlucky and have to search all the items before stumbling on the target. On average, she will have to search through about half the items on each trial before the search can be terminated. When no target is present, our observer will always need to search through all the items. This is just one possibility.

serial self-terminating search A search from item to item, ending when a target is found.

The inefficient search for a *T* among *L*s is nothing like the hardest search we could devise, of course. For starters, if we need to spend a lot of time

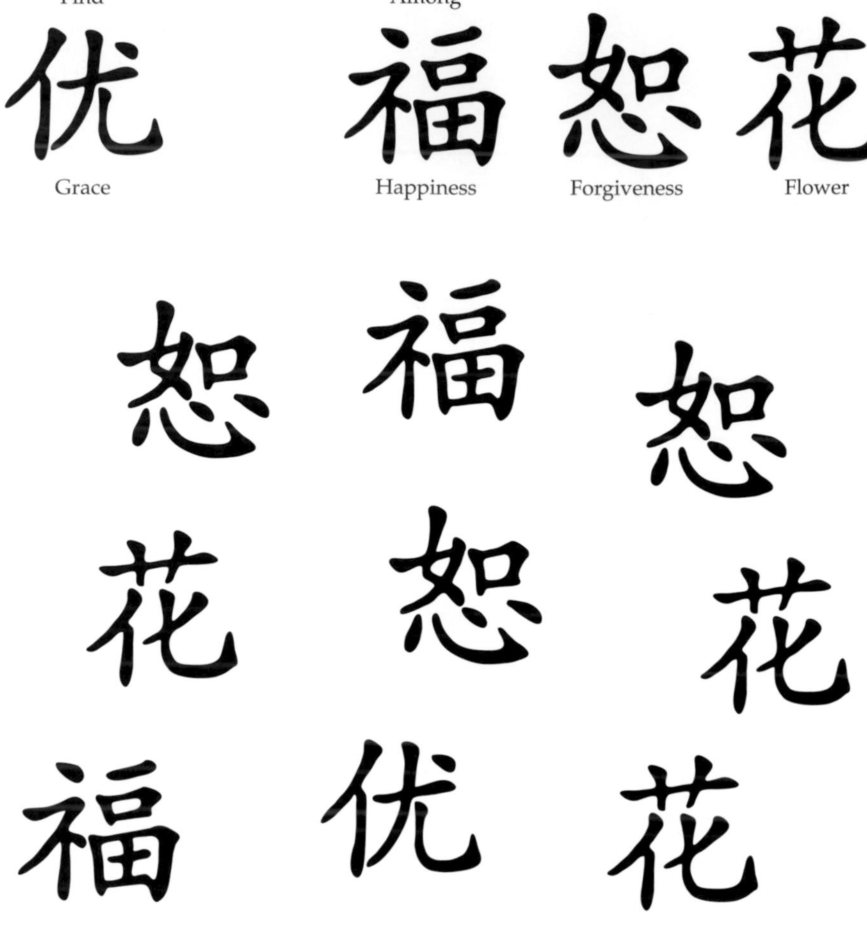

FIGURE 8.8 Search can be much more laborious if you're not familiar with what you're searching for. Here, the search for the Chinese character for "grace" will be much easier if you read Chinese.

with each item, search will be much slower, as it is in the search for a Chinese character in **Figure 8.8** (unless, of course, you happen to read Chinese). What makes searches like the *T*-among-*L*s search interesting is that they are inefficient, even though the items are easy to see and very familiar.

In Real-World Searches, Basic Features Guide Visual Search

In the real world, it would be very rare to have a true feature search for the only red item among homogeneous distractors. How often do you have to find the strawberry in the lime display? It is probably even rarer to have to search through a scene containing objects that all share the same basic features—perhaps the proverbial needle in the haystack. Usually, those basic features can be used to narrow down the search, even if they cannot eliminate all distractions. This is known as **guided search** (Wolfe, 1994; Wolfe, Cave, and Franzel, 1989). If you are looking for a tomato in **Figure 8.9**, you will be able to find it quite quickly, even though it is not the only red thing or the only round thing or, indeed, the only possessor of any unique feature. Tomatoes are distinguished from most of the distractors by a *conjunction* of several features. If you can guide your attention to red and round and large, you will have eliminated most of the competition.

guided search Search in which attention can be restricted to a subset of possible items on the basis of information about the target item's basic features (e.g., its color).

conjunction search Search for a target defined by the presence of two or more attributes (e.g., a *red*, *vertical* target among *red* horizontal and blue *vertical* distractors).

In the lab, we use **conjunction searches** like those in Figure 8.6*b*. In a conjunction search, no single feature defines the target. Instead, the target is defined by the conjunction—the co-occurrence—of two or more features. In this case we're looking for the red, vertical items. In terms of efficiency, the

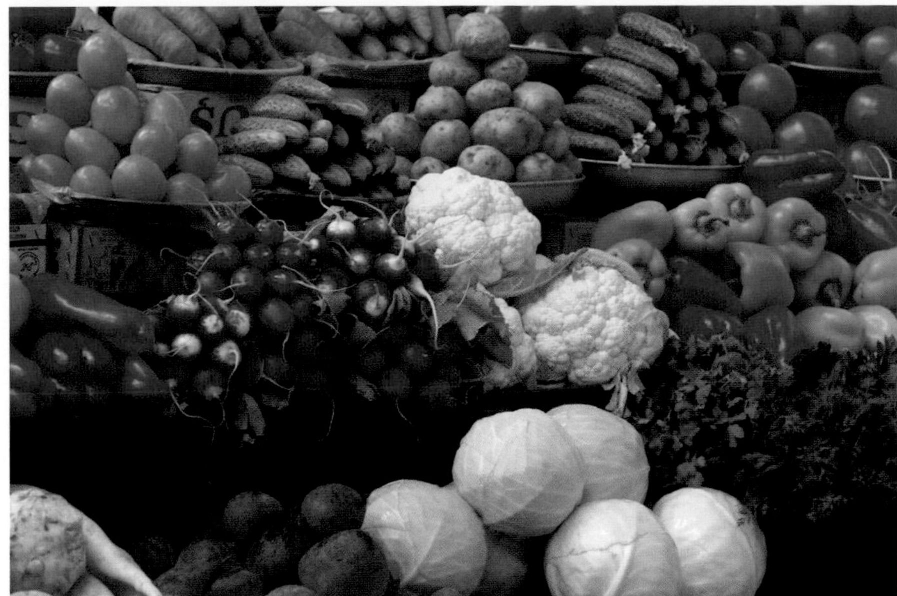

FIGURE 8.9 A real-world conjunction search: Find the big, round, red tomatoes among things that might be big or round or red, but do not have all three basic features.

two-feature conjunction searches tend to lie between the very efficient feature searches and the inefficient serial searches. We can make these conjunctions more complex in an effort to get closer to the real world of cats, vegetables, and so on. So, in **Figure 8.10**, the target is defined on six dimensions: the color, shape (straight, curved, jagged) and orientation of the whole object and the same three characteristics of the part within it. Each distractor shares two features with the target, but the target is still easy to find because we can guide our attention to the right conjunction of features (Wolfe, 1994; Wolfe, Cave, and Franzel, 1989).

Find

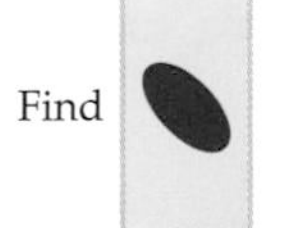

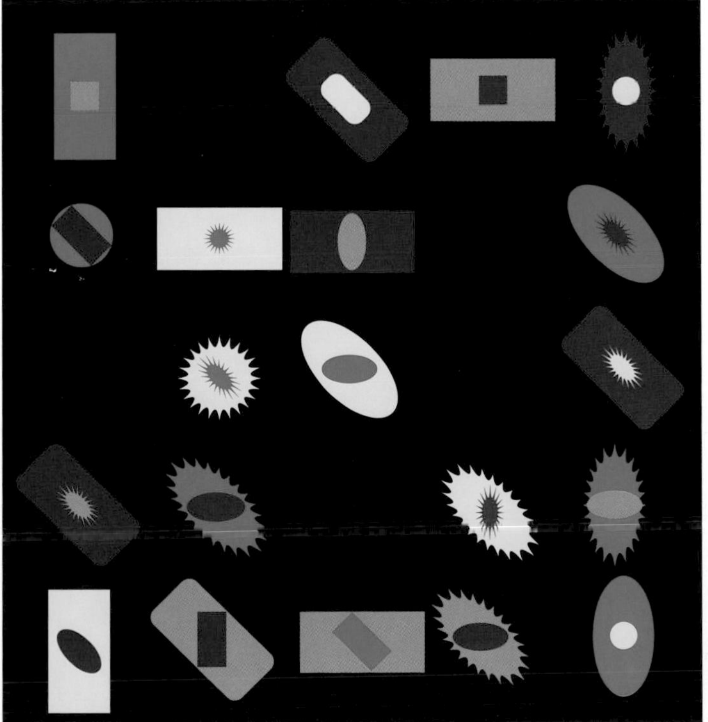

FIGURE 8.10 A six-dimensional conjunction. Suppose the task is to find the yellow, straight, vertical thing with the red, curved, oblique part among distractors, each of which shares two features with the target. The object in the lower right corner matches the target in three dimensions: straightness and verticalness of the whole, and curvature of the part. The one at lower left matches exactly.

The Binding Problem in Visual Search

One way to understand the need for attention is to consider what is known as the **binding problem** (Treisman, 1996; von der Malsburg, 1981), which is this: We might be able to analyze a collection of basic features in a **preattentive stage** of processing, but we won't know how those features are bound together until we attend to the object. Looking back at Figure 8.6*c*, the problem with *T*s and *L*s is that they both have vertical and horizontal features. It is the relationship of those features to each other that is critical. The point is made more forcefully in **Figure 8.11**. A quick glance tells us that we're looking at *pluses* whose components are red and blue and vertical and horizontal. To find the two items that have redness and verticalness bound together, we must direct attention to the individual items.

This idea that there is a preattentive stage of basic feature processing followed by a second, attention-demanding stage is the core of Anne Treisman's **feature integration theory** (Treisman and Gelade, 1980). The idea of guided search, mentioned earlier, fits into this framework. We can use some preattentive feature information to guide the choice of what should be attended and bound next. If we are searching for a *little, brown* mouse, we

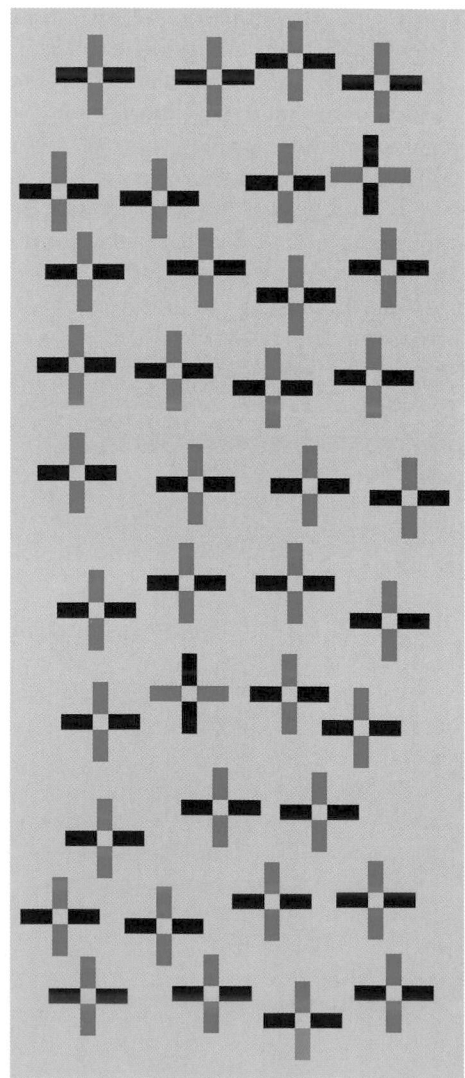

FIGURE 8.11 A conjunction search with a binding problem. In this image it is hard to find the red verticals (there are two of them) because all of the items have the features red and blue and vertical and horizontal.

binding problem The challenge of tying different attributes of visual stimuli (e.g., color, orientation, motion), which are handled by different brain circuits, to the appropriate object so that we perceive a unified object (e.g., red, vertical, moving right).

preattentive stage The processing of a stimulus that occurs before selective attention is deployed to that stimulus.

feature integration theory Anne Treisman's theory of visual attention, which holds that a limited set of basic features can be processed in parallel preattentively, but that other properties, including the correct binding of features to objects, require attention.

should guide our attention to little stuff and brown stuff and not devote attention to shiny, red or large, square things.

If attention is needed to bind features correctly, what happens if we don't have enough time to complete the job? We'll see something, but what? If it works for you, the demonstration in **Figure 8.12** (on the next page—but don't look yet) will provide part of the answer. What you must do is look quickly at the figure, then look away and write down as many of the letters and their colors as you can. Try that now.

If you compare your list to the actual figure, you may find that you matched the wrong color to a letter. For example, you might be quite sure that you saw a green *H*. If so, you have experienced an **illusory conjunction**, a false combination of the features from two or more different objects (Treisman and Schmidt, 1982). You are unlikely to think that you have seen a blue *H* or a green *T* because neither the color blue nor the letter *T* is present in the figure. We conjoin only those features that are actually in the display. When we can't complete the task of binding, we do the best we can with the information we have.

Attending in Time: RSVP and the Attentional Blink

So far in this chapter, we have concentrated on attentional selection in space. The *timing* of these acts of selection has been a secondary concern. We learn some interesting new bits of information if we make selection in time our object of study. Imagine the following situation: You're looking at a stream of letters that all appear at the same location in space. Showing the stimuli in this way is known as **rapid serial visual presentation** (**RSVP**). You're trying to decide if there is an *X* in the stream of letters. How fast can the characters be presented and still permit you to do the task with high accuracy? With fairly large, clearly visible stimuli, we can reliably pick an *X* out of letters when the characters are appearing at a rate of 8 to 10 items per second. Indeed, the task does not need to be limited to simple characters. If we're watching a stream of photographs flash by at this rate, we can monitor that stream for the appearance of a picnic photograph. We don't even need to know which particular picnic we're looking for. The general idea of "picnic" is adequate for the task (Potter, 1976). You can view scenes in an RSVP sequence yourself in **Web Activity 8.3: The RSVP Paradigm**.

Returning to simple letters, suppose we change the task a bit. Instead of looking for one target in a stream of letters, now we're looking for two. We can call the first T1 (for "target one") and the second T2. For instance, T1 might be a white letter in a stream of black letters and T2 might be an *X* (**Figure 8.13*a***). The *X* would be present in 50% of the trials. The critical variable is the interval between T1 and T2, and the somewhat surprising result is shown in Figure 8.13*b*. If T2 appears 200 to 300 ms after T1, and if T1 is correctly reported, we are very likely to miss T2. This phenomenon is known as **attentional blink** (Shapiro, 1994); it is as if our ability to visually attend to the characters in the RSVP sequence were temporarily knocked out, even though our eyes remain wide open. You'll find more on this topic in **Web Activity 8.4: The Attentional Blink and Repetition Blindness**.

To show that missing T2 in this scenario is an attentional problem, we can do a control experiment in which subjects report only T2. If subjects are asked to monitor the RSVP stream for the T2 *X*, they pay no particular attention to the now irrelevant white letter, and T2 performance is uniformly good at all delays between T1 and T2.

Somehow the act of attending to T1 makes it very hard to attend to T2 if T2 appears 200 to 300 ms later in the stream. What is happening? Marvin

illusory conjunction An erroneous combination of two features in a visual scene—for example, seeing a red *X* when the display contains red letters and *X*s but no red *X*s.

rapid serial visual presentation (RSVP) An experimental procedure in which stimuli appear in a stream at one location (typically the point of fixation) at a rapid rate (typically about eight per second).

attentional blink The difficulty in perceiving and responding to the second of two target stimuli amid a rapid stream of distracting stimuli if the observer has responded to the first target stimulus within 200 to 500 milliseconds before the second stimulus is presented.

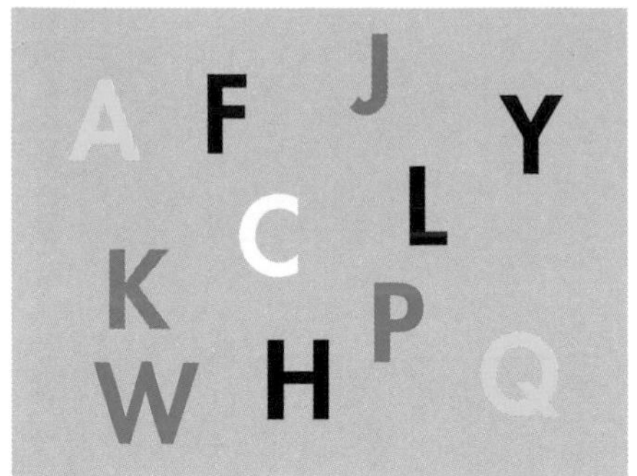

FIGURE 8.12 Illusory conjunctions. Look at this figure quickly and then try to recall the colors of the letters. You may know what colors were there and many of the letters, but you are quite likely to pair a color and a letter incorrectly.

Chun suggests the following metaphor: Imagine you're fishing with a net in a less-than-pristine stream, with boots and tires and the occasional fish floating or swimming by. You can monitor the stream and identify each item as it passes—boot, tire, boot, fish, boot, and so on. You can also dip your net in and catch a fish (**Figure 8.14***a*). Once you have a fish in the net, however, it takes some time before you can get the net back into the water to catch fish number 2. As a result, you might miss fish 2 if it swims by too soon after you've caught fish 1 (Figure 8.14*b* and *c*).

Looking back at Figure 8.13, notice that performance is quite good if T2 appears immediately after T1. In Chun's metaphorical account, these are

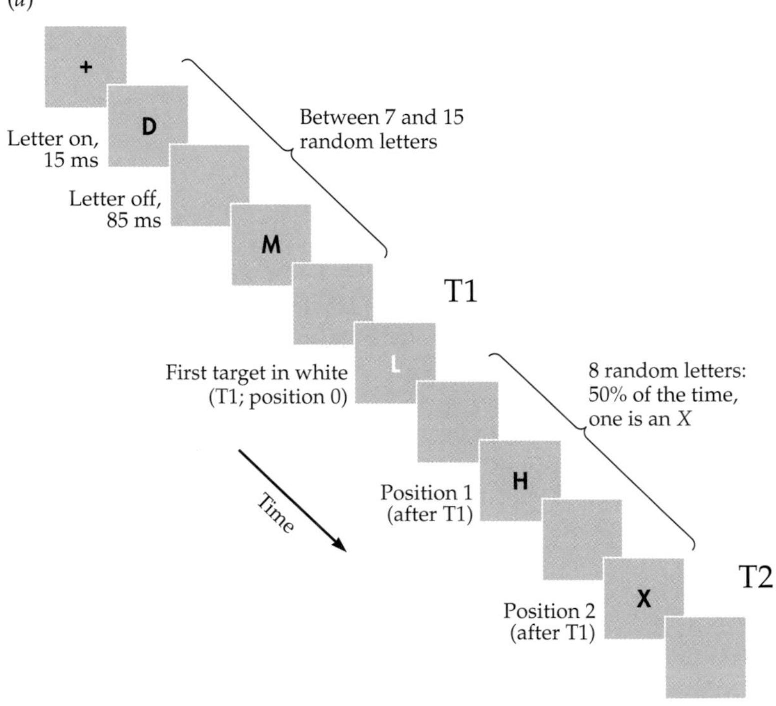

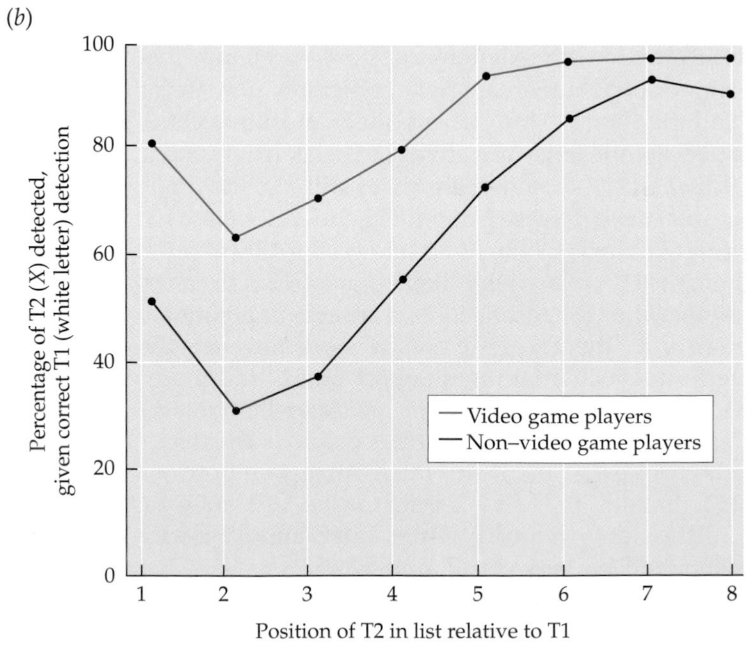

FIGURE 8.13 The attentional blink (AB) in video game and non–video game players. (*a*) In this AB task, observers try to report two targets; the white letter (T1) and whether there is an *X* (T2) in the stream after that white letter. Letters appear every 100 milliseconds. T2 can appear in various positions in the list after T1. Here T2 is in Position 2. (*b*) If the *X* appears within 500 milliseconds (positions 1–5 after T1), detection is impaired. That is the "attentional blink." Video game players show less of a blink.

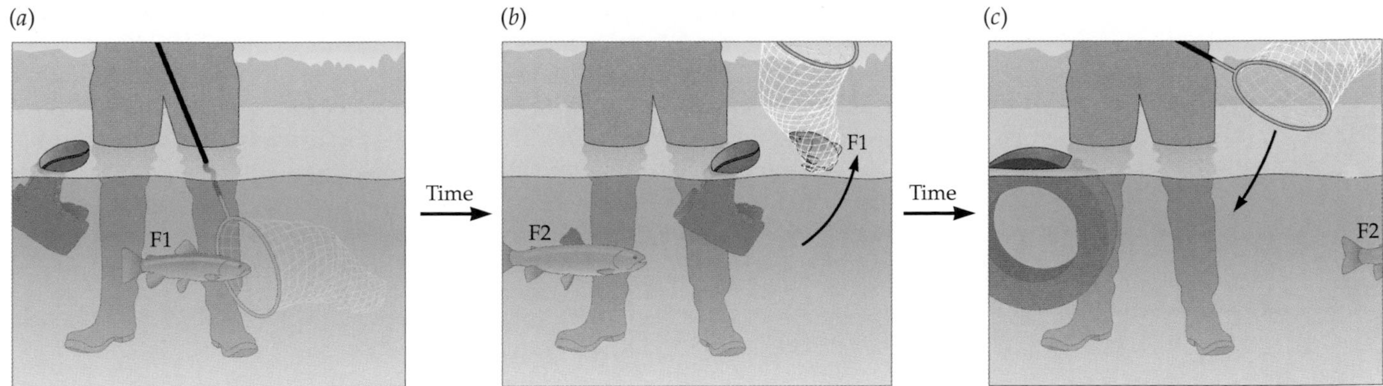

FIGURE 8.14 Marvin Chun's fishing metaphor for attentional blink. You can see all the stuff in the river as it drifts by. But if you commit to fishing out fish number 1 (F1), you will not be able to fish out fish number 2 (F2) if that second fish shows up while fish 1 is still in your net.

cases in which one scoop nets two fishes. This metaphor illustrates the idea that two processes are at work. A fast process can identify each object as it appears and disappears, and a slower process is required if the observer will actually respond to any particular item (Chun and Potter, 1995).

Figure 8.13*b* shows data from two groups of subjects who perform differently on the attentional blink task. Interestingly, the group that shows a smaller attentional blink consists of players of "first-person shooter" video games. Indeed, those gamers seem to do better on a range of attentional tasks (C. S. Green and Bavelier, 2003). Why? It could be that people who choose to play these video games have better attentional resources. To test this idea, Green and Bavelier (2003) took two groups of non–video game players. One group got experience with a first-person shooter game, and the other group played Tetris. The first-person shooter group improved on attentional tasks; the other group did not. Of course, this is not an endorsement of violent video games, but it does suggest that attentional abilities can be changed by training and that those first-person shooter video games produce change. If you visit the website, you can experience a related but not identical effect (Web Activity 8.4: The Attentional Blink and Repetition Blindness).

Suppose we present an RSVP stream and ask you if any item is repeated. If the items are reasonably close together, it turns out to be surprisingly difficult to determine if you have seen one or two of a letter, word, or picture. This deficit is known as **repetition blindness** (Chun, 1997; Kanwisher, 1987). To understand the problem with repetition, it is useful to think back to the recognition demons of pandemonium from Chapter 4. Suppose we show a stream of words including two instances of the word *cat*. The *cat* demon yells when the first *cat* appears. He is still yelling when the second *cat* comes along, and later processes, monitoring that demon, cannot tell the difference between one instance and two. If the *cat* instances are sufficiently separated in time, they can be individuated. This effect is so strong that it will cause us to make a meaningful sentence meaningless if the words come fast enough. If we show subjects the sentence "It was time to work because work needed to be done," they will often report back, "It was time to work because needed to be done," losing the second instance of *work*.

The Physiological Basis of Attention

In an oft-quoted passage, William James declared, "Everyone knows what attention is." This great nineteenth-century psychologist went on to say, "It is the taking possession by the mind, in clear and vivid form, of one out of what seem several simultaneously possible objects or trains of thought"

repetition blindness A failure to detect the second occurrence of a letter, word, or picture in a rapidly presented stream of stimuli when the second occurrence falls within 200 to 500 milliseconds of the first.

Subject A

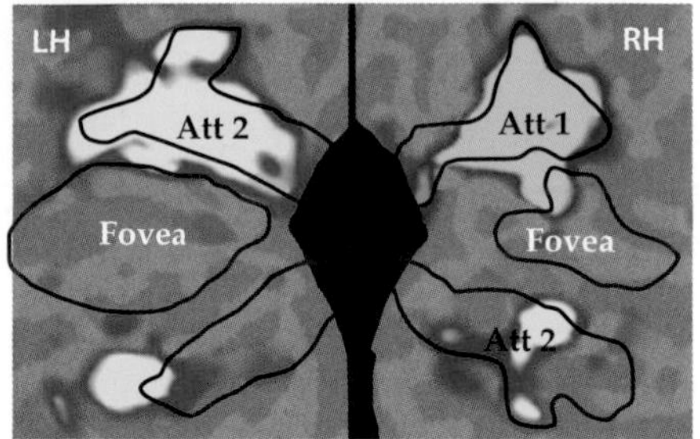

Subject B

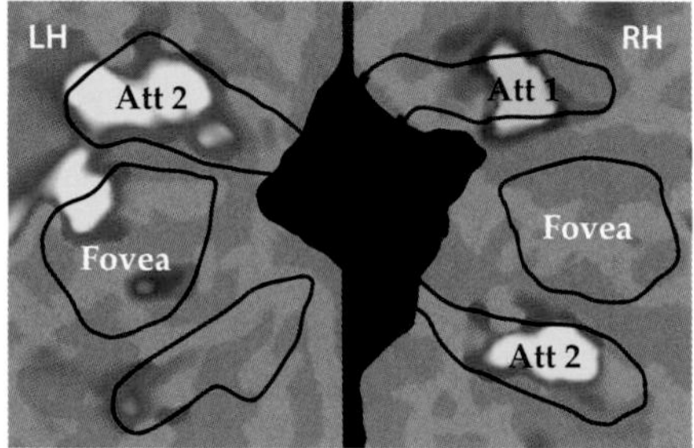

FIGURE 8.15 Spotlights of attention in the human brain. This fMRI image of human visual cortex (striate and some extrastriate) shows activity in the brain while subjects paid attention to one stimulus (Att 1) or two stimuli (Att 2). The stimuli were outside the fovea, so the regions of activity don't include the fovea. (From McMains and Somers, 2004.)

(James, 1890, Vol. 1, pp. 403–404). That seems fair enough, but what does it mean for the mind to take possession of a possible object? If we try to get specific, we discover that this attention that everyone "knows" can be rather difficult to pin down. In part, it is difficult to know what attention does because attention performs a variety of tasks, as already discussed. But we also need to deal with the physiological question of what the brain is actually doing when it selects one location in space, or one object, or one moment in time, for further processing. Let's consider some of the neural possibilities.

Attention Could Enhance Neural Activity

If we are asked to attend to one location in the visual field, as in a Posner cueing task (see Figure 8.3), the neurons that respond to stimuli in that part of the field will become more active. It used to be thought that this response did not apply to striate cortex, the first part of visual cortex to process visual input (see Chapter 3). However, fMRI experiments in humans, as well as electrophysiological studies of monkeys, have shown that even the first stages of cortical processing are influenced by attention (**Figure 8.15**) (Brefczynski and DeYoe, 1999; Gandhi, Heeger, and Boynton, 1998; Haenny and Schiller, 1988; McMains and Somers, 2004).

As we progress further into the visual areas of the cortex, even larger attentional effects are seen (Reynolds and Chelazzi, 2004). In fact, the effects seen at the early stages in the cortex are quite possibly the results of feedback from these later stages of processing (Martinez et al., 1999). That feedback may be a very important part of visual processing (Ahissar and Hochstein, 2004; Di Lollo, Enns, and Rensink, 2000).

Attention Could Enhance the Processing of a Specific Type of Stimulus

The mechanisms of attention described in the previous section might suffice if we want to keep watch "out of the corner of the eye" by enhancing activity in a specific region of visual cortex. But imagine picking pennies out of a change bowl (a real-world visual search task). Somehow the wish to find pennies makes the pennies more salient. If we switched to quarters, the pennies would recede in salience and the quarters would rise. In this case, we are attending not on the basis of spatial location, but on the basis of a stimulus property.

You can experience this attentional shift in the salience of different stimulus attributes in **Figure 8.16**. Without moving your eyes, you can select the red items or the blue items or the horizontal items. Each act of selection

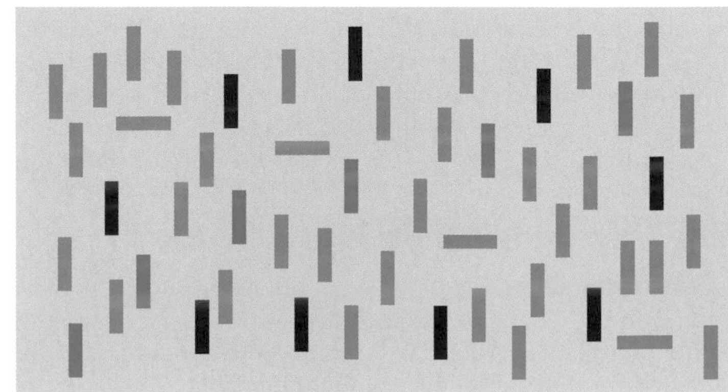

FIGURE 8.16 Attentional selection. First, attend to the red items and notice the rough oval that they form. Next, without moving your eyes, switch attention to the blue items or the horizontal items. Different aspects of the picture appear more prominent as you shift the property that you select to attend to.

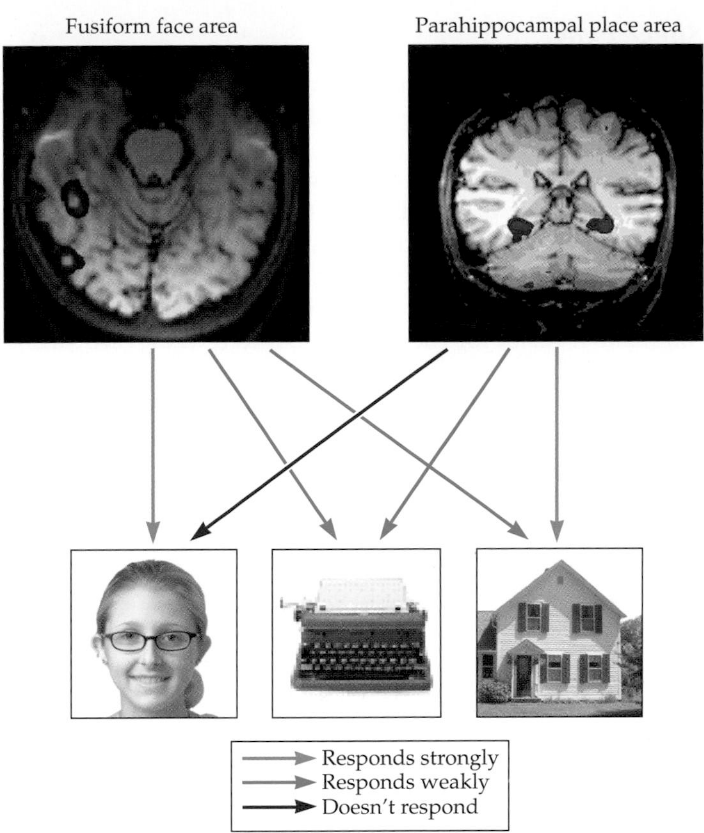

FIGURE 8.17 Functional MRI reveals that different pieces of the cortex are activated by faces and by places. This is true even when both stimuli are present at the same time (as in Figure 8.18) and the observer merely alters his mental set from faces to places. (MRIs courtesy of Nancy Kanwisher.)

seems to alter what you see, even as the stimulus remains physically unchanged. You may not have noticed, for example, that the blue items form a rough diagonal line until you attended to that color.

Attentional selection can also be used to perform one type of specialized processing rather than another. For instance, fMRI has shown that different parts of the human brain are especially important in the processing of faces (the **fusiform face area**; Kanwisher, McDermott, and Chun, 1997) and places (the **parahippocampal place area**; Epstein et al., 1999) (**Figure 8.17**). If subjects view an image of a face superimposed over an image of a house (**Figure 8.18**), the face area becomes more active when the subject is attending to the face, and the place area becomes more active when the subject is attending to the house (O'Craven and Kanwisher, 2000).

fusiform face area An area in the fusiform gyrus of human extrastriate cortex that responds preferentially to faces in fMRI studies.

parahippocampal place area A region of cortex in the temporal lobe of humans that appears to respond with particular strength to images of places (as opposed to isolated objects).

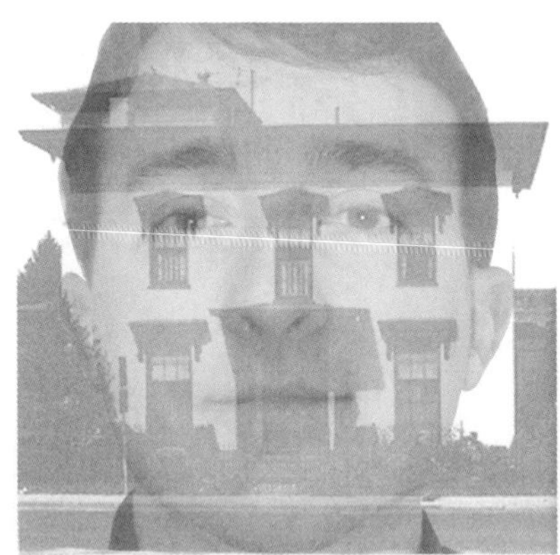

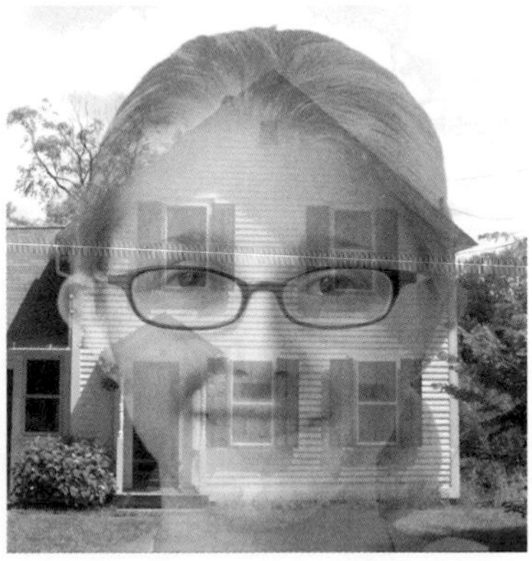

FIGURE 8.18 These images combine faces and houses. In both cases you can use attention to enhance the perception of one or the other. As you switch your attention from one type of object to the other, you also change the activation of different parts of the brain, as shown in Figure 8.17. (Left image from Downing, Liu, and Kanwisher, 2001.)

Attention and Single Cells

response enhancement An effect of attention on the response of a neuron in which the neuron responding to an attended stimulus gives a bigger response.

sharper tuning An effect of attention on the response of a neuron in which the neuron responds more precisely. For example, a neuron that responds to lines with orientations from –20° to +20° might come to respond to ±10-degree lines.

On a finer scale, we can ask how attention might change the responses of a single neuron. **Figure 8.19** shows one set of possibilities. Suppose a cell responded to a range of different orientations but was maximally responsive to vertical lines (see Chapter 3). Attention might make the cell more responsive across the board (see Figure 8.19*a*). This sort of **response enhancement** has been seen in visual cortex cells, but simple response enhancement seems like a rather indiscriminate change. Alternatively, a cell might become more precisely tuned. In the example in Figure 8.19*b*, **sharper tuning** would mean that attention could make it easier for the neuron to find a weak vertical signal amid the noise of other orientations (as seems to happen when we attend to the horizontal bars in Figure 8.16). Lu and Dosher (1998) have done elegant psychophysical experiments showing that attention does make it possible to exclude noise in this way, though some efforts to find physiological evidence for sharper tuning have turned up only response enhancement (Treue and Trujillo, 1999).

A more radical possibility is that attention changes the preferences of a neuron. As illustrated in Figure 8.19*c*, a cell that was initially tuned to vertical lines might come to respond better to a different orientation under the influence of attention. The best evidence for a change in the fundamental preferences of a neuron comes from studies of its preferences in space—that is, the size and shape of a neuron's receptive field (Moran and Desimone, 1985). **Figure 8.20** shows just such a change in a specific area of monkey cortex. When the monkey attends to one stimulus, the cell's sensitivity is

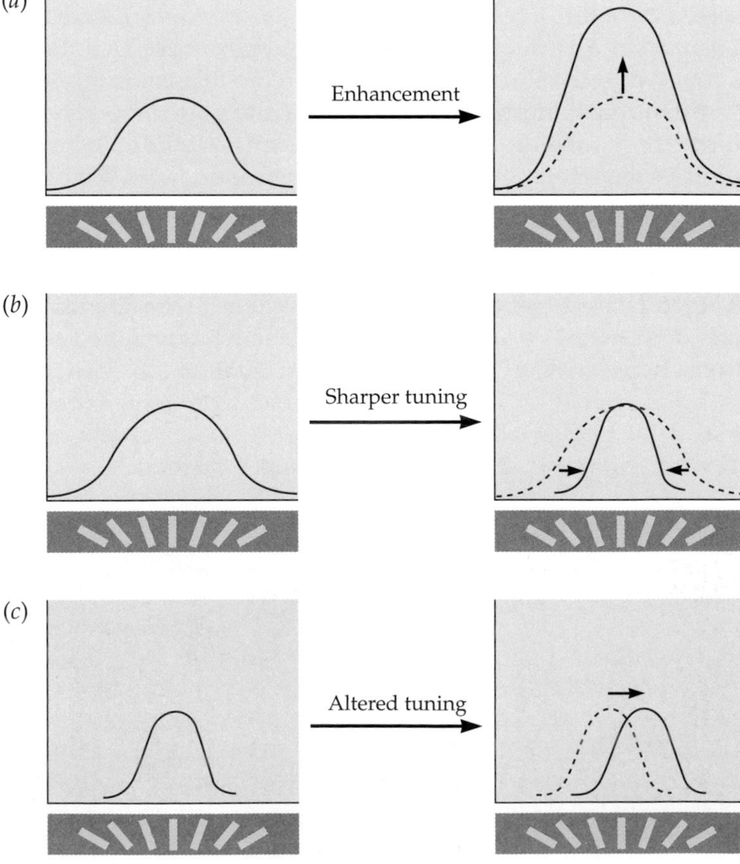

FIGURE 8.19 Three ways that the response of a cell could be changed as a result of attention: (*a*) enhancement, (*b*) sharper tuning, (*c*) altered tuning. In each row, the red line shows the response of a single cell to lines of different orientations, without attention (left column) and with attention (right column).

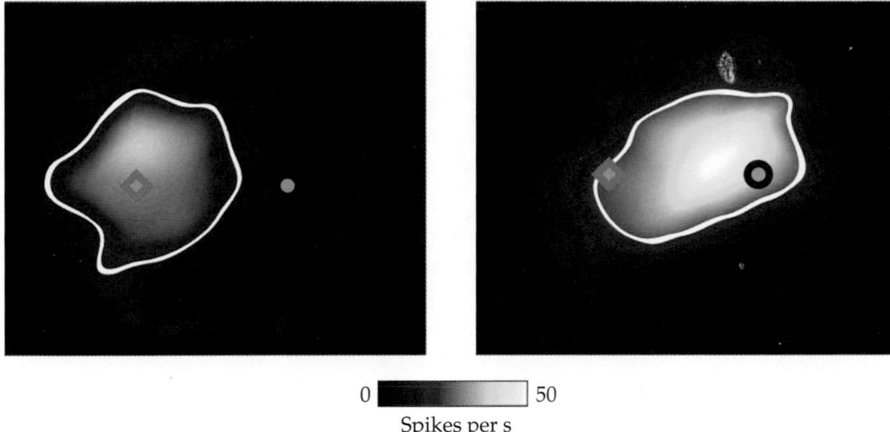

FIGURE 8.20 Each of these images is a map of part of the visual field. In this experiment, the investigators flashed little spots of light at different locations and measured the response of one cell. Brighter, whiter locations are areas of greater response. The only difference between the left and right maps is that on the left the monkey was attending to the location marked by the diamond, while on the right it attended to the location of the circle. This change in attention caused the receptive field of the cell to shrink-wrap itself around the attended stimulus location. (From Womelsdorf et al., 2006.)

enhanced around that location. When its attention is shifted to another location, the receptive field shifts too (Womelsdorf et al., 2006).

If cells are restricting their processing to the object of attention, then sensitivity to neighboring items might be reduced as resources are withdrawn from them. This prediction is borne out: mapping the effects of attention reveals inhibition surrounding the object of attention (Mounts, 2000).

The three hypotheses about the microcircuitry of attention discussed here are not mutually exclusive. Different neurons perform different parts of the task of attending, and each subtask may require a different type of change in neuronal responses. As a hypothetical example, simple response enhancement from one neuron might be the "command" that causes another neuron to sharpen its tuning and/or to change the shape of its receptive field.

visual-field defect A portion of the visual field with no vision or with abnormal vision, typically resulting from damage to the visual nervous system.

parietal lobe In each cerebral hemisphere, a lobe that lies toward the top of the brain between the frontal and occipital lobes.

Disorders of Visual Attention

What would happen if you could no longer pay attention? A complete inability to attend would be devastating. Because we cannot recognize objects or find what we're looking for without attention, complete inattention would be something near to functional blindness. Brain damage that produces a deficit this severe is very rare. More common is the attentional equivalent of a **visual-field defect**. As you may recall, if someone is unfortunate enough to lose primary visual cortex in the right hemisphere, that person will be blind on the opposite (left) side of visual space. Suppose, however, that the lesion was in the right **parietal lobe**. Patients with this sort of lesion (**Figure 8.21**) would have problems directing attention to objects and places on their left. These problems manifest themselves in a curious set of clinical symptoms, including neglect and extinction.

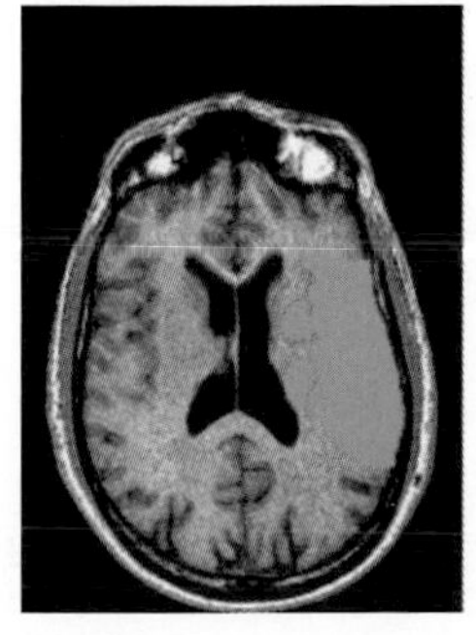
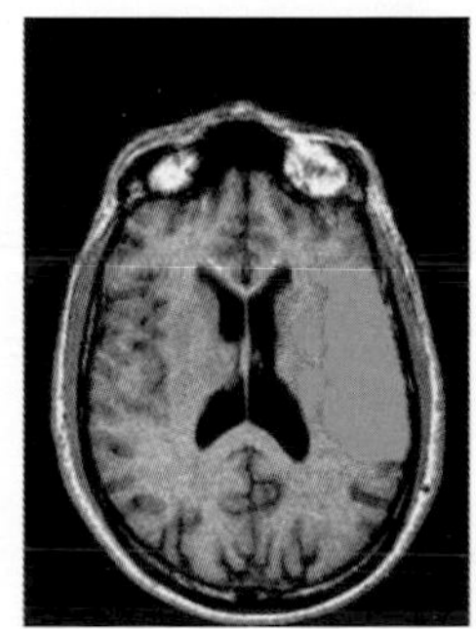
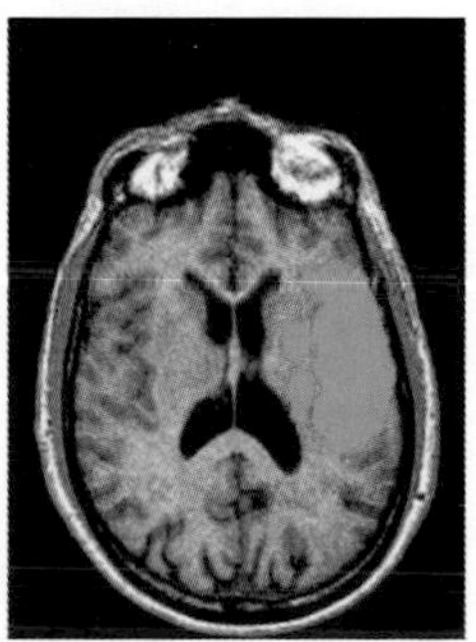
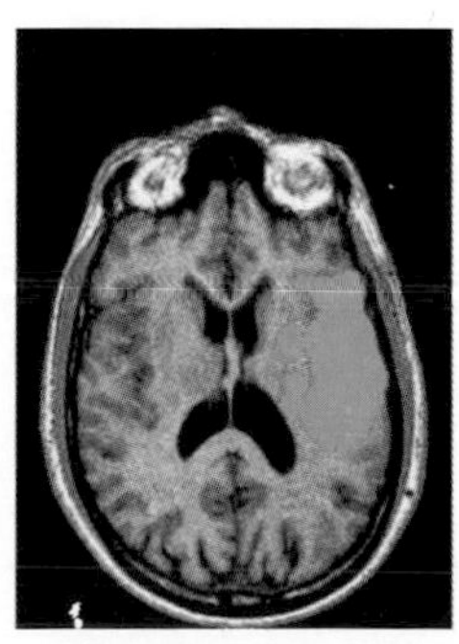
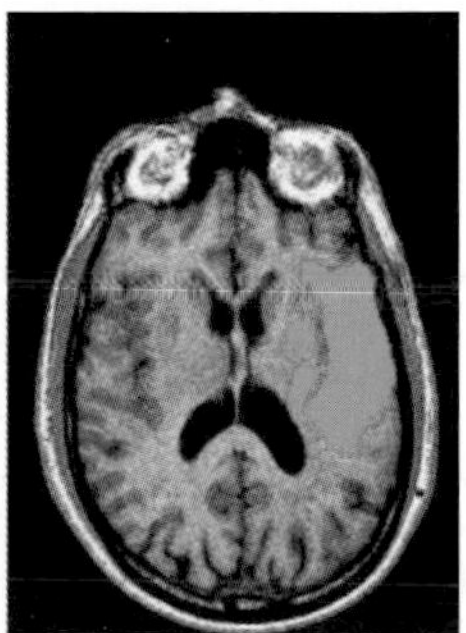

FIGURE 8.21 Five images through the brain of a neglect patient (viewed as though from above). The damage (shown here in yellow) includes the right parietal and frontal lobes. The patient neglects the left side of space. (Image courtesy of Lynn Robertson and Krista Schendel.)

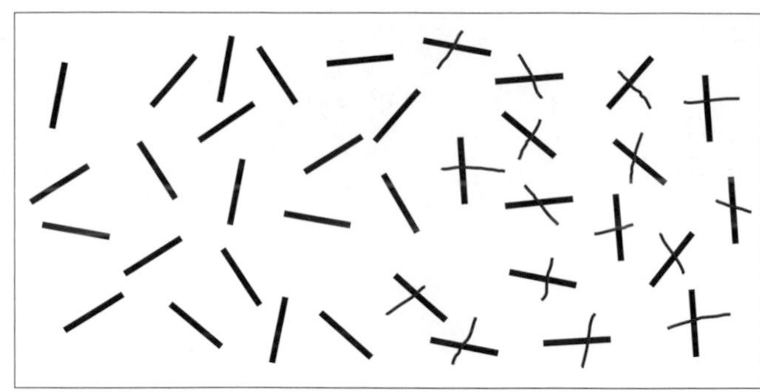

FIGURE 8.22 A neglect patient would produce this sort of result if asked to cross out all the lines on the page.

Neglect

neglect In visual attention, the inability to attend to or respond to stimuli in the contralesional visual field (typically, neglect of the left field after right parietal damage). Also, neglect of half of the body or half of an object.

contralesional field The visual field on the side opposite a brain lesion (e.g., points to the left of fixation are contralesional to damage to the right hemisphere of the brain).

Neglect patients behave as if part of the world were not there. Asked to describe what he is seeing, a patient experiencing neglect of the left visual field will tend to name objects to the right of fixation and ignore objects on the left. A "line cancellation test" is a more systematic way to assess this problem. The patient is given a piece of paper full of lines and asked to draw an intersecting line through each one. A neglect patient might produce something like **Figure 8.22**: the lines on one side (the right, in this case) are crossed out, but those on the other side (here, the left) are overlooked. **Figure 8.23** shows what might result if a neglect patient, again experiencing neglect of the left visual field, is asked to copy a picture. Again, the right side is reproduced fairly faithfully, but the left side is missing. Such a neglect patient might also eat only the right side of dinner or shave only the right side of his face.

It is not always clear if neglect affects one side of the visual world or one side of objects. Mostly likely, neglect can be either or both. In one elegant illustration of this point, Steve Tipper and Marlene Behrmann (1996) had neglect patients try to detect changes on one or the other side of a barbell. When the barbell had one ball in the left field and one in the right, patients were better on the right. Tipper and Behrmann's clever trick was to rotate the barbell, while the patient was watching, so that the left ball moved into the right field and the right ball moved into the left (**Figure 8.24**). Now the patients did better than they should have with the piece of the object in the normally neglected, **contralesional field** (the field on the side opposite the lesion). Apparently, they were neglecting half of the object, and the neglect somehow moved with the object.

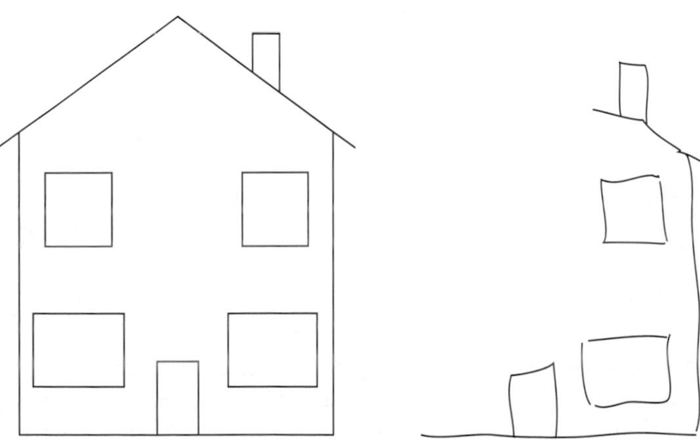

FIGURE 8.23 This is what can happen when a neglect patient tries to copy a drawing. This patient omitted the left side of the object.

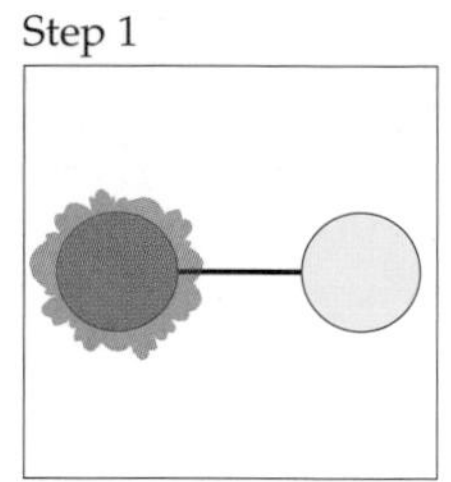

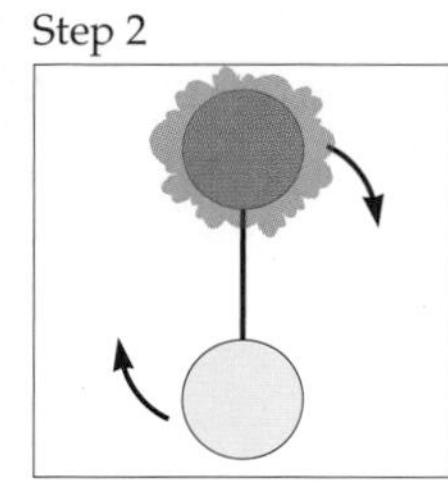

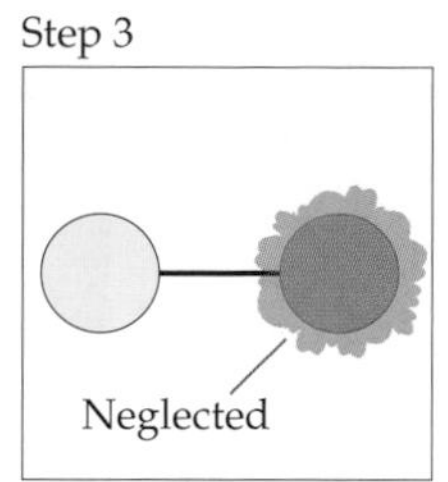

FIGURE 8.24 Tipper and Behrmann's (1996) experiment. Step 1: The patient neglected the left side of the barbell. Step 2: The barbell was rotated through 180 degrees. Step 3: The neglect rotated with the object in this example of object-centered neglect.

Extinction

The phenomenon of **extinction** is related to neglect; it might even be neglect in a milder form (Driver, 1998). A neurologist might test for neglect by having a patient fixate on her (the neurologist's) nose. She might then hold up a fork in the patient's good (in this case, right) visual field and ask, "What do you see?" "A fork," would come the reply. Next the neurologist might present a spoon in the bad (left) field. A patient with left-visual-field neglect would be nonplussed, but an extinction patient would be able to report the presence of the spoon. If the neurologist were to hold up a fork in one hand and a spoon in the other, however, the extinction patient would report only the object in the good field. The other object would be perceptually "extinguished."

In neglect, the patient may be entirely unable to deploy attention to the contralesional side of the world or the object. In extinction, the patient may be able to get attention to an object in the contralesional field if it is the only salient object. However, if there is competition from another similar object in the **ipsilesional field** (the same side as the lesion), then the two objects compete for attention and the ipsilesional object wins. Objects are always competing for our attention, but as a general rule, it is no great matter for us to redeploy attention from one object to the next. In extinction, the losing object loses the ability to attract attention far more completely than is the case normally.

Balint Syndrome

What happens if a patient is unfortunate enough to have *bilateral* lesions of the parietal lobes (that is, lesions in both hemispheres)? This condition is rare, but it does happen, and the result can be a disorder known as Balint syndrome (named for the doctor who described it in 1909). The disorder has three major symptoms (Driver, 1998):

1. Spatial localization abilities are greatly reduced. As a result, a patient with Balint syndrome may have a very hard time trying to reach to an object.
2. Patients with Balint syndrome don't move their eyes very much. They tend to gaze fixedly ahead.
3. Finally, and of most interest for present purposes, patients with Balint syndrome behave as if they can see only one object at a time. This deficit seems like an extreme form of extinction or neglect, in that attending to one object eliminates everything else. This inability to perceive more than one thing at a time is known as **simultagnosia**. (As noted in earlier chapters, agnosia is a failure to know something. Simultagnosia is a failure to know about more than one object at a time.)

As discussed earlier, even people who are neurologically normal can have some trouble binding features together. Remember those pluses in Figure 8.11 that were treated as bundles of red-and-blue-and-vertical-and-horizon-

extinction In visual attention, the inability to perceive a stimulus to one side of the point of fixation (e.g., to the right) in the presence of another stimulus, typically in a comparable position in the other visual field (e.g., on the left side).

ipsilesional field The visual field on the same side as a brain lesion.

simultagnosia An inability to perceive more than one object at a time. Simultagnosia is a consequence of bilateral damage to the parietal lobes (Balint syndrome).

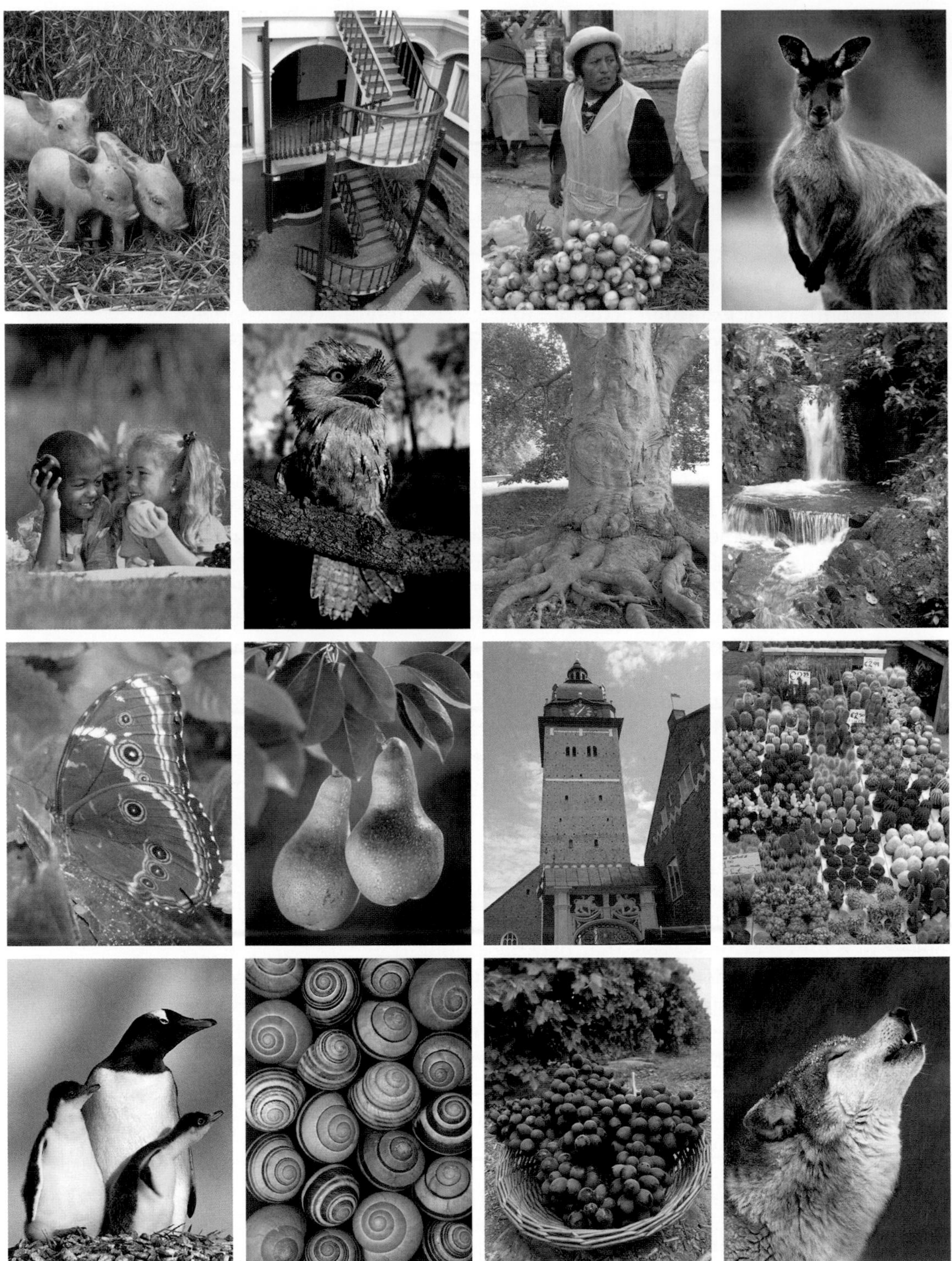

FIGURE 8.25 Spend a second or two looking at each of these pictures. Then move on to Figure 8.26.

tal until attention sorted out which color went with which orientation? Remember also the demonstration of illusory conjunction in Figure 8.12, where you may have been convinced that you saw a combination of color and form that was not present? Stacia Friedman-Hill, Lynn Robertson, and Anne Treisman found that binding errors of this sort were much more severe in one patient with Balint syndrome whom they tested (Friedman-Hill, Robertson, and Treisman, 1995). This makes sense if you think about combining simultagnosia with a spatial localization deficit. Not only does a patient with Balint syndrome see only one thing at a time, but the features of that "thing" may have come from several different locations in the world.

Perceiving and Understanding Scenes

Without attention, normal visual perception is not possible. Patients suffering from Balint syndrome make this point very dramatically: we can't function as visual animals if we can "see" only one object at a time. But what does it really mean to see more than one object? How do we perceive entire visual scenes? This is the topic we will explore in the remainder of this chapter. As we will see, there are surprising similarities between the impoverished perceptual world of a patient with Balint syndrome and the apparently rich world of normal visual perception.

Picture Memory and Change Blindness

Have a look at **Figure 8.25**. It contains photographs of 16 scenes. Spend about one second on each scene, and then flip the page to view **Figure 8.26**. There you will find another set of 16 scenes. Your job is to determine which 8 of the 16 in Figure 8.26 you saw in Figure 8.25. You probably won't need the answer key (it's in the figure caption). It is likely that you will correctly classify 14 or more of the images as "old" or "new." That's pretty quick learning of fairly complicated stimuli. Yet it is a mere fraction of what you could do if you had the time and we had the pictures. Roger Shepard (1967) conducted the original version of the test with 612 pictures and found that his observers were 98% correct. They were 90% correct when quizzed a week later. Standing, Conezio, and Haber (1970) got 85% accuracy after showing their observers 2500 pictures for 2 seconds apiece, and Standing (1973) later obtained similar results with 10,000(!) images. In these studies, Standing used a diverse collection of scenes clipped from magazines of the time.

What would happen if we restricted the "scenes" to single objects (an apple, a backpack), and what would happen if we included other examples of these objects in the test set (did I see *that* apple?) or, worse yet, the same object in a different pose (was that backpack lying down before?)? Aude Oliva and her students (Brady et al., 2008) tried this with 2500 objects. When asked to pick between an old item and a new one, their observers got 92% correct if the new item was an object of a type that had not been seen before in the experiment. Amazingly, observers were still 88% correct remembering which example of a category they had seen and 87% correct remembering which state of a specific object they had seen. If we tried the same experiment with a list of words, the accuracy would be far lower. People are spectacularly good at remembering pictures.

When we discussed attentional blink earlier in this chapter, we mentioned another set of experiments with pictures, conducted by Molly Potter and her colleagues. They presented pictures of scenes very rapidly and asked observers to say whether, for example, a picnic scene was present in the stream of images (Potter 1975, 1976). Once again, observers were remarkably good at this task. Helene Intraub (1981) took the paradigm a step further and showed that people could monitor a stream of stimuli for the one that was *not* an animal at rates of 8 images per second. That means that every image in the stream could be classified as "animal" or "not animal" after a mere 125 ms of exposure. By the way, at that rate, we cannot commit images to memory very effectively, but we do have a pretty clear idea of what we're seeing as it flashes by.

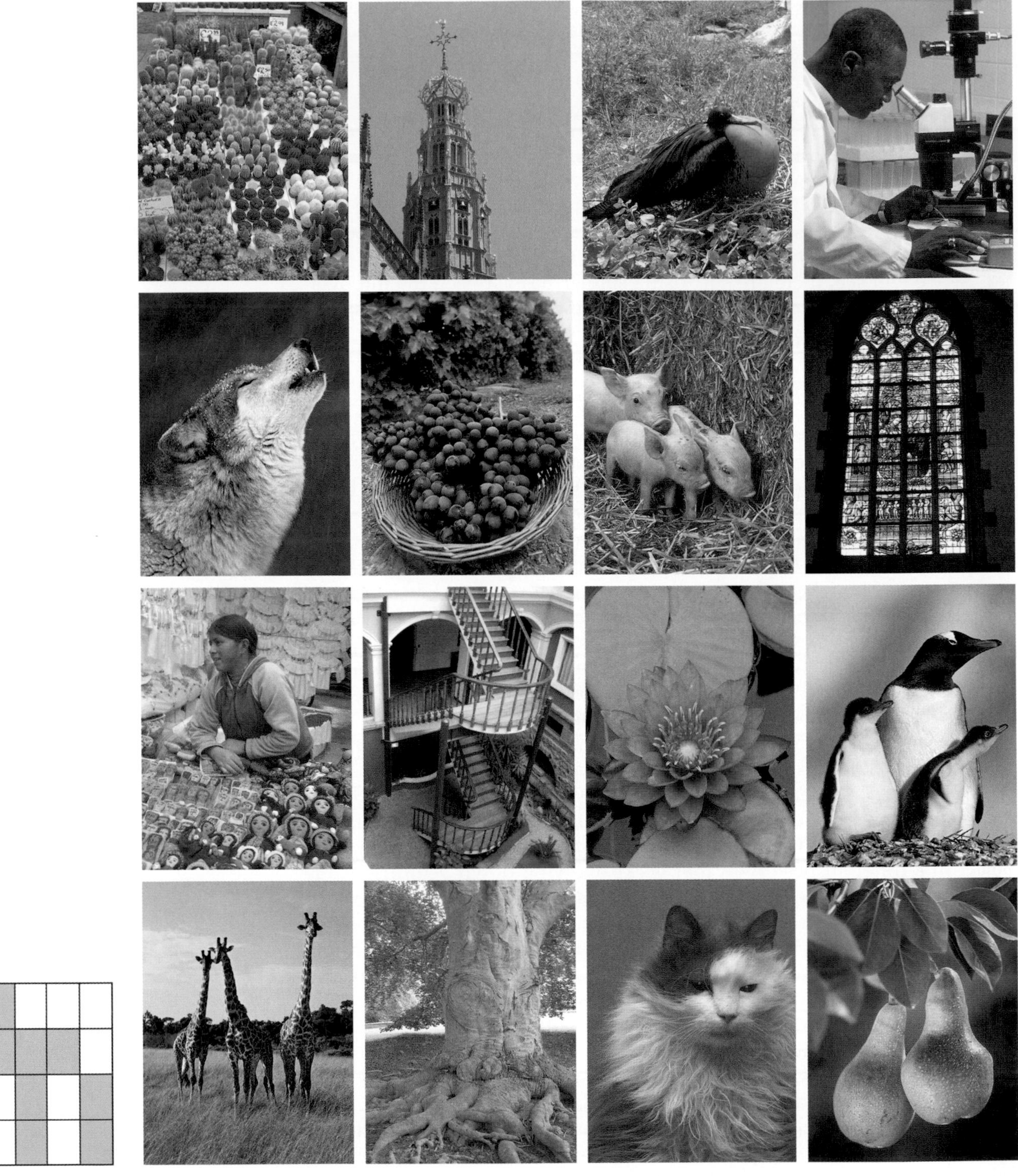

FIGURE 8.26 Which of these pictures did you see in Figure 8.25? Look at each one and label it as "old" or "new." You can check your answers on the grid to the left. The shaded squares show the locations of old pictures.

On the basis these findings, we could conclude that pictures can be understood very rapidly and that, given enough time, perhaps a second, we can code them into memory in sufficient detail to be able to recognize them days later. But don't endorse that conclusion too quickly. In the 1990s, Ron Rensink and his colleagues introduced a different sort of picture memory experiment (Rensink, O'Regan, and Clark, 1997). They showed observers

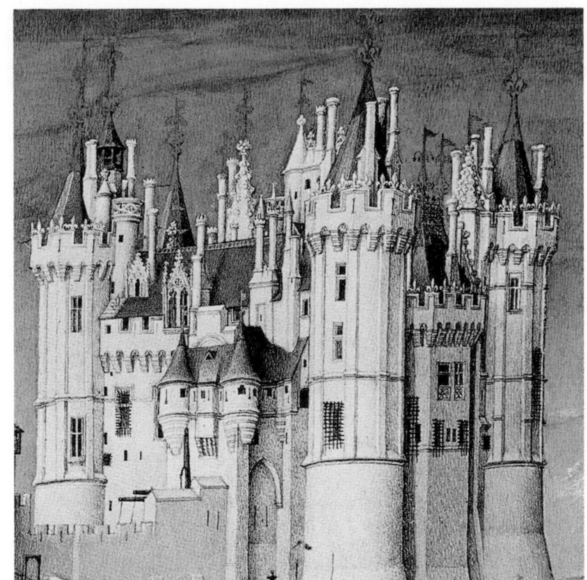

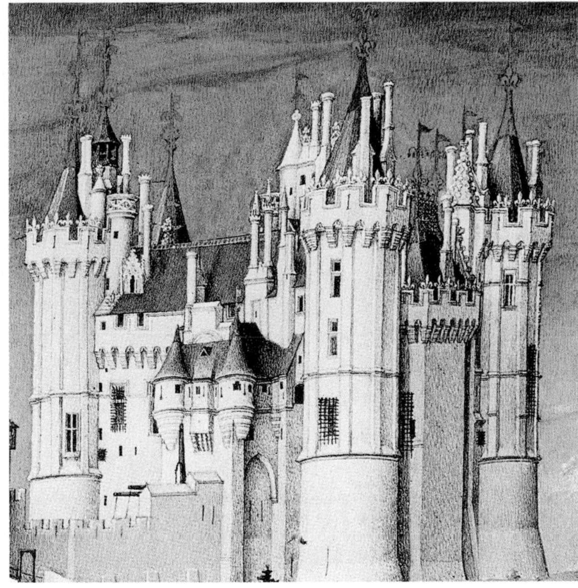

FIGURE 8.27 There are four differences between these two images. Can you find them?

just one picture at a time. The observers would look at the picture for a while, and then it would vanish for 80 ms (0.08 second) and would be replaced with a similar image. The observer's task was to determine what had changed. The two versions of the same image would flip back and forth, with a brief interval between the images in which a blank screen was presented, until the observer spotted the change or time ran out. A static version of the task is illustrated in **Figure 8.27**. Try to find the differences between the two pictures in this figure. The answers are in **Figure 8.28**. You can also try detecting changes in some flicker movies in Web Activity 8.5: Change Blindness.

It may have taken you a while to discover all four changes in Figure 8.27. The same thing happened in Rensink's experiment: participants took several seconds on average to find the changes, and some never managed at all. This phenomenon is known as **change blindness**. If the blank screen between the two images is removed, the changes are obvious because observers expe-

change blindness The failure to notice a change between two scenes. If the change does not alter the gist, or meaning, of the scene, quite large changes can pass unnoticed.

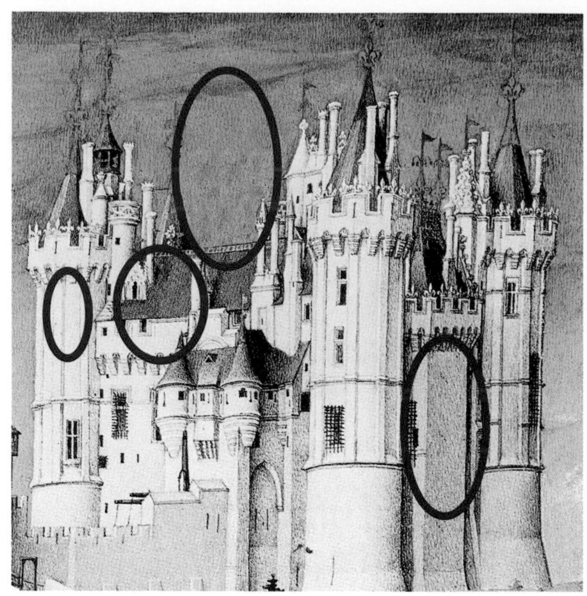

FIGURE 8.28 Here are the locations of the differences between the two images in Figure 8.27. When you go back to Figure 8.27 with this information, you will have no trouble seeing what was altered.

rience a kind of apparent motion effect (see Chapter 7) when an object changes position, disappears, or changes color. But once we've taken care of that low-level factor by inserting the blank screen, viewers can be quite oblivious to jet engines that vanish from airplanes, branches that jump from tree to tree, and boats that change color.

Actually, we can eliminate the need for a blank screen if the change is made while the eyes are moving. We are virtually blind during an abrupt (saccadic) eye movement. McConkie and Currie (1996) took advantage of this fact to make dramatic changes in a scene while an observer was just looking around. If they made the changes while the eye was in motion, observers often failed to notice.

It is not immediately obvious how these various facts can all be true of the same visual system. This is a topic of current controversy in the field. How can we remember thousands of objects after a mere second or two of viewing? And if we can do that, how can we fail to notice substantive change in a picture that is right in front of us? Does it make any sense that we remember the picture but seem oblivious to important details? Before we try to propose answers to these questions, let's step back a bit and look at the basic visual processes involved in recognizing scenes.

Local and Global Approaches to Scene Recognition

In Chapter 7 we learned that people execute a complex series of saccades when viewing a scene, moving their eyes around at a rate of about three or four times per second to examine objects of interest. Perhaps we assemble a representation of a scene from a collection of smaller snapshots taken after each saccade, rather like the David Hockney collage in **Figure 8.29**.

The first problem with this story is that, although we remember something from fixation to fixation (Hollingworth and Henderson, 2002), it is pretty clear that we cannot add the contents of one fixation to the contents of the next as though we were putting a puzzle together (Irwin, 1996; Irwin, Yantis, and Jonides, 1983).

The second problem is that the Potter and Intraub experiments established that we can recognize scenes (or at least categorize them as farm-

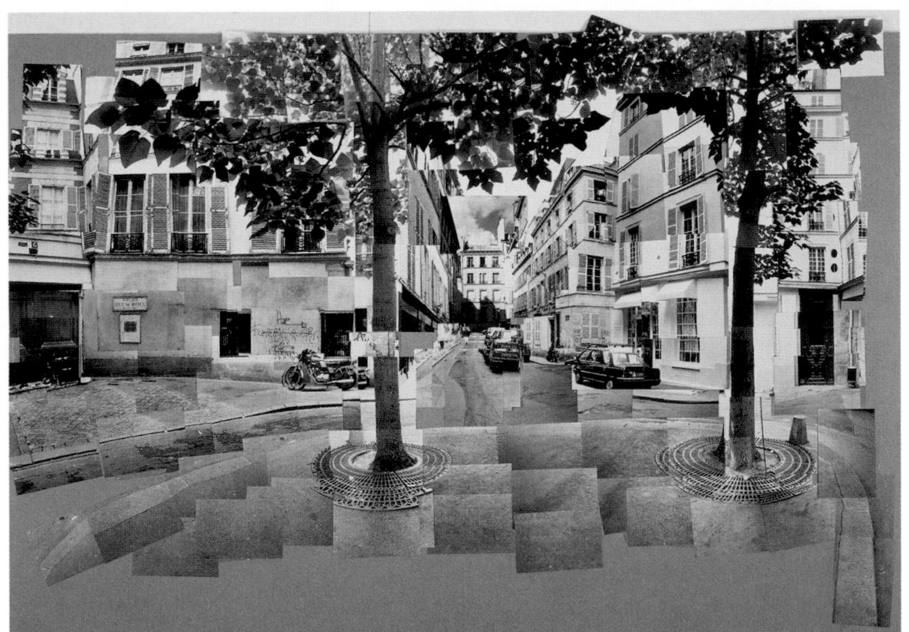

FIGURE 8.29 David Hockney's photo collage *Place Furstenberg, Paris, August 7, 8, 9, 1985 #1* might be a metaphor for the way we see scenes. Maybe, like a collage, our perception of scenes is put together from a set of "snapshots" over time.

yards, picnics, city streets, and so on) in an *eighth* of a second. We can't count on being able to make even one saccade in such a brief period of time. Maybe covert attention can save the day. Recall from the visual search experiments described earlier in this chapter that **covert attentional shifts** enable us to process something like 20 to 30 objects per second. This is much faster than the 3 to 4 objects per second that can be fixated with **overt** movements of the eyes. Covert attentional shifts don't change which part of the world falls on the fovea, so we wouldn't be fixating each of these objects. Nevertheless, we might be able to compile a list of three or four objects in the scene, as well as some rudimentary information about how the objects relate to each other (e.g., "the chicken is to the left of the cow and on top of the tractor").

Is recognizing this short list of objects the same as recognizing the scene? Introspection may not be the best guide to the processes of vision, but rapid scene interpretation does not *feel* like the rapid recognition of a few objects and their relations to each other. An isolated cow, chicken, and tractor are easily distinguishable from the same three objects embedded in a farmyard scene. What's the difference?

As already described, of course, the difference is the farmyard. It seems that the farmyard, or more generally, the **spatial layout** of the scene, is not just another object to be attended. By *spatial layout* we mean the overall structure of the scene. Is it wide open, like a prairie or closed like a closet? Is the scene empty like a parking lot after closing time or cluttered like a messy desktop? Where are the large surfaces, such as the ground, walls, and so on? How are they oriented?

For a long time, evidence has suggested that the spatial layout has special status in picture recognition. For example, Geoff Loftus (Loftus and Mackworth, 1978) found that observers responded differently to an object if it appeared in its natural setting than if it appeared in an unusual setting (e.g., an octopus in an underwater scene versus in a farmyard). The mystery has been how something as seemingly complicated as the meaning of a scene layout could be computed quickly enough to shape responses to simple objects.

covert attentional shift A shift of attention in the absence of corresponding movements of the eyes.

overt attentional shift A shift of attention accompanied by corresponding movements of the eyes.

spatial layout The description of the structure of a scene (e.g., enclosed, open, rough, smooth) without reference to the identity of specific objects in the scene.

FIGURE 8.30 A simple visual "scene" composed of two sinusoidal gratings.

An interesting potential answer comes from the work of Aude Oliva and Antonio Torralba (2001). Consider the very boring "scene" in **Figure 8.30**. It is composed of a vertically oriented low-spatial-frequency component (a broad, upright sine wave) combined with a diagonally oriented high-spatial-frequency component (a narrower sine wave that's tilted to the right). As we learned in Chapter 3, *any* image can be broken down like this into its spatial-frequency components, and in fact, the visual system appears to process images in exactly this way, via a set of spatial frequency–tuned channels.

If we further analyze the spatial-frequency components of scenes, we find that certain patterns of frequencies correspond to certain types of scenes. To take a fairly obvious example, wide-open scenes (beaches, prairies, parking lots, and so on) tend to have a lot of strong horizontal components (corresponding to the horizon). Oliva and Torralba called this dimension "openness" and defined a number of other dimensions, including "naturalness" (versus "man-made") and "roughness." For each of these dimensions they could measure the amount of openness or naturalness or roughness by looking at the sine waves that made up the stimulus.

When Oliva and Torralba measured the properties of thousands of scenes, they observed something very useful: scenes with the same meaning tended to be neighbors. Suppose we define a simple two-dimensional space using the dimensions of openness and expansion. **Figure 8.31** graphs a set of man-made scenes using these two dimensions. Look how the scenes organize themselves. The frontal views of buildings fall in the upper right (low openness, low expansion). Highways fall in the lower left (high openness, high expansion). The rules that made this picture don't know about buildings or highways, just sine waves. Nevertheless, scenes with the same "gist" tend to cluster together.

Remember that these dimensions are defined on the basis of a spatial-frequency analysis of the entire scene. There would be no need to shift our gaze or even our attentional focus—no need to bind features or recognize objects.

Oliva and Torralba's work shows how we might achieve a basic understanding of the meaning of a scene very quickly by analyzing the spatial-frequency components of the image. This analysis might tell us that we were looking at something that might be a highway, a building, or a farmyard. At this point, the local attention-dependent processes described earlier might kick in and fill in this generic description with the identities and relative locations of a few objects. Now we would have a scene description along the lines of "a farmyard with *this* chicken in *this* pose near *this* cow and *this* tractor." This combination of global and local information might create a representation rich enough to specify a particular scene and compact enough to be quickly stored in memory for later recognition.

What Do We Actually See?

We can now return to the change blindness phenomenon discussed earlier. In the 1990s, Dan Simons and Dan Levin (1997) did a weird experiment on the streets of Ithaca, New York. One experimenter asked an unsuspecting passerby for directions. While the passerby was giving those directions, a couple of other people carried a door down the street and between the passerby and the experimenter. While the door was moving by, the experimenter ducked down, sneaked away, and was replaced by a second experimenter. Then the door was gone down the street, and the critical question was whether the passerby would return to giving instructions. In many cases, he or she did just that, as if the change in experimenter were unnoticed. How could that be? Perhaps this change was undetected because it

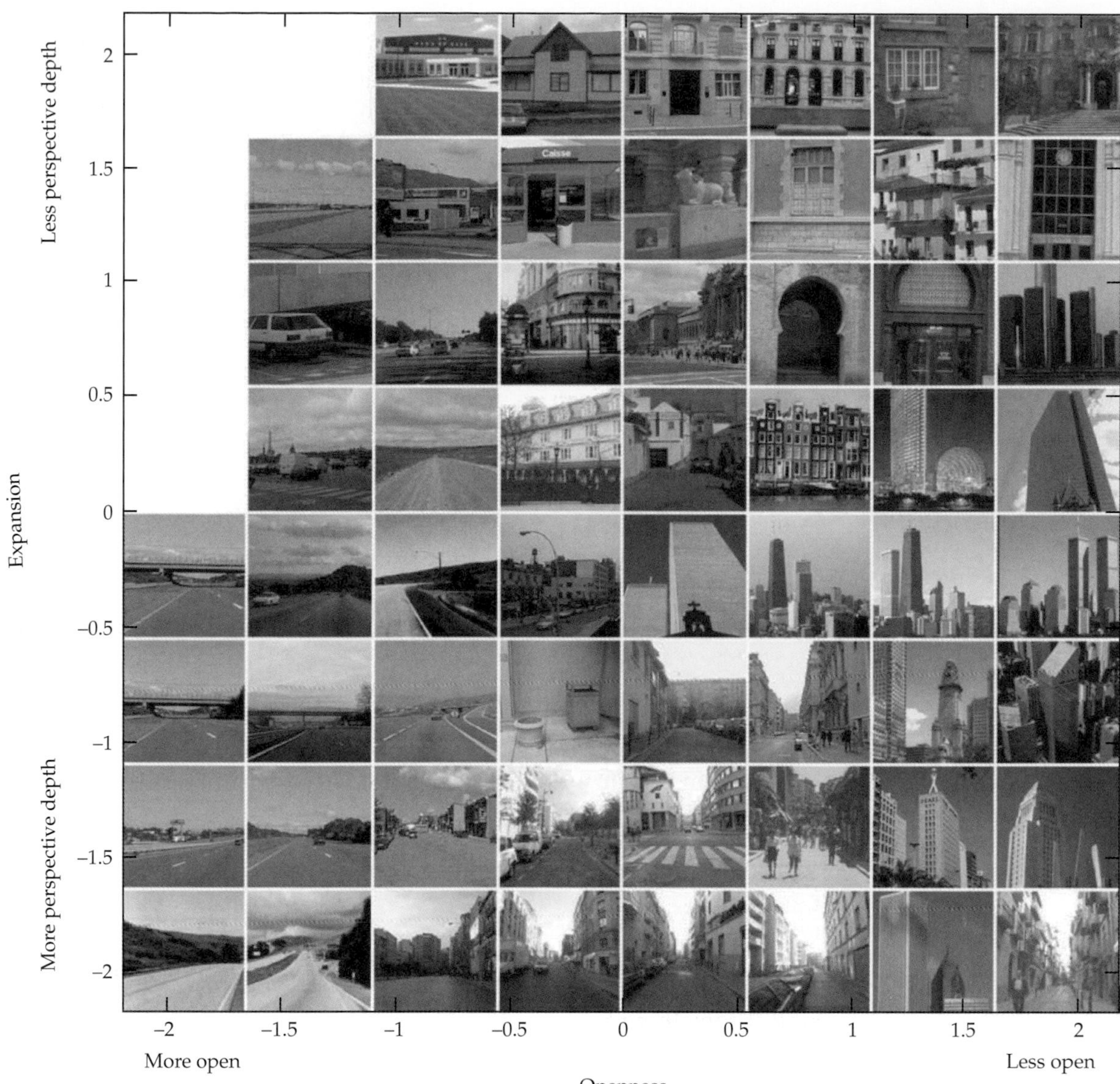

FIGURE 8.31 Spatial layout from global information. In this collection of urban scenes, the x-axis represents openness (from panoramic scenes to vertically structured scenes) and the y-axis represents expansion (capturing a sense of depth from perspective). (Courtesy of Aude Oliva.)

didn't change the "gist" of the scene. The observer might think, "I'm giving instructions to a guy. Now there is this weird door. Now I'm giving instructions to a guy again," and simply never register that the *guy* changed. See **Web Activity 8.5: Change Blindness** for another example.

In yet another experiment, which you can experience for yourself in **Web Activity 8.6: The Attentional Bottleneck**, participants observed a collection of red and green spots. While they watched, one of the spots suddenly got brighter, and on half the trials the enlarged spot also changed color. The change in brightness invariably attracted attention to the altered spot. All the observers had to do was determine if the spot had changed color. They performed horribly; they managed to get only 52% correct in a task where they could get 50% correct just by guessing. It seemed that unless the observers happened to be attending to the critical spot *before* the change occurred, they had no idea whether the color had changed (Wolfe, Reinecke, and Brawn, 2006).

How can we understand these inabilities to see (or, at least, to report on) what is going on right in front of our eyes? One possibility is that we really "see" only one thing at a time: the current object of attention. This appears to be the logical implication of the experiment with red and green dots. Perhaps attention constitutes a bottleneck between the visual world and our conscious perception of this world. If a stimulus doesn't make it through this bottleneck, we are effectively blind to it.

The problem with this view is that we *think* we see so much more. As we look around the world, we experience a full-color, in-focus, three-dimensional scene filled with clearly identifiable objects. We know, from the research described in earlier chapters, that this experience must be a construction of the mind, not an exact copy of the stimulus. We know from Chapter 2 that the world is decently focused only at the fovea and that high-resolution processing occurs only in the central 1 degree or so of the visual field. We know from Chapter 7 that the scene before us is smeared across the retina three to five times each second as we move our eyes. We know from Chapter 6 that we are actually getting two slightly different copies of the scene from our two retinas, and that both copies are really two-dimensional.

Over and over in this book, we say that a particular aspect of perception is an inference, a guess about the world. Our conscious experience of the world is the mother of all inferences or, more accurately, the sum of all those more intelligent guesses that we have made about color, shape, size, distance, and virtually every other aspect of our perception.

This realization is hard for us to accept because perception doesn't *feel* like an inference about what is. It feels like it must be showing us what is really out there. It feels like Truth. Phenomena like change blindness are important because they show us the gap between perception and reality. These experiments show us that we don't see what *is* there. Rather, we see what *was* there when we last paid attention, and even then we may not remember it perfectly (e.g., Irwin, Zacks, and Brown, 1990). See **Web Essay 8.1: Boundary Extension** for evidence that what we remember about a scene after the fact also does not correspond exactly to what we saw.

Outside the lab, the bottleneck between the world and our perception is not usually much of a problem, because the world is a pretty stable and predictable place—at least on a moment-to-moment basis. If you put your coffee mug down on the desk and turn your attention to the computer screen, the mug will be there when you choose to attend to it again. Only in the lab does the coffee mug vanish during an eye movement. This means that the physical world can serve as an external memory that backs up the perceptual world we create in our minds (O'Regan, 1992).

When the world does change, it usually changes in very predictable ways. If we have just driven past Second and Third avenues, we probably don't need to look at the next street sign to know that it says "Fourth." At a rate of about 20 objects per second, we can monitor the relevant items in this relatively stable world and be reasonably sure that we are up-to-date. And if something surprising does occur (a tiger leaps into the middle of Fourth Avenue, for example), the event will probably be marked by a visual transient that grabs our attention so that we can update our internal representation pretty quickly and maintain our grasp on reality (Yantis, 1993). (See **Web Essay 8.2: Attentional Capture**.)

Summary

1. Attention is a vital aspect of perception because we cannot process all of the input from our senses. The term *attention* refers to a large set of selective mechanisms that enable us to focus on some stimuli at the expense of others. Though this chapter talked almost exclusively about visual attention, attentional mechanisms exist in all sensory domains.
2. In vision, it is possible to direct attention to one location or one object. If something happens at an attended location, we will be faster to respond to it. It can be useful to refer to the "spotlight" of attention, though deployments of attention differ in important ways from movements of a spotlight.
3. In visual search tasks, observers typically look for a target item among a number of distractor items. If the target is defined by a salient basic feature, such as its color or orientation, search is very efficient and the number of distractors has little influence on the reaction time (the time required to find the target). If no basic feature information can guide the deployment of attention, then search is inefficient, as if each item needed to be examined one after the other. Search can be of intermediate efficiency if some feature information is available (e.g., if we're looking for a red car, we don't need to examine the blue objects in the parking lot).
4. Attention varies over time as well as space. In the attentional-blink paradigm, observers search for two items in a rapid stream of stimuli that appear at fixation. Attention to the first target makes it hard to find the second if the second appears within 200 to 500 ms of the first. When two identical items appear in the stream of stimuli, a different phenomenon, repetition blindness, makes it hard to detect the second instance.
5. The effects of attention manifest themselves in several different ways in the brain. In some cases, attention is marked by a general increase in neural activity. In other cases, attention to a particular attribute tunes cells more sharply for that attribute. And in still other cases, attention to a stimulus or location causes receptive fields to shrink so as to exclude unattended stimuli.
6. Damage to the parietal lobe of the brain produces deficits in visual attention. Damage to the right parietal lobe can lead to neglect, a disorder in which it is hard to direct attention into the contralesional (in this case, the left) visual field. Neglect patients may ignore half of an object or of their own body. Balint syndrome is the result of bilateral damage to the parietal lobe. Patients with this disorder may show simultagnosia, an inability to see more than one object at a time.
7. Picture memory experiments show that people can remember thousands of images after only a second or two of exposure to each. In contrast, change blindness experiments show that people can miss large changes in scenes if those changes do not markedly alter the meaning of the scene.
8. Perception of scenes may be the result of a combination of local attention to objects and a global ability to glean some information about, for example, the layout of a scene. We may see a sort of theory made up of the products of these two processes. Most of the time this fairly sketchy theory is adequate because we can rapidly check the world to determine if the chair, the book, and the desk are still there.

Refer to the
Sensation and Perception
website
(www.sinauer.com/wolfe2e)
for activities, essays, study questions, and other study aids.

CHAPTER 9

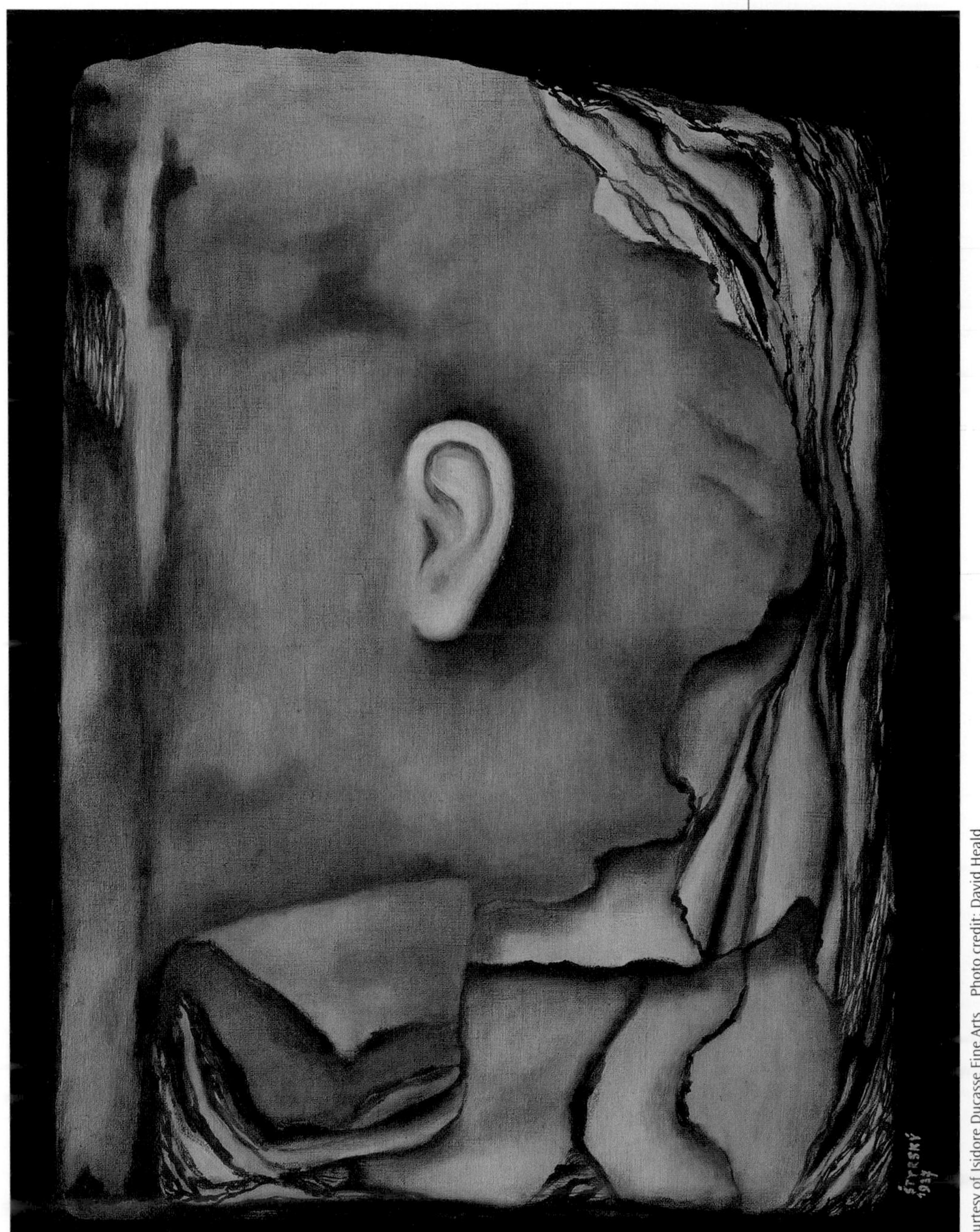

Courtesy of Isidore Ducasse Fine Arts Photo credit: David Heald

Jindřich Štyrský, *Gift (Dar)*, 1937

Hearing: Physiology and Psychoacoustics

It is often said that humans are visual animals. We are reminded of the importance of vision in our lives whenever we close our eyes or awaken in the night, because so much of what we sense and know about our environment is suddenly gone. In contrast, most people never get such reminders of the importance of hearing. Our ears are always open, and we can hear perfectly well in the dark. When we enter a theater just before the movie starts, we don't need to wait half an hour to be able to hear the soft strains of the opening theme. We can hear things when our nose is not pointed at the source of the sound, and we can even hear around obstacles and corners. For better or worse, we can often hear through walls that light cannot penetrate. For all these reasons, it is easy to take hearing for granted.

Try to imagine a world, though, where nothing makes a sound. You cannot hear a train coming, and the blast of its air horn simply escapes into the night. At a concert, musicians move deftly as the audience stands or jumps or claps, but the enthusiasm of both performers and spectators is only a curiosity. A person cries out, and you don't help because you cannot hear the cry. You cannot talk on the phone. Deafness deprives you of the most fundamental of human abilities: communication through speech. Without hearing, the world seems a more dangerous place in which you are relatively isolated by day and nearly totally isolated by night. At night your sense of vision, which may compensate for hearing loss when it's light out, is compromised by the fact that it's dark.

The Function of Hearing

For the next three chapters, you will be hearing all about hearing. In this chapter we cover the basics: the nature of sound, the anatomy and physiology of the auditory system, and how we perceive the two fundamental sound qualities—loudness and pitch. We conclude this chapter by looking at some of the ways in which hearing can be impaired and what we can do to ameliorate these impairments. In Chapter 10 we will move on to discuss some of the ways we use acoustic information to learn about our environment. Then, in Chapter 11, we will cover the higher-level auditory functions that come into play when we're listening to speech and music.

Many fundamental principles apply to vision, hearing, and all the other senses. However, each sense developed at different periods in our evolutionary history and in response to different environmental challenges. So, although you should find that much of what you have learned thus far will prove helpful for understanding hearing, you should also come to appreciate that biology has provided some very different (and very clever) solutions to the idiosyncratic problems involved in sensing and interpreting sound.

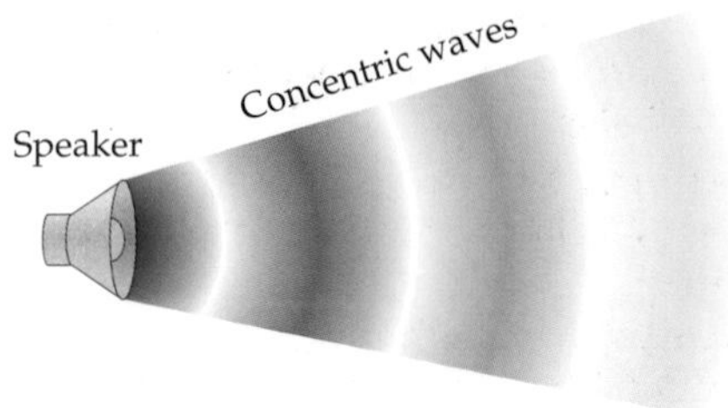

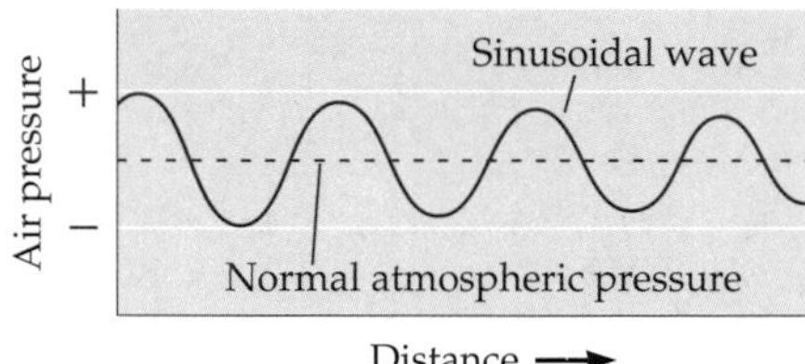

FIGURE 9.1 The pattern of pressure fluctuations of a sound stays the same as the sound wave moves away from the source, but the amount of pressure change decreases with increasing distance.

What Is Sound?

Sounds are created when objects vibrate. The vibrations of an object (the sound source) cause molecules in the object's surrounding medium (for humans, usually the Earth's atmosphere) to vibrate as well, and this vibration in turn causes pressure changes in the medium (**Figure 9.1**). These pressure changes are best described as waves, and they are similar to the waves on a pond that are caused when we drop a rock into the water. The water molecules displaced by the rock do not themselves travel very far, but the *pattern* of displacement will move outward from the source until something (the shore, a boat, a swimming duck, or anything else) gets in the way. Although the patterns of pond and sound waves do not change as they spread out, the initial amount of pressure change is dispersed over a larger and larger area as the wave moves away, so the wave becomes less prominent as it gets farther from its source.

Sound waves travel at a particular speed depending on the medium, moving faster through denser substances. For example, the speed of sound through air is about 340 meters per second, depending on the humidity level (sounds travel a bit faster on muggy days), but the speed of sound through water is about 1500 meters per second. Light waves move through air almost a million times faster than sound waves, accounting for the lag between seeing lightning and hearing thunder.

In the 1950s, there was a great race to fly an airplane faster than the speed of sound (over 760 miles per hour), and more recently a jet car exceeded the speed of sound on land. When an object such as a jet plane travels faster than the speed of sound, the plane catches up to and passes the fronts of the sound waves it is creating. As a result, the sound waves combine into a shock wave, or a huge pressure fluctuation. When this shock wave reaches the ground and we hear it, it is called a "sonic boom."

amplitude The magnitude of displacement (increase or decrease) of a sound pressure wave or of a head movement (e.g., angular velocity, linear acceleration, tilt).

intensity The amount of sound energy falling on a unit area (such as a square centimeter).

Basic Qualities of Sound Waves: Frequency and Amplitude

As we've seen, the sound waves that we hear are simply fluctuations in air pressure across time. The magnitude of the pressure change in a sound wave—the difference between the highest pressure area and the lowest pressure area—is called the **amplitude** or **intensity** of a wave (**Figure 9.2**). Pressure fluctuations can be very close together, or they can be spread apart over longer periods. For light waves, we usually describe the pattern of fluctua-

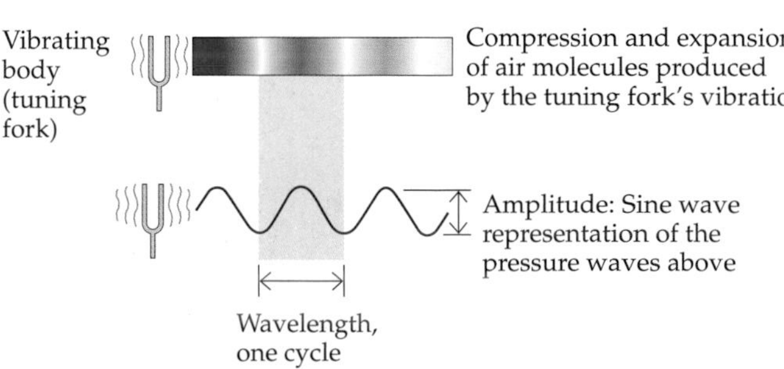

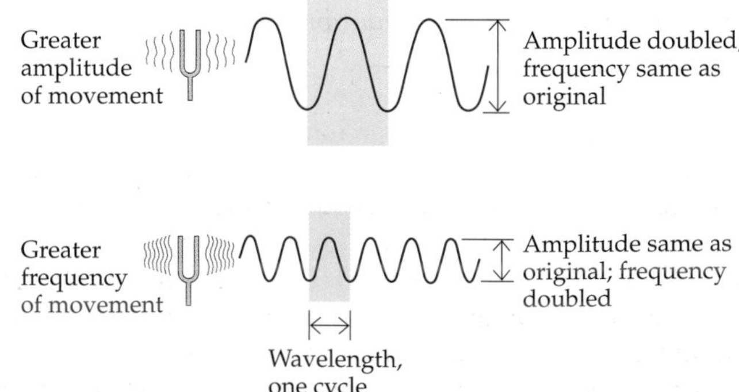

FIGURE 9.2 Sound waves are described by the frequency and amplitude of pressure fluctuations. Here, changes in frequency and amplitude are shown for sine waves, the simplest kind of sound wave.

tions by measuring the distance between peaks in the waves—the wavelength. Although sound waves also have wavelengths, we more typically describe their patterns by noting how quickly the pressure fluctuates; this rate of fluctuation is known as the **frequency** of the wave (see Figure 9.2). To see an example of frequency, dangle a thread in front of a stereo. As the speaker creates fluctuations in air pressure, the thread will wave back and forth. The speed of this waving is the thread's frequency. Sound wave frequencies are measured in **hertz (Hz)**, where 1 Hz equals one cycle per second. For example, the pressure in a 500-Hz wave goes from its highest point down to its lowest point and back up to its highest point 500 times every second.

Just as the amplitude and wavelength of light waves correspond to perceptual qualities in vision (brightness and color, respectively), the amplitude and frequency of sound waves are highly correlated with auditory characteristics. Amplitude is associated with the perceptual quality of **loudness**: the more intense a sound wave is, the louder it will sound. Frequency is associated with **pitch**: low-frequency sounds correspond to low pitches (e.g., low notes played by a tuba) and high-frequency sounds corresponding to high pitches (e.g., the high notes from a piccolo). We will have much more to say about the relationships between amplitude and loudness and between frequency and pitch later in this chapter.

frequency For sound, the number of times per second that a pattern of pressure change repeats.

hertz (Hz) A unit of measure for frequency. One hertz equals one cycle per second.

loudness The psychological aspect of sound related to perceived intensity or magnitude.

pitch The psychological aspect of sound related mainly to the fundamental frequency.

decibel (dB) A unit of measure for the physical intensity of sound. Decibels define the difference between two sounds as the ratio between two sound pressures. Each 10:1 sound pressure ratio equals 20 dB, and a 100:1 ratio equals 40 dB.

As Chapter 1 described, visible light makes up only a small portion of the much broader range of electromagnetic energy. Similarly, human hearing uses a limited range of the frequencies present in environmental sounds. If you are relatively young and you have been careful about your exposure to loud sounds, you may be able to detect sounds that vary from about 20 to 20,000 Hz (**Figure 9.3**). Some animals hear sounds that have lower and higher frequencies than those heard by humans. Elephants hear vibrations at very low frequencies that help them detect the presence of large animals, such as other elephants. Dogs can be called with whistles that emit sounds at frequencies too high for humans to hear, and the sonar systems used by some bats utilize sound frequencies above 60,000 Hz.

Humans hear across a very wide range of sound intensities: the ratio between the faintest sound humans can detect and the loudest sounds that do not cause serious damage to ears is more than one to a million. To describe differences in amplitude across such a broad range, sound levels are measured on a logarithmic scale using units called **decibels (dB)**. Decibels define the difference between two sounds in terms of the ratio between sound pressures. Each 10:1 sound pressure ratio is equal to 20 decibels (dB), so a 100:1 ratio is equal to 40 decibels. The equation for defining decibels is

$$\text{dB} = 20 \log(p/p_0)$$

The variable p corresponds to the pressure (intensity) of the sound being described. The constant term p_0 is a reference pressure and is typically defined in auditory research contexts to be 0.0002 dyne/cm^2, and levels are defined as dB SPL (sound pressure level). This level (0.0002 dyne/cm^2) is close to the minimum pressure that can be detected at frequencies for which hearing is most sensitive, and decibel values greater than zero describe the ratio between a sound being measured and 0.0002 dyne/cm^2.

Using a reference value such as p_0 is common to many measuring systems. For example, 0°C is defined as the tem-

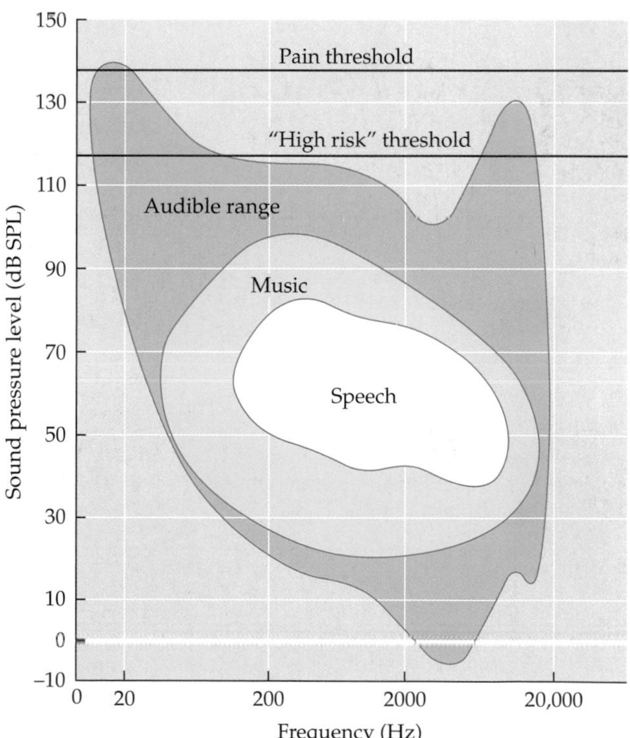

FIGURE 9.3 Humans can hear frequencies that range from about 20 to 20,000 Hz across a very wide range of intensities.

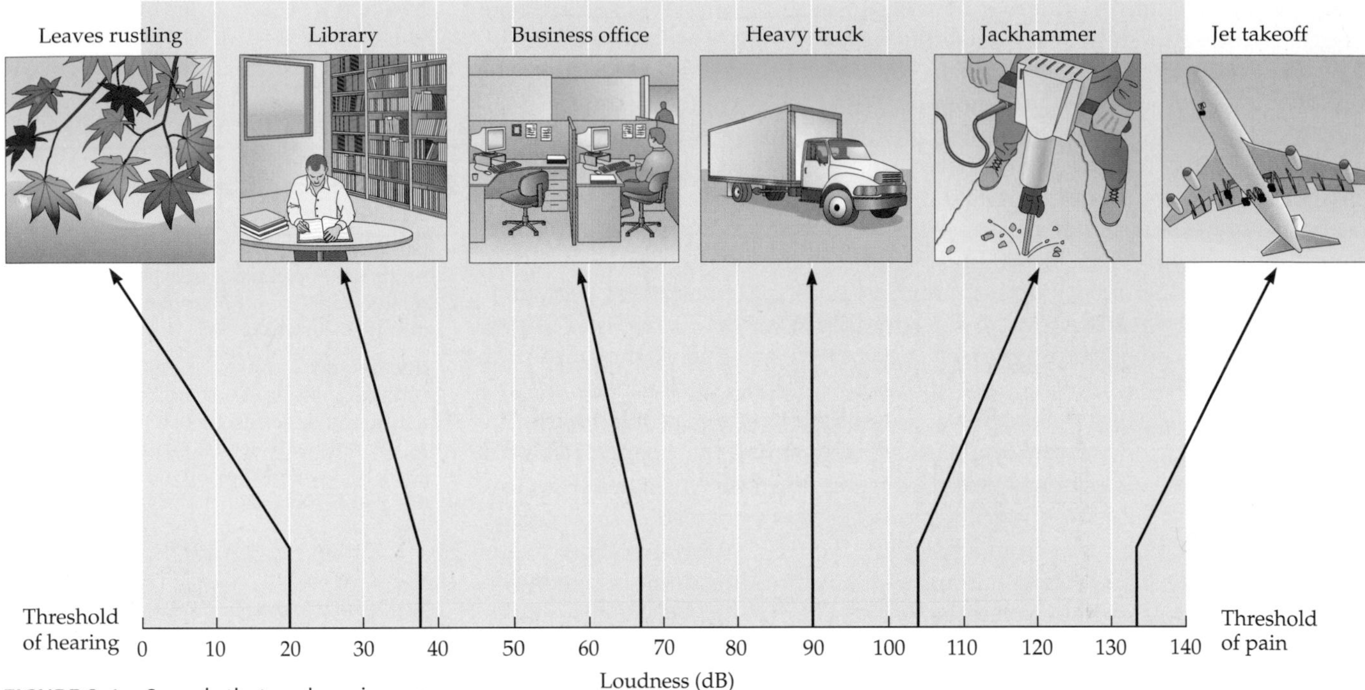

FIGURE 9.4 Sounds that we hear in our daily environments vary greatly in intensity.

perature at which water freezes, and 100°C is the temperature at which water boils. If the pressure of the sound that you're measuring (p) is equal to 0.0002 dyne/cm^2, then dB = 20 log(1). Because the log of 1 is zero, a sound pressure that low would be equal to 0 dB SPL. Sounds with amplitudes even smaller than p_0 have negative decibel levels, just as substances colder than the freezing point of water have negative centigrade temperatures.

An important thing to remember about logarithmic scales such as decibels is that relatively small decibel changes can correspond to large physical changes. For example, an increase of 6 dB corresponds to a doubling of the amount of pressure. **Figure 9.4** shows the decibel levels of some common sound sources.

Sine Waves, Complex Tones, and Fourier Analysis

sine wave (or pure tone) The waveform for which variation as a function of time is a sine function.

period The time (or space) required for one cycle of a repeating waveform.

phase The relative position of two or more sine waves. For sounds, the phase is the relative position in time.

One of the simplest kinds of sounds is a **sine wave**, or **pure tone**. (See Web Activity 9.1: What We Hear.) The air pressure in a sine wave changes continuously (sinusoidally) at the same frequency (**Figure 9.5**). The time taken for one complete cycle of a sine wave is the **period** of the sine wave, and there are 360 degrees of **phase** across one period. Thus, the undulation of the sine wave over time is described in degrees in the same way that rotations around a circle would be described.

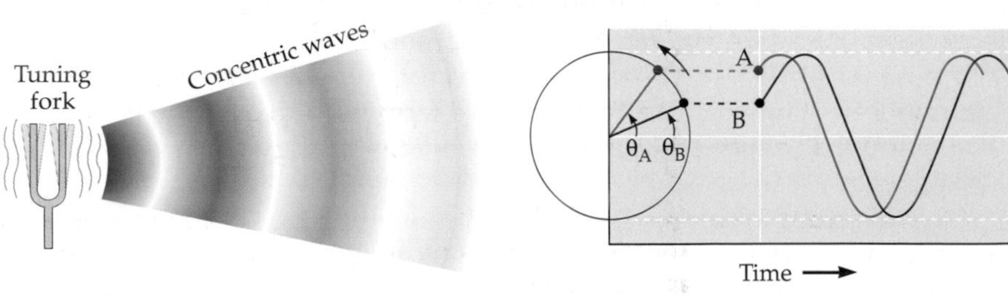

FIGURE 9.5 A sine wave is a circular motion extended over time. The two sine waves here have the same frequency but different phases. At any point in time, A is at one phase angle in the cycle, θ_A, and B is at another phase angle, θ_B.

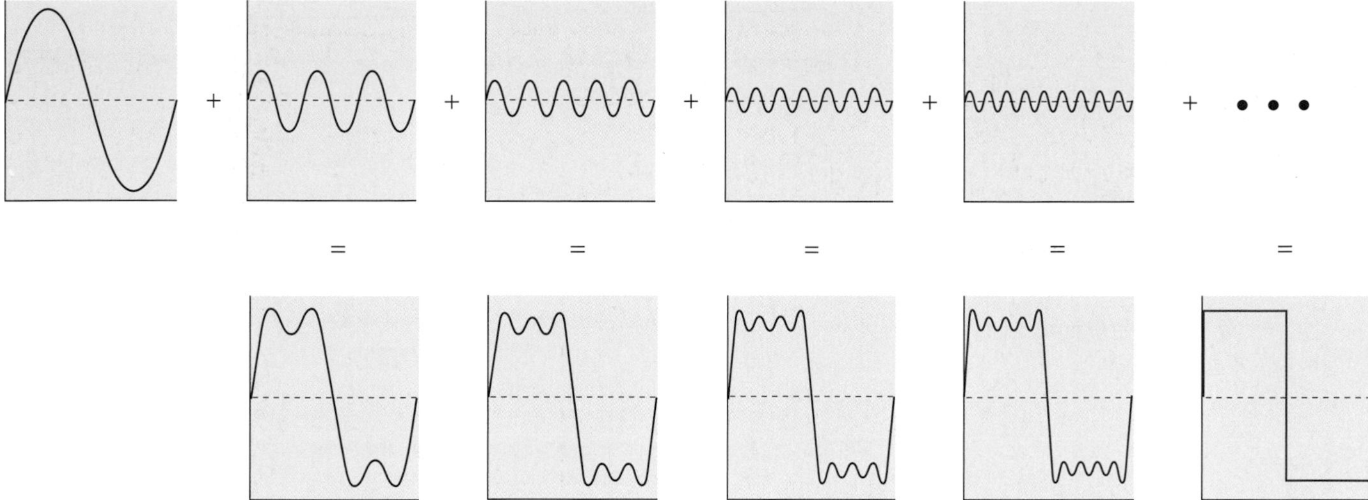

FIGURE 9.6 Every complex sound wave can be analyzed as a combination of sine waves, each with its own frequency, amplitude, and phase. Here, multiple sine waves are added together to form more complex waveforms. When infinitely more sine waves with even higher frequencies are added, a square wave (bottom right) can be constructed.

Sine waves are not common, everyday sounds, because few vibrations in the world are so pure. If you have taken a hearing test or used tuning forks, you may have heard sine waves. Flutes can produce musical notes that are close to pure tones, but other musical instruments, human voices, birds, cars, and almost all other sound sources in the world produce **complex tones**.

If pure tones are so uncommon, you may wonder why we're bothering to discuss them. It turns out that all sounds, no matter how complex, can be described as a combination of sine waves (**Figure 9.6**). Even the cacophony of a room full of people talking or the swelling sound of a full orchestra can be broken down into combinations of sine waves at many different frequencies with different amplitudes and phases. The individual sine wave components of a complex sound can be described by a process called **Fourier analysis**. We can summarize the results of a Fourier analysis with a graph, called a **spectrum**, that shows the intensity of each sine wave frequency found in the complex tone (**Figure 9.7**). (See Web Activity 9.2: Fourier Analysis.)

Sounds with **harmonic spectra**, illustrated in Figure 9.8, are typically caused by a simple vibrating source, such as the string of a guitar or the reed of a saxophone. Each frequency component in such a sound is called a "harmonic." The first harmonic, called the **fundamental frequency**, is the lowest-frequency component of the sound. All the other harmonics have frequencies that are integer multiples of the fundamental.

The shape of the Fourier spectrum is one of the most important qualities that distinguish different sounds. The properties of sound sources determine the spectral shapes of sounds; thus these shapes can help us identify sound sources. For example, **Figure 9.8** illustrates spectra from three musical instruments. Each instrument is producing a tone with the same fundamental frequency (262 Hz, which corresponds to the note C_4, or middle C) and the same harmonics (524 Hz, 786 Hz, 1048 Hz, and so on). However, the shapes of the spectra (the pattern of amplitudes for each harmonic) vary. **Timbre** (pronounced "tamber," like "amber") is a term used to describe the quality of a sound that depends, in part, on the relative energy levels of harmonic components.

We will return to harmonics, timbre, and other aspects of complex sounds in Chapter 10. For this chapter, we will stick mainly to the story of how the auditory system perceives simple sounds such as sine wave tones.

complex tone A sound wave consisting of more than one sinusoidal component of different frequencies.

Fourier analysis A mathematical theorem by which any sound can be divided into a set of sine waves. Combining these sine waves will reproduce the original sound.

spectrum A representation of the relative energy (intensity) present at each frequency.

harmonic spectrum The spectrum of a complex sound in which energy is at integer multiples of the fundamental frequency.

fundamental frequency The lowest-frequency component of a complex periodic sound.

timbre The psychological sensation by which a listener can judge that two sounds with the same loudness and pitch are dissimilar. Timbre quality is conveyed by harmonics and other high frequencies.

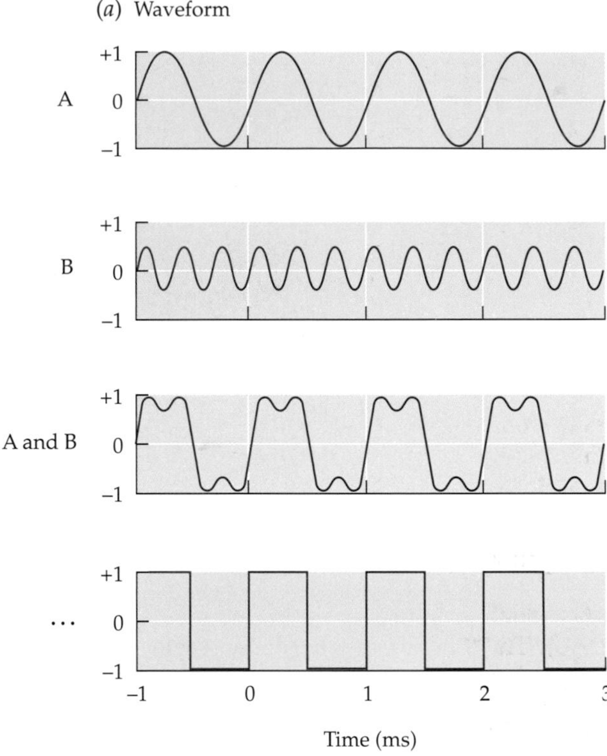

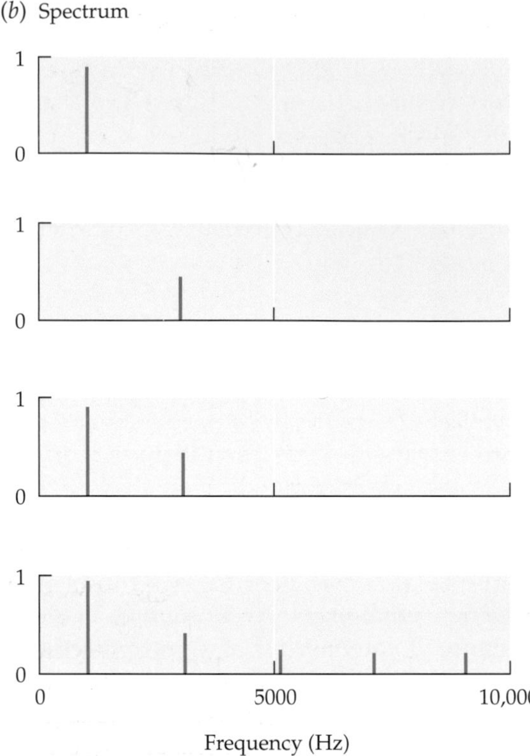

FIGURE 9.7 A spectrum displays the amplitude for each frequency present in a sound wave. Each signal is shown as a waveform (*a*) and as a spectrum (*b*).

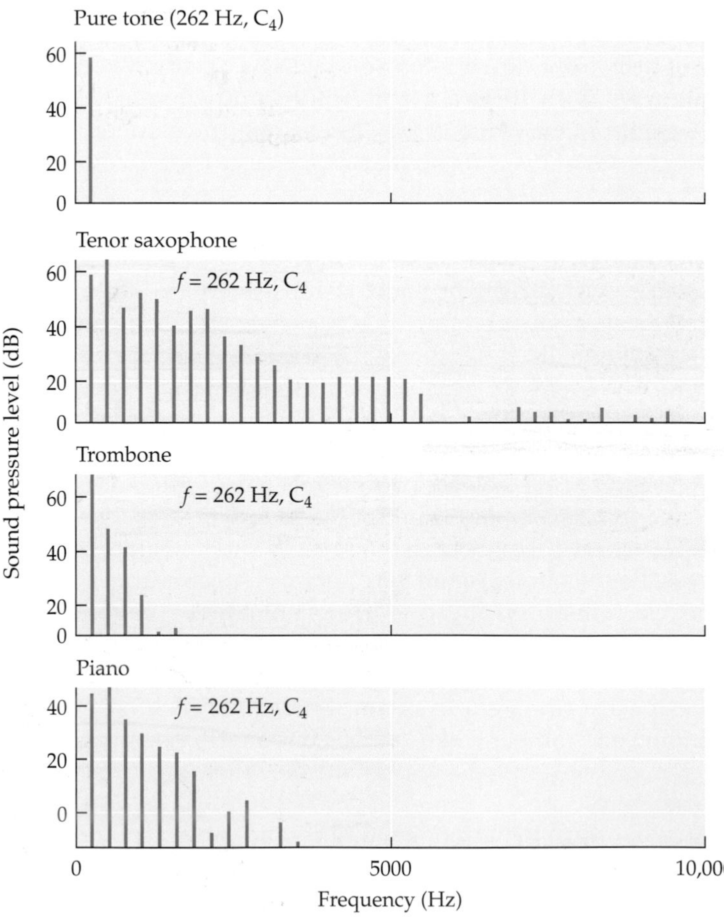

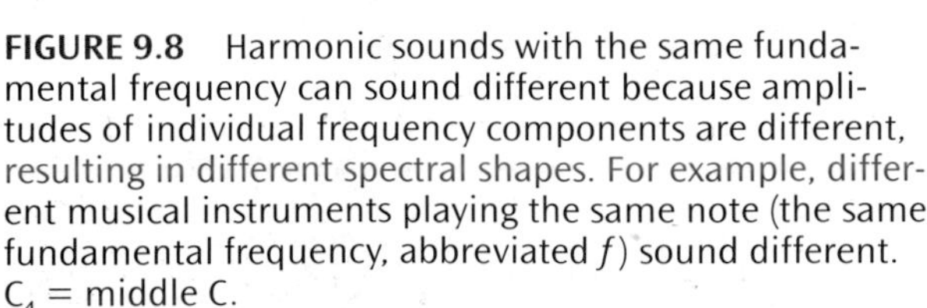

FIGURE 9.8 Harmonic sounds with the same fundamental frequency can sound different because amplitudes of individual frequency components are different, resulting in different spectral shapes. For example, different musical instruments playing the same note (the same fundamental frequency, abbreviated f) sound different. C_4 = middle C.

Basic Structure of the Mammalian Auditory System

Now that you know what sound is, we can examine how sounds are detected and recognized by the auditory system. The sense of hearing has evolved over millions of years to be able to do some pretty amazing things. We are about to describe quite a few anatomical structures that are essential for understanding how sequences of tiny air pressure changes are turned into meaningful sound perception. The discussion may occasionally be a bit confusing, but if you consult the figures and Web Activity 9.3: Structure of the Auditory System often, you will soon know the parts and how they fit together.

pinna The outer, funnel-like part of the ear.

ear canal The canal that conducts sound vibrations from the pinna to the tympanic membrane and prevents damage to the tympanic membrane.

tympanic membrane The eardrum; a thin sheet of skin at the end of the outer ear canal. The tympanic membrane vibrates in response to sound.

Outer Ear

Sounds are first collected from the environment by the **pinna** (plural *pinnae*), the curly structure on the side of the head that we typically call an ear. Only mammals have pinnae, which vary wildly in shape and size across species and vary somewhat less dramatically across individuals within species (**Figure 9.9**). As we will see in Chapter 10, the particular shapes of the pinnae play an important role in our ability to localize sound sources.

Sound waves are funneled by the pinna into and through the **ear canal**, which extends about 25 millimeters (mm) into the head (**Figure 9.10**). The length and shape of the ear canal enhance sound frequencies between about 2000 and 6000 Hz, but the main purpose of the canal is to insulate the structure at its end, the **tympanic membrane** (eardrum), from damage. The tympanic membrane is a thin sheet of skin that moves in and out in response to the pressure changes of sound waves.

It is a common myth that puncturing your eardrum will leave you deaf. In fact, in most cases a damaged tympanic membrane will heal itself, just as other parts of the skin do. However, it is possible to damage the tympanic membrane beyond repair, so it's a good idea to follow your mother's advice and refrain from sticking things in your ear.

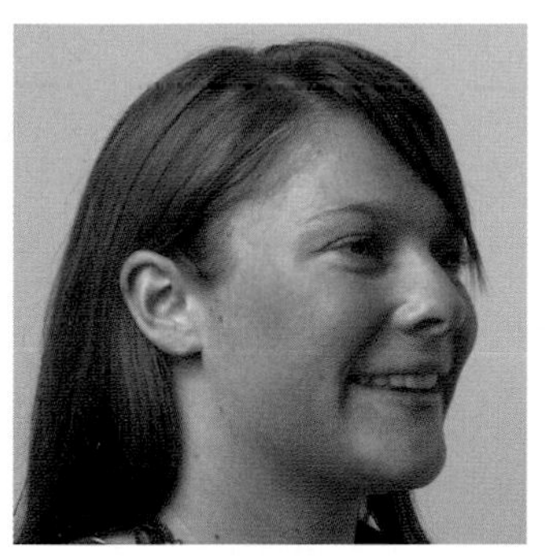
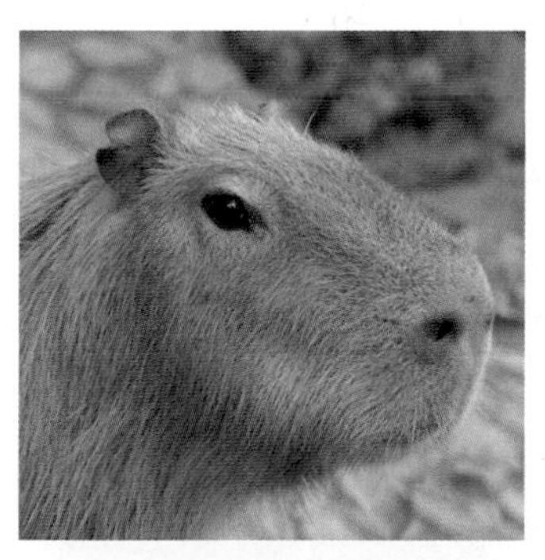
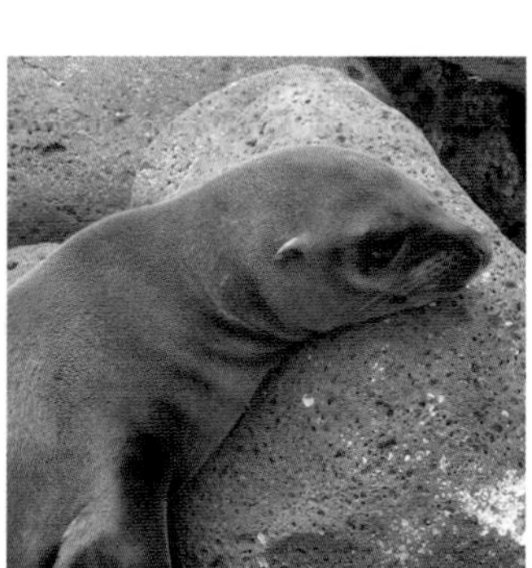
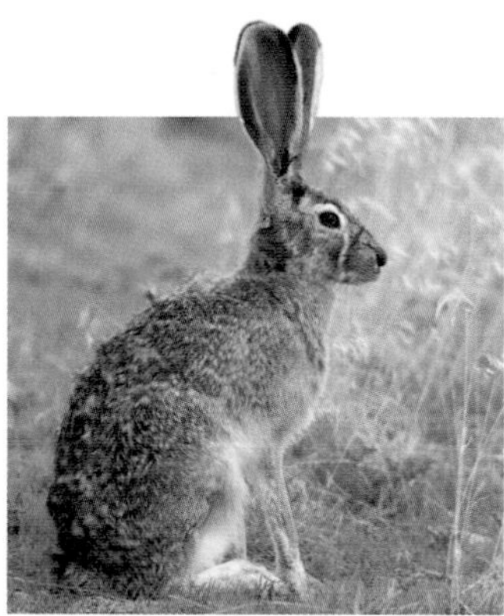
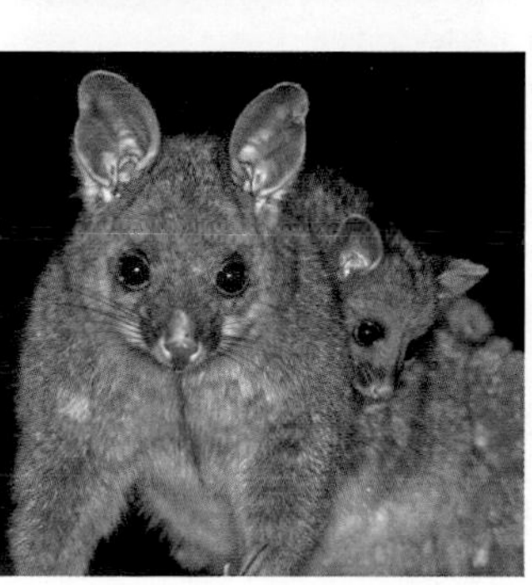
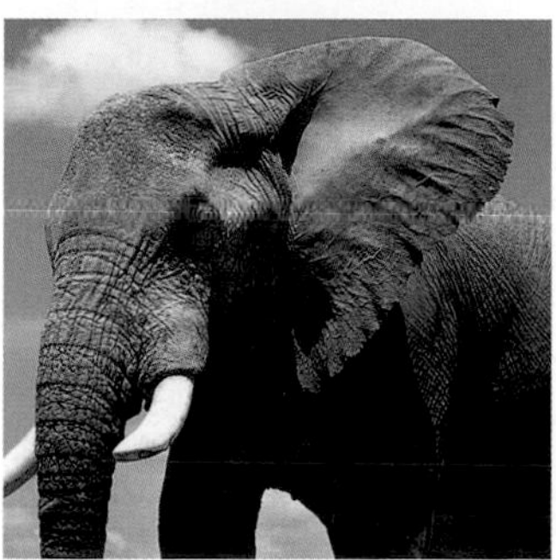
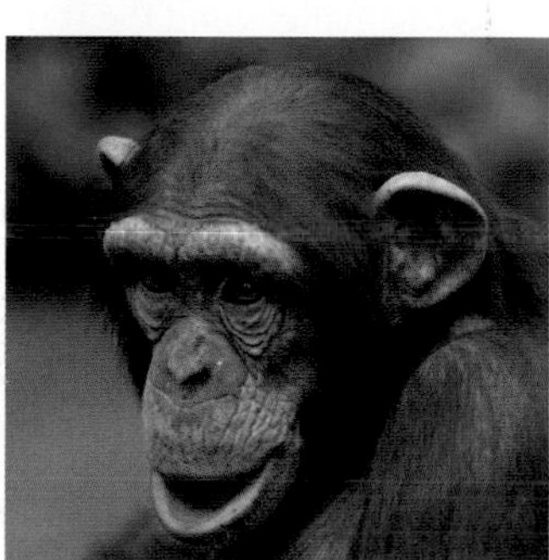

FIGURE 9.9 Pinna size and shape vary greatly among mammals.

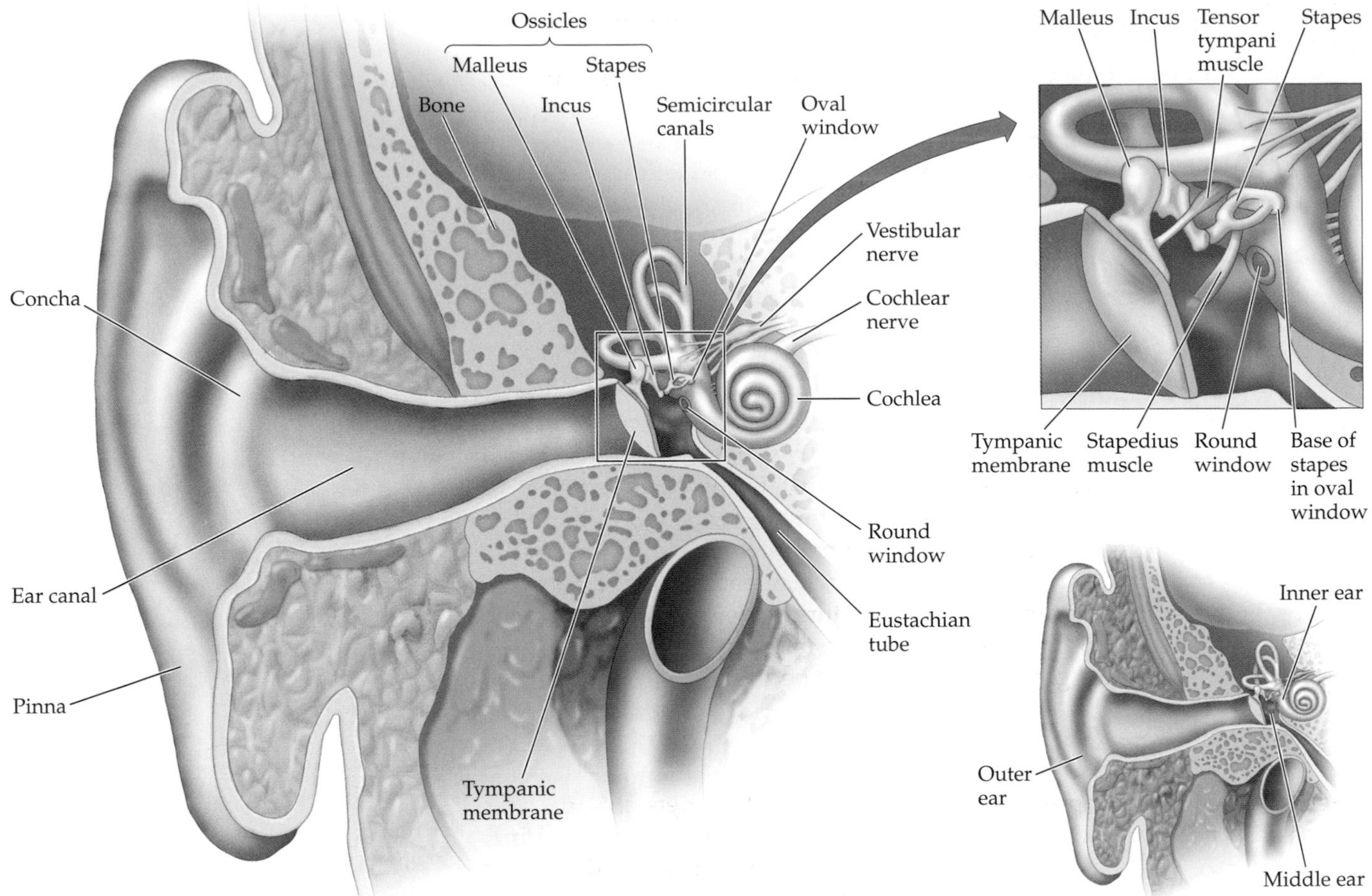

FIGURE 9.10 Structures of the human ear. Note that the tympanic membrane has about 18 times as much surface area as the oval window beneath the stapes.

outer ear The external sound-gathering portion of the ear, consisting of the pinna and the ear canal.

middle ear An air-filled chamber containing the middle bones, or ossicles. The middle ear conveys and amplifies vibration from the tympanic membrane to the oval window.

ossicles Three tiny bones of the middle ear: malleus, incus, and stapes.

malleus One of the ossicles. The malleus receives vibration from the tympanic membrane and is attached to the incus.

incus The middle ossicle. The incus connects the malleus and the stapes.

stapes One of the ossicles. Connected to the incus on one end, the stapes presses against the oval window of the cochlea on the other end.

oval window The flexible opening to the cochlea through which the stapes transmits vibration to the fluid inside.

inner ear A hollow cavity in the temporal bone of the skull, and the structures within this cavity: the cochlea and vestibular canals.

Middle Ear

Together, the pinna and ear canal make up a division of the auditory system called the **outer ear** (see Figure 9.10). The tympanic membrane is the border between the outer ear and the **middle ear**, which consists of three tiny bones, the **ossicles**, that amplify sound waves. The first ossicle, the **malleus**, is connected to the tympanic membrane on one side and to the second ossicle, the **incus**, on the other. The incus is connected in turn to the **stapes**, which transmits the vibrations of sound waves to the **oval window**, another membrane, which forms the border between the middle ear and the **inner ear**.

The ossicles, which are the smallest bones in the human body, amplify sound vibrations in two ways. First, the joints between the bones are hinged in a way that makes them work like levers: a modest amount of energy on one side of the fulcrum (joint) becomes larger on the other. This lever action increases the amount of pressure change by about a third.

The second way the ossicles increase the energy transmitted to the inner ear is by concentrating energy from a larger to a smaller surface area: The tympanic membrane, which moves the malleus, is about 18 times as large as the oval window, which is moved by the stapes (see Figure 9.10). Therefore, the pressure on the oval window is magnified 18 times relative to the pressure on the tympanic membrane. This is the same principle that makes snowshoes effective for keeping feet from sinking in the snow and makes stiletto heels a danger to wood floors (think of the tympanic membrane as the heel of the foot and the oval window as the tip of the stiletto).

Amplification provided by the ossicles is essential to our ability to hear faint sounds because the inner ear, as we will see in a moment, is made up of a collection of fluid-filled chambers. Because it takes more energy to move liquid than it does to move air, this fluid creates an impedance mismatch: if sound waves were transmitted to the oval window directly, many would simply bounce back without moving the oval window at all.

The ossicles play an important role for loud sounds too. The middle ear has two muscles: the **tensor tympani** (attached to the malleus) and the **stapedius** (attached to the stapes) (see Figure 9.10). As might be expected, given that the ossicles are the smallest bones in the body, the tensor tympani and the stapedius are the smallest muscles in the body. Their main purpose is to tense when sounds are very loud, restricting the movement of the ossicles and thus muffling pressure changes that might be large enough to damage the delicate structures in the inner ear. Unfortunately, this **acoustic reflex** follows the onset of loud sounds by about one-fifth of a second. So although it helps in environments that are loud for sustained periods, the acoustic reflex cannot protect against abrupt loud sounds, such as the firing of a gun. The muscles of the middle ear can also be tensed during swallowing, talking, and general body movement, helping to keep the auditory system from being overwhelmed by sounds generated by our own bodies.

Inner Ear

The inner ear is an impressive feat of evolution. It is here that the fine changes in sound pressure available in the environment are translated into neural signals that inform the listener about the world. The function of the inner ear with respect to sound waves in hearing is thus roughly analogous to that of the retina with respect to light waves in vision: it translates the information carried by the waves into neural signals.

COCHLEAR CANALS AND MEMBRANES The major structure of the inner ear is the **cochlea** (from the Greek *kochlos*, "snail"), a tiny coiled structure embedded in the temporal bone of the skull (see Figure 9.10). Rolled up, the cochlea is the size of a baby pea, about 4 mm in diameter in humans. Uncoiled, it would be a tube about 35 mm long. The cochlea is filled with watery fluids in three parallel canals (**Figure 9.11**): the **tympanic canal** (or *scala tympani*), the **vestibular canal** (or *scala vestibuli*), and the **middle canal** (or *scala media*). The tympanic and vestibular canals are connected by a small opening, the **helicotrema**, and these two canals are effectively wrapped around the middle canal. Think of the tympanic and vestibular canals as one long balloon (the kind clowns use to make hats and animals), blown up and folded back on itself. The middle canal is another long balloon that is squeezed, lengthwise, between the two halves of the first balloon.

The three canals of the cochlea are separated by two membranes (see Figure 9.11): **Reissner's membrane**, between the vestibular canal and the middle canal; and the **basilar membrane**, between the middle canal and the tympanic canal. Strictly speaking, the basilar membrane is not really a membrane, because it is not a thin pliable sheet like the tympanic membrane, the oval window, or Reissner's membrane. Rather, it is a plate made up of fibers that have some stiffness. The basilar membrane forms the base of the **cochlear partition**, a complex structure through which sound waves are transduced into neural signals.

Vibrations transmitted through the tympanic membrane and middle-ear bones cause the stapes to push and pull the flexible oval window in and out

tensor tympani The muscle attached to the malleus; tensing the tensor tympani decreases vibration.

stapedius The muscle attached to the stapes; tensing the stapedius decreases vibration.

acoustic reflex A reflex that protects the ear from intense sounds, via contraction of the stapedius and tensor tympani muscles.

cochlea A spiral structure of the inner ear containing the organ of Corti.

tympanic canal One of three fluid-filled passages in the cochlea. The tympanic canal extends from the round window at the base of the cochlea to the helicotrema at the apex. Also called *scala tympani*.

vestibular canal One of three fluid-filled passages in the cochlea. The vestibular canal extends from the oval window at the base of the cochlea to the helicotrema at the apex. Also called *scala vestibuli*.

middle canal One of three fluid-filled passages in the cochlea. The middle canal is sandwiched between the tympanic and vestibular canals and contains the cochlear partition. Also called *scala media*.

helicotrema The opening that connects the tympanic and vestibular canals at the apex of the cochlea.

Reissner's membrane A thin sheath of tissue separating the vestibular and middle canals in the cochlea.

basilar membrane A plate of fibers that forms the base of the cochlear partition and separates the middle and tympanic canals in the cochlea.

cochlear partition The combined basilar membrane, tectorial membrane, and organ of Corti, which are together responsible for the transduction of sound waves into neural signals.

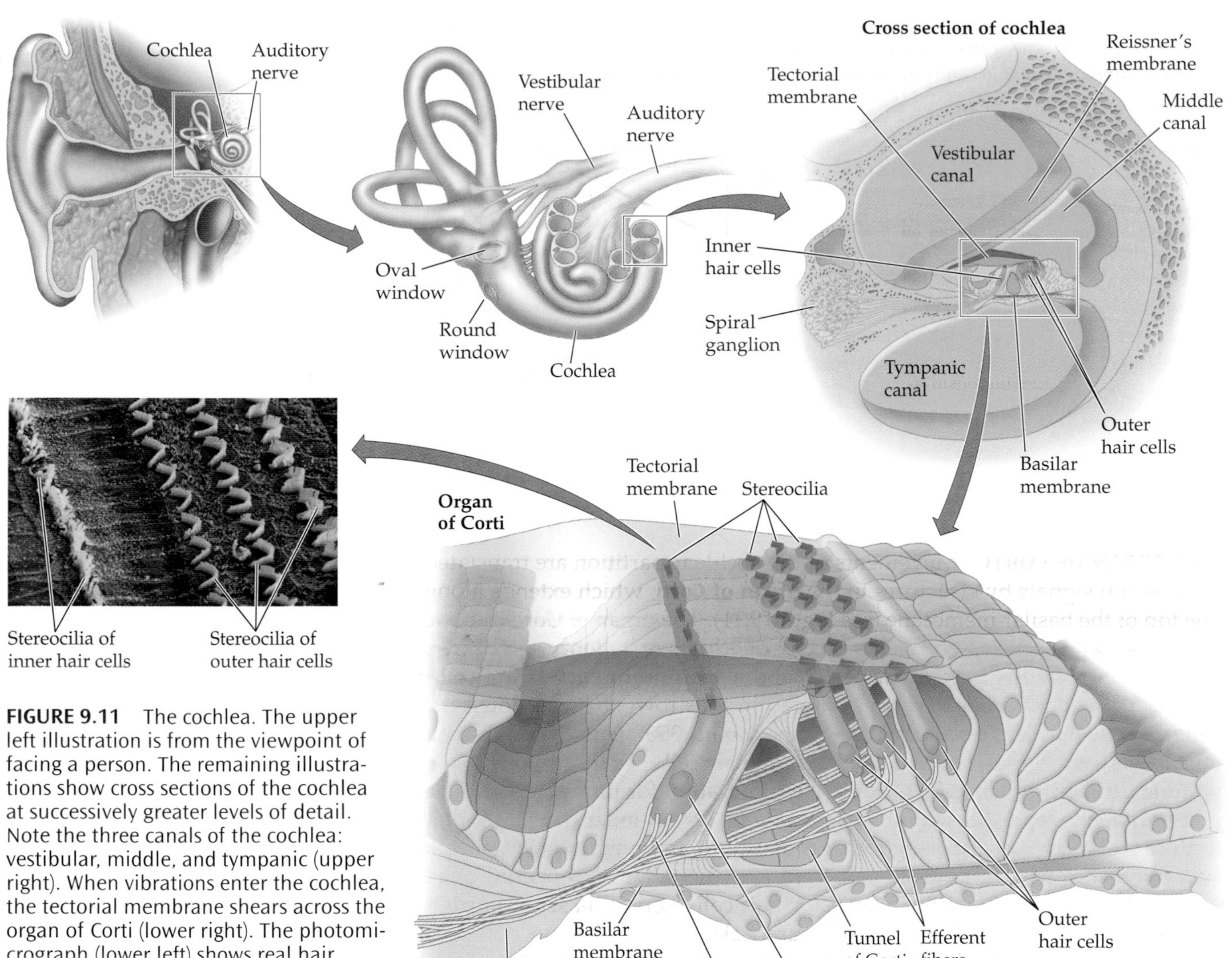

FIGURE 9.11 The cochlea. The upper left illustration is from the viewpoint of facing a person. The remaining illustrations show cross sections of the cochlea at successively greater levels of detail. Note the three canals of the cochlea: vestibular, middle, and tympanic (upper right). When vibrations enter the cochlea, the tectorial membrane shears across the organ of Corti (lower right). The photomicrograph (lower left) shows real hair cells: the single row of inner hair cells (left) and three rows of outer hair cells (right). (Micrograph from Kessel and Kardon, 1979.)

of the vestibular canal at the base of the cochlea. This movement of the oval window causes waves of pressure changes, called "traveling waves," to flow through the fluid in the vestibular canal, in much the same way that the membrane of a loudspeaker initiates sound waves in the air. Because the cochlea is a closed system, however, the pressure changes cannot spread out in all directions, as they do in the atmosphere. Instead, a displacement, or "bulge," forms in the vestibular canal and travels from the base of the cochlea down to the apex. By the time the traveling wave reaches the apex, its displacement has mostly dissipated (see Figure 9.14). If sounds are extremely intense, any pressure that remains is transmitted through the helicotrema and back to the cochlear base through the tympanic canal, where it is absorbed by yet another membrane, called the **round window** (see Figure 9.11).

Because the vestibular and tympanic canals are wrapped tightly around the middle canal, when the vestibular canal bulges out it puts pressure on the middle canal. This pressure has the effect of displacing the cochlear partition (which, recall, lies at the bottom of the middle canal), moving the partition down as the vestibular canal bulge comes through, and back up as the bulge passes by.

round window A soft area of tissue at the base of the tympanic canal that releases excess pressure remaining from extremely intense sounds.

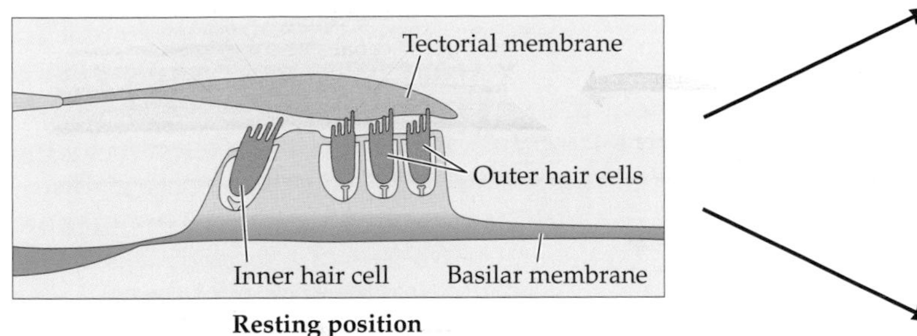

Sound-induced vibration

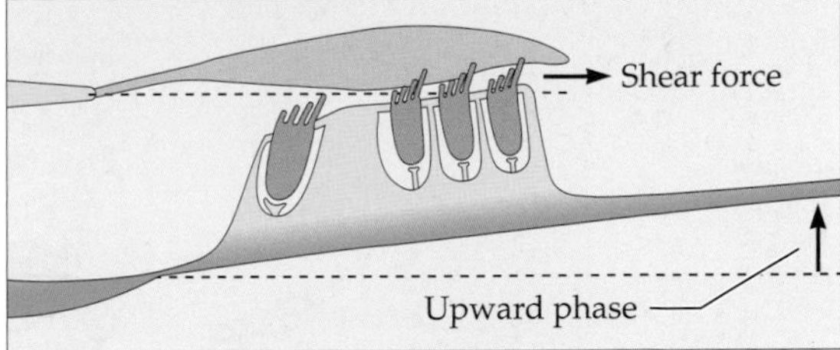

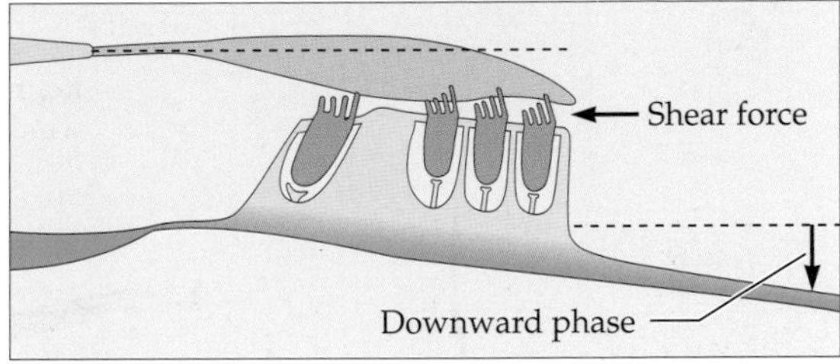

FIGURE 9.12 When vibration causes a displacement along the cochlear partition, the tectorial membrane and hair cells move in opposite directions (shear), and the deflection of stereocilia during this action results in the release of neurotransmitters.

THE ORGAN OF CORTI Movements of the cochlear partition are translated into neural signals by structures in the **organ of Corti**, which extends along the top of the basilar membrane (see Figure 9.11). The organ of Corti is made up of specialized neurons called **hair cells**, dendrites of **auditory nerve fibers** that terminate at the base of hair cells, and a scaffold of supporting cells. Hair cells in each human ear are arranged in four rows that run down the length of the basilar membrane: one row of about 3500 inner hair cells and three rows with a total of about 10,500 outer hair cells.

Inner and outer hair cells provide the foundation for minuscule hairlike bristles called **stereocilia** (singular *stereocilium*). On an inner hair cell, stereocilia are arranged as if posing for a group photo, in several nearly straight rows with the shorter stereocilia in front and the taller ones peering over their shoulders in the back. On an outer hair cell, stereocilia stand in rows that form the shape of a *V* or *W* (see Figure 9.11).

The **tectorial membrane** extends atop the organ of Corti. Like the basilar membrane, it isn't really a membrane. Rather, it is a gelatinous flap that is attached on one end and floats above the outer hair cells on the other end. Taller stereocilia of outer hair cells are embedded in the tectorial membrane, and the cilia of inner hair cells are nestled against it. Because the tectorial membrane is attached on only one end, it shears across the width of the cochlear partition whenever the partition moves up and down. This shearing motion in turn causes the stereocilia of both inner and outer hair cells to bend back and forth (**Figure 9.12**).

INNER AND OUTER HAIR CELLS Like photoreceptors in the retina, hair cells are specialized neurons that transduce one kind of energy (in this case, sound pressure) into another form of energy (neural firing). Deflection of a hair cell's stereocilia causes a change in voltage potential that initiates the release of neurotransmitters, which in turn encourages firing by auditory nerve fibers that have dendritic synapses on hair cells. However, it is the differences between photoreceptors and hair cells that are most interesting. While the retina has almost 100 million photoreceptors, the cochlea has only about 14,000 hair cells. And the stereocilia of hair cells blow away the competition when it comes to speed and sensitivity. As we'll see in Chapter 10, hair cells must be capable of responding so fast that we can detect time differences of as little as 10 millionths of a second (microseconds, μs) in order to

organ of Corti A structure on the basilar membrane of the cochlea that is composed of hair cells and dendrites of auditory nerve fibers.

hair cells Cells that support the stereocilia that transduce mechanical movement in the cochlea and vestibular labyrinth into neural activity sent to the brain stem; some hair cells also receive inputs from the brain.

auditory nerve fibers A collection of neurons that convey information from hair cells in the cochlea to (afferent) and from (efferent) the brain stem. This collection also includes neurons for the vestibular system.

stereocilia Hairlike extensions on the tips of hair cells in the cochlea that initiate the release of neurotransmitters when they are flexed.

tectorial membrane A gelatinous structure, attached on one end, that extends into the middle canal of the ear, floating above inner hair cells and touching outer hair cells.

tip link A tiny filament that stretches from the tip of a stereocilium to the side of its neighbor.

know the direction from which a sound arrives. In contrast, when we watch a movie, pictures shown at 24 frames per second appear continuous to the visual system. Hair cells are not only extremely fast, but also extremely sensitive. It may take 30 minutes for our eyes to fully adjust to a dark theater, but our ears are always ready for the slightest sound.

Recall that the shortest stereocilia are in front of slightly taller stereocilia that are in front of still-taller stereocilia (**Figure 9.13**). Each stereocilium is connected to its taller neighbor by a tiny filament called a **tip link**, so each set of stereocilia connected by tip links bends together when deflected by the shearing motion of the tectorial membrane. When a stereocilium deflects, the tip link pulls on the taller stereocilium in a way that opens an ion pore somewhat like opening a gate for just a tiny fraction of a second. This action permits potassium (K^+) ions to flow rapidly into the hair cell, causing rapid depolarization. In turn, depolarization leads to a rapid influx of calcium ions (Ca^{2+}) and initiation of the release of neurotransmitters from the base of the hair cell to stimulate dendrites of the auditory nerve (Fettiplace and Hackney, 2006; Hudspeth, 1997).

The opening of ion pores that results from the direct connection between stereocilia via tip links is the only known example of mechanoelectrical transduction (MET), which is responsible for both the extreme speed and the sensitivity of hair cells. Unlike the case in vision, depolarization in hearing does not await a cascade of biochemical processes such as those in photoactivation. MET is also extremely sensitive: ion pores open when deflection is

(a)

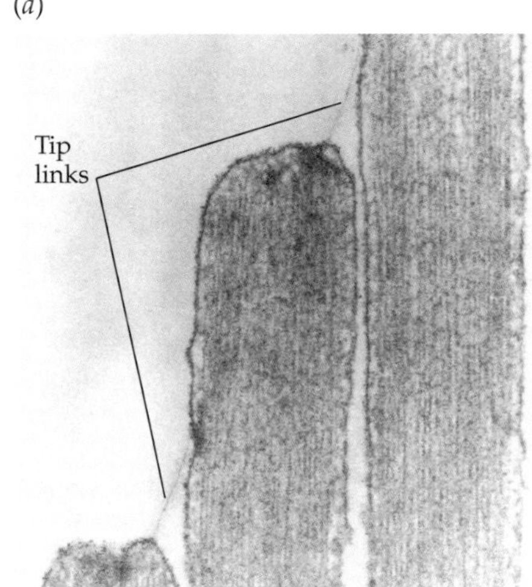

(b)

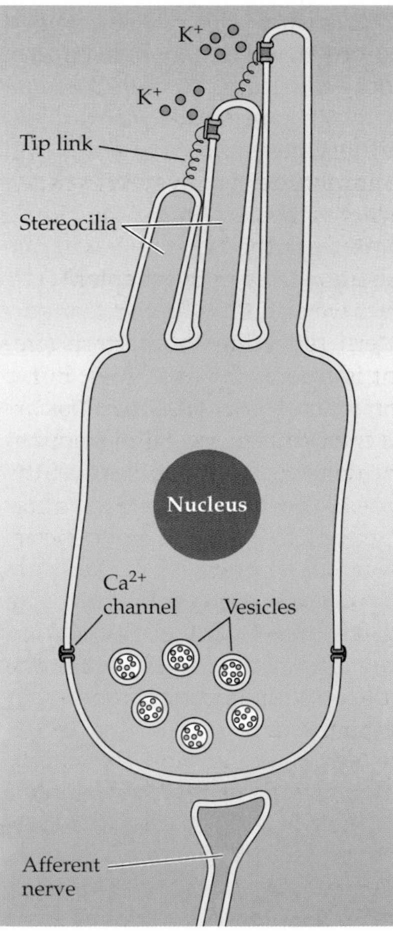

(c)

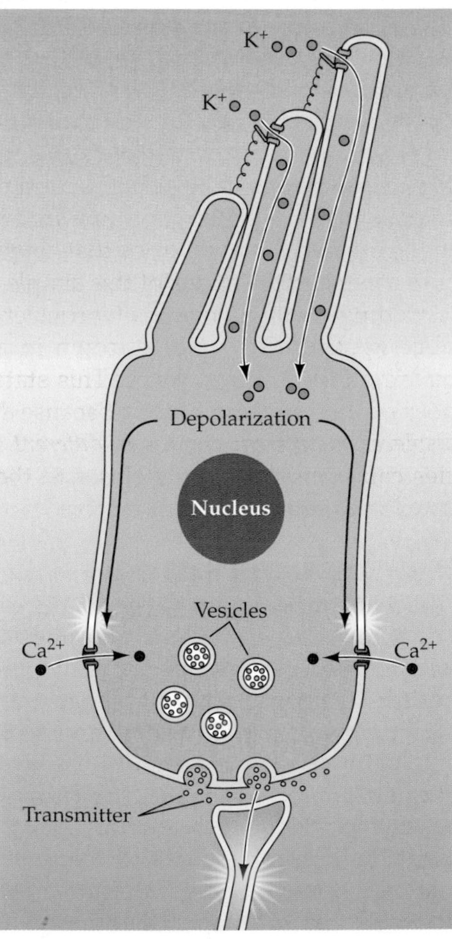

FIGURE 9.13 Stereocilia regulate the flow of ions into and out of hair cells. *(a)* This photomicrograph shows the threadlike tip links that connect the tip of each stereocilium to its taller neighbor. *(b,c)* Bending the stereocilia atop a hair cell opens the ion pore, permitting a rapid influx of potassium (K^+) ions into the hair cell, and this depolarization opens channels that allow Ca^{2+} to enter the base of the hair cell, causing release of neurotransmitter into the synapse between the hair cell and an afferent auditory nerve (AN) fiber.

as little as 1 nanometer (nm), roughly the diameter of a single atom. This deflection is equivalent to the top of the 324-meter (1063-foot) Eiffel Tower swaying by only about half an inch (Goldberg, 2008).

The firing of the auditory nerve fibers finally completes the process of translating sound waves into patterns of neural activity. Here's a brief summary of the whole process: An air pressure wave is funneled by the pinna through the auditory canal to the tympanic membrane, which vibrates back and forth in time with the sound wave. The tympanic membrane moves the malleus, which moves the incus, which moves the stapes, which pushes and pulls on the oval window. The movement of the oval window causes pressure bulges to move down the length of the vestibular canal, and these bulges in the vestibular canal displace the middle canal up and down. This up-and-down motion forces the tectorial membrane to shear across the organ of Corti, moving the stereocilia atop hair cells back and forth. The flexing of the stereocilia initiates rapid depolarization that results in the release of neurotransmitters into synapses between the hair cells and dendrites of auditory nerve fibers. These neurotransmitters initiate action potentials in the auditory nerve fibers that are carried back to the brain. And that's all there is to it!

CODING OF AMPLITUDE AND FREQUENCY IN THE COCHLEA Now let's return to the bulging vestibular canal and undulating middle canal to see how the two fundamental characteristics of sound waves—amplitude and frequency—are encoded by the cochlea.

As the amplitude of a sound wave increases, the tympanic membrane and oval window move farther in and out with each pressure fluctuation. The result is that the bulge in the vestibular canal becomes bigger, which causes the cochlear partition to move farther up and down, which causes the tectorial membrane to shear across the organ of Corti more forcefully, which causes the hair cells to bend farther back and forth, which causes more neurotransmitters to be released, which causes the auditory nerve fibers to fire action potentials more quickly. Thus, sound wave amplitude is conveyed in much the same way as light wave amplitude: the larger the amplitude, the higher the firing rate of the neurons that communicate with the brain. (We will discuss some complications of this simple explanation later in the chapter.)

Coding for frequency is a bit trickier. Earlier we said that the cochlear partition is displaced up and down in a pattern reflecting the pattern (frequency) of the sound wave. This statement is true as far as it goes, but it does not tell the whole story, because *different parts of the cochlear partition are displaced to different degrees by different sound wave frequencies*. High frequencies cause displacements closer to the oval window, near the base of the cochlea; lower frequencies cause displacements nearer the apex. In other words, different parts of the cochlea are "tuned" to different frequencies. This tuning is known as the **place code** for sound frequency.

Cochlear tuning to frequency is caused, in large part, by the way the structure of the basilar membrane changes along the length of the cochlea (**Figure 9.14**). The cochlea as a whole narrows from base to apex, but the basilar membrane actually widens toward the apex. In addition, the basilar membrane is thick at the base and becomes thinner as it widens. As a result, the cochlea separates frequencies along its length like an acoustic prism. Higher frequencies bend the narrower, stiffer regions of the basilar membrane near the base more, and lower frequencies cause greater displacements in the wider, more flexible regions near the apex.

In addition to this passive, structural way of being tuned to frequency, active processes sharpen the tuning. Remember that there are two different

place code Tuning of different parts of the cochlea to different frequencies, in which information about the particular frequency of an incoming sound wave is coded by the place along the cochlear partition that has the greatest mechanical displacement.

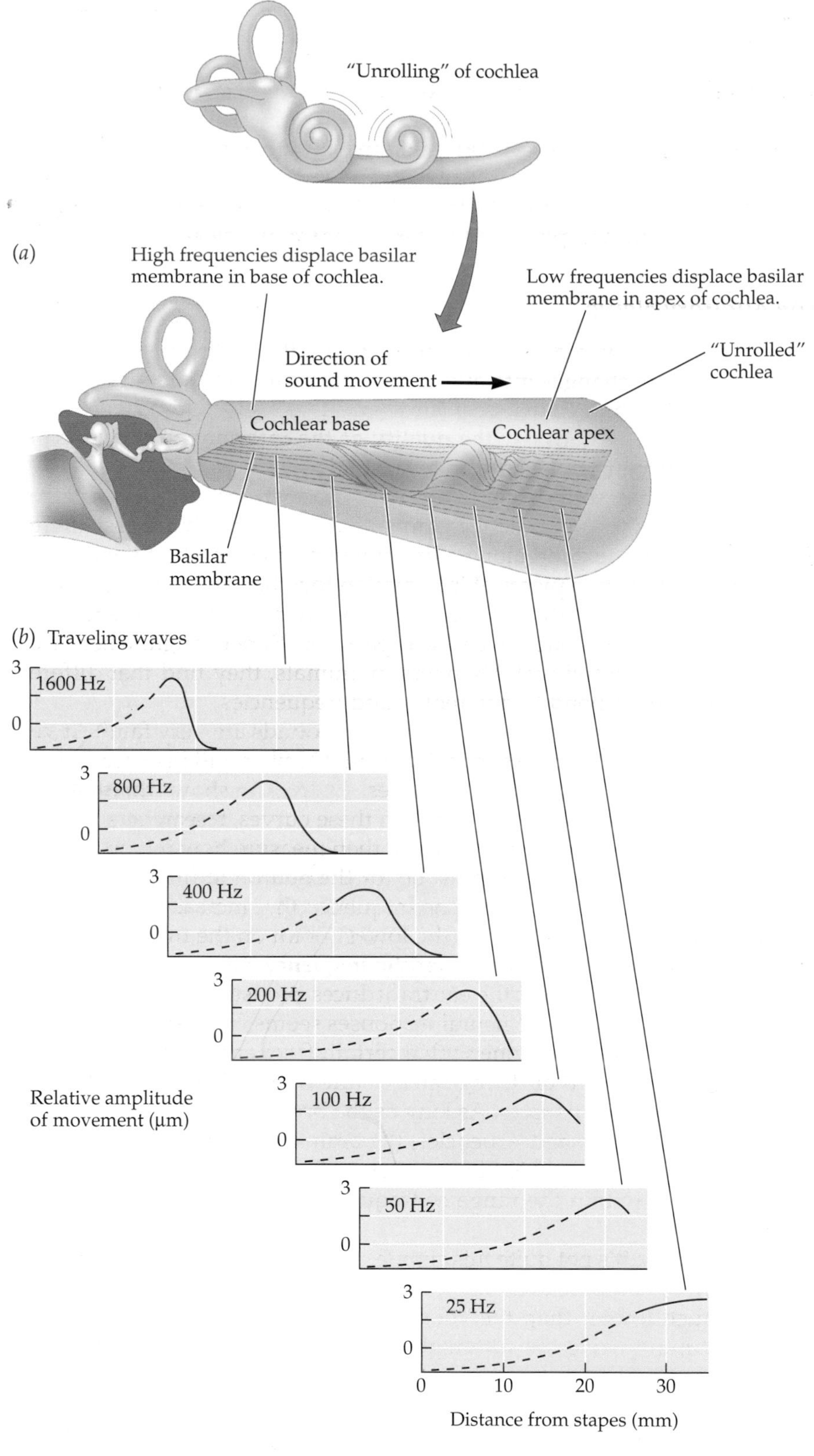

FIGURE 9.14 The cochlea is tuned to different frequencies. The narrower end of the basilar membrane toward the base is stiffer and most sensitive to higher frequencies. The wider, more flexible end toward the apex is most sensitive to lower frequencies. Here the cochlea is illustrated as if it were uncoiled (*a*), and the shapes of the traveling waves for different frequencies of vibration are shown (*b*).

types of hair cells: inner hair cells and outer hair cells. Over 90% of the **afferent fibers** in the auditory nerve—fibers that take information *to* the brain—synapse on the 3500 inner hair cells (10 to 30 auditory nerve fibers listen to each inner hair cell). If the inner hair cells are conveying almost all the information about sound waves to the brain, then what are the 10,500 outer hair cells for? It turns out that most of the nerve fibers that synapse with the

afferent fiber A neuron that carries sensory information to the central nervous system.

outer hair cells are **efferent fibers**, conveying information *from* the brain. When these efferent fibers become active, outer hair cells with which they synapse become physically longer, making the nearby cochlear partition stiffer (Fettiplace and Hackney, 2006). By making some parts of the cochlear partition stiffer than other parts, the outer hair cells make the cochlea more sensitive and more sharply tuned to particular frequencies.

efferent fiber A neuron that carries information from the central nervous system to the periphery.

threshold tuning curve A map plotting the thresholds of a neuron or fiber in response to sine waves with varying frequencies at the lowest intensity that will give rise to a response.

characteristic frequency (CF) The frequency to which a particular auditory nerve fiber is most sensitive.

The Auditory Nerve

Now that we've covered the mechanics of how the auditory system translates air pressure changes into auditory nerve firing, let's discuss what we know about the characteristics of these auditory nerve (AN) fibers. More specifically, we will consider the quality of the information conveyed by afferent AN fibers from the cochlea to the brain.

Remember that sounds with different frequencies displace different regions of the cochlear partition, and inner hair cells, on which most afferent AN fibers synapse, extend along a line traveling the length of the cochlear partition. Put these two pieces of information together, and we can infer that the responses of individual AN fibers to different frequencies should be related to their place along the cochlear partition. Sure enough, when scientists record from individual AN fibers in animals, they find that different fibers selectively respond to different sound frequencies.

This frequency selectivity is clearest when sounds are very faint. At very low intensity levels (even less than 0 dB), an AN fiber will increase firing to only a very restricted range of frequencies. **Figure 9.15** shows **threshold tuning curves** for several AN fibers. To graph these curves, researchers insert an electrode very close to a single AN fiber, then measure how intense the sine waves of different frequencies must be for the neuron to fire faster than its normal, spontaneous firing rate. The frequency that increases the neuron's firing rate at the lowest intensity (the lowest point on the threshold tuning curve) is called the neuron's **characteristic frequency (CF)**.

Up to this point, the way the ear transduces acoustic energy at different frequencies into a pattern of neural responses seems fairly straightforward. A low-intensity sine wave tone with a certain frequency will cause certain AN fibers to increase their firing rates, while other AN fibers continue to fire at their spontaneous rates. As long as the brain knows which AN fibers have which characteristic frequencies, the brain can interpret the pattern of firing rates across all the AN fibers to determine the frequency of any tone (as long as it is within the range of frequencies picked up by the human cochlea).

Unfortunately, it's not quite this simple. Almost all sounds in the environment are more complex than single sine waves, and most sounds we hear are also much louder than the very quiet sound waves used to measure threshold tuning curves. So although the previous paragraph captures the gist of how AN fibers code for sound frequencies, we have to do a bit more work to understand how higher-intensity, complex sounds are encoded in the auditory nerve. We will consider two of the specific complications we have to deal with; then we'll look at one additional mechanism that the auditory system uses to convey low-frequency components of sound waves.

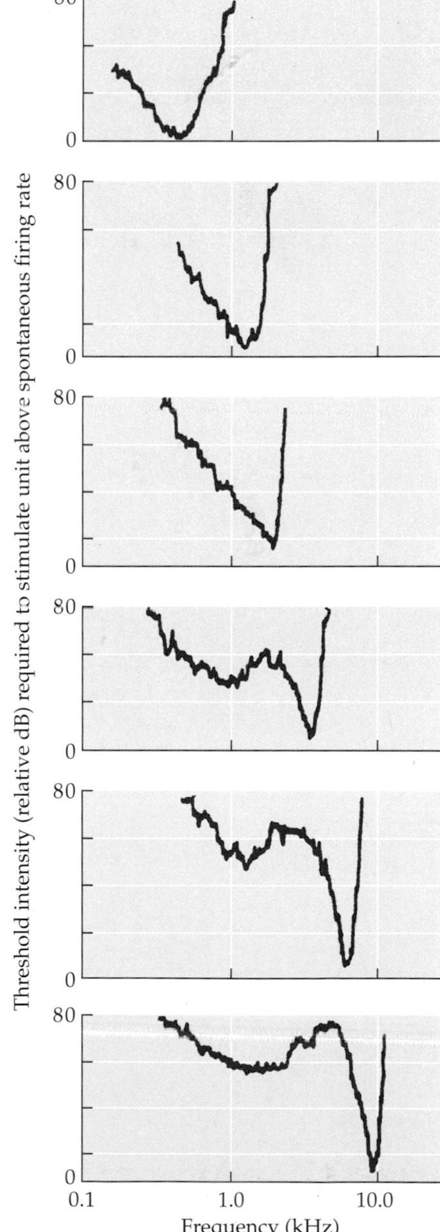

FIGURE 9.15 Threshold tuning curves for six auditory nerve fibers, each tuned to a different frequency. Curves define the lowest intensity necessary for the neuron to fire above its spontaneous rate at each frequency. The characteristic frequency for each of these six nerve fibers is at the lowest point of the tuning curve.

FIGURE 9.16 Two-tone suppression. The threshold tuning curve (dark red) is for one auditory nerve fiber with a characteristic frequency of 8000 Hz. Whenever a second tone is played at the frequencies and levels within the light red areas to each side, the response of this AN fiber to an 8000-Hz tone is reduced (suppressed).

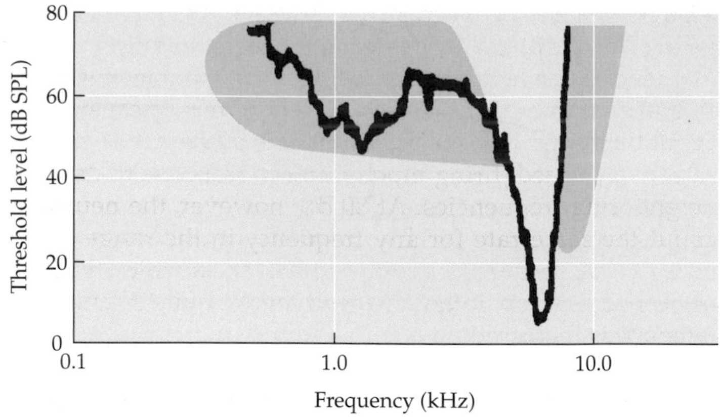

two-tone suppression A decrease in the firing rate of one auditory nerve fiber due to one tone, when a second tone is presented at the same time.

isointensity curve A map plotting the firing rate of an auditory nerve fiber against varying frequencies at varying intensities.

TWO-TONE SUPPRESSION The rate at which an AN fiber responds changes when energy is introduced at nearby frequencies. In particular, when a second tone of a slightly different frequency is added, the rate of neural firing for the first tone actually decreases—a phenomenon called **two-tone suppression**. As **Figure 9.16** shows, suppression effects are particularly pronounced when the second (suppressor) tone has a lower frequency than the first tone. In other words, if we are recording from an AN fiber whose CF is 8000 Hz and we use an 8000-Hz test tone, a 1000-Hz suppressor tone has a greater effect on the neuron's firing rate than a 15,000-Hz suppressor tone has.

The suppression effect appears to be caused by mechanical changes to the basilar membrane (Rhode and Cooper, 1993). The important point for our purposes is that understanding the response of the whole auditory nerve to complex sounds (that is, frequency combinations) is more complicated than simply adding up the responses of individual AN fibers to individual pure tones.

RATE SATURATION The sounds that matter most to listeners—most conversational speech, for example—are usually heard at intensities that comfortably exceed the threshold for just detecting sounds. Are AN fibers as selective for their characteristic frequencies at levels well above threshold as they are for the barely audible sounds used to chart threshold tuning curves?

To answer this question, we can look at **isointensity curves**, which we chart by measuring an AN fiber's firing rate to a wide range of frequencies, all presented at the same intensity level. **Figure 9.17** shows a family of isointensity curves for one AN fiber with a CF of 2000 Hz. The bottom curve shows the average firing rate (number of action potentials per second) of the neuron in response to 20-dB tones

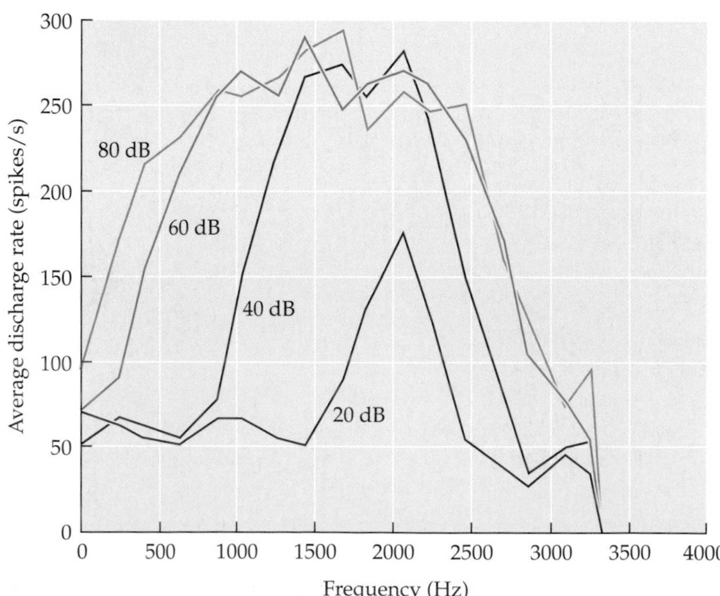

FIGURE 9.17 Isointensity functions for one auditory nerve fiber with a characteristic frequency of 2000 Hz. Tones of varying frequencies are presented at 20, 40, 60, and 80 dB. The neuron fires vigorously to a wider range of frequencies (mostly lower) when intensity is increased. Note that the 20-dB curve resembles an upside-down threshold tuning curve (compare to Figure 9.15) because 20 dB is almost as low as the intensities at which thresholds are measured.

with frequencies between 50 and 3300 Hz. The other curves track firing rates for 40-dB, 60-dB, and 80-dB tones over the same frequency range (for higher frequencies, the neuron always fires at its spontaneous rate).

We learn from these curves that for relatively quiet, 20-dB sounds (this is about the sound level of leaves rustling in the wind), the neuron is still quite selectively tuned, firing much faster in response to its CF (2000 Hz) than to neighboring frequencies. At 80 dB, however, the neuron appears to fire at about the same rate for any frequency in the range of 800 to 2500 Hz. In other words, frequencies such as 1000 Hz, to which the AN fiber had almost no response at low intensity levels, evoke quite substantial responses when intensity is increased.

The phenomenon behind this broadening of frequency selectivity is called **rate saturation**. Remember that AN fibers fire in response to the bending of stereocilia on hair cells, and that, in general, the farther they bend, the faster the firing rate is. For a 20-dB tone at 1000 Hz, the stereocilia on the hair cell feeding the AN fiber featured in Figure 9.17 will not bend at all, so the fiber's firing rate remains at its resting level. The firing rate rises above this resting level when the frequency of the 20-dB tone is increased to 1700 Hz, and it reaches its highest level at the AN fiber's characteristic frequency, 2000 Hz.

When the intensity is increased to 40 dB, however, the bulge in the vestibular canal is so large that stereocilia start bending even to a 1000-Hz tone (see Figure 9.17). If we increase the frequency to 1250 Hz, the firing rate increases, and it increases even more at 1500 Hz. The problem is that at about 1500 Hz, the fiber's firing rate maxes out (saturates). The stereocilia are bending as much as they can at this point, so increasing the frequency of the tone has no additional effect on the AN fiber's firing rate until we increase the frequency above the fiber's CF and the firing rate starts dropping again. For 80-dB tones, the fiber maxes out at even lower and higher frequencies relative to the CF of 2000 Hz.

For moderately intense tones, then, the brain cannot rely on a single AN fiber to determine the frequency of the tone. For example, we can't use the rule "if an AN fiber with a characteristic frequency of 2000 Hz is firing very fast, the sound must be 2000 Hz" because, as Figure 9.17 illustrates, this neuron will fire at its maximum rate to a 1000-Hz tone if the sound wave has a large enough amplitude.

One way the auditory system gets around this problem is to use AN fibers with different spontaneous firing rates. **Figure 9.18** shows **rate–intensity functions** for six fibers, all of which listen to the same hair cell (remember that dendrites from 10 to 30 auditory neurons synapse with each inner hair cell). To plot these curves, the intensity level of a tone at the AN fiber's CF is slowly raised from 0 dB up to 90 dB. As you can see, the resting rates of some fibers (whose functions are plotted in red) are less than 10 spikes per second. These neurons are

rate saturation The point at which a nerve fiber is firing as rapidly as possible and further stimulation is incapable of increasing the firing rate.

rate–intensity function A map plotting the firing rate of an auditory nerve fiber in response to a sound of constant frequency at increasing intensities.

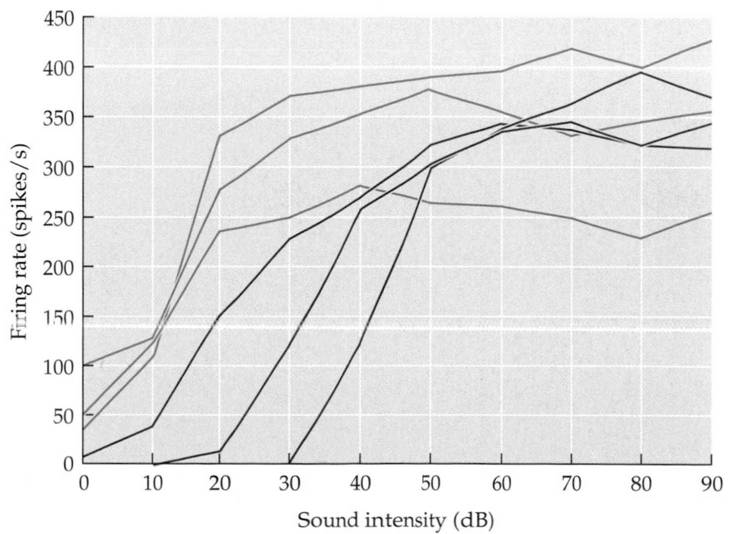

FIGURE 9.18 Firing rate plotted against sound intensity for six auditory nerve fibers: three low-spontaneous (red) and three high-spontaneous (blue). Firing rates for all six neurons increase with increasing sound level. Low-spontaneous neurons require higher-intensity sounds before they begin to fire, and they continue to increase firing rate to higher sound levels.

low-spontaneous fibers Auditory nerve fibers with low rates (less than 10 per second) of spontaneous firing; low-spontaneous fibers require relatively intense sound before firing at higher rates.

high-spontaneous fibers Auditory nerve fibers with high rates (more than 30 per second) of spontaneous firing; high-spontaneous fibers increase their firing rate in response to relatively low levels of sound.

mid-spontaneous fibers Auditory nerve fibers with medium rates (10–30 per second) of spontaneous firing. The characteristics of mid-spontaneous fibers are intermediate between low- and high-spontaneous fibers.

phase locking Firing of a single neuron at one distinct point in the period (cycle) of a sound wave at a given frequency. (The neuron need not fire on every cycle, but each firing will occur at the same point in the cycle).

temporal code Tuning of different parts of the cochlea to different frequencies, in which information about the particular frequency of an incoming sound wave is coded by the timing of neural firing as it relates to the period of the sound.

low-spontaneous fibers. The blue lines plot firing rates for **high-spontaneous fibers**, which fire 30 or more times per second, even in silence. **Mid-spontaneous fibers** have resting rates between these levels.

High-spontaneous auditory nerve fibers are somewhat analogous to rods in the retina: they are especially sensitive to low levels of sound, responding at rates above resting level even when decibel levels are quite low. The trade-off is that the firing rate of these fibers quickly reaches saturation, so their frequency selectivity is relatively poor when intensity is relatively high. Low-spontaneous fibers are more like cones, requiring more energy (higher-intensity sound waves) to start responding, but retaining their frequency selectivity over a broader range of intensity.

In addition to deploying different AN fibers with different spontaneous rates, the auditory system accurately determines the frequency of incoming sound waves by integrating the information across a broad range of AN fibers, and using the *pattern* of firing rates across all these fibers. Remember that in the visual system, we use the pattern of firing across our three types of cones to calculate the wavelength of light. The auditory system uses the same principle, but it has some 14,000 auditory nerve fibers in each ear to discern acoustic frequency. Consequently, the frequency sensitivity of the human auditory system as a whole is exquisite across a wide range of intensity levels, despite the coarse selectivity of individual auditory nerve fibers.

THE TEMPORAL CODE FOR SOUND FREQUENCY In addition to the cochlear place code, the auditory system has another way to encode frequency. As **Figure 9.19** illustrates, many auditory nerve fibers tend to fire action potentials at one particular point in the phase of a sound wave—a phenomenon called **phase locking**. Phase locking may occur because AN fibers fire when the stereocilia of hair cells move in one direction (e.g., as the basilar membrane moves up toward the tectorial membrane) but do not fire when the stereocilia move in the other direction. Recall from our discussion of mechanoelectrical transduction in stereocilia that the encoding of time is extremely accurate.

The existence of phase locking means that the firing pattern of an AN fiber carries a **temporal code** for the sound wave frequency. For example, if the AN fiber fires an action potential 100 times per second, then downstream neurons listening to the AN fiber can infer that the sound wave includes a frequency component of 100 Hz.

As measured in the auditory nerve, temporal coding becomes inconsistent for frequencies higher than 1000 Hz and is virtually absent above 4000 or 5000 Hz. In large part, this inconsistency is due to the refractory period of the AN fiber. For high frequencies, the fibers simply cannot produce action potentials quickly enough to fire on every cycle of the sound. However, mul-

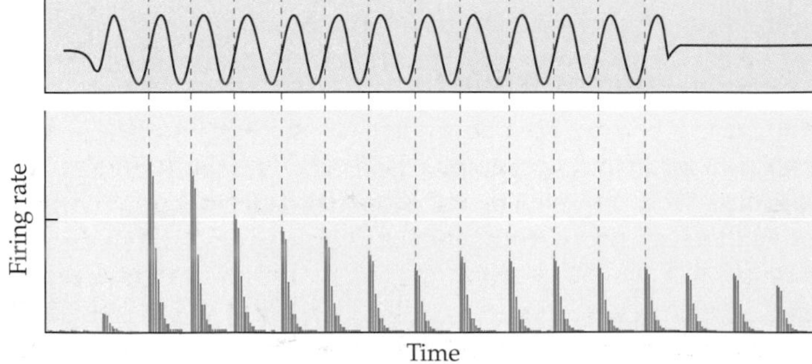

FIGURE 9.19 The histogram (bottom) shows neural spikes for an auditory nerve fiber in response to the same low-frequency sine wave (top) being played many times. Note that the neuron is most likely to fire at one particular phase of each cycle of the sine wave. This phase locking provides a temporal code to sound frequency.

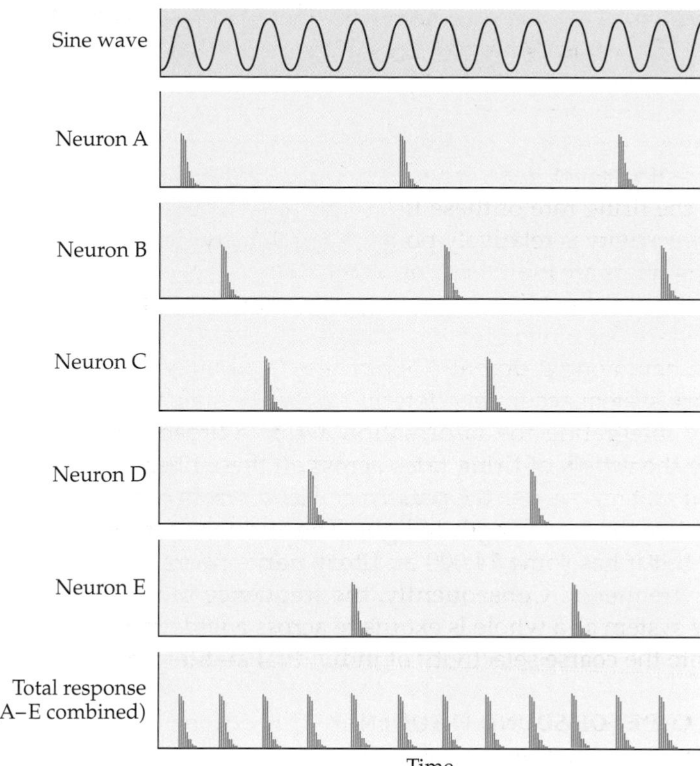

FIGURE 9.20 The volley principle. Even if one neuron cannot fire in response to every cycle of a higher-frequency tone, multiple auditory nerve fibers together can provide a temporal code for frequency if different neurons (A, B, C, D, E) each fire at different periods of the sine wave.

tiple neurons could, in principle, encode higher frequencies as a group. For example, four neurons could each fire only once every fourth cycle of a 2000-Hz sound. If the four neurons "took turns," each would have to fire only 500 times per second to fully encode the 2000-Hz sound in their joint temporal pattern. This idea has a long history (Wever, 1949), and it is referred to as the **volley principle** (Figure 9.20). According to this hypothesis, neurons sustain a temporal pattern of firing much like the pattern of Revolutionary War–era soldiers firing guns from the front line of a formation while the second and third lines took time to reload.

Interestingly, even AN fibers with relatively high-frequency CFs encode lower-frequency energy in the temporal pattern of their responses. For example, if you are listening to a fairly loud sound that is a combination of 200- and 8000-Hz sine wave tones, a neuron near the base of the cochlea that becomes wildly excited by the 8000-Hz component of the sound will also tend to be phase-locked to the 200-Hz component. This neuron thus carries information both about the high-frequency component (via place coding, because the brain knows the neuron's CF) and the low-frequency component (via temporal coding).

Auditory Brain Structures

The auditory nerve, also known as cranial nerve VIII, carries signals from the cochlea to the brain stem, where all AN fibers initially synapse in the **cochlear nucleus** (Figure 9.21). The cochlear nucleus contains many different types of specialized neurons. Some of these are especially sensitive to just the onsets of sound at particular frequencies. Some are sensitive to the coincidence of onsets across many frequencies (that is, they fire when multiple frequencies are initially heard, but stop firing if the sound continues playing). Some

volley principle An idea stating that multiple neurons can provide a temporal code for frequency if each neuron fires at a distinct point in the period of a sound wave but does not fire on every period.

cochlear nucleus The first brain stem nucleus at which afferent auditory nerve fibers synapse.

FIGURE 9.21 Pathways in the auditory system. Not all pathways are shown in this schematic. Although there are two parallel pathways, information from both ears comes together very early in the auditory system, at the superior olives.

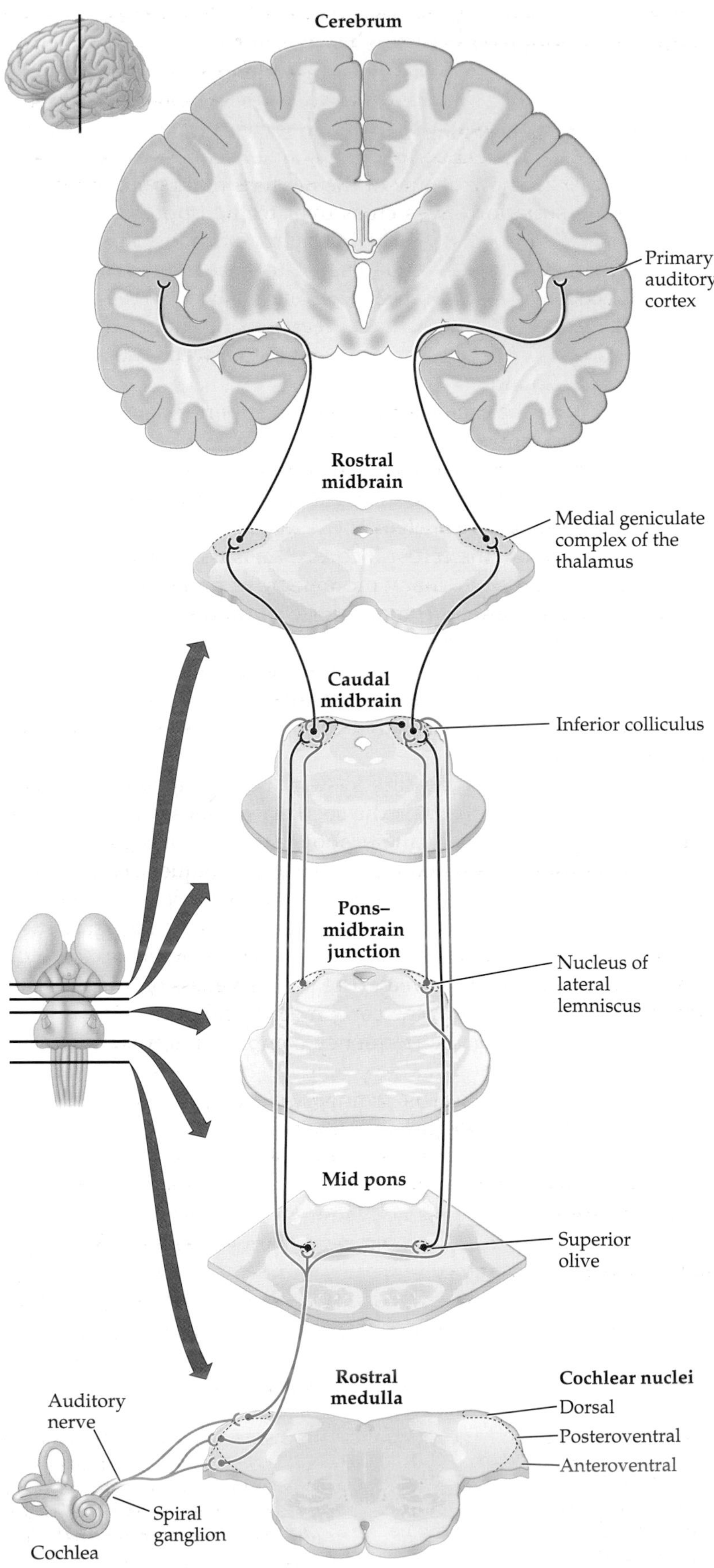

cochlear nucleus neurons use lateral inhibition to sharpen the tuning to one frequency by suppressing nearby frequencies—a mechanism reminiscent of that used by retinal ganglion cells to respond to spots of light instead of broad fields of light. Others respond in exactly the same way as the AN fibers that feed them. Some neurons appear to serve as little more than quick relays from the cochlea to the **superior olive**, another brain stem nucleus.

As Figure 9.21 shows, some of the neurons that project from the cochlear nuclei to the superior olives cross over to the opposite side of the brain. Thus, unlike the visual system, where inputs from each visual field remain separate until they have extended a fair distance in the visual cortex, signals from both cochleas reach both sides of the brain after only a single synapse. As we will see in Chapter 10, this direct relay of information from both ears is essential to using tiny timing differences between the two ears to detect the source of a sound.

Neurons from the cochlear nucleus and superior olive travel up the brain stem to the **inferior colliculus**. Most (but not all) of the input to each inferior colliculus comes from the opposite (contralateral) ear; that is, the left inferior colliculus listens primarily to the right ear, and vice versa.

The **medial geniculate nucleus** of the thalamus is the last stop in the auditory pathway before the cerebral cortex. As is the case in the lateral geniculate of the visual system, many more neurons project from the cortex to the medial geniculate (efferent) than project from the medial geniculate to the cortex (afferent.) These efferent connections, some of which presumably convey information back to lower stages of the auditory system, provide further anatomical evidence that sensory systems are two-way streets, in which feedback from the brain is tightly integrated with sensory information flowing up to the brain.

All structures of the auditory system, beginning with the basilar membrane and continuing through the cochlear nucleus, superior olive, inferior colliculus, and medial geniculate, show a consistent organizational pattern in which neurons are aligned respective to the frequencies to which they are most sensitive. That is, neurons most responsive to low-frequency energy lie on one edge of each structure, neurons responding to high frequencies lie on the other edge, and neurons responding to other frequencies are spread out in an orderly fashion in between. The pervasiveness of this **tonotopic organization** pattern reflects both the early mechanical properties of transduction and the importance of the frequency composition of sounds for auditory perception.

Tonotopic organization is maintained in the **primary auditory cortex**, which is referred to as **A1**, just as primary visual cortex is called V1. Neurons from A1 project to the surrounding **belt area** of cortex, and neurons from this belt synapse with neurons in the adjacent **parabelt area** (**Figure 9.22**). Just about any sound will cause activation in some part of A1. In the belt and parabelt areas, referred to as "secondary" or "associational" auditory areas, simple sounds such as sine waves and white noise elicit less activity, particularly if the stimuli have limited temporal structure. Thus we see that, as in other sensory systems, processing proceeds from simpler to more complex

superior olive An early brain stem region in the auditory pathway where inputs from both ears converge.

inferior colliculus A midbrain nucleus in the auditory pathway.

medial geniculate nucleus The part of the thalamus that relays auditory signals to the temporal cortex and receives input from the auditory cortex.

tonotopic organization An arrangement in which neurons that respond to different frequencies are organized anatomically in order of frequency.

primary auditory cortex (A1) The first area within the temporal lobes of the brain responsible for processing acoustic information.

belt area A region of cortex, directly adjacent to the primary auditory cortex (A1), with inputs from A1, where neurons respond to more complex characteristics of sounds.

parabelt area A region of cortex, lateral and adjacent to the belt area, where neurons respond to more complex characteristics of sounds, as well as to input from other senses.

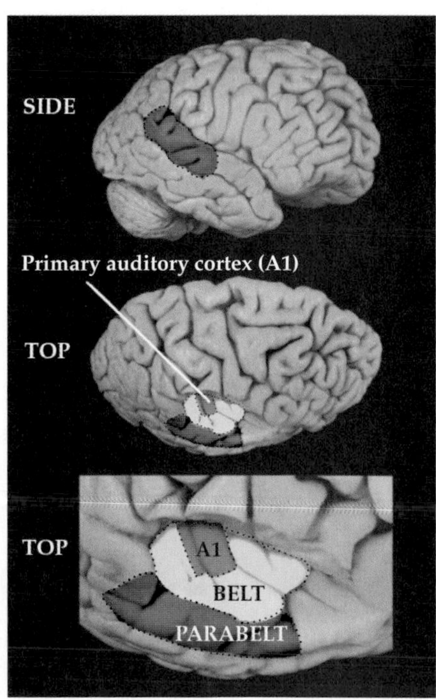

FIGURE 9.22 The first stages of auditory processing begin in the temporal lobe in areas within the Sylvian fissure. The top picture is from the side of the brain, and the lower two pictures are looking down at the brain with the parietal cortex cut away. Primary auditory cortex (A1) is in the center. It is surrounded by belt regions, and parabelt regions extend past the belt to the front and side. (From Brugge and Howard, 2002.)

stimuli as we move farther along the auditory pathway. We also find greater evidence of cross-modal processing (e.g., combining acoustic and optic information), particularly in parabelt areas.

Comparing the overall structure of the auditory and visual systems shows that a relatively large proportion of the processing in the auditory system is done before A1, whereas the majority of the most important visual processing occurs in cortical areas V1 and beyond. This difference may be a by-product of the evolutionary history of the two senses. The earliest mammals were small animals that were probably prey favored by dinosaurs and early birds. They were also nocturnal, so hearing, smell, and touch were their primary senses. Survival may have required these mammals to become proficient listeners with primarily brain stem processes to rely on, because the stem was just about all there was to the brain in those days. The shift of some mammals to a diurnal lifestyle coincided evolutionarily with an enormous expansion of the cortex, so it makes sense that the new visual capabilities that arose later in mammals developed largely in the cortex. Interestingly, one auditory capability that we know to be a very recent evolutionary advance—speech processing—is subserved almost entirely by cortical areas. We will return to the role of the cortex in auditory processing when we discuss speech and music perception in Chapter 11.

Basic Operating Characteristics of the Auditory System

Up to this point we have discussed the anatomy of the auditory system and the physiology of how the system encodes the two basic physical attributes of sound waves: amplitude (intensity) and frequency. As we've seen, these issues are investigated by direct observation of the anatomical structures: scientists examine basilar membranes, record from auditory nerve fibers, dissect various brain structures, and so on.

We turn now to the findings of researchers who have approached the auditory system from a different perspective. Instead of playing a sound and trying to determine how one particular neuron responds, we can instead play the sound and ask actual human listeners—each of whom is the sum total of a great many neurons—what they hear. When human listeners are asked to report their auditory sensations, their answers are due partly to the acoustic properties of the sound signal and partly to their own psychological characteristics. This method of investigation is thus called **psychoacoustics**.

Scientists who study psychoacoustics (psychoacousticians) are always careful to distinguish between the physical characteristics of sounds and the impressions of these sounds for listeners. As we noted earlier, whereas frequency, measured in hertz, is a physical description of the spectral composition of a sound, the subjective attribute of frequency for listeners is *pitch*. Sounds are measured with respect to frequency, but listeners hear pitch. Similarly, the intensity of sound is measured as sound pressure in decibels, but listeners hear *loudness*. If the auditory system operated exactly the same as electronic measuring devices do, we could treat the terms *frequency* and *pitch* and the terms *intensity* and *loudness* interchangeably. As we will see, however, biological auditory systems do not work exactly as electronic measuring devices work. For example, one sound wave may be heard as quite a bit louder than another, even though the two waves have exactly the same amplitude. Careful study of the differences between the responses of mechanical listening devices (sound-level meters and spectrum analyzers) and biological listening devices (human beings) provides great insight into how the human auditory system works.

psychoacoustics The study of the psychological correlates of the physical dimensions of acoustics; a branch of psychophysics.

Intensity and Loudness

The bottom curve in **Figure 9.23** shows the human **audibility threshold**, which graphs the lowest sound pressure level that can be reliably detected across the frequency range of human hearing (20–20,000 Hz). Note that the best (lowest) absolute thresholds for human hearing are between 2000 and 6000 Hz (2–6 kHz; remember that these frequencies are enhanced by the physical properties of the auditory canal). Thresholds rise on both sides of this range, meaning that higher- and lower-frequency sound waves must have larger amplitudes in order to be heard.

audibility threshold The lowest sound pressure level that can be reliably detected at a given frequency.

equal-loudness curve A graph plotting sound pressure level (dB SPL) against the frequency for which a listener perceives constant loudness.

temporal integration The process by which a sound at a constant level is perceived as being louder when it is of greater duration. The term also applies to perceived brightness, which depends on the duration of light.

The other lines in Figure 9.23 are **equal-loudness curves**. We obtain these curves by asking listeners to equate the loudness of sounds with different frequencies. The starting point for each curve is always 1000 Hz, so the curve marked "40" tracks the amplitude necessary to make tones at other frequencies sound exactly as loud as a 1000-Hz, 40-dB tone; the curve marked "60" represents the decibel levels necessary to match a 1000-Hz, 60-dB tone; and so on. As the figure shows, the same pattern of frequency-dependent sensitivity that we see in the audibility curve extends to sounds above threshold. (See Web Activity 9.4: Equal-Loudness Curves.)

The two orange tick marks in Figure 9.23 indicate that a 100-Hz tone presented at 60 dB sounds about as loud as a 1000-Hz tone presented at 50 dB (that is, both points fall on the equal-loudness curve marked "50"), whereas a 4000-Hz tone presented at 80 dB sounds louder than a 1000-Hz tone presented at the same level (purple tick marks). These observations demonstrate the inequality of sound pressure level and loudness: equal-amplitude sounds can be perceived as softer or louder than each other, depending on the frequencies of the sound waves.

Another way to track the relationship between amplitude and loudness is to pick one frequency, steadily raise the intensity of the sound, and ask a listener to judge how the loudness increases. Experiments of this type show, once again, that the relationship between intensity and loudness is far from perfect. Doubling the perceived loudness of a sound requires more than a doubling in the amount of acoustic energy present in a sound wave, especially above 40 dB. The same kind of relationship holds in vision: the number of photons must be more than doubled to double the perceived brightness of a light. These power functions extend the limited range of biological sensory systems across wider ranges of physical energy in the environment.

The loudness of a sound also depends on how long the sound is: within limits, longer sounds are heard as being louder. Again, the same thing happens in vision: flashes of light appear brighter when they are longer. The reason for this general phenomenon is that the perception of loudness or brightness depends on the summation of energy over a brief, but noticeable, period of time—a process called **temporal integration**. For hearing, temporal integration occurs over an interval of 100 to 200 milliseconds

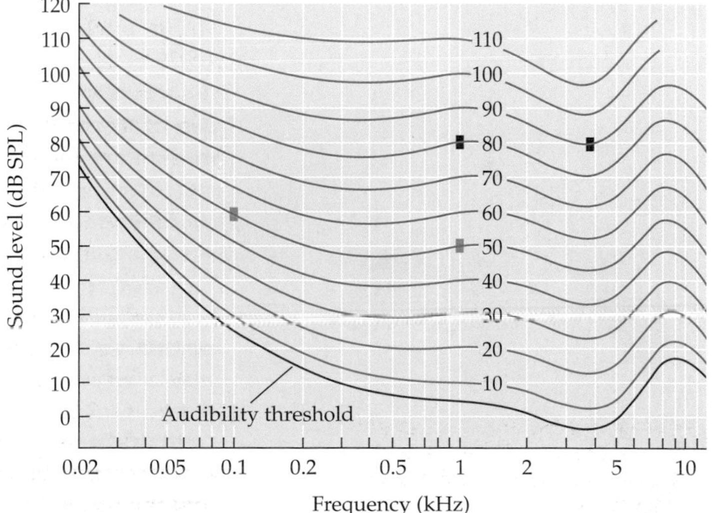

FIGURE 9.23 The lowest curve (red) illustrates the threshold for hearing sounds at varying frequencies. The curves labeled 10, 20, 30, and so on are equal-loudness curves. For a single contour, tones of different frequencies have different physical intensities, but they sound equally loud.

(ms). So if a sound is presented for less than 100 ms, it will be perceived as softer than the same amplitude and frequency presented for 300 ms. However, there will be little difference in loudness perception if the duration of the sound is increased from 300 to 1000 ms or longer.

In addition to studying absolute loudness judgments, psychoacousticians have been interested in how proficient humans are at discriminating between the loudness levels of two sounds. There are several different ways to measure the smallest differences in intensity that can be detected, and many measures show sensitivity to changes of less than 1 dB. This ability is quite impressive, given the wide range of sound intensities (from 0 to about 100 dB) that humans can perceive and the fact that, unlike the visual system, the auditory system is always sensitive to this entire range (remember that, to achieve maximum visual sensitivity, we need time to adapt to lower or higher ambient light levels). Although the ability to discriminate between subtle loudness differences might not seem all that important to survival, we will see in Chapter 10 how the auditory system uses differences between the intensity levels of sounds reaching the left and right ears to determine *where* sound sources are located.

For a time, it was difficult to understand how listeners could be sensitive to such small differences in loudness over such a large range. As we noted earlier, sound wave intensity is generally signaled by the firing rate of auditory nerve fibers: larger intensities (loud sounds) correspond to higher firing rates, and smaller intensities (quiet sounds) correspond to lower firing rates. When researchers recorded from individual AN fibers, however, they found that the difference between the intensity at which a neuron just starts firing and the intensity at which the neuron's firing rate saturates is typically less than 30 dB—a much smaller window than the 100-dB range over which humans can detect loudness differences.

The auditory system has a number of ways to get around this limitation. Perhaps most important, intensity thresholds vary from one AN fiber to the next. For example, one fiber might selectively respond to the range of amplitudes between 0 and 25 dB, another might span the range of 15 to 40 dB, a third might cover 38 to 65 dB, and so on (see Figure 9.18). A population of neurons with different thresholds can then encode a much broader range of intensities than is possible with any single neuron. In addition, remember that neurons become responsive to a broader range of frequencies when intensity is higher. One result is that, as sounds become more intense, many more AN fibers become excited.

Frequency and Pitch

The tonotopic organization of the auditory system, from basilar membrane to primary auditory cortex, is a very big hint that frequency composition is a fundamental determinant of how we hear sounds. More than anything else, psychoacousticians have studied how listeners perceive pitch, the psychological counterpart to frequency. As was the case with intensity and loudness, the frequency of a sound is related to, but not perfectly correlated with, the perceived pitch of the sound. For any given frequency increase (that is, an increase of 50 Hz), listeners will perceive a greater rise in pitch for lower frequencies than they do for higher frequencies. For example, listeners perceive a greater pitch difference when a tone shifts from 500 to 1000 Hz than when a tone shifts from 5000 to 5500 Hz.

Research done using pure tones (sounds composed of a single sine wave) indicates that humans are remarkably good at detecting very small differences in frequency. For example, listeners can discriminate between tones of 999 Hz and 1000 Hz—a difference of only one-tenth of 1%! Pitch discrimination at the lower and higher ends of the auditory system's frequency range is not quite as good, but it is still impressive. Part of the reason that discriminability decreases for high pitches appears to be that the temporal code for frequencies starts breaking down above 1000 Hz and is relatively nonfunctional above 5000 Hz. Performance thus suffers because the auditory system has to rely exclusively on place coding (the pattern of AN fiber responses from different parts of the cochlea).

Psychoacousticians have also used **masking** experiments to investigate frequency selectivity. In the research described in the previous paragraph, listeners never hear more than one sound frequency at a time. In a masking experiment, multiple frequencies are combined, and we see how well listeners can pick out certain components. That is, we look at how effective one sound—the masker—is at hiding another sound. We already discussed a phenomenon of two-toned suppression, in which an auditory nerve's response to one frequency can be disrupted by a second frequency. If place coding underlies pitch perception, we should expect to see the same kind of phenomenon in masking experiments.

In the classic approach to measuring frequency selectivity using masking, a single sine wave tone is placed in the middle of a band of acoustic noise (Fletcher, 1940). **White noise** is a signal that includes equal energy of every frequency in the human auditory range (20–20,000 Hz), just as white light includes light rays of all frequencies in the visible spectrum. A more limited band of noise might include all frequencies in the range of 500 to 1500 Hz; an even smaller band could span 500 to 510 Hz.

In a typical experiment, we might start with a 2000-Hz sine wave test tone presented along with a very narrow band of noise—say, 1975 to 2025 Hz (see Figure 9.24). We would then adjust the intensity of the test tone until listeners could just hear it over the noise. Next, we would increase the bandwidth of the noise, perhaps from 50 to 100 Hz, so that now the noise would include frequencies between 1950 and 2050 Hz. As we might expect, the listener would need to increase the intensity of the test tone to be able to hear it over this broader range of noise frequencies.

If we keep widening the bandwidth, however, we will eventually reach a point at which adding more energy to the noise stops affecting the detectability of the test tone. The size of the noise band at this point is called the **critical bandwidth** (**Figure 9.24*a***). For the experimental data plotted in Figure 9.24*b*, the critical bandwidth is 400 Hz. In this case, to pick out a 2000-Hz tone from the background noise, listeners must increase the intensity of the tone when the bandwidth is widened from 50 to 100 to 200 to 400 Hz, but going from a 400-Hz noise band to an 800-Hz band does *not* require the listener to make the test tone any louder. In fact, the 400-Hz noise band is

masking Using a second sound, frequently noise, to make the detection of another sound more difficult.

white noise Noise consisting of all audible frequencies in equal amounts. White noise in hearing is analogous to white light in vision, for which all wavelengths are present.

critical bandwidth The range of frequencies conveyed within a channel in the auditory system.

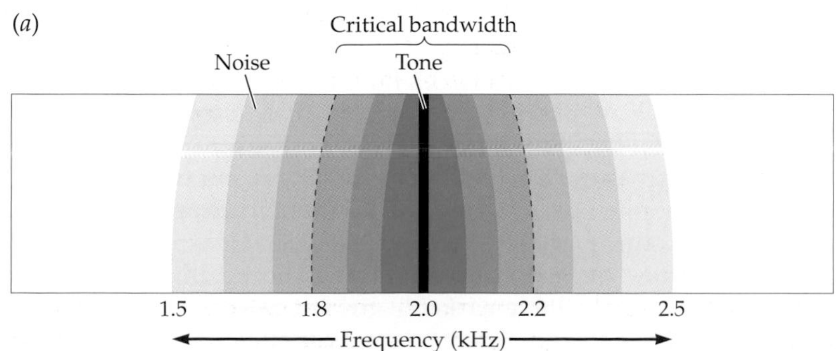

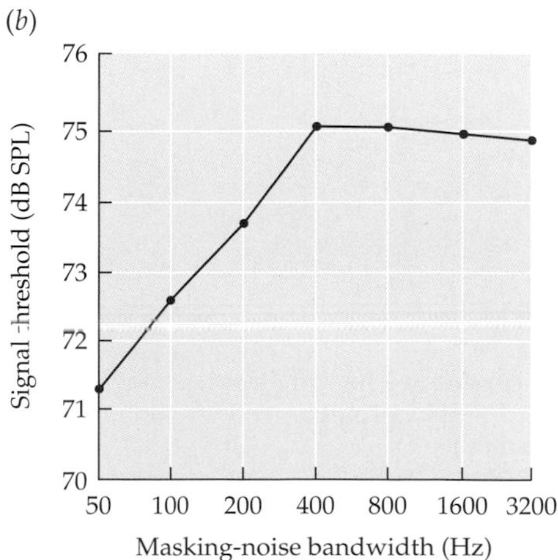

FIGURE 9.24 Critical bandwidth and masking. (*a*) To measure the width of a critical band, subjects listen for a tone in the center of a band of noise of constant intensity. It is harder to detect the tone as the band of noise widens up to a point, when further widening has no effect on detecting the tone. This point defines the critical bandwidth. (*b*) For this plot of bandwidth data, a 2000-Hz tone was used (Schoonevelt and Moore, 1989). The bandwidth of the noise had no effect on detection of the tone when it exceeded 400 Hz, so 400 Hz is the width of the critical band at 2000 Hz.

just as effective a masker as white noise covering the entire spectrum of human hearing.

Results from the masking paradigm have helped cement the role of place coding in pitch perception by revealing similarities between perceptual effects and physiological findings. First of all, the width of the critical bandwidth changes depending on the frequency of the test tone, and these widths correspond to the physical spacing of frequencies along the basilar membrane. For example, we know that a greater proportion of the basilar membrane vibrates in response to low frequencies, and that higher-frequency ranges vibrate smaller portions of the membrane. Correspondingly, masking studies show that the critical bandwidths for low frequencies are smaller than the critical bandwidths for high frequencies because the spacing between low frequencies is larger on the basilar membrane.

Another important finding is that masking effects are asymmetrical. More specifically, for a mask whose bandwidth is below the critical bandwidth of a test tone, the mask is more effective if it is centered on a frequency *below* the test tone's frequency—a phenomenon called the "upward spread of masking." This phenomenon may seem counterintuitive, but a look back at Figure 9.14 shows how displacement of the basilar membrane (the traveling wave) extends from the high-frequency base to the low-frequency apex. Displacement for low-frequency energy sounds toward the apex leaves a trail of displacement across high-frequency regions toward the base. In addition, two-tone suppression experiments indicate that suppression is greater if the suppressor tone is slightly below an AN fiber's characteristic frequency than if the suppressor tone is slightly above the fiber's characteristic frequency (see Figure 9.16).

Hearing Loss

Roughly 30 million Americans suffer some form of hearing impairment. When we talk about hearing loss, we typically do not mean the total loss of all hearing (deafness), but rather the elevation of sound thresholds. For example, frequencies that used to be audible at 20 dB may become inaudible unless they are presented at 40 or 60 dB. Of course, in the end we do not just need to detect sounds; the term *hearing* really refers to using spectral and temporal differences between sounds in order to learn something about events going on in the environment. As we will see, common forms of hearing loss affect the ability to interpret sounds, even when the sounds are loud enough to be detectable.

Hearing can be impaired by damage to any of the structures along the chain of auditory processing from the outer ear all the way up to the auditory cortex. The simplest way to introduce some hearing loss is to obstruct the ear canal, thus inhibiting the ability of sound waves to exert pressure on the tympanic membrane. Many people do this on purpose by wearing earplugs. A less intentional hearing loss can be created by the excessive buildup of ear wax (cerumen) in the ear canal. This problem is easy to remedy, as long as the effort to clear out the ear canal does not damage the tympanic membrane.

Another type of hearing impairment, called **conductive hearing loss**, occurs when the middle-ear bones lose (or are impaired in) their ability to freely convey (conduct) vibrations from the tympanic membrane to the oval window. Such impairment occurs most often when the middle ear fills with mucus during ear infections—a condition known as **otitis media**. The oval window usually still vibrates under these conditions; but, without the amplifying power of the ossicles, hearing thresholds can be raised by as much as 50 dB (that is, sounds need to be 50 dB louder in order to be heard).

conductive hearing loss Hearing loss caused by problems with the bones of the middle ear.

otitis media Inflammation of the middle ear, commonly in children as a result of infection.

Thankfully, for the millions of young children who suffer ear infections, normal hearing returns after mucus is absorbed back into surrounding tissues; however, this reabsorption can take up to several months. A more serious type of conductive loss, **otosclerosis**, is caused by abnormal growth of the middle-ear bones, most typically around the oval window next to the stapes. Surgery can free the stapes from these bone growths and improve hearing.

By far the most common, and most serious, form of auditory impairment is **sensorineural hearing loss**, which most commonly occurs inside the cochlea, and sometimes as a result of damage to the auditory nerve. Most often, sensorineural hearing loss occurs when hair cells are injured. For example, certain antibiotics and cancer drugs are **ototoxic**, meaning that they kill hair cells directly. In part, the reason for this effect is that ion pores on stereocilia that have been opened through mechanoelectrical transduction (MET) are not especially selective about what they permit to flow into the hair cell. Physicians are well aware of these dangers and typically avoid using such drugs, but sometimes a patient faces the decision of life with deafness versus no life at all.

A more common cause of hearing loss is damage to the hair cells by excessive exposure to noise. Those exquisitely fast and sensitive hair cells are also very vulnerable to damage from excessive sound levels. It is fairly well known that shooting a gun without ear protection can cause hearing loss. Extended exposure to loud sounds such as the noise of factory equipment also causes hearing loss. It is no coincidence that so many aging rock stars and race car drivers wear hearing aids. (It is ironic, but wise, that many heavy-metal music fans now wear ear protection at concerts.) And evidence suggests that cumulative exposure to even everyday noises present in the environments of industrialized countries can cause hearing loss. In one study (Goycoolea et al., 1986), middle-aged and elderly residents of Easter Island who stayed almost exclusively on their quiet island their whole lives were compared to other Easter Islanders, who made more frequent trips to the noisier outside world. As **Figure 9.25***a* shows, the more time people spent off the island, the more hearing loss they experienced.

Hearing loss is a natural consequence of aging for many people, and it is difficult to separate a person's age from the amount of exposure to noise. Typically, age-related hearing loss first affects the perception of high frequencies (Figure 9.25*b*). The 20- to 20,000-Hz frequency range for human hearing really applies only to young people; by the time most of us reach college age, we may have already lost the ability to hear frequencies above

otosclerosis Abnormal growth of the middle-ear bones that causes hearing loss.

sensorineural hearing loss Hearing loss due to defects in the cochlea or auditory nerve.

ototoxic Producing adverse effects on organs or nerves involved in hearing or balance.

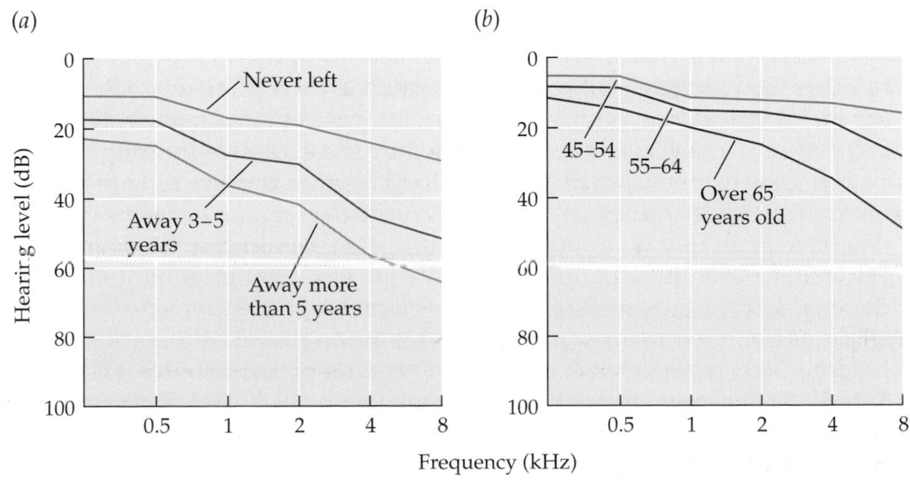

FIGURE 9.25 Environmental noise affects hearing. (*a*) The more people are exposed to noise in their environment, the more their hearing deteriorates. Easter Island residents who spent more years off of the relatively quiet island had relatively worse hearing. (*b*) Hearing becomes less sensitive with age, particularly for high frequencies. (After Goycoolea et al., 1986.)

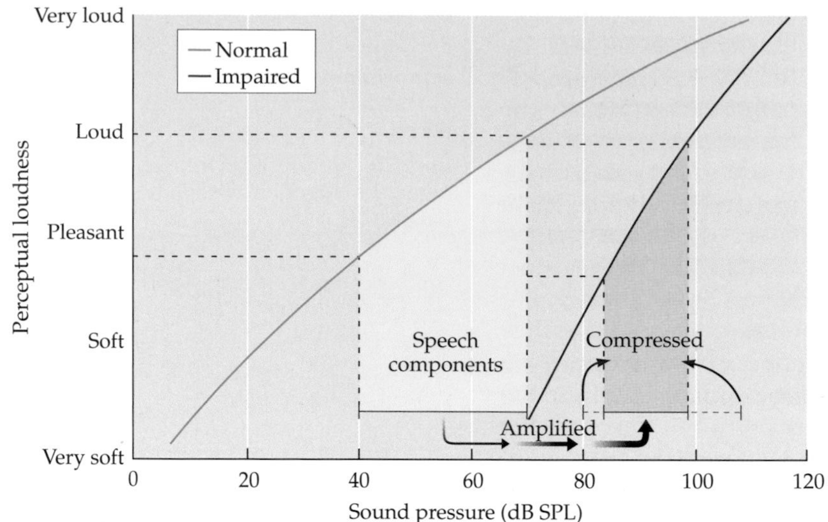

FIGURE 9.26 When thresholds are increased by hearing impairment, it takes more energy to hear a sound, but loudness increases faster than it does with healthy ears. When a hearing aid is used to increase the intensity of sounds, all variation in sound levels must be compressed into a smaller range of intensity because very loud sounds can be just as painful for listeners with hearing impairment as they are for listeners with healthy hearing. (After C. D. Geisler, 1998.)

15,000 Hz. The decrease in the ability to hear higher-frequency sounds continues throughout life, with the highest audible frequency becoming lower and lower as we get older. Fortunately, many of the auditory stimuli that people care most about, including speech and music, are composed predominantly of lower frequencies.

The earliest devices for helping people with hearing loss were simple horns. The small end of the horn would be held at the entry to the ear canal, and the wide end would be used to funnel more acoustic energy toward the listener's ear. Although effective, these horns were obviously somewhat cumbersome. Electronic hearing aids are much more convenient, but they must be designed to do more than simply amplify all sounds, because extremely loud sounds (above 100 dB) are just as annoying (or painful) for impaired listeners as they are for listeners with normal hearing. For a person who cannot hear sounds until they are at least 70 dB intense, compared to about 0 dB for healthy hearing, sounds that could normally vary between 0 and 100 dB must be squeezed between 70 and 100 dB (**Figure 9.26**). Nearly all modern hearing aids use some means to amplify the signal while also compressing intensity differences to keep the highest intensities within a comfortable listening level. Hearing aids can also be tuned to provide the greatest amplification only for frequencies in the region of greatest loss (for most people, higher frequencies will need to be amplified more).

One advantage of the old horns over electronic hearing aids was that they permitted listeners to direct their hearing toward the sound source they were most interested in. We may think about hearing aids as amplifying the voice to which one is listening, but they also amplify all the other sounds in the environment. The background noise in a car, or even the sound of a refrigerator, can become loud enough to compete with the sound of a person's voice. When the entire range of hearing is compressed from 100 dB to only 30 dB, a 10-dB difference between the rumbling of the car's engine and the voice of the person in the passenger seat becomes compressed into only a 3-dB difference.

Hearing aids are improving all the time, and they have provided relief to millions of Americans, including Ronald Reagan and Bill Clinton. However, despite researchers' many clever innovations for improving the signal that arrives at the tympanic membrane, damage to the mechanisms that transduce sound waves into neural signals is proving difficult or impossible to overcome completely. The best advice is to never need a hearing aid: protect your hair cells by avoiding exposure to loud sounds and by using hearing protection such as earplugs or muffs when necessary.

Modern medical science and engineering are providing some degree of hearing to thousands of people who are deaf. Cochlear prosthetics, more commonly known as cochlear implants (**Figure 9.27***a*), are tiny flexible coils with about two dozen miniature electrode contacts along their lengths. Surgeons delicately thread these electrode arrays through the round window as far toward the apex of the cochlea as possible. The electrode array is connected to a tiny radio receiver under the scalp, and signals are transmitted from a small microphone device on the outside of the head behind the ear

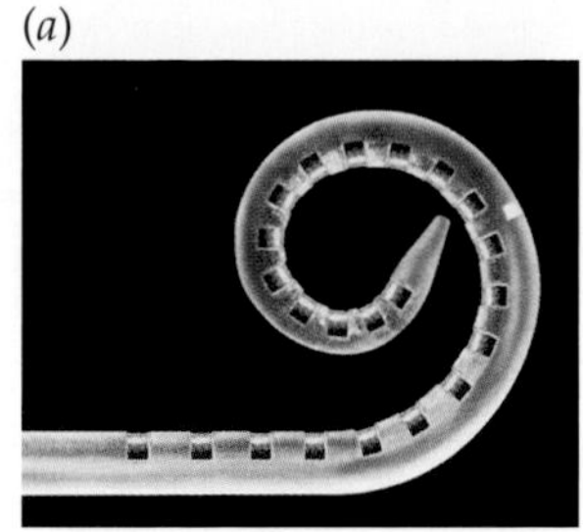

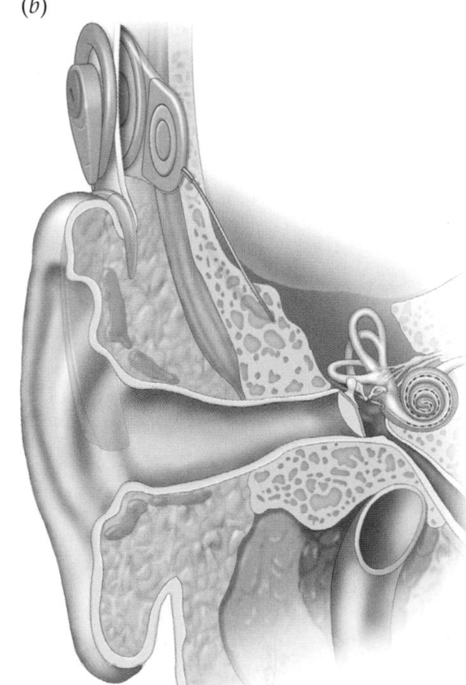

FIGURE 9.27 Cochlear implants give some people who are deaf the ability to hear. (*a*) The cochlear implant electrode array. The flexible array of electrodes is inserted through the round window as far as possible toward the apex of the cochlea. (*b*) The electrode array is connected to a small receiver beneath the scalp, and a small microphone and transmitter are placed over the receiver on the outside of the head.

(Figure 9.27*b*). Signals coming in from the microphone activate the miniature electrodes at appropriate positions along the cochlear implant, which in turn stimulates associated auditory nerve fibers.

Although cochlear implants are a modern medical miracle, they cannot provide hearing that equals what nature provides. But it is not surprising that a handful of electrodes cannot replace the function of 14,000 hair cells. Some people benefit more than others from receiving implants, and many adults with electrical hearing converse flawlessly over the phone. Young children, receiving implants as young as age 1 or 2, do best of all because young brains are particularly plastic. Children's brain circuitry develops to get the most information possible from their electronic ears.

Summary

1. Sounds are fluctuations of pressure. Sound waves are defined by the frequency, intensity (amplitude), and phase of fluctuations. Sound frequency and intensity correspond to our perceptions of pitch and loudness, respectively.
2. Sound is funneled into the ear by the outer ear, made more intense by the middle ear, and transformed into neural signals by the inner ear.
3. In the inner ear, cilia on the tops of inner hair cells are flexed by pressure fluctuations in ways that provide information about frequency and intensity to the auditory nerve and the brain. Auditory nerve fibers convey information through both the rate and the timing patterns with which they fire.
4. Different characteristics of sounds are processed at multiple places in the brain stem before information reaches the cortex. Information from both ears is brought together very early in the chain of processing. At each stage of auditory processing, including primary auditory cortex, neurons are organized in relation to the frequencies of sounds (tonotopically).
5. Humans and other mammals can hear sounds across an enormous range of intensities. Not all sound frequencies are heard as being equally loud, however. Hearing across such a wide range of intensities is accomplished by the use of many auditory neurons. Some neurons respond across certain levels of intensity; others span different levels of intensity. In addition, more neurons overall respond when sounds are more intense.
6. Series of channels (or filters) process sounds within bands of frequency. Depending on frequency, these channels vary in how wide (many frequencies) or narrow they are. Consequently, it is easier to detect differences between some frequencies than between others. When energy from multiple frequencies is present, lower-frequency energy makes it relatively more difficult to hear higher frequencies.
7. Hearing loss is caused by damage to the bones of the middle ear, to the hair cells in the cochlea, or to the neurons in the auditory nerve. Although hearing aids are helpful to listeners with hearing impairment, they cannot restore hearing as well as glasses can improve vision.

Refer to the
Sensation and Perception
website
(www.sinauer.com/wolfe2e)
for activities, essays, study questions, and other study aids.

CHAPTER 10

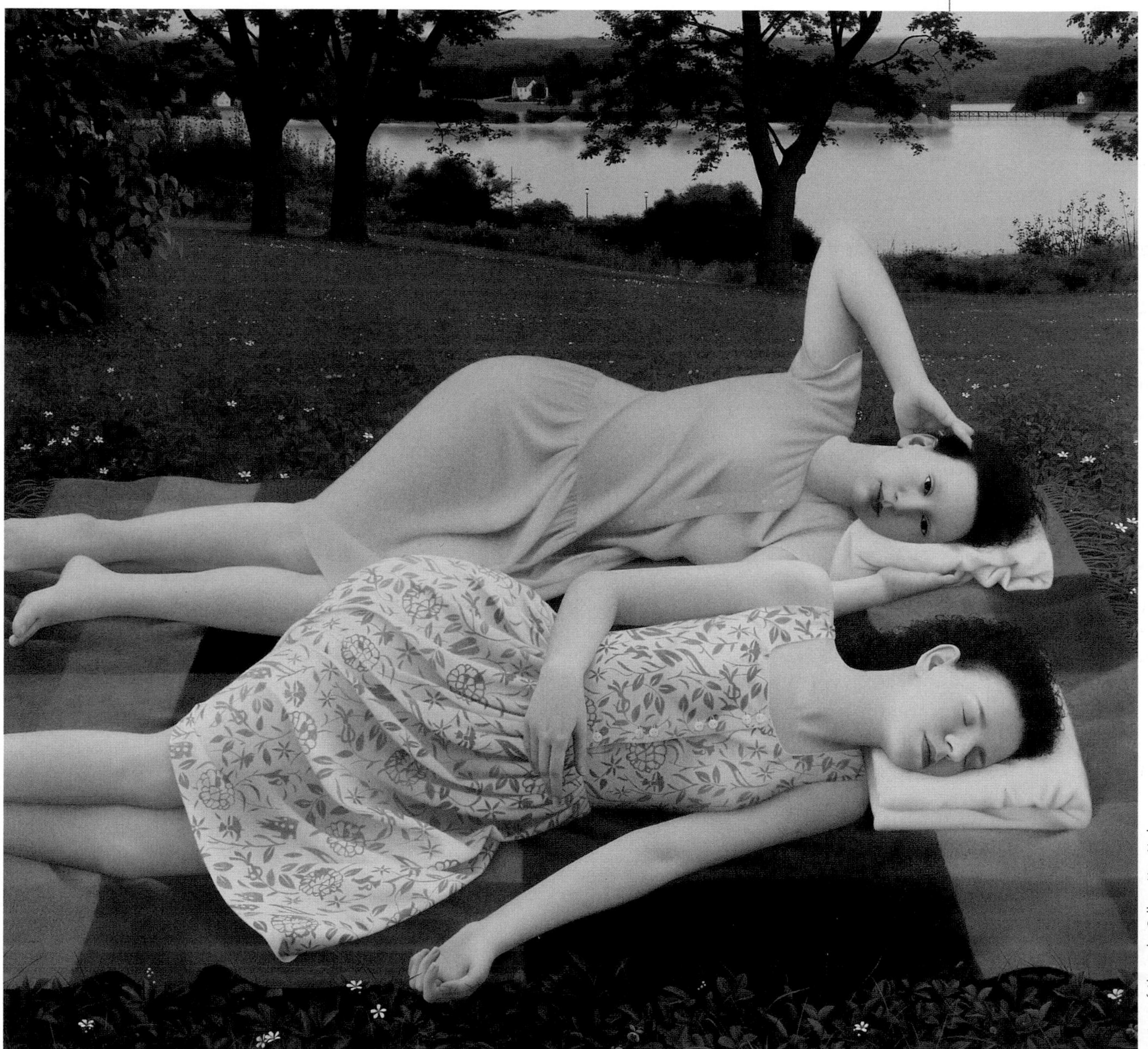

Courtesy of Alexandre Gallery, New York

Brett Bigbee, *Two Women*, 1990–1992

Hearing in the Environment

The auditory system's ability to transform tiny air pressure changes into a rich perceptual world is quite amazing. From the funneling of sound waves by the pinnae, to the mechanics of middle-ear bones, to the tiny perturbations of the basilar partition and hair cells, to the sophisticated neural encoding in the brain stem and cerebral cortex—some remarkable mechanisms have evolved for the receipt of auditory information about the world around us.

Research revealing these inner workings of the auditory system, described in the previous chapter, typically uses very simple stimuli under constrained situations—often isolated pure tones heard through headphones by listeners sitting in an otherwise perfectly quiet laboratory. Although this research is invaluable for understanding how the auditory system functions, this is obviously not the way we experience auditory stimuli in our daily lives. In this chapter we get "outside the head" to investigate how hearing helps us learn about the real-world environment.

We start by looking at how it is possible to determine the location of a sound source. As we will see, in many respects sound localization parallels visual depth perception, described in Chapter 6. We then turn from *where* to *what*, describing some important perceptual aspects of complex sounds, which are composed of simpler sounds in much the same way that visual representations of objects are built up from simple features (see Chapter 4). The third part of the chapter deals with auditory scene analysis, where we will see how some sounds group together, while separating from others, in ways that resemble the Gestalt principles introduced in Chapter 4. In the fourth and last portion of the chapter, we consider the auditory analog of visual object occlusion (see Chapter 6), and see how the auditory system seamlessly fills in gaps to form a complete and coherent "picture" of our auditory environment.

Sound Localization

Suppose you were out camping in your local state park one mild summer night, enjoying the last embers of your campfire, when suddenly an owl began hooting somewhere in front of you. You would instantly know whether the owl was perched to the left, to the right, or directly behind the fire pit. Moreover, if you were willing to leave the comfort of the fire, and if the owl were cooperative enough to sit still and keep hooting, you could easily walk to the exact source of the sound, even though you wouldn't be able to see the owl until you were very close to it.

When you think about it a bit, you will realize that this feat of auditory localization is quite different from determining the location of a visual object. If you could see the owl in front of you, you would know that it was

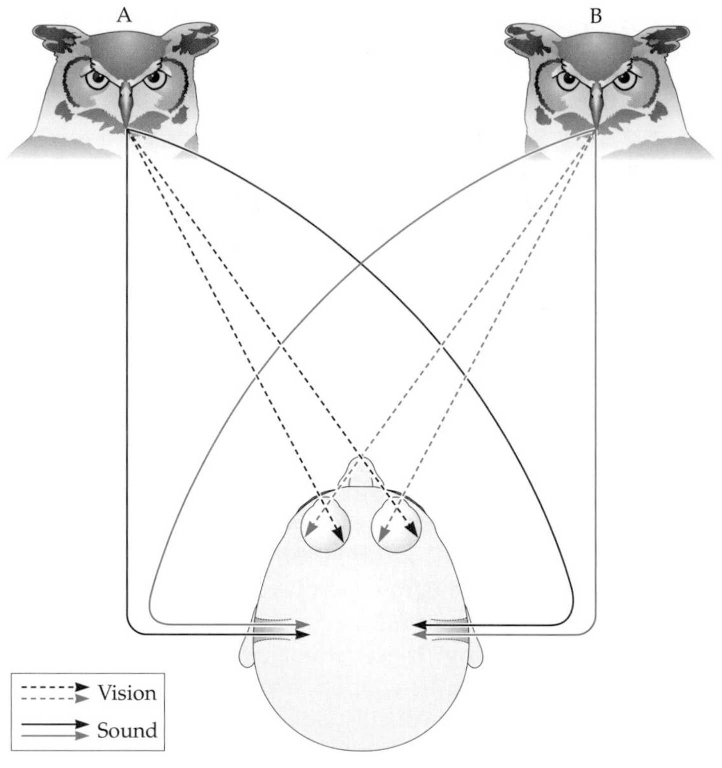

FIGURE 10.1 The position of the owl is easily encoded by the visual system because the owl's image falls on different parts of the retina (and thus activates different receptors) depending on whether it is to the left (A) or to the right (B) of the observer. In the auditory system, however, the same receptors are activated regardless of the owl's position.

to the left or the right of your fovea because its image would appear on the right or left side of your retina (**Figure 10.1**). But the owl's hoots enter your ears in exactly the same place (funneled through the pinnae into the middle and inner ear) regardless of where the owl is.

You may recall that we face a similar dilemma when trying to determine how far away a visual object is. For example, if you hold your right and left index fingers in front of your face, with your right finger closer than your left, the location of the two images on your retinas will not tell you anything about which finger is closer to you. As we saw in Chapter 6, visual depth perception involves processing and integrating a set of "cues"—stimulus aspects that provide indirect evidence about how far away an object is. The auditory system uses a similar approach to determine the location in space from which a sound is coming. (See **Web Activity 10.1: Auditory Localization Cues.**)

Just as having two eyes turned out to be one of the keys to determining visual depth relations, having two ears is crucial for determining auditory locations. For most positions in space, the sound source will be closer to one ear than to the other. Thus, there are two potential types of information for determining the source of a sound (**Figure 10.2**). First, even though sound travels very fast, the pressure wave will not arrive at both ears at the same time. Sounds arrive sooner, albeit very slightly, at the ear closer to the source. Second, the intensity of a sound is greater at the ear closer to the source. These are our first two auditory localization cues.

Interaural Time Difference

interaural time difference (ITD) The difference in time between a sound arriving at one ear versus the other.

Let's first consider what we can learn from the **interaural time difference**, or **ITD**. If the source is to the left, the sound will reach the left ear first. If it is to the right, it will reach the right ear first. Thus, we can tell whether a sound

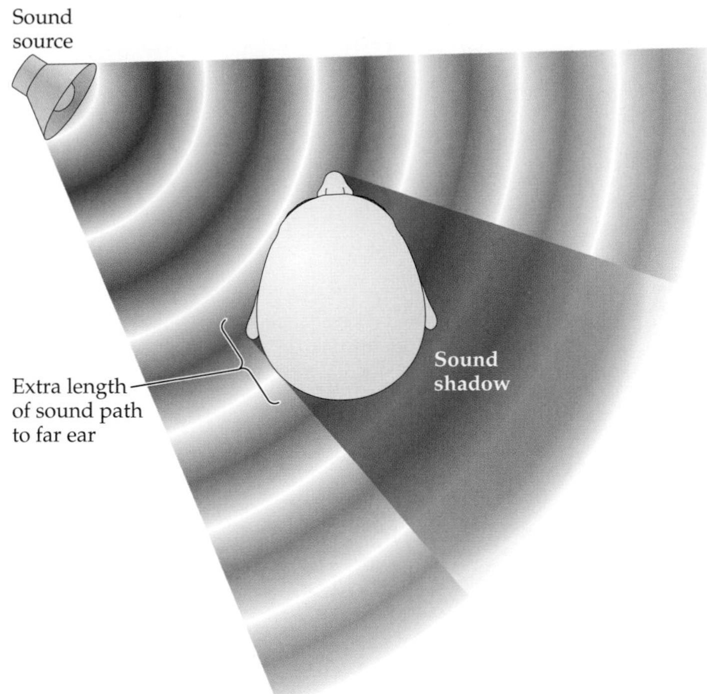

FIGURE 10.2 The two ears receive slightly different inputs when the sound source is located to one side or the other. For frequencies greater than 1000 hertz, the head blocks some of the energy from reaching the opposite ear.

is coming from our right or left by determining which ear receives the sound first (**Figure 10.3**). The term used to describe locations on an imaginary circle that extends around us—front, back, left, and right—in a horizontal plane is **azimuth**.

azimuth The angle of a sound source on the horizontal plane relative to a point in the center of the head between the ears. Azimuth is measured in degrees, with 0 degrees being straight ahead. The angle increases clockwise toward the right, with 180 degrees being directly behind.

A more detailed analysis of the ITD can tell us even more. See if you can answer the following questions, which require no knowledge of ear physiology to evaluate: Where would a sound source need to be located to produce the maximum possible ITD? What location would lead to the minimum possible ITD, and what would the ITD be in this case? Finally, what would happen at intermediate locations?

Figure 10.4 illustrates the answers to these questions. The ITDs for sounds coming from various angles are represented by colored circles. Red

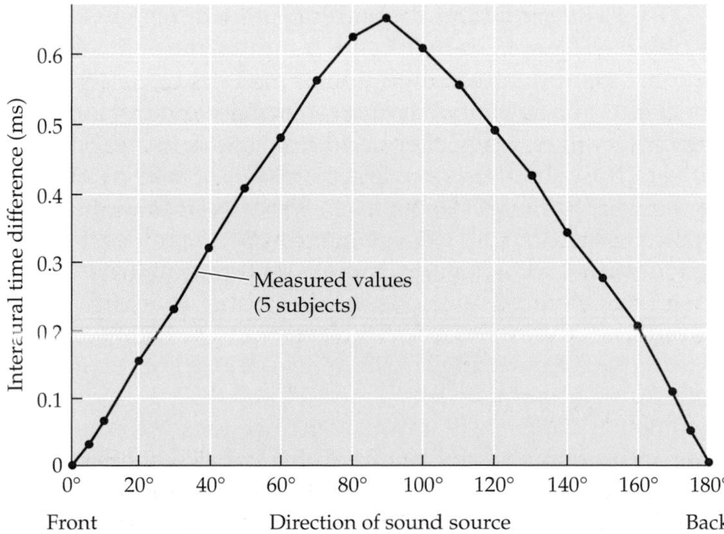

FIGURE 10.3 Interaural time differences for sound sources varying in azimuth from directly in front of listeners (0 degrees) to directly behind (180 degrees). The amount of difference in the times when the sound reaches each ear depends on where a sound comes from in space. (Data from Fedderson et al., 1957.)

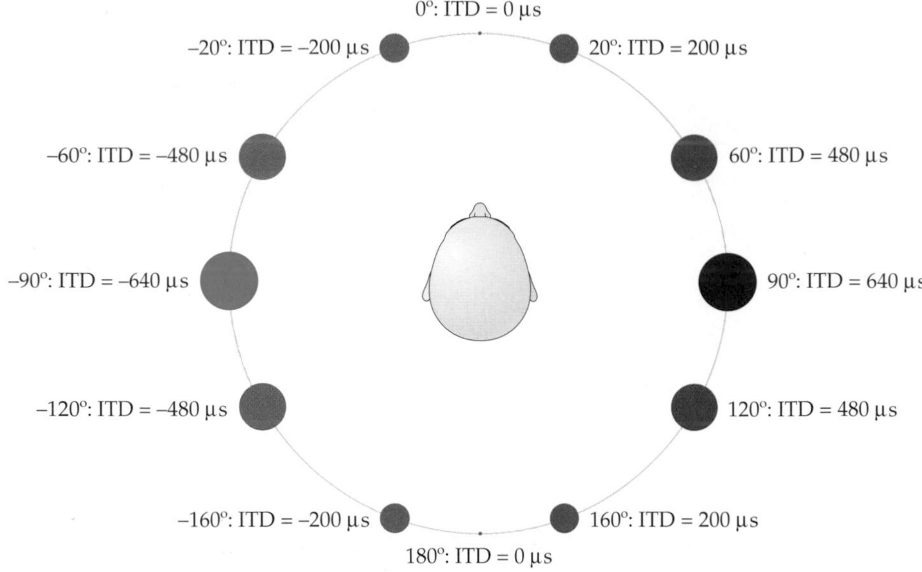

FIGURE 10.4 Interaural time differences for different positions around the head. Blue indicates locations from which sound reaches the left ear first; red indicates locations from which sound reaches the right ear first. (Data from Fedderson et al., 1957.)

circles indicate positions from which a sound will reach the right ear before the left ear; blue circles show positions from which a sound will reach the left ear first. The size and brightness of each circle represent the magnitude of the ITD.

As you can see, ITDs are largest, about 640 microseconds (millionths of a second, abbreviated µs) when sounds come directly from the left or directly from the right, although this value varies somewhat depending on the size of your head. A sound coming from directly in front of or directly behind the listener produces an ITD of 0; the sound reaches both ears simultaneously. For intermediate locations, the ITD will be somewhere between these two values. Thus, a sound source located at an angle of 60 degrees will always produce an ITD of 480 µs, and a sound coming from –20 degrees will always produce an ITD of –200 µs. That might not seem like much of a time difference, but studies have shown that listeners can detect interaural delays of as little as 10 µs (Klumpp and Eady, 1956), which is good enough to detect the angle of a sound source to within 1 degree.

PHYSIOLOGY OF ITDs The portion of the auditory system responsible for calculating ITDs obviously needs to be receiving input from both ears. As we saw in Chapter 8, binaural input enters almost every stage of the auditory nervous system after the auditory nerve. As information moves upward through the system, however, with every additional synapse the timing between the two ears is likely to become less precise. The **medial superior olives (MSOs)** are the first places in the auditory system where inputs from both ears converge (**Figure 10.5**), so this is a natural place to look for ITD detectors. Sure enough, T. C. T. Yin and Chan (1990) found neurons in the MSOs whose firing rates increase in response to very brief time differences between inputs from the two ears of cats.

medial superior olive (MSO) A relay station in the brain stem where inputs from both ears contribute to detection of the interaural time difference.

ITD detectors form their connections from inputs coming in from the two ears during the first few months of life (Brand et al., 2002; Kapfer et al., 2002). The developmental sequence is similar to the one for the formation of binocular neurons in the visual cortex, and it probably has a similar cause. The interpretation of ITDs (e.g., associating a given ITD with a given angle, as shown in Figure 10.4) is critically dependent on the size of the head. If

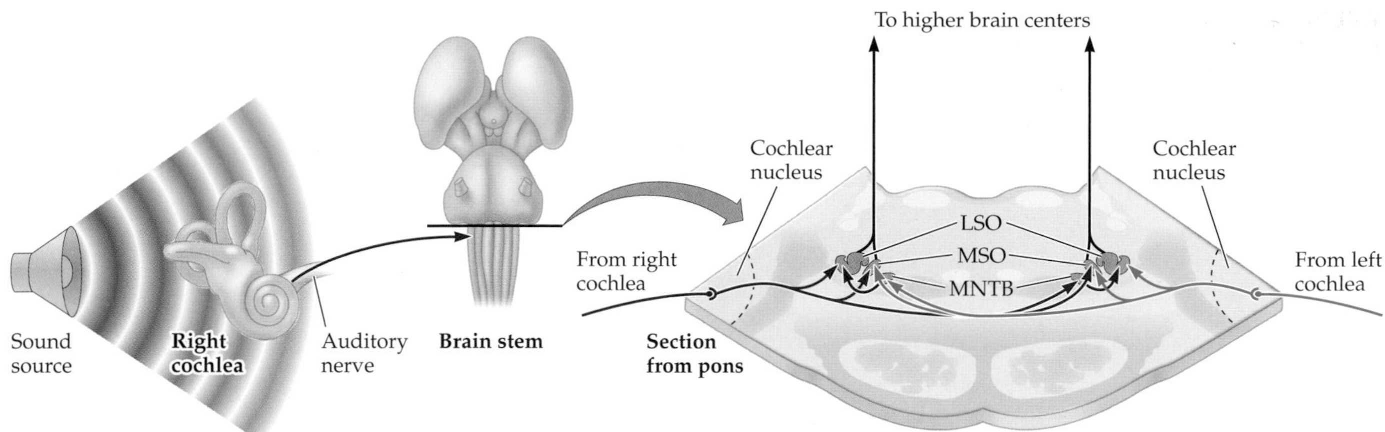

FIGURE 10.5 After only a single synapse in the cochlear nucleus, information from each ear travels to both the medial superior olive (MSO) and the lateral superior olive (LSO) on each side of the brain stem. MNTB = medial nucleus of the trapezoid body.

babies came out of the womb with their ITD interpretation mechanisms prewired to the size of their infant heads, their sound localization abilities would steadily decline as their ears moved farther and farther apart as a result of the growth of their heads during childhood and adolescence.

Interaural Level Difference

The second cue to sound localization is called the **interaural level difference**, or **ILD**, in sound intensity. Sounds are more intense at the ear closer to the sound source because the head partially blocks the sound pressure wave from reaching the opposite ear. The properties of the ILD relevant for auditory localization are similar to those of the ITD:

- Sounds are more intense at the ear that is closer to the sound source, and less intense at the ear farther away from the source.
- The ILD is largest at 90 and –90 degrees, and it is nonexistent at 0 degrees (directly in front) and 180 degrees (directly behind).
- Between these two extremes, the ILD generally correlates with the angle of the sound source, but because of the irregular shape of the head, the correlation is not quite as great as it is with ITDs.

Although the general relationship between ILD and sound source angle is almost identical to the relationship between ITD and angle, there is an important difference between the two cues: the head blocks high-frequency sounds much more effectively than it does low-frequency sounds. This is because the long wavelengths of low-frequency sounds "bend around" the head in much the same way that a large ocean wave crashes over a piling near the shore. Thus, as shown in **Figure 10.6**, ILDs are greatest for high-frequency tones, and the ILD cue provides the best information about sound source location. ILDs are greatly reduced for low frequencies, becoming almost nonexistent below 1000 hertz (Hz).

PHYSIOLOGY OF ILDs Neurons that are sensitive to intensity differences between the two ears can be found in the **lateral superior olives (LSOs)**, which receive both excitatory and inhibitory inputs. Excitatory connections to the LSOs come from the ipsilateral ear (that is, excitatory connections to the left LSO originate in the left cochlea, and excitatory connections to the right LSO come from the right cochlea). Inhibitory inputs come from the contralateral ear (the ear on the opposite side of the head) via the medial nucleus of the trapezoid body (MNTB).

interaural level difference (ILD) The difference in level (intensity) between a sound arriving at one ear versus the other.

lateral superior olive (LSO) A relay station in the brain stem where inputs from both ears contribute to the detection of the interaural level difference.

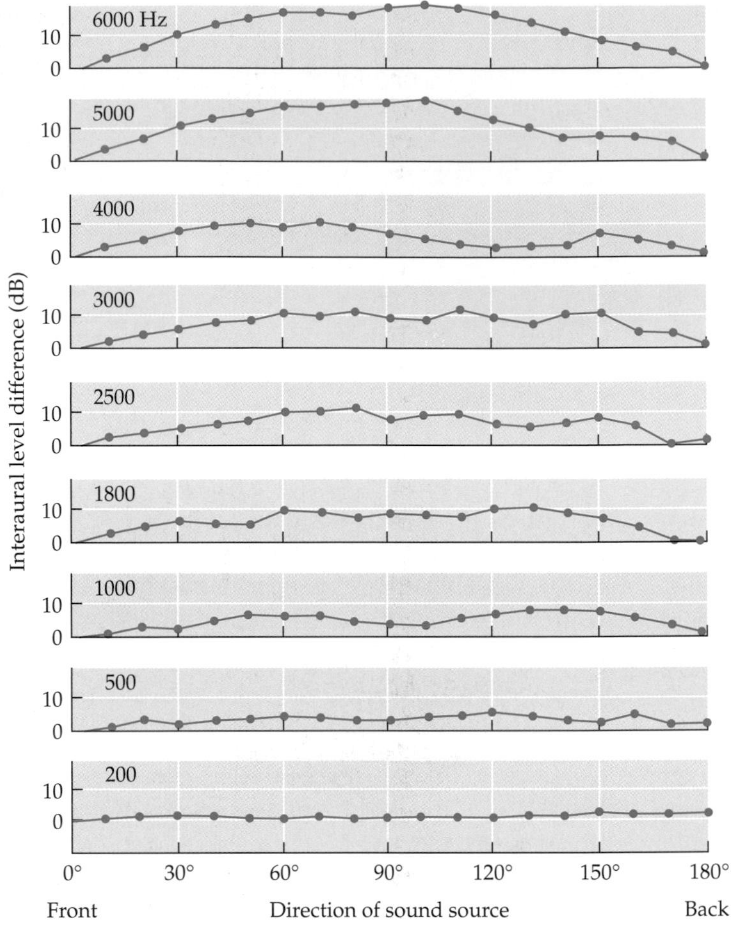

FIGURE 10.6 Interaural level (intensity) differences (ILDs) for tones of different frequencies presented at different positions around the head. Note that the biggest differences are for frequencies greater than 1000 Hz, at which point the head creates a shadow. The curves are not symmetrical toward the front and back, because of filtering characteristics of the pinnae. (Data from Fedderson et al., 1957.)

What makes neurons in the LSOs so sensitive to differences in intensity across the two ears is the competition between excitatory inputs from one ear (ipsilateral) and inhibitory inputs from the other ear (contralateral). When the sound is more intense at one ear, connections from that ear are both better at exciting LSO neurons on that side and better at inhibiting LSO neurons on the other side.

Cones of Confusion

If you examine Figures 10.4 and 10.6 for a bit, you should see a potential problem with using ITDs and ILDs for sound localization: An ITD of –480 μs arises from a sound source that is located at either an angle of –60 degrees from the line of sight (ten o'clock in Figure 10.4) or an angle of –120 degrees (eight o'clock). Adding information from intensity differences does not help us here, because the ILDs for these two angles are also identical. If we also consider the elevation of a sound source (how far above or below our head the sound source is—a factor we've been ignoring up to now), we find that a given ITD or ILD could arise from any point on the surface of a **cone of confusion** that extends perpendicularly from the left or right ear (**Figure 10.7**).

cone of confusion A region of positions in space where all sounds produce the same time and level (intensity) differences (ITDs and ILDs).

Although many books speak of a single cone of confusion, actually an infinite number of cones are nested inside one another. In fact, the widest "cone" is really a circle extending from directly in front of you, up to directly over your head, back to directly behind the back of your head, and continu-

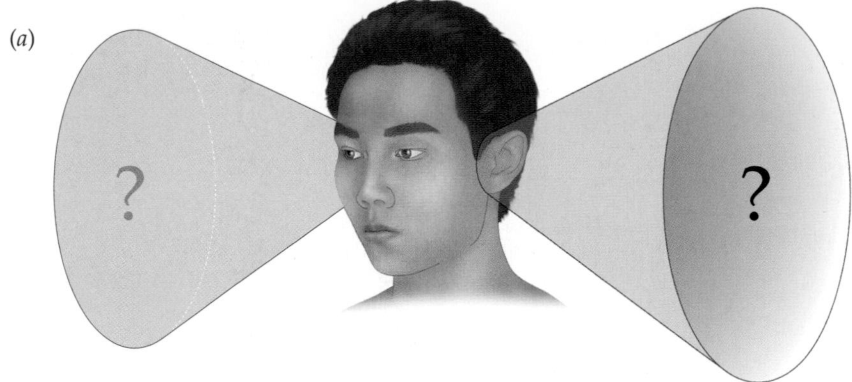

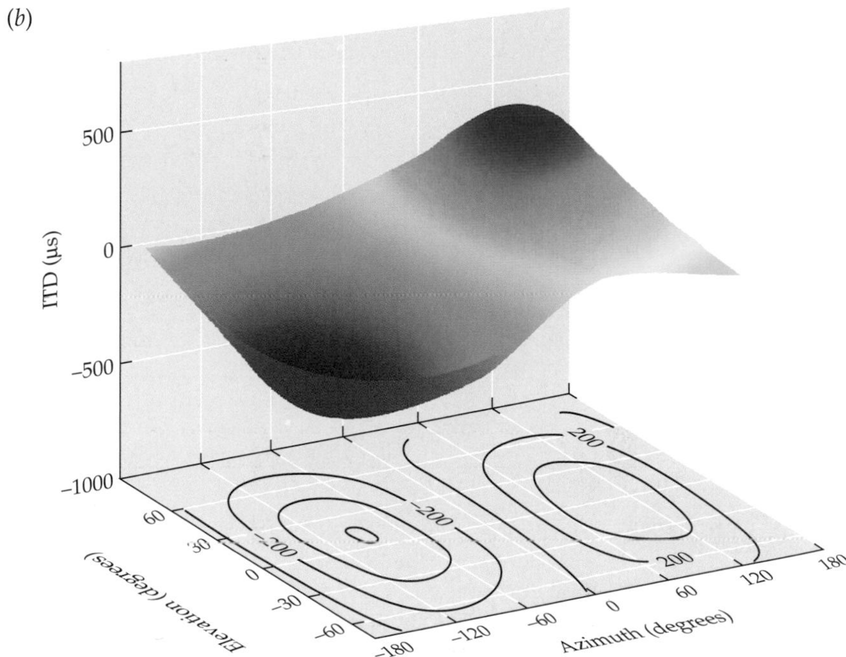

FIGURE 10.7 Elevation adds another dimension to sound localization. (*a*) Cones of confusion. (*b*) Interaural time differences (ITDs) are plotted here across azimuth and elevation. A sound with zero azimuth and elevation is directly in front of a listener's head. All of the locations in space that share the same color provide exactly the same ITDs. Red contours plotted beneath the colored surface illustrate how all the locations on the red line give rise to the same ITD. (Part *b* after Wightman and Kistler, 1998.)

ing to directly below you. As strange as it may seem, this widest cone is the most confusing of the cones.

This point was vividly demonstrated in experiments by Wallach (1940). Try to imagine yourself as a subject in these experiments. Your head position is fixed as your chin sits within a cupped chin rest, and you are surrounded by a vertically oriented, cylindrical screen covered with vertical stripes. The cylinder now starts rotating around your head. Assuming you don't get motion sickness, you will soon experience an induced motion effect, in which you will perceive the screen to be stationary and yourself to be rotating. Now the experimenter activates a sound source located directly in front of your nose. What location do you perceive as the source of the sound? The answer is that you hear the sound as coming from either directly above or directly below you because these are the only two points from which the ITD and ILD of a sound remain constant while your body moves constantly around.

Experiments like the one just described establish that cones of confusion are real perceptual phenomena, not just theoretical problems for the auditory system. In the real world, however, our heads are not held in a fixed position. As soon as you move your head, the ITD and ILD of a sound source shift, and only one spatial location will be consistent with the ITDs and ILDs perceived at both head positions (**Figure 10.8**).

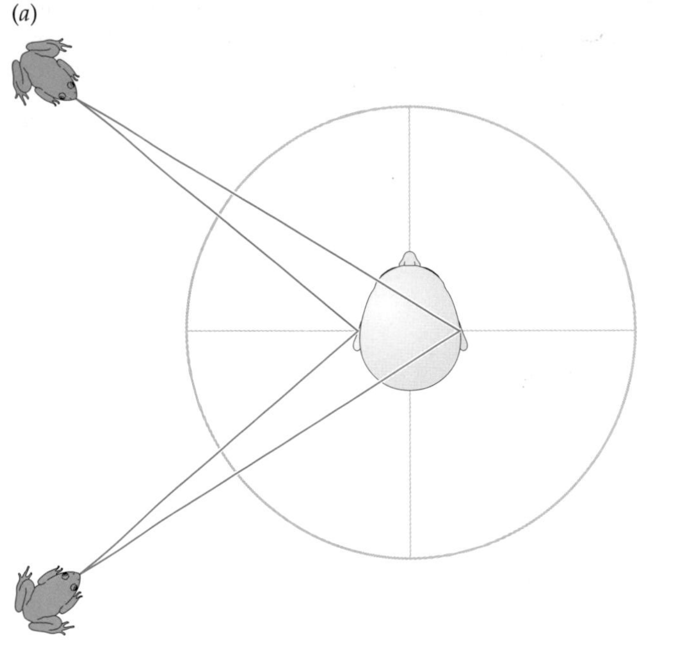

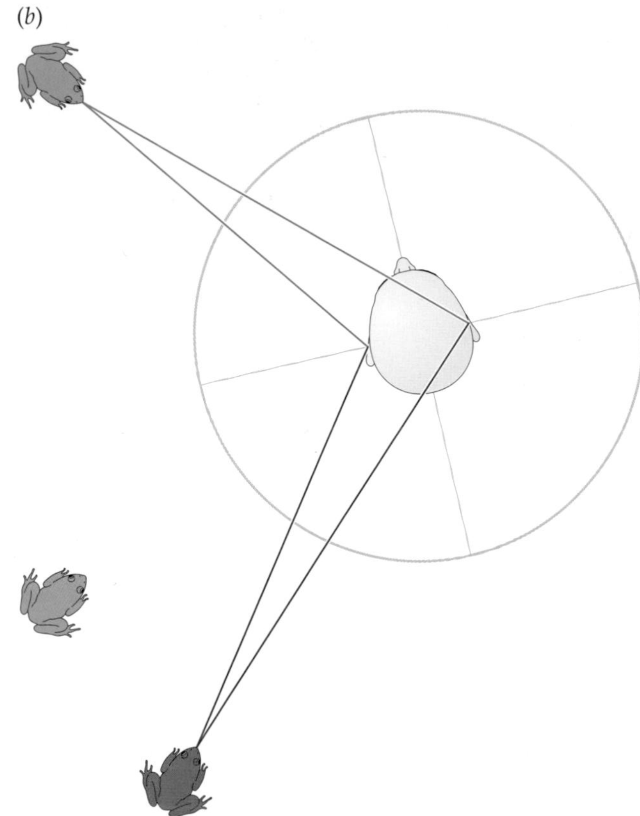

FIGURE 10.8 Evaluating ITDs and ILDs from two different head positions helps in sound localization. (*a*) At first, a sound source coming from the blue frog will lead to an ITD and ILD that would also be consistent with a sound coming from the green frog. (*b*) If the head is rotated slightly counterclockwise, the ITD/ILD will no longer be consistent with the location of the green frog. There will still be an ambiguity, however. Now the ITD/ILD will be consistent with the red frog as well as the blue frog. But only the blue location is consistent with both the first and the second sets of ITDs and ILDs.

Pinna and Head Cues

Another reason why cones of confusion are not major practical problems for the auditory system is that time and intensity differences are not the only cues for hearing the location of sound sources. Take a look at one of your pinnae (or, more realistically, take a look at a friend's pinna, since you can't get a good look at the side of your own head without an elaborate mirror setup). You'll see that the shape of the pinna is quite complex, with lots of idiosyncratic nooks and crannies (**Figure 10.9**). Remember that the pinnae serve to funnel sound energy into the ear canal. But because of their complex shapes, the pinnae funnel certain sound frequencies more efficiently than others. Furthermore, the intensity of each frequency varies slightly according to the direction of the sound. This variation provides us with another auditory localization cue.

Here's a simple example to illustrate how the effects of pinna shape are measured. Suppose you are in an anechoic room, a room in which the walls are padded so that very little sound enters from the outside and very little sound reverberates off the walls. The room is full of speakers at many locations up, down, and all around you. Tiny microphones are inserted inside your auditory canals, right next to your eardrums. These microphones can measure just how much energy from different frequencies actually reaches your eardrums from different locations around you. **Figure 10.10***a* shows the measurements at the eardrum for sounds played over a speaker 30 degrees to the left of a listener in an experimental setup like the one just described and 12 degrees up from the listener's head. Although energy at all frequencies was equally intense coming from the speaker, you can see that energy at all frequencies is not equally intense at the eardrum. Some frequencies, such

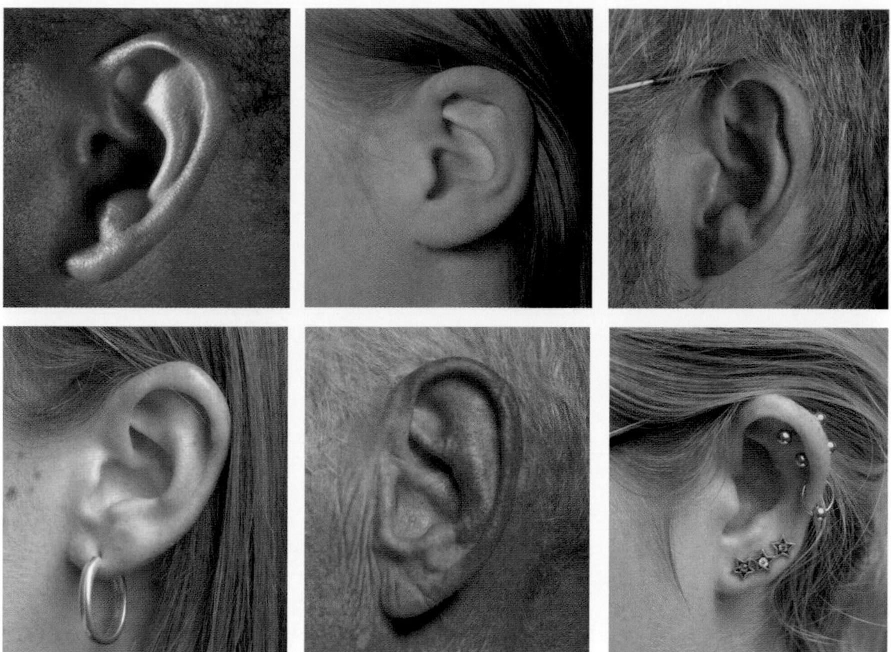

FIGURE 10.9 Pinna shapes vary quite a lot between people. Listeners learn how their personal pinnae affect how they hear sounds from different places in the environment.

as 5000 Hz, have higher intensity when they arrive at the eardrum; others, such as 800 Hz, have less intensity.

So far, we've shown how the pinnae alter the "spectral shapes" of complex sounds, but we haven't shown how spectral shapes provide cues to auditory localization. Figure 10.6 showed how the relative intensities of different frequencies change depending on azimuth, and illustrated that those curves are not symmetrical toward the front and back, because of filtering characteristics of the pinnae. For the final piece of the puzzle, look at Figure 10.10*b*, which shows the sound recorded by in-ear microphones when the speaker is moved up and down in elevation. As you can see, the relative intensities of different frequencies continuously change with changes in elevation as well as azimuth. The sum total of these intensity shifts can be measured and combined to determine the **head-related transfer function** (usually referred to by its acronym, **HRTF**) for a set of pinnae.

The importance of the HRTF in sound localization is easily understood if we consider the difference between hearing a concert live versus through a set of headphones. In person, we perceive the sound of the French horns as coming from one side of the orchestra and the sound of the flutes as coming from the other side. But when we wear headphones (especially the type inserted directly inside the auditory canals), sounds are delivered directly to the eardrums, bypassing the pinnae. Auditory engineers can use multiple microphones to simulate the ITDs and ILDs that result from the musicians' different locations (the Beatles were early users of this type of technology), but the HRTFs cannot be simulated. As a result, we may be able to get some sense of direction when listening to the concert through headphones, but the sounds will seem to come from inside the skull, rather than out in the world. The situation is akin to that of visual depth perception. Pictorial cues can give a limited sense of depth, but to get a true perception of three-dimensionality, we really need binocular-disparity information that normally we get only when we're seeing real objects.

Actually, just as stereoscopes can be designed to simulate binocular disparity, it is possible to simulate HRTFs. Instead of using two camera lenses

head-related transfer function (HRTF) A function that describes how the pinna, ear canal, head, and torso change the intensity of sounds with different frequencies that arrive at each ear from different locations in space (azimuth and elevation).

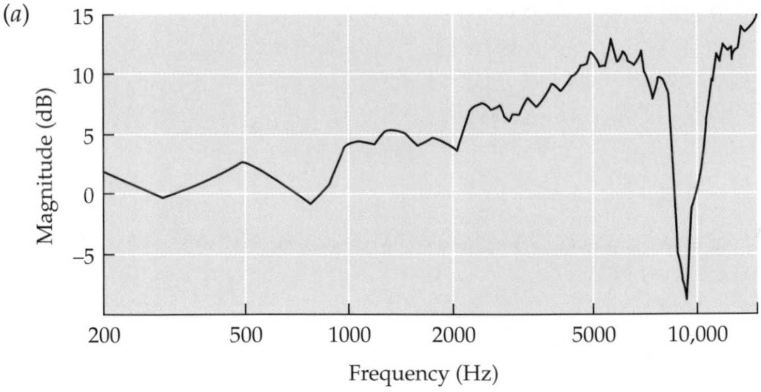

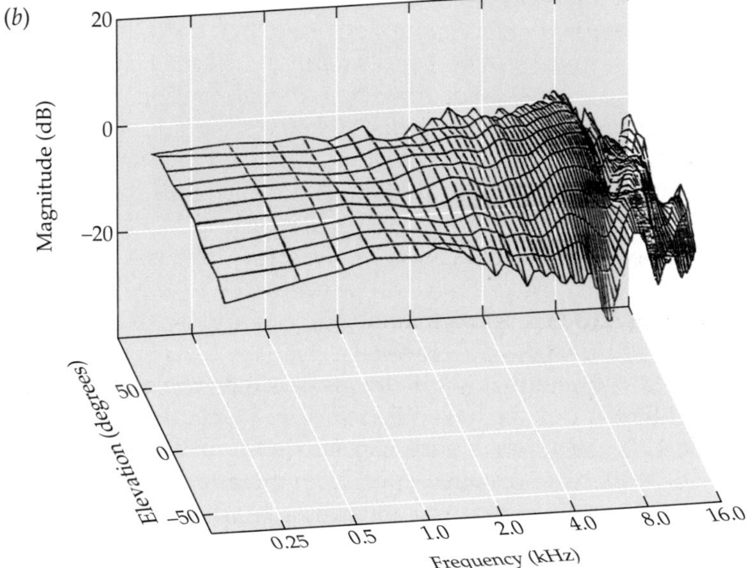

FIGURE 10.10 Head-related transfer functions (HRTFs). (*a*) Differences in intensity at the eardrum for sounds of varying frequency are plotted in this HRTF for a single point in space. (*b*) The series of HRTFs plotted here is for the same azimuth, but at different elevations. (*a* from Kistler and Wightman, 1992; *b* from Wightman and Jenison, 1995.)

in place of two eyes, two microphones are placed near the eardrums as described earlier. Then the sound source, such as a concert, is recorded from these two microphones. If this special stereo recording, called a "binaural recording," is played over headphones, the listener experiences the sounds as if they were back out in the world where they belong. Unfortunately, however, every set of pinnae is different (see Figure 10.9), so for this simulation to work, all listeners need their own individual recordings.

Just as heads (and their corresponding ITDs and ILDs) grow to be larger, ears grow and change during development and are often subject to mutilations of varying degrees (e.g., piercings). Research suggests that listeners learn about the way HRTFs relate to places in the environment through their extensive experience listening to sounds, while other sources of information, such as vision, provide feedback about location (Wightman and Kistler, 1998). This learning through experience suggests that children may update the way they use HRTF information during development, and it appears that such learning can continue into adulthood. Hofman and colleagues (Hofman, Van Riswick, and Van Opsal, 1998) inserted plastic molds into folds of adults' pinnae. As expected, listeners immediately became much poorer at localizing sounds. After 6 weeks of living with these molds in their ears, however, the subjects' localization abilities greatly improved. Somewhat surprisingly, these listeners also remained quite good at localizing with their "old ears" when the molds were removed. It would be interesting to know how well Leonard

Nimoy (who played Spock in the original *Star Trek* series) could localize sounds with his Vulcan ear molds. The experience of listeners in this study suggests that switching between human and Vulcan pinnae everyday may have become just a normal part of Spock's auditory life.

Auditory Distance Perception

How do listeners know how far away a sound is? Although it is important to know what direction a sound is coming from, none of the cues we've discussed so far (ITD, ILD, HRTF) provide much information concerning the distance between a listener and a sound source that is much more than an arm's length away.

The simplest cue for judging the distance of a sound source is the *relative intensity* of the sound: Because sounds become less intense with greater distance, listeners have little difficulty perceiving the relative distances of two identical sound sources—for example, a pair of croaking bullfrogs. The louder croaks must be coming from the closer frog. Unfortunately, this cue suffers from the same problem as relative size in depth perception. Interpreting the cue requires one to make assumptions about the sound sources that may turn out to be false (e.g., the softer frog might be very close, but its croaks muffled by surrounding vegetation).

Furthermore, the effectiveness of relative intensity decreases substantially as distance increases because sound intensity decreases according to the **inverse-square law**. When sound sources are close to the listener, a small difference in distance can produce a relatively large intensity difference. For example, a sound that is 1 meter away is 6 decibels (dB) more intense than a sound that is 2 meters away. But the same 1-meter difference between sound sources 39 and 40 meters away produces an intensity change of only a fraction of 1 dB. As one might expect from these facts, listeners are fairly good at using intensity differences to determine distance when sounds are presented within 1 meter of the head (Brungart, Durlach, and Rabinowitz, 1999), but listeners tend to consistently underestimate the distance to sound sources farther away, and the amount of underestimation is larger for longer distances (Zahorik, 2002).

Intensity works best as a distance cue when the sound source or the listener is moving. If a frog starts hopping toward you, you will know it because its croaks will become louder and louder. Listeners also get some information about how far away a source is when they move through the environment. This is because, in a manner akin to motion parallax in the perception of visual depth, sounds that are farther away do not seem to change direction in relation to the listener as much as nearer sounds do.

Another possible cue for auditory distance is the *spectral composition* of sounds. The sound-absorbing qualities of air dampen high frequencies more than low frequencies, so when sound sources are far away, higher frequencies decrease in energy more than lower frequencies as the sound waves travel from the source to the ear. Thus, the farther away a sound source is, the "muddier" it sounds. This change in spectral composition is noticeable only for fairly large distances, greater than 1000 meters. You experience the change in spectral composition when you hear thunder from near your window to far away. Nearby, you hear a loud "crack," but farther away the sound is more like a "boom." Note that this auditory cue is analogous to the visual depth cue of aerial perspective (see Chapter 6; more distant objects look more blurry).

A final distance cue stems from the fact that, in most environments, the sound that arrives at the ear is some combination of direct energy (which arrives directly from the source) and reverberant energy (which has bounced

inverse-square law A principle stating that as distance from a source increases, intensity decreases faster such that decrease in intensity is the distance squared. This general law also applies to optics and other forms of energy.

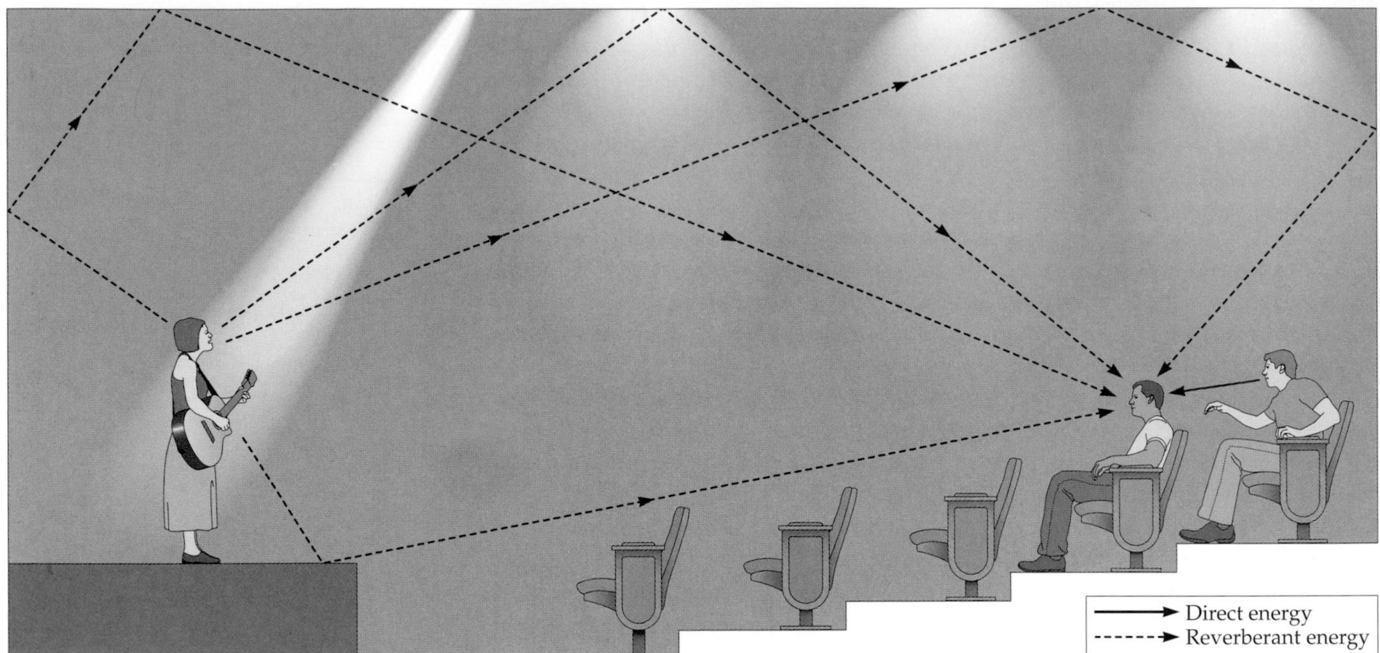

FIGURE 10.11 The relative amounts of direct and reverberant energy coming from the listener's neighbor and the singer will inform the listener of the relative distances of the two sound sources.

off surfaces in the environment). The *relative amounts of direct versus reverberant energy* inform the listener about distance because when a sound source is close to a listener, most of the energy reaching the ear is direct, whereas reverberant energy provides a greater proportion of the total when the sound source is farther away. Suppose you're attending a concert. The intensities of the musician's song and your neighbor's whispered comments might be identical, but the singer's voice will take time to bounce off the concert hall's walls before reaching your ear, whereas you will hear only the direct energy from the whispers (**Figure 10.11**). (See **Web Essay 10.1: Reverberations and the Precedence Effect.**)

Complex Sounds

Simple sounds like sine waves and bands of noise are very useful for exploring the fundamental operating characteristics of auditory systems, just as sinusoidal contrast gratings and single-wavelength light sources are crucial tools for vision researchers. But pure sine wave tones, like pure single-wavelength light sources, are rare in the real auditory world, where objects and events that matter to listeners are more complex, more interesting, and therefore more challenging for researchers to study.

Harmonics

Many environmental sounds, including the human voice and musical instruments, have harmonic structure (**Figure 10.12**). In fact, harmonic sounds are among the most common types of sounds in the environment. The lowest frequency of a harmonic spectrum is the **fundamental frequency**. With natural vibratory sources (as opposed to pure tones produced in the laboratory), there is also energy at frequencies that are integer multiples of the fundamental frequency. For example, a female speaker may produce a vowel sound with a fundamental frequency of 250 Hz. The vocal cords will produce the greatest energy at 250 Hz, less at 500 Hz, less still at 750 Hz,

fundamental frequency The lowest-frequency component of a complex periodic sound.

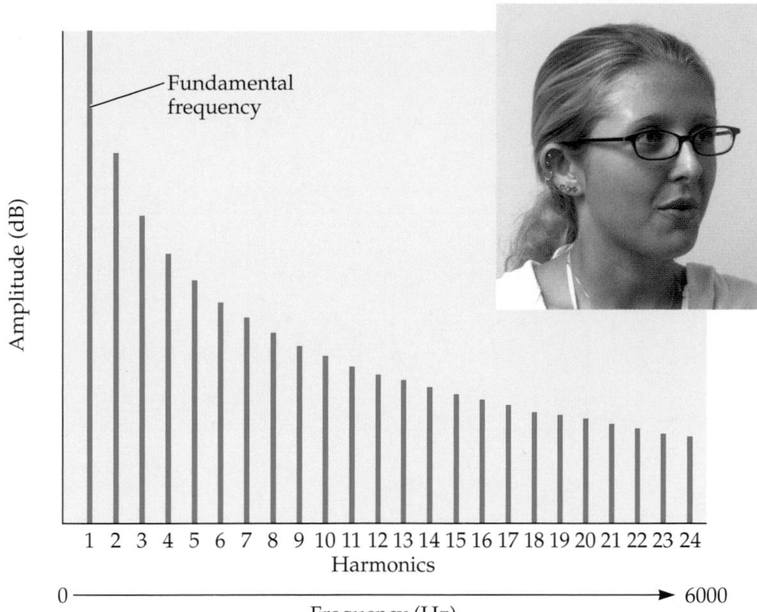

FIGURE 10.12 Many environmental sounds, including voices, are harmonic. The lowest frequency of a harmonic sound is the fundamental frequency, and there are peaks of energy at integer multiples of the fundamental.

even less at 1000 Hz, and so on. In this case, 500 Hz is the second harmonic, 750 Hz is the third harmonic, and 1000 Hz is the fourth harmonic. For harmonic complexes, the perceived pitch of the complex is determined by the fundamental frequency, and the harmonics (often called "overtones" by musicians) add to the perceived richness of the sound.

The auditory system is acutely sensitive to the natural relationships between harmonics. In fact, if the first harmonic (fundamental frequency) is removed from a series of harmonics as shown in **Figure 10.13**, and only the others (second, third, fourth, and so on) are presented, the pitch that listeners hear corresponds to the fundamental frequency—even though it is not part of the sound! Listeners hear the *missing fundamental*. (See **Web Activity 10.2: The Missing-Fundamental Effect**.) It is not even necessary to have all the other harmonics present in order to hear the missing fundamental; just a few will do.

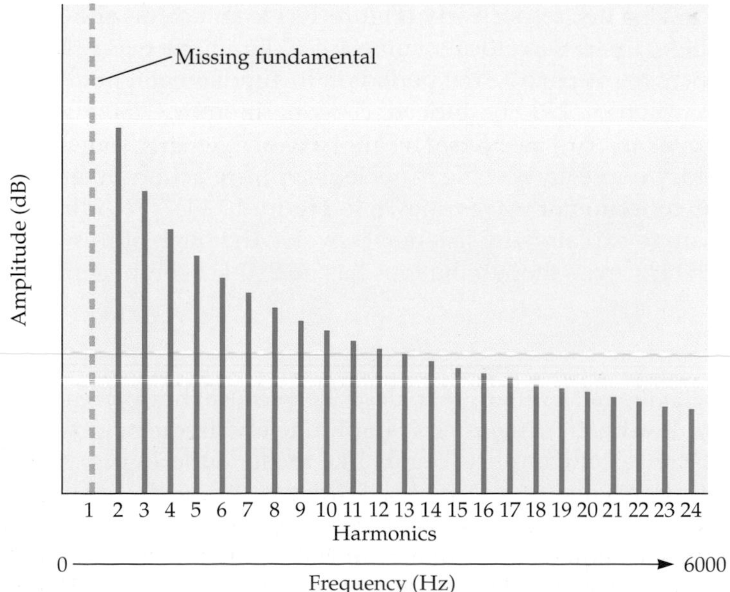

FIGURE 10.13 If the fundamental (lowest frequency) of a harmonic sound is removed, listeners still hear the pitch of this "missing fundamental."

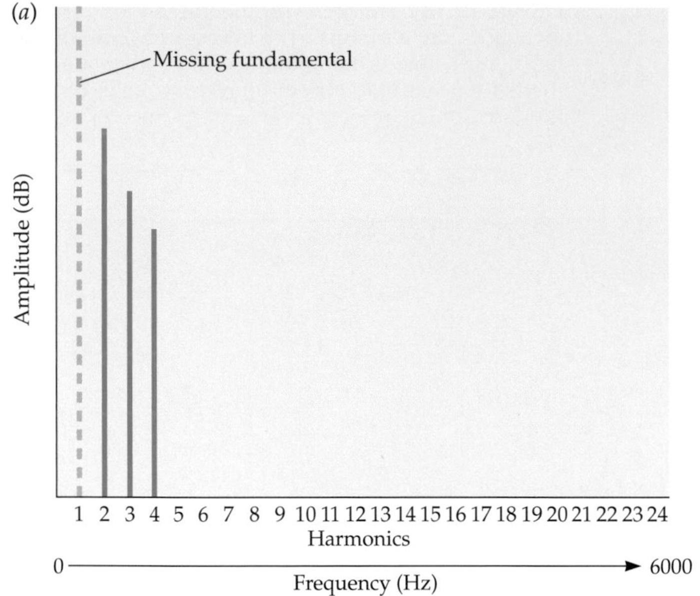

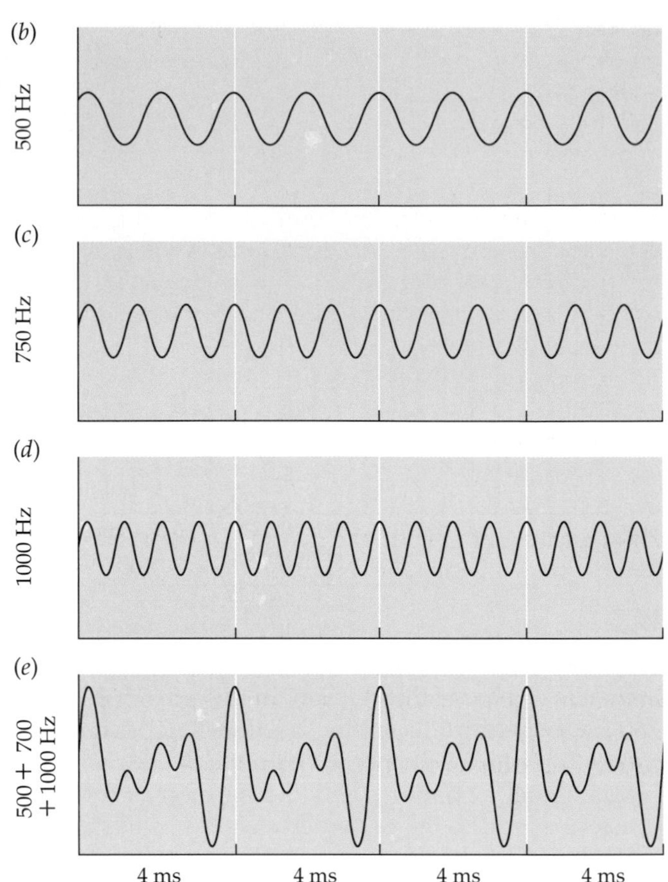

FIGURE 10.14 When only three harmonics of the same fundamental frequency are presented (*b–d*), listeners still hear the pitch of the missing fundamental frequency (*a*) because the harmonics share a common energy fluctuation every 4 ms, the period of a 250-Hz signal (*e*).

The most straightforward explanations of the missing-fundamental effect involve the temporal code for pitch discussed in Chapter 9. One thing that all harmonics of a fundamental have in common is fluctuations in sound pressure at regular intervals corresponding to the fundamental frequency. For example, the waveform for a 500-Hz tone has a peak every 2.0 milliseconds (ms) (**Figure 10.14***b*). The waveforms for 750- and 1000-Hz tones have peaks every 1.3 and 1.0 ms, respectively (Figure 10.14*c* and *d*). As shown in Figure 10.14*e*, these three waveforms come into alignment every 4 ms, which, conveniently, happens to be the period of the fundamental frequency for these three harmonics, 250 Hz. Indeed, *every* harmonic of 250 Hz will have an energy peak every 4 ms. Researchers have shown that some neurons in the auditory nerve and cochlear nucleus will fire action potentials every 4 ms to the collection of waves shown in Figure 10.14*e*, providing an elegant mechanism to explain why listeners perceive the pitch of this complex tone to be 250 Hz, even though the tone has no 250-Hz component.

Timbre

Loudness and pitch are relatively easy to describe because they correspond fairly well to simple acoustic dimensions (amplitude and frequency, respectively). But the richness of complex sounds like those found in our world depends on more than simple sensations of loudness and pitch. For example, a trombone and a tenor saxophone might play the same note (that is, a note with exactly the same fundamental frequency) at exactly the same loudness (the sound waves have identical intensities), but we would have no trouble discerning that two different instruments were being played. The perceptual quality that differs between these two musical instruments, as well as between vowel sounds such as those in the words *hot*, *heat*, and *hoot*, is known as **timbre**. (See Web Activity 10.3: Timbre.)

timbre The psychological sensation by which a listener can judge that two sounds with the same loudness and pitch are dissimilar. Timbre quality is conveyed by harmonics and other high frequencies.

What exactly is timbre? You won't find an answer to this question in the dictionary, because the official definition of *timbre* is "the quality that makes listeners hear two different sounds even though both sounds have the same pitch and loudness" (American Standards Association, 1960). However, differences in timbre between musical instruments or vowel sounds can be estimated closely by comparison of the extent to which the overall spectra of two sounds overlap (Plomp, 1976). Perception of visual color depends on the relative levels of energy at different wavelengths (see Chapter 5), and very similarly, perception of timbre is related to the relative energy of different acoustic spectral components. For example, the trombone and tenor saxophone notes shown in **Figure 10.15** share the same fundamental frequency (middle C, 262 Hz). However, note that the trombone's third (786-Hz) component is stronger than its fourth (1048-Hz) component, whereas for the saxophone, the relationship between the energies of these two components is reversed.

Perception of timbre depends on the context in which a sound is heard. Different environments change sounds in different ways. For example, higher frequencies tend to be reinforced by hard surfaces such as tile floors and concrete walls, but they are dampened by soft surfaces such as thick carpet and drapes or curtains. This is much like the problem of maintaining

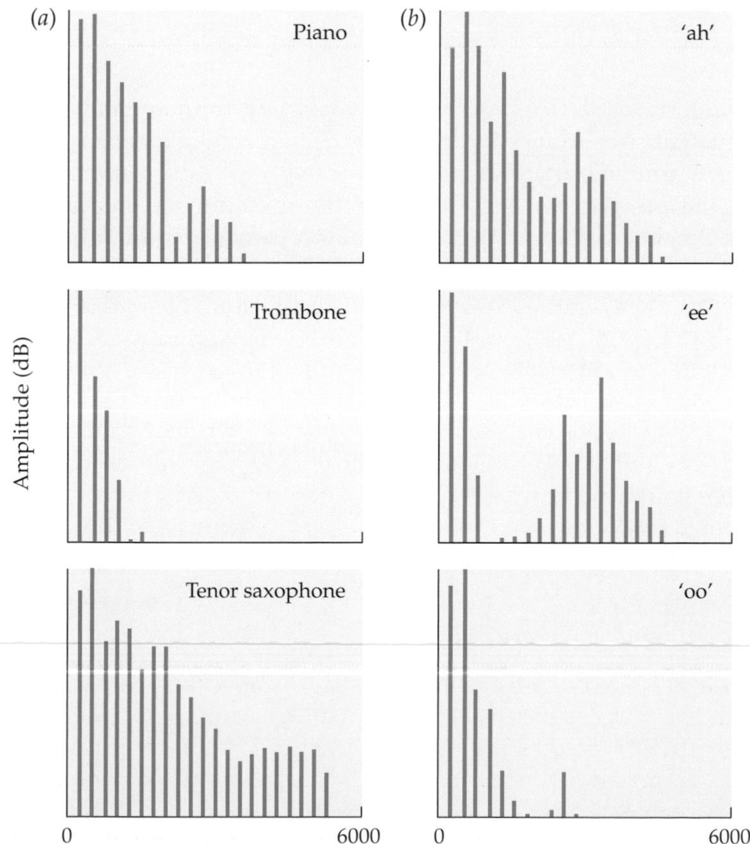

FIGURE 10.15 Timbre. (*a*) Three different musical instruments playing the same note (middle C, 262 Hz) sound different because they have different spectral shapes. (*b*) Three vowels produced by the same female talker, also with a fundamental frequency of 262 Hz, sound very different to listeners.

color constancy when different illuminants alter the composition of wavelengths that reach the eyes. Kiefte and Kluender (2008) used the different spectral shapes of the vowel sounds 'ee' and 'oo' to learn how our ears calibrate for changes in listening environment. They took advantage of the fact that the spectra for 'ee' and 'oo' differ in two important ways (**Figure 10.16***a*). The vowel sound 'ee' has a relatively flat spectrum with almost as much energy in high frequencies as in low frequencies. In contrast, energy in 'oo' is dominated by low frequencies that have less and less energy as frequency increases. We can say that the "tilt" of the 'ee' spectrum is much flatter than the tilt of 'oo.' The sounds 'ee' and 'oo' differ also in terms of where their spectra show peaks. The second peak in the 'ee' spectrum is at a higher frequency than the second peak in the 'oo' spectrum. Listeners use both tilt and the frequency of this second peak to tell 'ee' from 'oo' (Figure 10.16*b*) (Kiefte and Kluender, 2005).

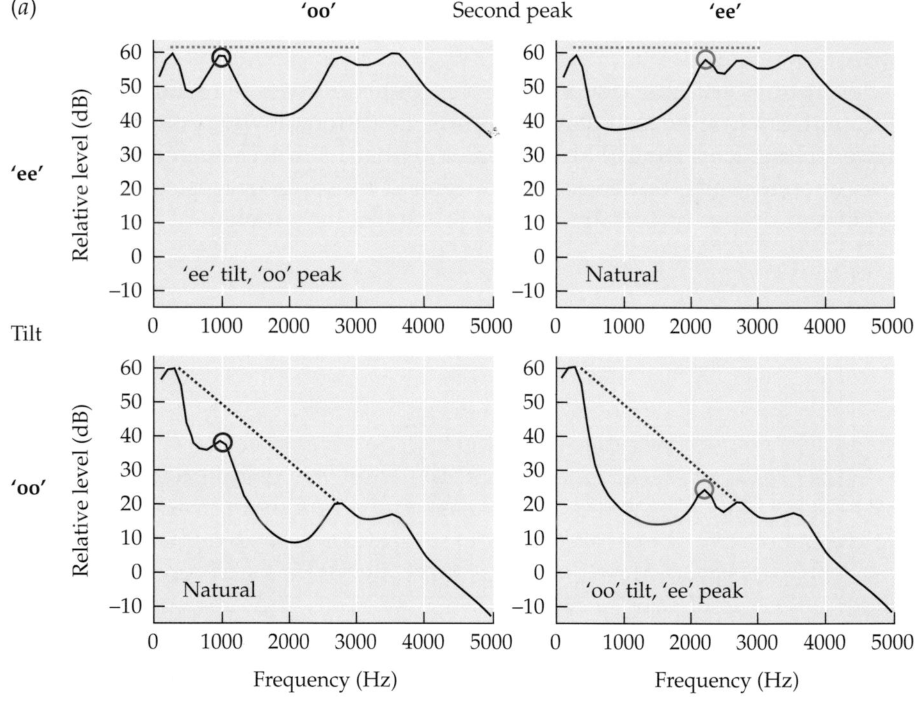

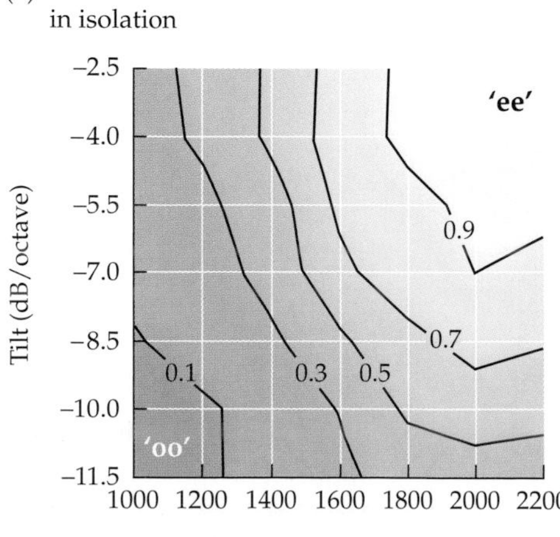

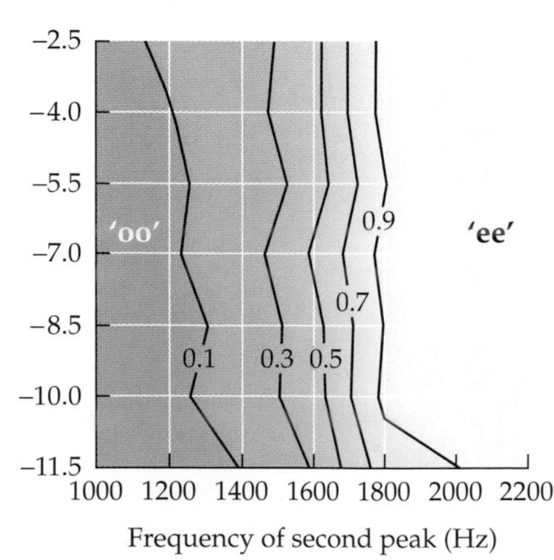

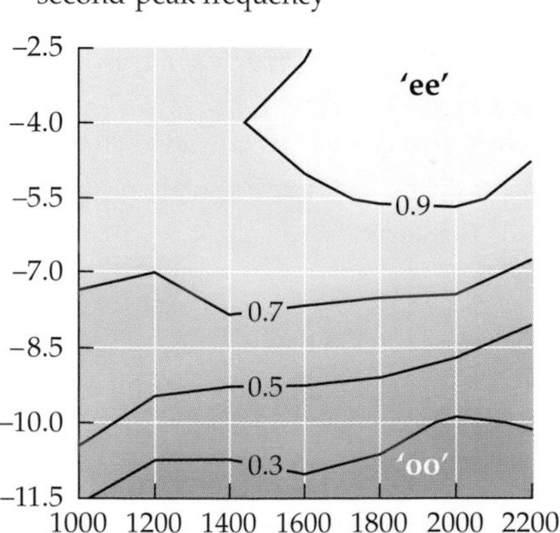

FIGURE 10.16 Listeners use both spectral tilt and the frequencies of spectral peaks to identify vowels. (*a*) Spectra of natural 'ee' and 'oo' are shown in the upper right and lower left, respectively. The vowel 'ee' has a relatively flat spectrum, and 'oo' has a tilted spectrum, such that there is much less energy at higher frequencies. The second spectral peak is lower in frequency for 'oo' than for 'ee.' Experimentally manipulated vowel sounds are also shown with the tilt of 'ee' and second peak of 'oo' in the upper left, and the tilt of 'oo' and second peak of 'ee' in the lower right. (*b*) Listeners use both tilt and frequency of the second peak to identify vowels. Lighter areas correspond to sounds that subjects hear as 'ee' and darker areas are sounds that listeners hear as 'oo.' (*c*) Upon hearing vowels after a sentence that has the same tilt as the following vowel, listeners use only the frequency of the second peak to identify the vowel. (*d*) However, when the preceding sentence includes a peak at the same frequency as the second peak in the vowel, listeners use mostly tilt to identify the vowel.

In order to learn how the auditory system adjusts for listening context, Kiefte and Kluender (2008) created stimuli that changed in both tilt and frequency of the second peak. Then, they had listeners identify these vowels following a sentence like "you will now hear the vowel" but with an interesting twist. They created some sentences so that the overall tilt of the sentence was the same as the tilt of the following vowel. To other sentences they added a peak in the spectrum all the way through the sentence at the same frequency as the second peak in the vowel that listeners would identify. Listeners heard these vowels in dramatically different ways depending on the spectral composition of the sentence that preceded them. When tilt stayed the same for both the preceding sentence and the vowel, listeners used only the frequency of the second peak to identify the vowel (Figure 10.16*c*). When the second peak was present all the way through the preceding sentence, listeners relied mostly on tilt to identify the vowels (Figure 10.16*d*).

Listeners calibrate for reliable spectral characteristics of a listening context much as observers calibrate for the spectral composition of illuminating light when perceiving color. When a particular spectral tilt is heard as a property of the context in which a sound is heard, listeners ignore tilt of the vowel as if it were a characteristic of the listening environment, not of the vowel. The same is true for the second spectral peak. More broadly, auditory color constancy is an example of the general principle that perceptual systems respond most robustly to change. When tilt or the added spectral peak is unchanging between sentence and vowel, it is ignored perceptually.

Attack and Decay

Another very important quality of a complex sound is the way it begins (the **attack** of the sound) and ends (the sound's **decay**). Our auditory systems are very sensitive to attack and decay characteristics. For example, as you will learn in Chapter 11, important contrasts between speech sounds in the words *bill* versus *will* or the words *cheat* versus *sheet* relate to differences in how quickly sound energy increases at the onset (the speed of attack).

The same musical instrument can have quite different attacks, from the rapid attack of a plucked violin string to the gradual attack of a bowed string (**Figure 10.17***a* and *b*). How quickly a sound decays depends on how long it takes for the vibrating object creating the sound (e.g., the violin string) to dissipate energy and stop moving. One of the more challenging aspects of designing music synthesizers that could mimic real musical instruments was learning how to mimic the attacks and decays of the instruments.

To appreciate the importance of attack and decay in sound quality, explore Web Activity 10.3: Timbre, where you will first hear a normal piano recording. The sound of a piano note is caused by a small hammer hitting a string. The amplitude of the resulting sound increases very quickly before more gradually dissipating. If a recording of a piano note is played backward, the sound no longer even remotely resembles that of a piano. Instead, the backward piano note sounds more like the same note played on an accordion.

Auditory Scene Analysis

The acoustic environment can be a busy place. In most natural situations, the sound source to which one is listening is not the only source present. Consider, for example, conversing with a friend at a party where many other people are talking, music is playing, chips are being munched, the door is being opened and closed, and so on. Now consider simpler environments,

attack The part of a sound during which amplitude increases (onset).

decay The part of a sound during which amplitude decreases (offset).

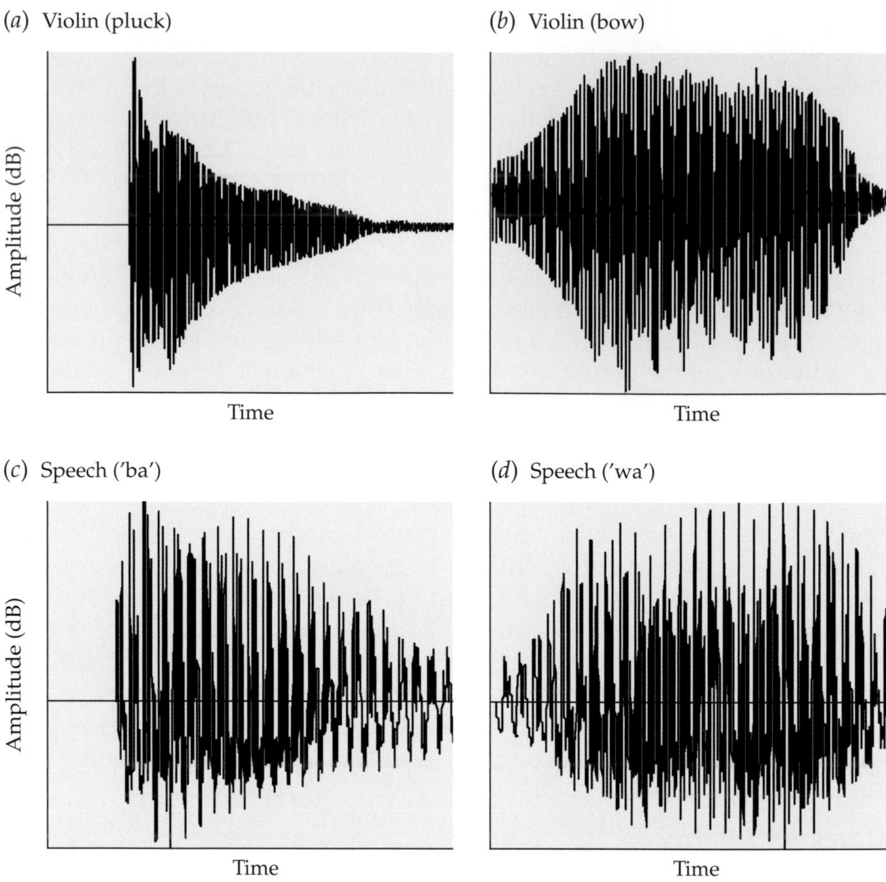

FIGURE 10.17 We use the onsets of sounds (attacks) to identify them. Attacks are quite different when a violin string is plucked (*a*) versus bowed (*b*). Similarly, different speech sounds, such as 'ba' (*c*) and 'wa' (*d*), have different attacks.

such as those you choose for studying. To read this chapter, you probably chose the spot where you are right now because it was relatively quiet, but stop and listen carefully. Is there the hum of a heater, air conditioner, computer, refrigerator, or some combination of these devices in the background? Can you hear people talking somewhere in the vicinity? Are chair legs sliding across floors? Places with only a single sound source are very uncommon. Indeed, there are few truly quiet places outside the laboratories of hearing scientists and the testing chambers of audiologists.

Environments with multiple sound sources are the rule, not the exception. How does the auditory system sort out these sources? Note that the visual system also has to contend with a busy world, but eyes can be directed to any part of the scene of interest to the visual system. Moreover, the rods and cones on the right side of the retina always see the objects on the left, politely leaving the receptors on the other side of the retina to collect data about objects on the right. For an auditory scene, the situation is greatly complicated by the fact that all the sound waves from all the sound sources in the environment are summed together in a single complex sound wave (**Figure 10.18**). You can move your ears around all you want, but everyone's voice at the party still has to be picked up by the same two sets of cochlear hair cells.

Somehow, however, the auditory system contends quite well with the situation: our perception is typically of a world with easily separable sounds. We can understand the conversation of a dance partner at a party, and we can pick out a favorite instrument in the band. This distinction of auditory events or objects in the broader auditory environment is commonly referred to as **source segregation** or **auditory scene analysis**.

source segregation (or auditory scene analysis) Processing an auditory scene consisting of multiple sound sources into separate sound images.

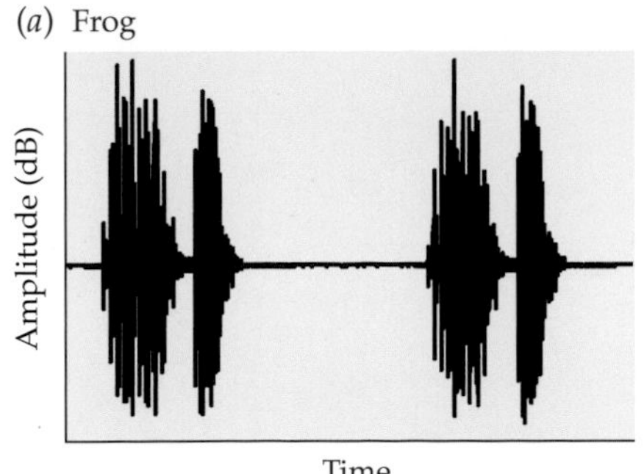

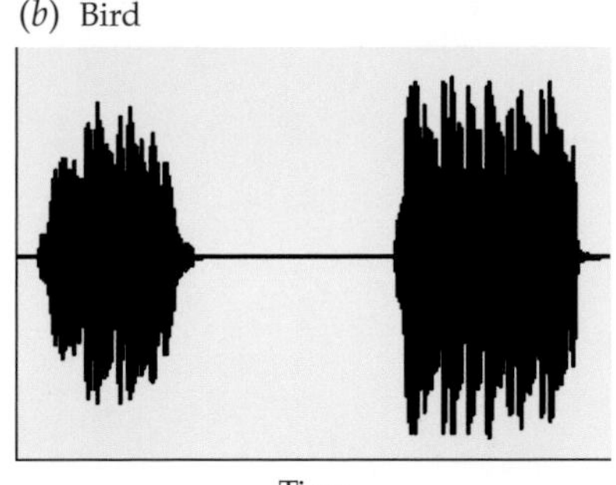

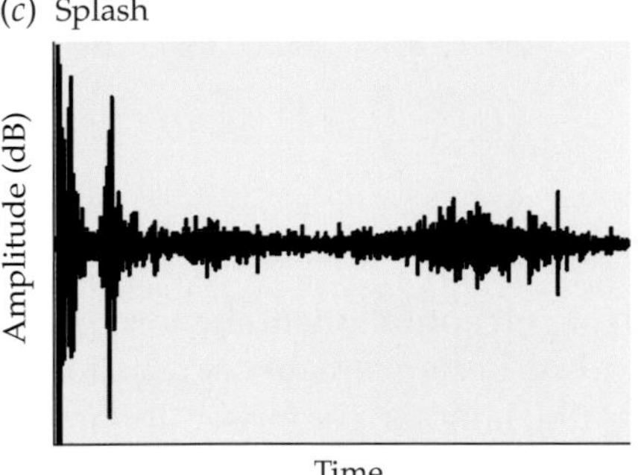

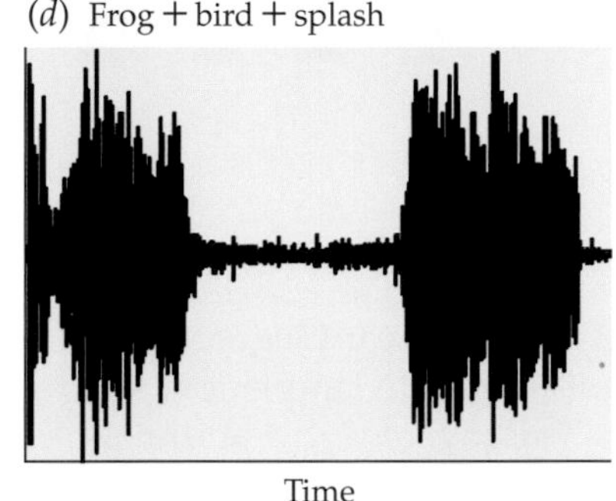

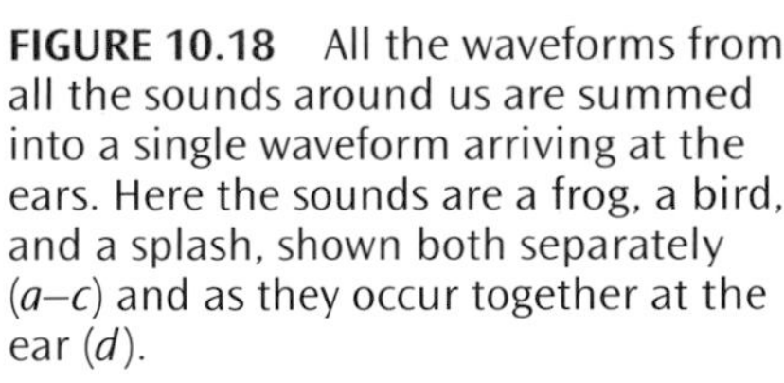

FIGURE 10.18 All the waveforms from all the sounds around us are summed into a single waveform arriving at the ears. Here the sounds are a frog, a bird, and a splash, shown both separately (*a–c*) and as they occur together at the ear (*d*).

Spatial, Spectral, and Temporal Segregation

The auditory system uses a number of strategies to segregate sound sources. One of the most obvious strategies is to use *spatial separation* between sounds. Sounds that emanate from the same location in space can typically be treated as if they arose from the same source. Moreover, in a natural environment in which sound sources move, a sound that is perceived to move in space can more easily be separated from background sounds that are relatively stationary. Listeners move too, so if a sound stays in the same place relative to the path of a listener, it will be easier for that sound to be sorted out from other sounds.

In addition to location, sounds can be segregated on the basis of their spectral or temporal qualities. For example, sounds with the same or similar pitch are more likely to be treated as coming from the same source and to be segregated from other sounds. Sounds that are perceived to emanate from the same source are often described as being part of the same *auditory stream*, and dividing the auditory world into separate auditory objects is known as **auditory stream segregation**.

A very simple example of auditory stream segregation involves two tones with similar frequencies that are alternated (see **Figure 10.19***a* and Web Activity 10.4: Auditory Stream Segregation). This sequence sounds like a single coherent stream of tones that warble up and down in frequency. But if the alternating tones are markedly different in frequency (Figure 10.19*b*), two streams of tones are heard—one higher in pitch than the other (G. A. Miller and Heise, 1950).

One way to measure whether a series of sounds has been broken into separate streams is to ask listeners to report the order of the tones. For example, Bregman and Campbell (1971) asked listeners to report the order of high (H) and low (L) tones—for example, HLHLHL or HHLLHH—for different sequences of tones with frequencies of 2500, 2000, 1600, 550, 430, and 350 Hz. When tones were presented rapidly (10 per second), listeners could not identify the order. Indeed, the majority of listeners actually reported hearing two separate streams of all high (2500, 2000, 1600) or all low (550, 430, 350) tones.

auditory stream segregation The perceptual organization of a complex acoustic signal into separate auditory events for which each stream is heard as a separate event.

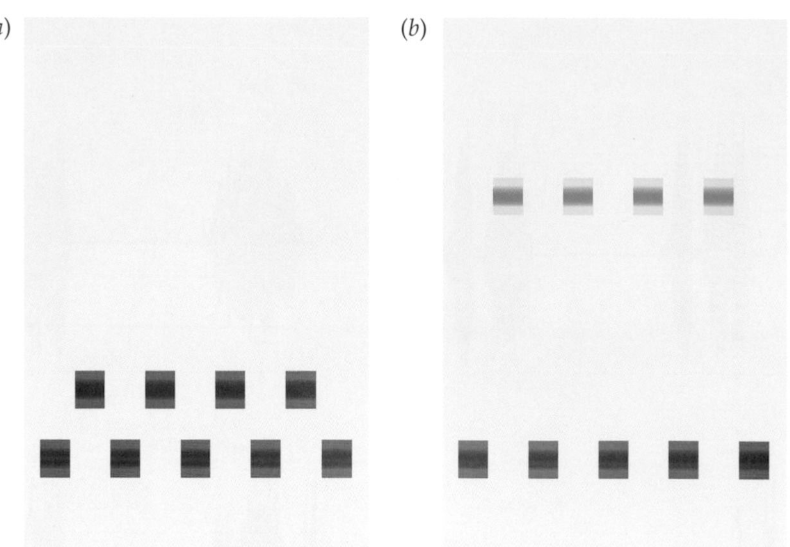

FIGURE 10.19 When tones that are close in frequency occur in rapid succession, they are heard as a single warbling stream (*a*), but when successive tones have very different frequencies, they are heard as two separate streams (*b*).

Auditory stream segregation is a powerful perceptual phenomenon that is not limited to simple tones in the laboratory. Before stream segregation was "discovered" by auditory scientists, the famous composer Johann Sebastian Bach exploited these auditory effects in his compositions (**Figure 10.20**). The same instrument, such as a pipe organ, would rapidly play interleaved sequences of low and high notes. Even though the musician played a sequence in the order H1L1H2L2H3L3, listeners heard two melodies—one high (H1H2H3) and one low (L1L2L3). (See **Web Activity 10.4: Auditory Stream Segregation**.) This bit of knowledge about auditory perception was known not only to Bach, but also to other Baroque composers of the seventeenth and early eighteenth centuries.

When thinking about auditory scene analysis, it is sometimes useful to describe effects using Gestalt principles such as those described for vision in Chapter 4. Instances of auditory stream segregation described in this section can be described as applications of the Gestalt principle of *similarity* (see Figure 4.10*a* in Chapter 4): sounds that are similar to each other tend to be grouped together into streams.

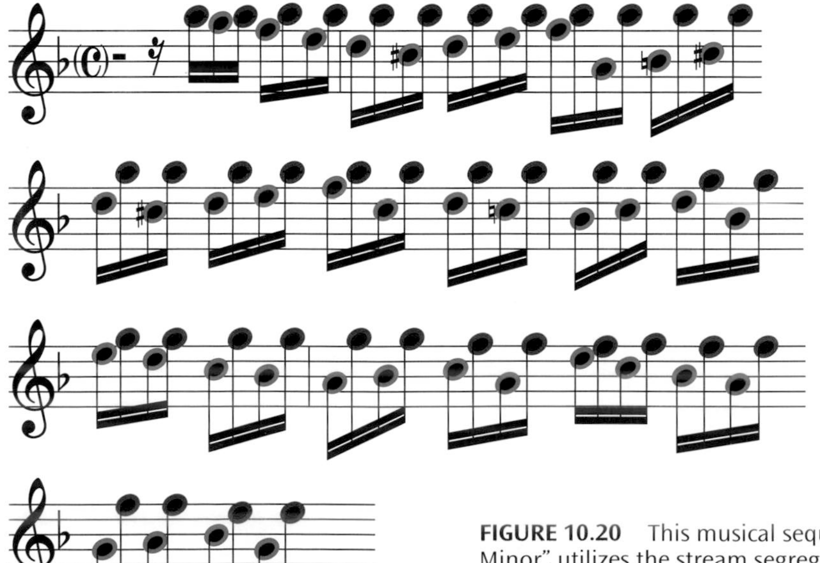

FIGURE 10.20 This musical sequence from J. S. Bach's "Toccata and Fugue in D Minor" utilizes the stream segregation principles "discovered" by auditory researchers in the twentieth century. When played in rapid succession, the higher notes (red) are heard as one melody separate from the lower notes (blue).

Grouping by Timbre

When a sequence of tones that have increasing and decreasing frequencies is presented (**Figure 10.21***a*), tones that deviate from the rising/falling pattern are heard to "pop out" of the sequence (Heise and Miller, 1951). What happens when two patterns overlap in frequency—one increasing then decreasing in frequency, and one decreasing then increasing in frequency (Figure 10.21*b*)? If the tones are simple sine waves, two streams of sound are heard without overlapping pitches (Figure 10.21*b*, left); one stream includes all the

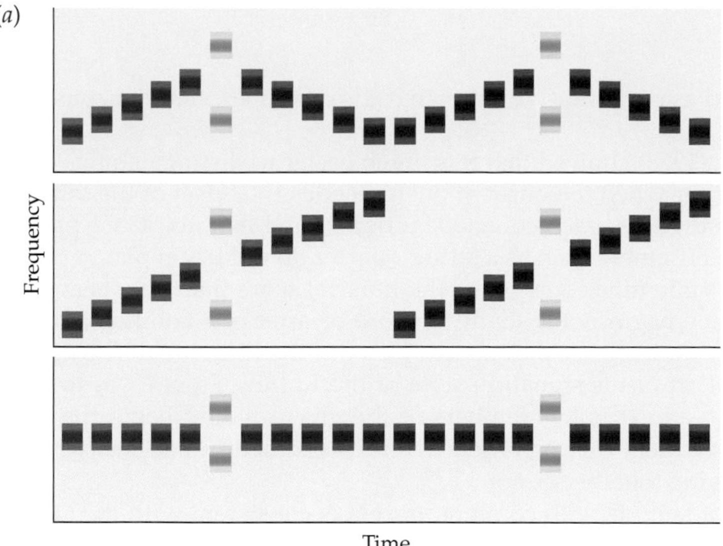

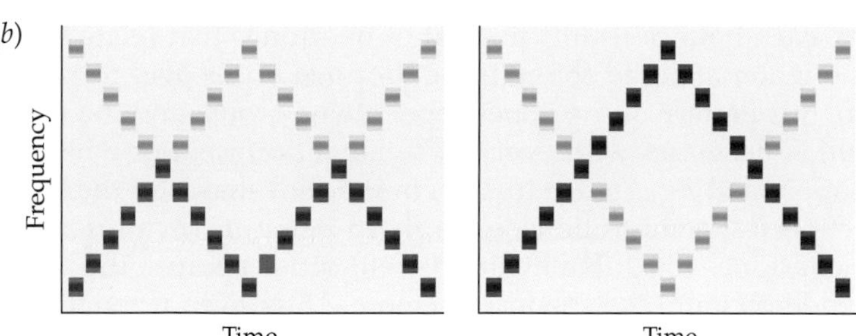

FIGURE 10.21 Timbre affects how sounds are grouped. (*a*) Individual tones (green) "pop out" of a stream if they do not fit the patterns of rising or falling frequency for the other tones (red). (*b*) Sounds that share the same timbre group together. When sounds in a succession all share the same timbre (left), they are heard as streams according to similar frequency. However, if sounds have different timbres (right), they will separate according to timbre, even if their frequencies cross another pattern with a different timbre.

high tones and one includes all the low tones. However, if harmonics are added to one of the sequences, thus creating a richer timbre, two overlapping patterns are heard as distinct (Figure 10.21*b*, right) (van Noorden, 1975).

Auditory stream segregation on the basis of groups of notes with similar timbres can be seen as another example of the principle of similarity at work. Grouping by timbre is a particularly robust application of this principle because sounds with similar timbre usually arise from the same sound source. This principle thus helps listeners pick out the melody played on a single instrument—a trombone, for example—even when another instrument, such as a saxophone, plays a different or even opposite sequence of notes (Wessel, 1979).

Neural processes that give rise to stream segregation can be found throughout the auditory system, from the first stages of auditory processing to primary auditory cortex (A1), as well as secondary areas of auditory cortex such as belt and parabelt areas (J. S. Snyder and Alain, 2007). There is neural evidence of stream segregation, based on simple cues such as frequencies of tones, in the brain stem; but segregation based on more sophisticated perceptual properties of sounds is more likely to take place in the cortex.

Grouping by Onset

In addition to timbre, sound components that begin at the same time, or nearly the same time, such as the harmonics of a music or speech sound, will also tend to be heard as coming from the same sound source. One way in which this phenomenon helps us is by grouping different harmonics into a single complex tone. Frequency components with different onset times are less likely to be grouped. For example, if a single harmonic of a vowel sound is made to begin before the rest of the harmonics of the vowel, it is less likely to be perceived as part of the vowel than if the onsets are simultaneous (C. J. Darwin, 1984).

R. A. Rasch (1978) showed that it is much easier to distinguish two notes from one another when the onset of one precedes the onset of the other by only three-hundredths of a second (30 ms). He noted that musicians playing together in an ensemble such as a string quartet do not begin playing notes at exactly the same time, even when the musical score instructs them to do so. Instead, they begin notes slightly before or after one another, and this staggered start probably helps listeners pick out the individual instruments in the group. Part of the signature style of the Rolling Stones was to carry this practice to an extreme. Members of the group would begin the same beat with such widely varying onsets that it was sometimes unclear whether they were playing together or not.

Grouping of sounds with common onsets is consistent with the Gestalt law of *common fate*. Consider the consequences of dropping a bottle on a hard surface and listening for whether or not the bottle breaks. When any object bounces, each bounce results in a set of overtones that relate to the size, shape, and material of the object. If the dropped bottle does not break (**Figure 10.22***a*), this pattern of overtones repeats as a group, and the intensity of the sounds decreases with every additional bounce. But when the bottle breaks upon landing (Figure 10.22*b*), individual shards of the bottle have different spectral compositions, each shard being its own resonator. Onsets of the overtones for different shards will differ because the pieces bounce independently until they bounce no more. Thus, even when the initial burst of noise is removed from the sound of the bouncing and breaking bottles, listeners can use patterns of onsets to accurately determine whether the bottle broke (W. H. Warren and Verbrugge, 1984).

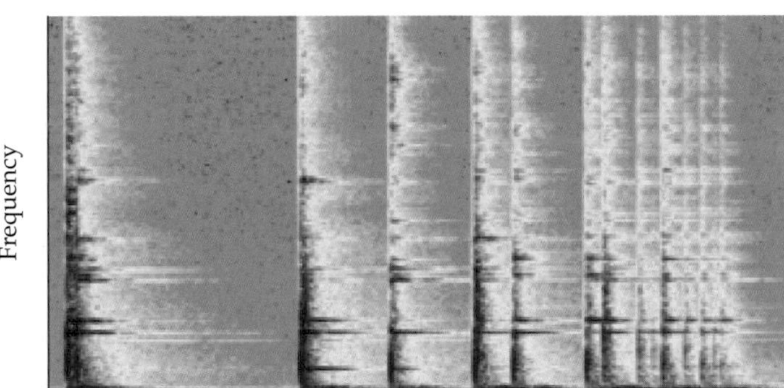

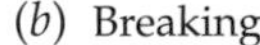

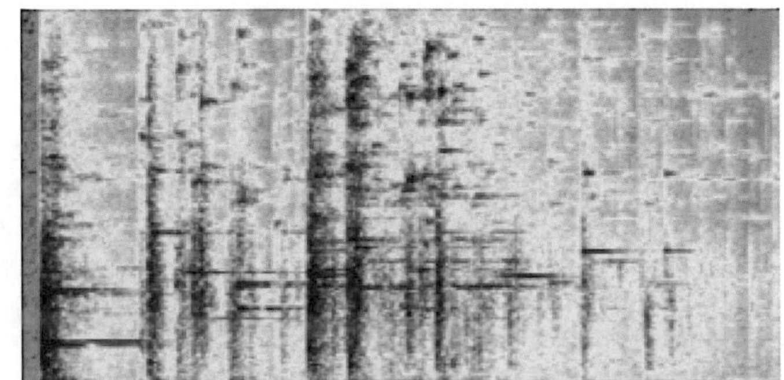

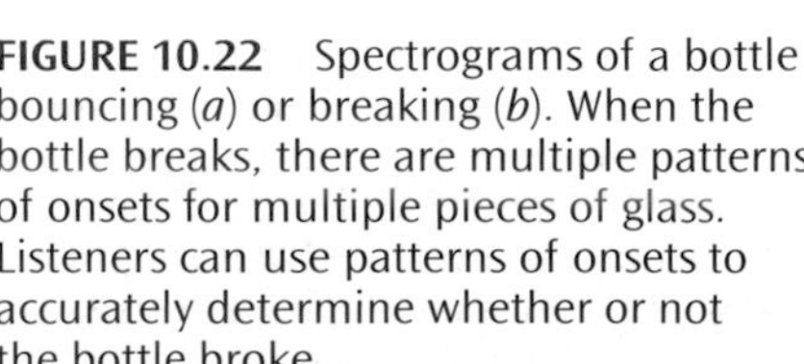
FIGURE 10.22 Spectrograms of a bottle bouncing (*a*) or breaking (*b*). When the bottle breaks, there are multiple patterns of onsets for multiple pieces of glass. Listeners can use patterns of onsets to accurately determine whether or not the bottle broke.

Continuity and Restoration Effects

As already discussed, the sound we're trying to listen to at any given time is usually not the only sound in the environment. In addition to dealing with overlapping auditory streams, we also often have to deal with the total masking of one sound source by another for brief periods. Suppose you're listening on your cell phone as a friend gives you directions to the restaurant where you're to meet for lunch. A car may honk, a baby may cry, or your cell phone may produce a short burst of static, but if you are paying attention and the interruption is not too long, you will probably be able to "hear through" the interruption. This effect is consistent with the Gestalt principle of *good continuation* (see Figure 4.7): the continuous auditory stream is heard to continue behind the masking sound. Auditory researchers have labeled the phenomena "continuity effects" or "perceptual restoration effects"—the latter label arising because the auditory system appears to restore the portion of the continuous stream that was blocked out by the interrupting sound (R. M. Warren, 1984). In this sense, auditory restoration is analogous to the visual system's filling in the portions of a background object that is sitting behind an occluding object.

Continuity effects have been demonstrated in the laboratory with a wide variety of target sounds and interrupting sounds. The simplest version of such an experiment is to delete portions of a pure tone and replace them with noise (**Figure 10.23***a*). The tone will sound continuous if the noise is intense enough to have masked the tone, had it been present (R. M. Warren, 1984).

How do we know that listeners really hear a sound as continuous in experiments such as this? One of the best ways to determine what people really perceive is to use a signal detection task. Kluender and Jenison (1992) utilized signal detection methodology with a slightly more complex version of the continuity effect (Figure 10.23*b*). In their experiments, listeners heard tone *glides*, in which a sine wave tone varies continuously in frequency over time (the resulting sound is similar to that of a slide whistle). When intense noise is superimposed over part of the glide, listeners report hearing the glide continue behind the noise. (See **Web Activity 10.5: Continuity and Restoration Effects**.) Kluender and Jenison prepared stimuli in which the middle portion of the glide either was present with the noise or was completely removed. In trials in which the noise was shortest and most intense, the signal detection measure of discriminability (d') dropped to 0. For these trials, then, perceptual restoration was complete: listeners had no idea whether or not the glide was actually present with the noise.

The compelling nature of perceptual restoration suggests that at some point the restored missing sounds are encoded in the brain as if they were

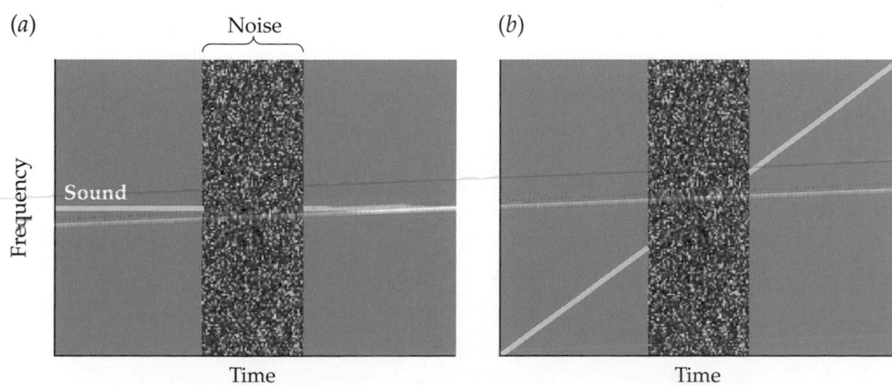

FIGURE 10.23 When a sound is deleted and replaced with a loud noise, listeners will hear the sound as if it continues through the noise. This is true when a tone maintains the same frequency (*a*) and when the tone steadily increases or decreases in frequency (*b*).

actually present in the signal. Imaging studies of humans, who can report when they do and do not hear the tone through the noise, show activity in primary auditory cortex (A1) that is consistent with what listeners report hearing, whether or not the tone is present (Riecke et al., 2007). Neurons that show similar responses to real and restored frequency glides have been found in A1 of cats. Sugita (1997) trained cats to respond according to whether or not there was a gap in a tonal glide. He then added noise across the gap and found that, when the noise was sufficiently more intense than the glide, the cats became less accurate in their responses. In A1, some neurons are particularly responsive to sounds that change in frequency. When Sugita played glides with gaps, the response of these neurons decreased. However, when noise more intense than the tones filled these gaps, the neurons responded as vigorously as they had for intact glides with no gaps.

These data from the auditory cortex cannot tell us whether restoration of the glides occurred in the cortex or at an point earlier in auditory processing. However, they make it easier to understand why perceptually restored sounds really sound present.

Restoration of Complex Sounds

Perceptual restoration also occurs for complex sounds such as music and speech. When Sasaki (1980) played familiar piano melodies with one or two notes excised and replaced by noise, listeners perceived the missing notes as having been present. Restoration was so complete that listeners could not report which notes had been removed and replaced with noise.

Just as compelling, if not more so, is perceptual restoration in speech. R. M. Warren and Obusek (1971) played the sentence "the state governors met with their respective legi*latures convening in the capital city" with the first *s* in *legislatures* removed and replaced by silence, a cough, a burst of noise, or any of a few other sounds. Despite the missing *s*, listeners heard the sentence as if it were intact and complete. Even when listeners were explicitly warned that a small part of the sentence had been removed and replaced with silence or another sound, they were unable to accurately report where the sentence had been changed, except when the missing *s* was replaced with silence.

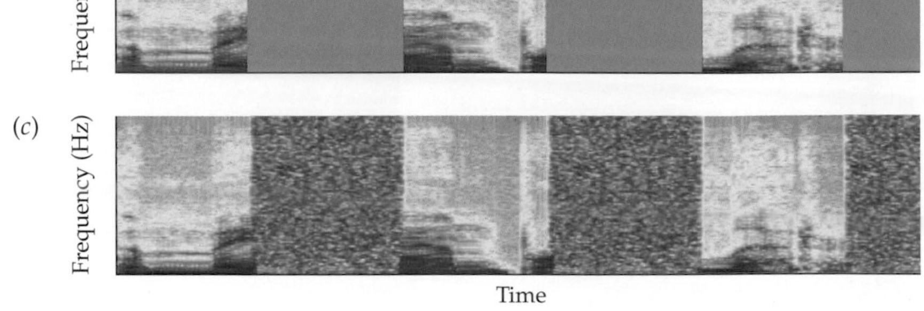

FIGURE 10.24 Adding noise improves comprehension. (*a*) Spectrogram of the sentence "the mailman brought a letter." (*b*) Listeners have great difficulty understanding the sentence when intervals are removed and replaced with silence. (*c*) When the same intervals are replaced by noise, however, it becomes easier to understand the sentence, because of perceptual restoration. (After Bashford and Warren, 1987.)

Listening to familiar melodies and to real speech sentences, as opposed to simple sounds such as sine waves and tonal glides, permits listeners to use more than just auditory processing to fill in missing information. Clearly, these "higher-order" sources of information are used for listening to sources in the face of other acoustic clutter. In a particularly compelling example, listeners restored a missing sound on the basis of linguistic information that followed the deletion (R. M. Warren and Sherman, 1974). For example, Warren and Sherman played utterances such as "The *eel fell off the car" and "The *eel fell off the table" (the asterisk represents a patch of noise). Listeners were much more likely to report hearing "wheel" in the former utterance and "meal" in the latter, even though the context information came well after the missing phoneme in the sentences. (See **Web Activity 10.5: Continuity and Restoration Effects**.) As this result hints, meaningful sentences actually become more intelligible when gaps are filled with intense noise than when gaps are left silent (**Figure 10.24**). Think about this: adding noise improves comprehension!

Summary

1. Listeners use small differences, in time and intensity, across the two ears to learn the direction in the horizontal plane (azimuth) from which a sound comes.
2. Time and intensity differences across the two ears are not sufficient to fully indicate the location from which a sound comes. In particular, time and intensity differences are not sufficient to indicate whether sounds come from the front or the back, or from higher or lower (elevation).
3. The pinna, ear canal, head, and torso alter the intensities of different frequencies for sounds coming from different places in space, and listeners use these changes in intensity across frequency to identify the location from which a sound comes.
4. Perception of auditory distance is similar to perception of visual depth because no single characteristic of the signal can inform a listener about how distant a sound source is. Listeners must combine intensity, spectral composition, and relative amounts of direct and reflected energy of sounds to estimate distance to a sound source.
5. Many natural sounds, including musical instruments and human speech, have rich harmonic structure with energy at integer multiples of the fundamental frequency, and listeners are especially good at perceiving the pitch of harmonic sounds.
6. Important perceptual qualities of complex sounds are timbre, conveyed by the relative amounts of energy at different frequencies, and onset and offset properties of attack and decay, respectively.
7. Because all the sounds in the environment are summed into a single waveform that reaches each ear, a major challenge for hearing is to separate sound sources in the combined signal. This general process is known as auditory scene analysis. Sound source segregation succeeds by using multiple characteristics of sounds, including spatial location, similarity in frequency and timbre, and onset properties.
8. In everyday environments, sounds to which a person is listening often are interrupted by other, louder sounds. Perceptual restoration is a process by which missing or degraded acoustic signals are perceptually replaced.

Refer to the
Sensation and Perception
website
(www.sinauer.com/wolfe2e)
for activities, essays, study questions, and other study aids.

CHAPTER 11

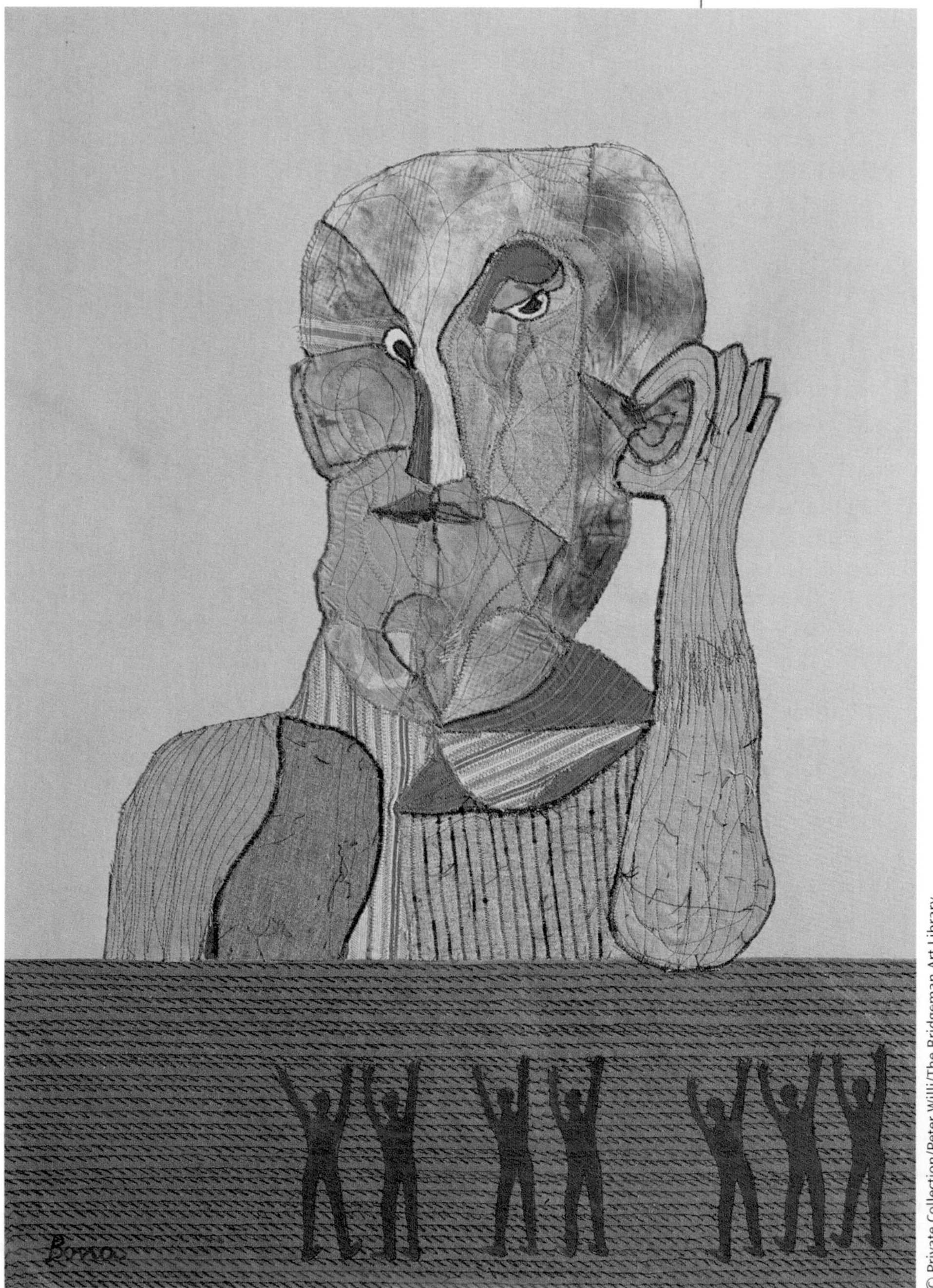

Bona de Mandiargues, *Personnage se Tenant la Tete*

Music and Speech Perception

An ear can break a human heart
As quickly as a spear
We wish the ear had not a heart
So dangerously near

— "The Saddest Noise, the Sweetest Noise," by Emily Dickinson

Sounds from musical instruments and human vocal tracts obey the same laws of physical acoustics as all other sounds. Guitar strings and human vocal folds are vibratory structures, with similarities to rubber bands and suspension bridges. Trombones and vocal tracts act as resonators following the same laws as empty bottles and hollow logs. In this sense, spoken words and musical notes are nothing more than very familiar, complex sounds.

In other ways, however, music and speech can be distinguished from most other environmental sounds. Much like visual art such as paintings and sculpture, music and speech are created with perceivers in mind. Music and speech both serve to communicate, and both can convey emotion and deeper meanings. In song, music and speech conspire to move the listener. Although birds, whales, and other animals do share acoustic messages and even sing to one another, there is no question that the depth and breadth of human communication by music and language has no rival in the acoustic world. In this chapter we delve into these communicative aspects of hearing: music and speech.

Music

People have been using music as a way to express themselves and influence the thoughts and emotions of others at least as far back as the Shang dynasty of China (1600–1100 BCE). You probably know the great ancient Greek scholar Pythagoras (c.580–c.500 BCE) from the Pythagorean theorem in high school geometry. To say that Pythagoras was obsessed with numbers would be an understatement. And the numbers that he and his followers cared about most were those found in musical scales. They were convinced that the musical intervals they found most pleasing should provide the greatest insights, not only to mathematics, but also to the universe as a whole.

Although music may not actually explain the known universe, we all appreciate how important music is to culture and, perhaps, to personal cultural identity. Music can be used to tell a story, as you may recall from hearing *Peter and the Wolf* when you were young. Listening to music affects people's moods (Eich, 1995; Pignatiello, Camp, and Rasar, 1986) and emotions (Sloboda, 1999). When listeners hear pleasant-sounding chords preceding a word, they are faster to respond that a word such as *charm* is positive, and

pitch The psychological aspect of sound related mainly to the fundamental frequency.

they are slower to respond that a word such as *evil* is negative (Sollberger, Reber, and Eckstein, 2003). Given the powerful effects of music on mood and emotion, some clinical psychologists practice music therapy, through which people sing, listen, play, and move to music in efforts to improve mental and physical health.

Music also has been shown to have deep physiological effects. High levels of the neurotransmitter serotonin (which is targeted by many antidepressant drugs, such as Prozac) are responsible for negative aspects of emotion and mood. When people must listen to disagreeable music, their levels of serotonin actually rise (Evers and Suhr, 2000). When people listen to highly pleasurable music, they experience changes in heart rate, muscle electrical activity, and respiration; and blood flow increases in brain regions that are thought to be involved in reward and motivation (Blood and Zatorre, 2001). Music is a powerful human invention indeed.

Musical Notes

From Chapter 9 you know that one of the most important characteristics of any acoustic signal is frequency. You also know that brain structures for processing sounds are tonotopically organized to correspond to frequency. The psychological quality of perceived frequency is **pitch**. When you imagined pitch while reading Chapter 9, you probably imagined musical pitch. **Figure 11.1** illustrates the extent of the frequency range of musical sounds in relation to human hearing.

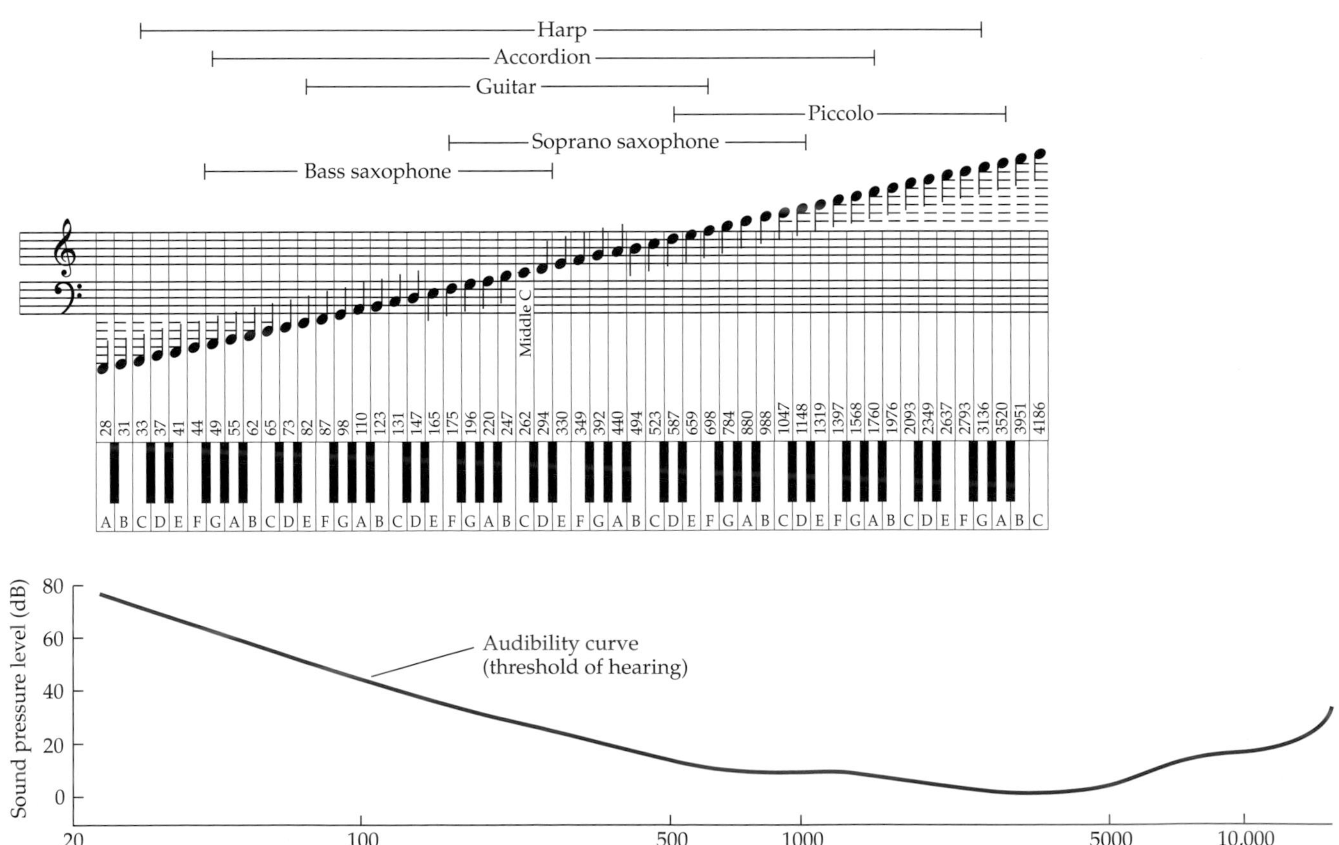

FIGURE 11.1 The sounds of music extend across a frequency range from about 25 to 4200 Hz.

TONE HEIGHT AND TONE CHROMA Musical pitch is one of the characteristics of musical notes, the sounds that comprise melodies. A very important concept in understanding musical pitch is the **octave**. When we described pitch (or psychoacoustic pitch) before, it seemed clear that the nearer any two sounds were in frequency, the nearer they were in pitch. Here is where octaves come in. When one of two periodic sounds is double the frequency of the other, those two sounds are one octave apart. For example, middle C (or C_4) has a fundamental frequency of 261.6 Hz. Notes that are one octave below and above middle C are 130.8 Hz (C_3) and 523.2 Hz (C_5), respectively. Not only do these three sounds have the same names on the musical scale (C), but they also sound similar. In fact, C_3 (130.8 Hz) sounds more similar to middle C (C_4, 261.6 Hz) than to a sound with a closer frequency—for example, E_3 (164.8 Hz)! Clearly there is more to musical pitch than just frequency.

In the preceding example, called "just intonation," frequencies of sounds are in simple ratios with one another (e.g., 2:1 for an octave). But in typical Western music, the frequencies of notes are adjusted slightly from simple ratios so that combinations of notes will sound equally good when played in higher or lower frequency ranges (keys). The set of notes (scale) used commonly in Western music is called "equal temperament."

Because of these octave relations, musical pitch is typically described as having two dimensions. The first is **tone height**, which relates to frequency in a fairly straightforward way. The second dimension, related to the octave, is **tone chroma** (from *chroma*, the Greek word for "color") (Bachem, 1950). You can visualize musical pitch as a helix. Frequency and tone height increase with increasing height on the helix, as shown in **Figure 11.2**. The circular laps around the helix correspond to changes in tone chroma. At the same point along each lap around the helix, a sound lies on a vertical line, and all sounds along that line share the same tone chroma and are separated by octaves. (See **Web Activity 11.1: Notes, Chords, and Octaves.**)

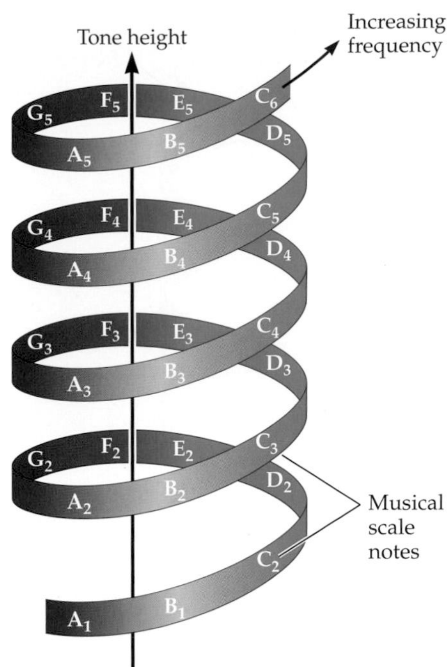

FIGURE 11.2 This helix illustrates the two characteristics of musical pitch: tone height and tone chroma.

In the early years of your schooling, you probably learned to sing the notes of the musical scale: do, re, mi, fa, sol, la, ti, do. Perhaps you even tested how many times you could sing the scale at increasingly higher pitches. In that case you were actually singing your way up the musical helix. Your pitch traveled a full turn upward with each repetition of a particular note—for example, do or re.

In Chapter 9 you learned that both a place code and a temporal code can be used in the perception of pitch. Neurons in the auditory nerve signal frequency both by their location in the cochlea (place) and by the timing of their firing (temporal). For frequencies greater than 5 kilohertz (kHz), temporal coding does not contribute to the perception of pitch, and pitch discrimination becomes appreciably worse because only place coding can be used. Most musical instruments generally produce notes that are below 4 kHz. Could tone chroma somehow be related to the temporal encoding of pitch (Moore, 2003)? We do not know. We do know that a sequence of pure tones with frequencies greater than 5 kHz does not convey a melody very well (Attneave and Olson, 1971), and listeners have great difficulty perceiving octave relationships between tones when one or both tones have a frequency greater than 5 kHz (Ward, 1954).

CHORDS Music is further defined by richer complex sounds called **chords**, which are created when three or more notes are played simultaneously. (The simultaneous playing of two notes is called a "dyad.") The major distinction between chords is whether they are *consonant* or *dissonant*. Perceived to be most pleasing, consonant chords are combinations of notes in which the

octave The interval between two sound frequencies having a ratio of 2:1.

tone height A sound quality corresponding to the level of pitch. Tone height is monotonically related to frequency.

tone chroma A sound quality shared by tones that have the same octave interval.

chord A combination of three or more musical notes with different pitches played simultaneously.

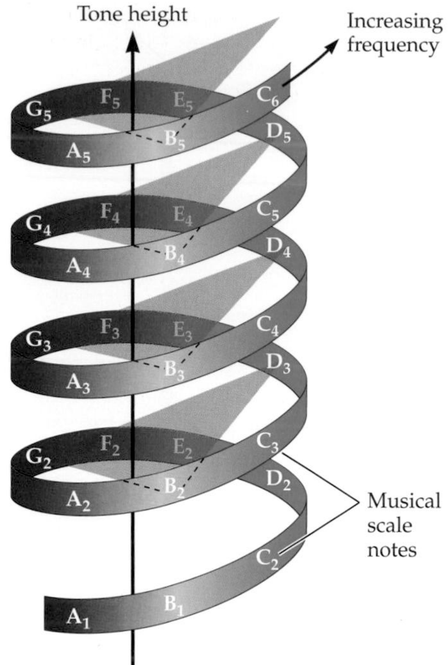

FIGURE 11.3 Chords are made up of three or more notes and can be played with different tone heights while their chromatic relationships are maintained. Here, the G-major chord is shown being played with different heights.

ratios between the note frequencies are simple. This is why Pythagoras was so taken by the relationship between pleasantness and mathematics. You already know one of the consonant relationships, the octave, in which the frequencies of the two notes are in the simple ratio of 2:1. Other major consonant intervals are the perfect fifth (3:2) and the perfect fourth (4:3). Dissonant intervals are defined by less elegant ratios. For example, the minor second (16:15) and the augmented fourth (45:32) do not sound very pleasing. Indeed, during the Middle Ages the augmented fourth was called the "devil in music" (Seay, 1975).

Because chords are defined by the ratios of the note frequencies combined to produce them, they are named the same no matter what octave they are played in. For example, the G-major chord consists of G, B, and D, and it can be played as $G_2+B_2+D_3$, $G_4+B_4+D_5$, $G_6+B_6+D_7$, or in any other octave, provided the ratios remain the same. Note that in the musical helix in **Figure 11.3**, the relationships between the notes of the chord on the helix stay the same as in Figure 11.2; all that changes is the pattern's height.

CULTURAL DIFFERENCES Any discussion of musical notes and chords would be incomplete if we didn't note that the vast majority of research on music perception has focused on the Western tradition. Musical scales and intervals vary widely across cultures. Although potent relationships between notes such as octaves are relatively universal, different musical traditions use different numbers of notes and spaces between notes within an octave. In addition, some notes are much more loosely tuned than are notes in the Western scale, so a wider range of pitches could qualify for a given note. For example, the Javanese *sléndro* and *pélog* scales have fewer notes within an octave, and there is greater variation in a note's acceptable frequencies.

Because people around the world have very different listening experiences, you might expect them to hear musical notes in different ways. In fact, when Javanese and Western musicians hear intervals between notes, their estimates of the intervals vary according to how well those notes correspond to Javanese versus Western scales, respectively (Perlman and Krumhansl, 1996). Furthermore, infants seem equipped to learn whatever scale is used in their environment. Lynch and Eilers (1990) tested the degree to which 6-month-old infants noticed inappropriate notes within both the traditional Western scale and the Javanese *pélog* scale. The infants appeared to be equally good at detecting such "mistakes" within both Western and Javanese scales, but adults from Florida were reliably better at detecting deviations from the Western scale.

Making Music

Notes or chords can form a **melody**, a sequence of sounds perceived as a single coherent structure. The notes of a familiar melody, such as "Twinkle, Twinkle, Little Star" (a.k.a. "Now I Know My ABCs," "Baa Baa Black Sheep," and Variation K.265 [300e] by Wolfgang Amadeus Mozart), "belong together" perceptually because they form this melody. Note that a melody is defined by its contour—the pattern of rises and declines in pitch—rather than by an exact sequence of sound frequencies (Handel, 1989).

melody An arrangement of notes or chords in succession.

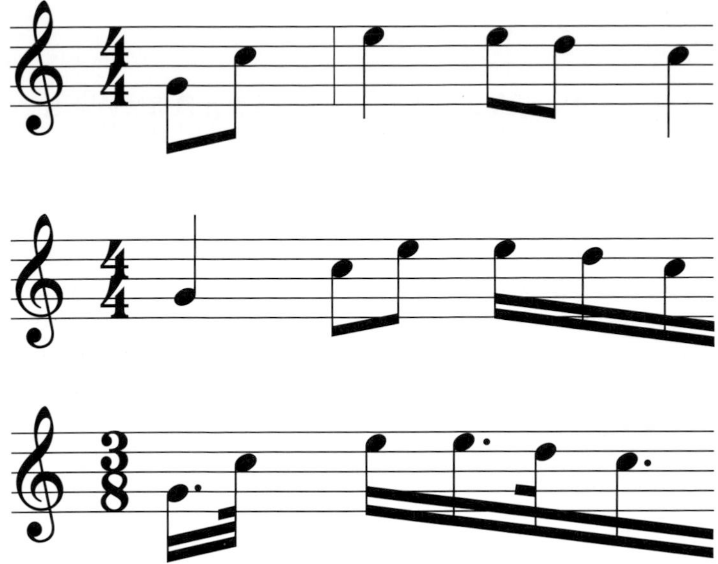

FIGURE 11.4 The pattern of increasing and decreasing pitches can remain the same, but the melody will change if notes have different durations. Here, three series of notes with the same melody contour are shown with notes that differ only in duration.

You have already learned one simple way in which melody is not a sequence of specific sounds: shift every note of a melody by one octave and the resulting melody is the same. When you sing with other people possessing higher or lower voices, they sing the same melody at very different pitches. Even within a single octave, the same melody will be heard from different notes if the steps between notes stay the same. The fact that variation in pitch matters more than absolute pitch should remind you of the general rule we've seen throughout this book: all perception is particularly sensitive to change. For example, your visual system is most attuned to changes in luminance, not to the exact number of photons bouncing off the objects in front of you. A scene may be lit dimly or brightly, yet the luminance contours remain the same, so you perceive the scene the same way in either case.

In addition to varying in pitch, notes and chords vary in duration. The average duration of a set of notes in a melody defines the music's **tempo**. Any melody can be played at either a fast or a slow tempo. But the relative durations within a sequence of notes are a critical part of the melodies themselves. If the notes of a given sequence are played with different durations, we will hear a completely different melody (**Figure 11.4**).

RHYTHM In addition to varying in speed, music varies in rhythm. The fact that music has rhythm should go without saying. After all, how else would we dance to it? Less obvious, perhaps, is that many—or even most—activities have rhythm. Walking and galloping have rhythm. So do finger tapping, waving, and swimming. Perhaps it is the very commonness of rhythm that causes us to hear nearly all sounds as rhythmic, even when they're not!

In the late 1800s, Bolton (1894) conducted experiments in which he played a sequence of identical sounds perfectly spaced in time; they had no rhythm. Nevertheless, his listeners readily reported that the sounds occurred in groups of two, three, or four. Moreover, they reported hearing the first sound of a group as "accented," or "stressed," while the remaining sounds were unaccented, or unstressed. When you've ridden in a train or a car, you've probably had a similar experience. Even though a train travels over junctions in the rails at nearly equal intervals, you hear the sound as "CLICK click CLICK click." When you ride in a car at a steady speed, you hear "THUMP thump THUMP thump" as your tires roll over cracks in a concrete road.

As Bolton's studies show, listeners are predisposed to group sounds into rhythmic patterns. Several qualities contribute to whether sounds will be

tempo The perceived speed of the presentation of sounds.

FIGURE 11.5 When two rhythms are played together and one rhythm (in this case, Aaa) is dominant, listeners tend to perceive the timing of beats in the nondominant rhythm (Bbbb) adjusted to conform with the dominant rhythm.

A a a A a a A a a A a a A a a A a a A a a A a a A a a

B b b b B b b b B b b b B b b b B b b b B b b b B b b b

← → ← →

heard as accented (stressed) or unaccented (unstressed). Sounds that are longer, louder, and higher in pitch all are more likely to be heard as leading their group (Woodrow, 1909). The timing relationship between one sound and the others in a sequence also helps determine accent. For example, we are more likely to hear a series of three sounds as Aaa–Aaa–Aaa than as aAa–aAa–aAa.

One particularly interesting example of musical rhythmic grouping is syncopation—or, more precisely, "syncopated auditory polyrhythms." When two different rhythms are overlapped, their rhythms can collide in interesting ways. For example, if one rhythm is based on three beats (Aaa–Aaa–Aaa–Aaa) and the other on four (Bbbb–Bbbb–Bbbb), the first accented sound for both rhythms will coincide only once every 12 beats. Across the 11 intervening beats, the two rhythms will be out of sync. When we listen to syncopated polyrhythms, one of the two rhythms becomes the dominant or controlling rhythm, and the other rhythm tends to be perceptually adjusted to accommodate the first (**Figure 11.5**). In particular, the accented beat of the subordinate rhythm shifts in time (Handel and Oshinsky, 1981). Thus, syncopation is the perception that beats in the subordinate rhythm have actually traveled backward or forward in time!

These findings reveal that rhythm is, in large part, psychological. We can produce sequences of sounds that are rhythmic and are perceived as such. But we also hear rhythm when it does not exist, and notes effectively travel in time to maintain the perception of consistent rhythm.

MELODY DEVELOPMENT Melody is also essentially a psychological entity (Handel, 1989). There is nothing about the particular sequence of notes in "Twinkle, Twinkle, Little Star" that makes them a melody. Rather it is our experience with a particular sequence of notes or with similar sequences that helps us perceive coherence.

Studies of 8-month-old listeners reveal that learning of melodies begins quite early in life. Saffran et al. (1999) created six simple and deliberately novel "melodies" composed of sequences of three tones. Infants sat on a parent's lap while hearing only 3 minutes of continuous random repetitions of the melodies. Next, infants heard both the original melodies and series of new three-tone sequences. These new sequences contained the same notes as the originals, but one part of the sequence was taken from one melody and another part from another melody. Because the infants responded differently to the new melodies, we can deduce that they had learned something about the original melodies.

This ability to learn new melodies is not limited to simple sequences of tones. In a study with 7-month-old infants, parents played a recording of two Mozart sonata movements to their infants every day for 2 weeks (Saffran, Loman, and Robertson, 2000). After another 2 weeks had passed, the infants were tested in a laboratory to see whether they remembered the movements. Infant listeners responded differently to the original movements than to similar Mozart movements introduced to them for the first time in the laboratory.

Speech

Most people who listen to speech also produce speech. Talkers speak so that they can be understood, and the relationship between production and perception of speech is an especially intimate one. Therefore, it is important to know some things about speech production before trying to understand speech perception.

vocal tract The airway above the larynx used for the production of speech. The vocal tract includes the oral tract and nasal tract.

One initial observation is that humans are capable of producing an incredible range of distinct speech sounds (the 5000 or so languages across the world use over 850 different speech sounds) (Maddieson, 1984). We owe this flexibility to the unique structure of the human **vocal tract** (**Figure 11.6**) (Lieberman, 1984). Unlike that of other animals, the human larynx is positioned quite low in the throat. One notorious disadvantage of such a low larynx is that humans are more susceptible to choking than any other animal. Another disadvantage is that, beyond infancy, we cannot swallow and breathe at the same time. The fact that these life-threatening anatomical liabilities were evolutionarily trumped by the survival advantage of oral communication is a testament to the importance of language to human life.

Speech Production

The production of speech has three basic components: respiration (lungs), phonation (vocal cords), and articulation (vocal tract) (see Figure 11.6). Speaking fluently requires an impressive degree of coordination among these components.

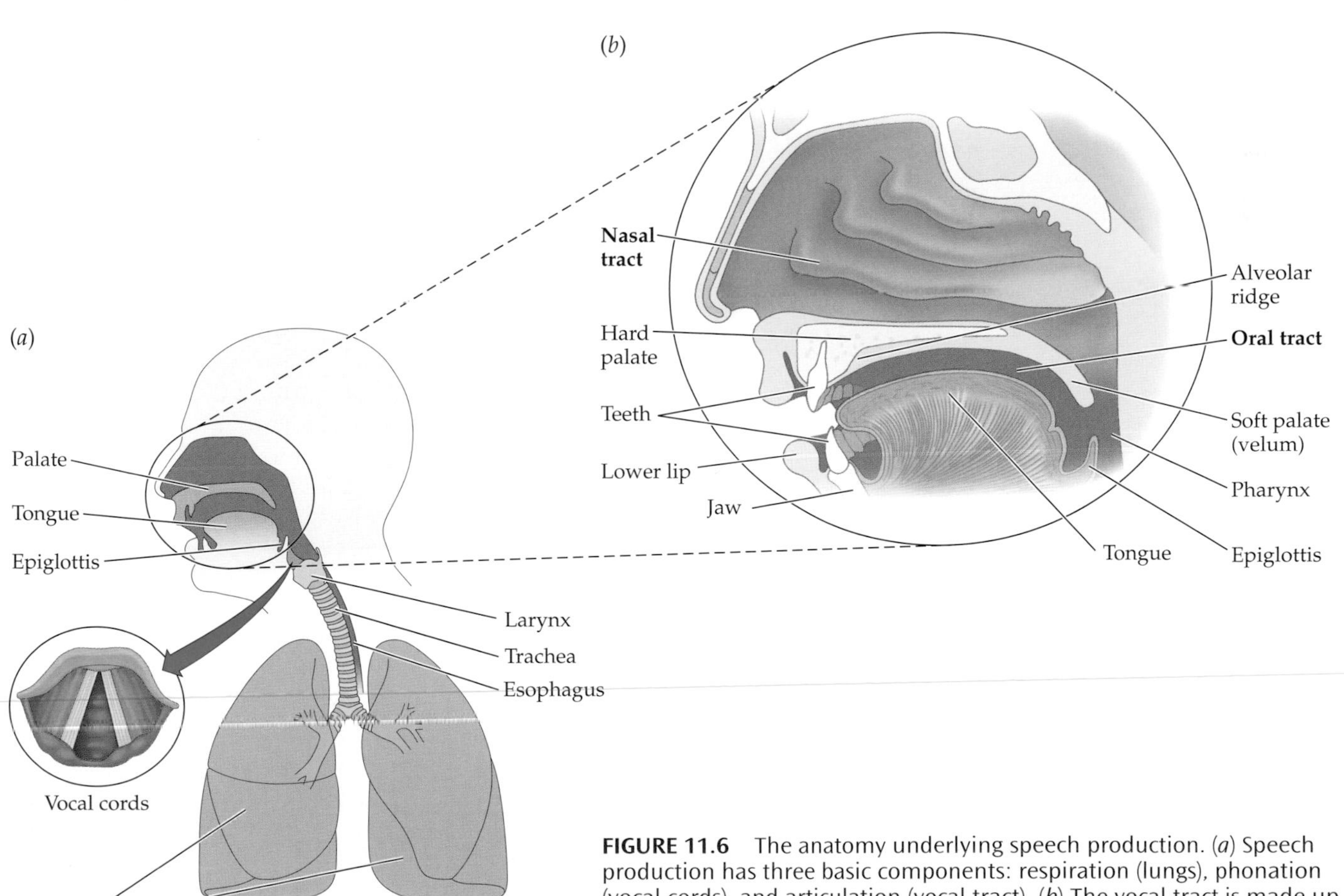

FIGURE 11.6 The anatomy underlying speech production. (*a*) Speech production has three basic components: respiration (lungs), phonation (vocal cords), and articulation (vocal tract). (*b*) The vocal tract is made up of the oral and nasal tracts.

RESPIRATION AND PHONATION To initiate a speech sound, the diaphragm pushes air out of the lungs, through the trachea, and up to the larynx. At the larynx, air must pass through the two vocal folds, which are made up of muscle tissue that can be adjusted to vary how freely air passes through the opening between them. These adjustments are described as types of phonation.

The rate at which vocal folds vibrate depends on their stiffness and mass. Consider guitar strings as an analogy. As in tuning a guitar string, more tension on vocal folds makes them stiffer and increases the rate of vibration, creating sounds with higher pitch. The pitch of a guitar string also depends on its thickness or mass. Thinner guitar strings vibrate more quickly and create higher-pitched sounds. Similarly, children, who have relatively small vocal folds, have high-pitched voices. Adult men generally have lower-pitched voices than women have, because one of the effects of testosterone during puberty is to increase the mass of the vocal folds. By varying the tension of vocal folds (stiffness) and the pressure of airflow from the lungs, individual talkers can vary the fundamental frequency of voiced sounds.

If we were to measure the sound right after the larynx, we would see that vibration of the vocal folds creates a harmonic spectrum as described in Chapter 10 and illustrated in **Figure 11.7***a*. If we could listen to just this part

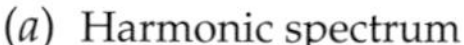

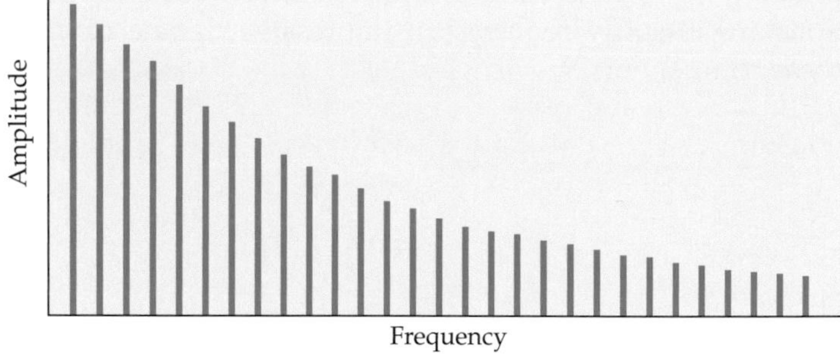

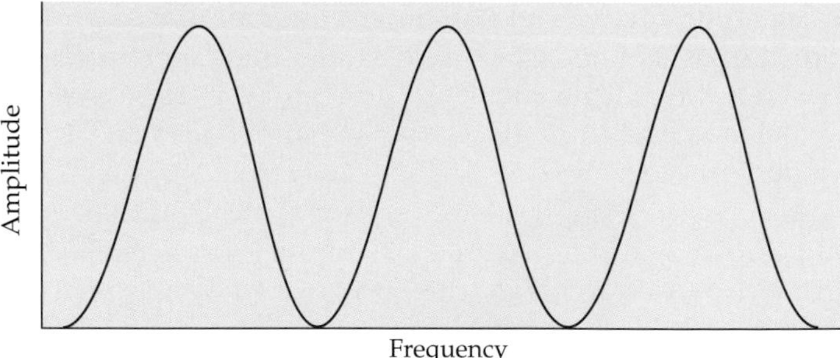

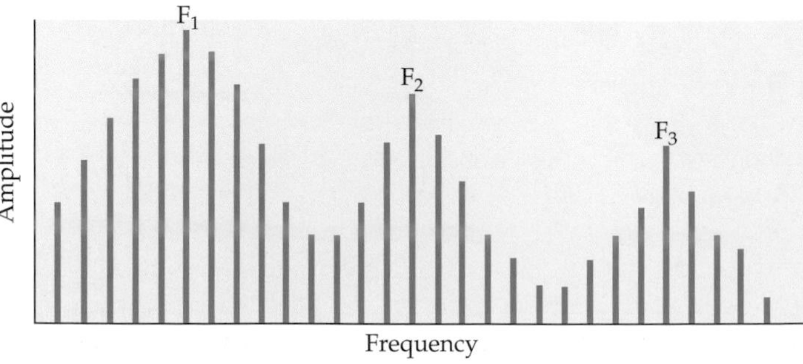

FIGURE 11.7 The spectrum of sound coming from the vocal folds is a harmonic spectrum (*a*). After passing through the vocal tract, which has resonances based on its shape at the time (*b*), there are peaks (formants) and troughs of energy at different frequencies in the sounds that come out of the mouth (*c*).

of speech, it would sound like a buzz. The first harmonic corresponds to the actual rate of physical vibration of the vocal folds, the fundamental frequency. Talkers can make interesting modifications in the way their vocal folds vibrate—creating breathy or creaky voices, for example—and singers can vary vocal-fold tension and air pressure to sing notes with widely varying frequencies. However, the really extraordinary part of producing speech sounds occurs above the larynx and vocal folds.

ARTICULATION The area above the larynx—the oral tract and nasal tract combined—is referred to as the "vocal tract." Humans have an unrivaled ability to change the shape of the vocal tract by manipulating the jaw, lips, tongue body, tongue tip, velum (soft palate), and other vocal-tract structures. These manipulations are referred to as **articulation**. As you will recall from Chapter 9, changing the size and shape of the space through which sound passes increases and decreases energy at different frequencies. We call these effects "resonance characteristics," and the spectra of speech sounds are shaped by the way people configure their tracts as resonators. Figure 11.7*b* illustrates the filtering effects of the vocal tract for the vowel sound 'ah,' as in *father*. Figure 11.7*c* portrays the net result of passing the periodic energy from the larynx through the vocal tract (see Figure 11.6*b*).

Peaks in the speech spectrum are referred to as **formants**, and formants are labeled by number, from lowest frequency to highest (F_1, F_2, F_3). These concentrations in energy occur at different frequencies depending on the length of the vocal tract. For shorter vocal tracts (children and short adults), formants are at higher frequencies than for longer vocal tracts. Because absolute frequencies change depending on who's talking, listeners must use the relationships between formant peaks to perceive speech sounds. Only the first three formants are depicted in Figure 11.7*c*. For the most part, we can distinguish almost all speech sounds on the basis of energy in the region of these lowest three formants. However, additional formants do exist, at higher frequencies with lower amplitudes.

In the previous two chapters, most of the sounds that we discussed had constant frequency spectra. That is, if the sound started with a 50-dB, 100-Hz component and a 60-dB, 200-Hz component, these frequencies continued at these amplitudes for the duration of the sound. One of the most distinctive characteristics of speech sounds is that their spectra change over time. To represent this third dimension (time) in addition to the dimensions of frequency and amplitude represented in frequency spectrum graphs of static sounds, auditory researchers use a type of display called a **spectrogram**. In a sound spectrogram, frequency is represented on the y-axis, time is tracked on the x-axis, and amplitude is indicated by the color of any point on the graph (**Figure 11.8**). Formants show up clearly in spectrograms as bands of acoustic energy that undulate up and down, depending on the speech sounds being produced.

CLASSIFYING SPEECH SOUNDS Speech sounds are most often described in terms of articulation. This is because, in the early days of studying speech, people did not have electronic recording or the ability to analyze sounds. Instead, they paid close attention to their own vocal tracts and described speech sounds in terms of the articulations necessary to produce them. You will get the most out of the following discussion if you "sing along" just as these early speech researchers did, producing the speech sounds yourself and feeling the various articulatory maneuvers necessary to speak them.

Vowel sounds are all made with a relatively open vocal tract, and they vary mostly in how high or low and how far forward or back the tongue is placed

articulation The act or manner of producing a speech sound using the vocal tract.

formant A resonance of the vocal tract. Formants are specified by their center frequency and are denoted by integers that increase with relative frequency.

spectrogram A pattern for sound analysis that provides a three-dimensional display plotting time on the horizontal axis, frequency on the vertical axis, and intensity on a color or gray scale.

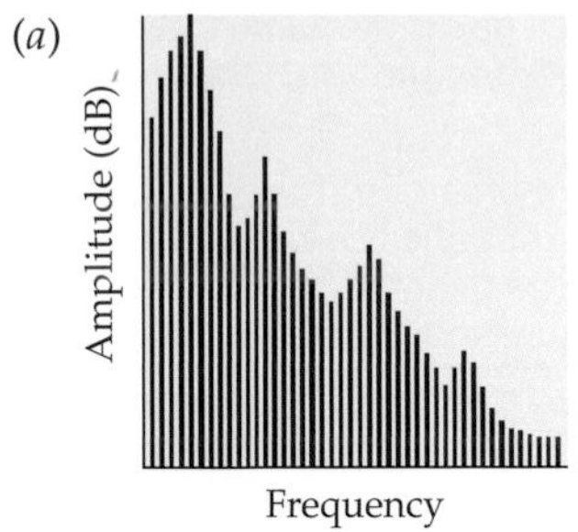

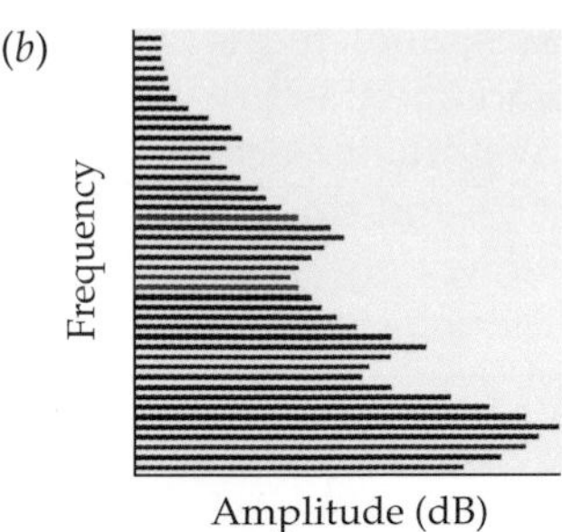

FIGURE 11.8 For sounds that do not vary over time, frequency spectra can be represented by graphs that plot amplitude on the y-axis and frequency on the x-axis (*a*). To graphically show sounds whose spectra change over time, we rotate the graph so that frequency is plotted on the y-axis (*b*); and then we plot time on the x-axis (*c*), with the amplitude of each frequency during each time slice represented by color (redder showing greater intensity). The spectrogram in part (*c*) shows the acoustic signal produced by a male uttering the sentence, "We were away a year ago."

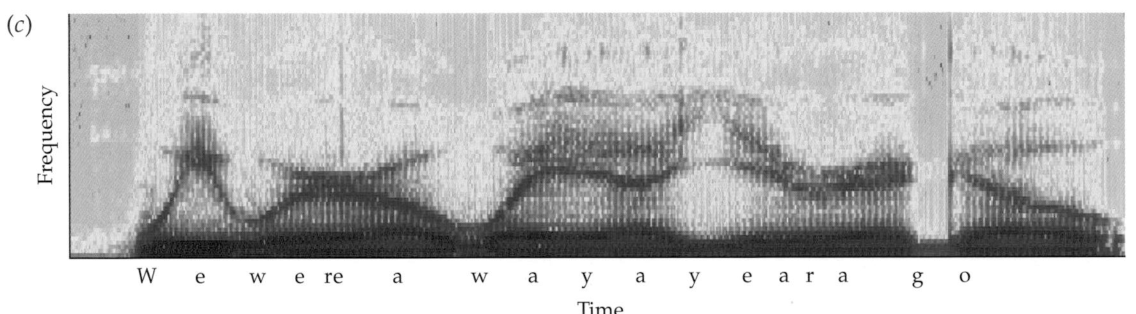

in the oral tract, along with whether or not the lips are rounded. We produce the 'ee' sound in the word *beet* by placing the tongue up and forward, the 'aw' in *bought* by moving the tongue down and back, and the 'oo' in *boot* by moving the tongue up and back while rounding the lips (**Figure 11.9**).

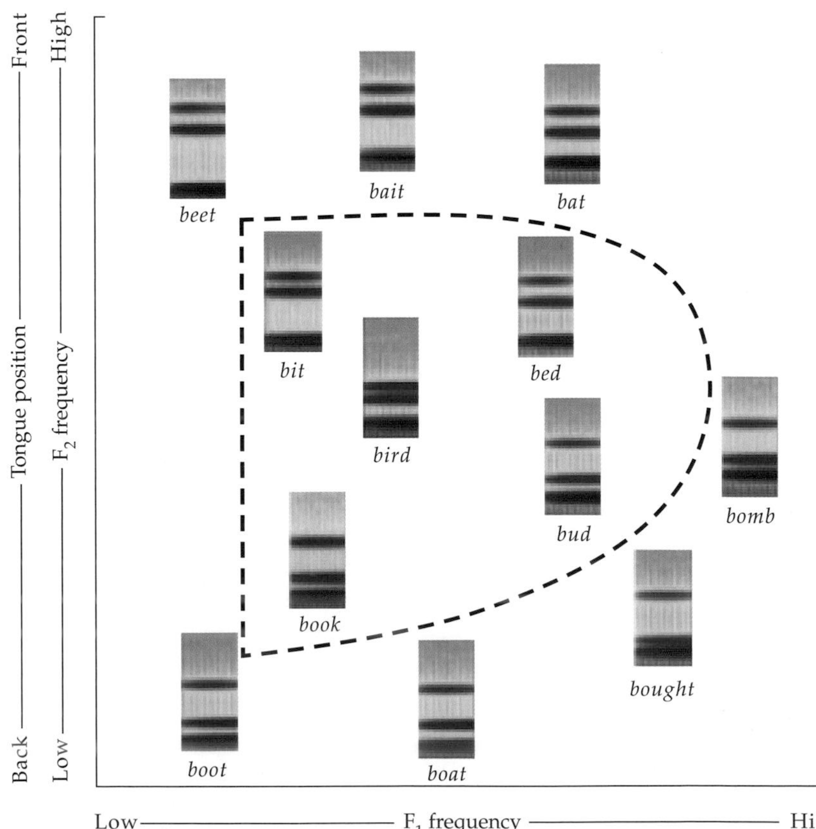

FIGURE 11.9 Vowel sounds of English, showing how the frequencies of the first (F_1) and second (F_2) formants relate to how high or low (F_1) and how far forward or back (F_2) the tongue is. The dashed line illustrates limits on how far the tongue moves when vowels are produced. For example, the vowels 'ee' and 'oo' are produced with the tongue very high in the mouth. In the case of 'ee,' the tongue is far forward; but for 'oo,' the tongue is far back.

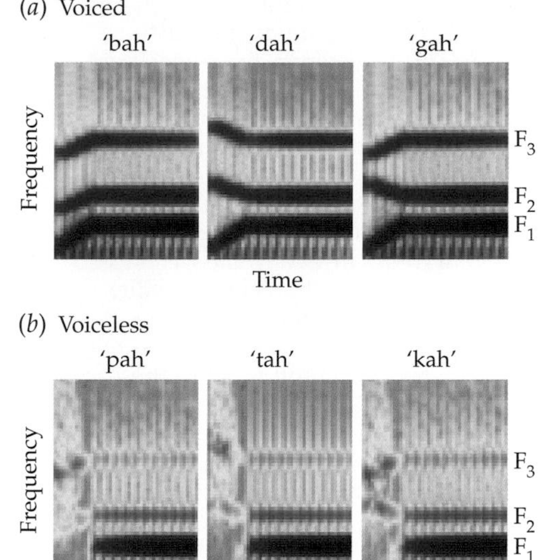

FIGURE 11.10 English stop consonants may be voiced (*a*), as in 'bah,' 'dah,' and 'gah'; or voiceless (*b*), as in 'pah,' 'tah,' and 'kah.' The main articulatory difference between voiced and voiceless stop consonants is that, for the latter, talkers delay vibration of the vocal folds by about one-twentieth of a second after opening the vocal tract to begin the sound.

We produce consonants by obstructing the vocal tract in some way, and each consonant sound can be classified according to three articulatory dimensions:

1. *Place of articulation* (see Figure 11.6*b*). Airflow can be obstructed
   - At the lips (*bilabial* speech sounds—'b,' 'p,' 'm')
   - At the alveolar ridge just behind the teeth (*alveolar* speech sounds—'d,' 't,' 'n')
   - At the soft palate (*velar* speech sounds—'g,' 'k,' 'ng')
2. *Manner of articulation*. Airflow can be
   - Totally obstructed (*stops*—'b,' 'd,' 'g,' 'p,' 't,' 'k') (see Figure 11.10)
   - Partially obstructed (*fricatives*—'s,' 'z,' 'f,' 'v,' 'th,' 'sh')
   - Only slightly obstructed (*laterals*—'l,' 'r'; and *glides*—'w,' 'y')
   - First blocked, then allowed to sneak through (*affricates*—'ch,' 'j')
   - Blocked at first from going through the mouth, but allowed to go through the nasal passage (*nasals*—'n,' 'm,' 'ng')
3. *Voicing*—(**Figure 11.10**). Whether the vocal cords
   - Are vibrating (*voiced* consonants—'b,' 'm,' 'z,' 'l,' 'r'; put your finger on your larynx as you say these consonants out loud and you will feel the vocal cords vibrating)
   - Are not vibrating (*voiceless* consonants—'p,' 's,' 'ch')

These speech sounds used in English are only a small sample of the sounds used by languages around the world. Most individual languages use fewer consonants and vowels than are used in English. Some sounds are quite common across languages, and others such as English 'th' and 'r,' are fairly uncommon around the world. When many or most languages include particular speech sounds, often the reason is that the differences between them are particularly easy to perceive. Humans must communicate in difficult environments where the listener is far away or there are many competing sounds. To be effective, speech sound repertoires of languages have developed over generations of individuals to include only sounds that are relatively easy to tell apart.

In addition to using relatively easily distinguishable sounds, another reason speech communicates well is that all distinctions between vowels and consonants are signaled with multiple differences between sounds. Because more than one acoustic property can be used to tell two sounds apart, distinctions are signaled redundantly, and this redundancy helps listeners. The speech signal is so redundant that, if we remove all energy below 1800 Hz, listeners will still perceive speech nearly perfectly, and the same is true if all energy is removed above 1800 Hz (**Figure 11.11**).

Speech Perception

Speech production is very fast. In a casual conversation, we produce about 10 to 15 consonants and vowels per second, and if we're in a hurry, we can as much as double this rate. To achieve this acoustic feat, our articulators (tongue, lips, jaw, and so on) must do many different things very quickly.

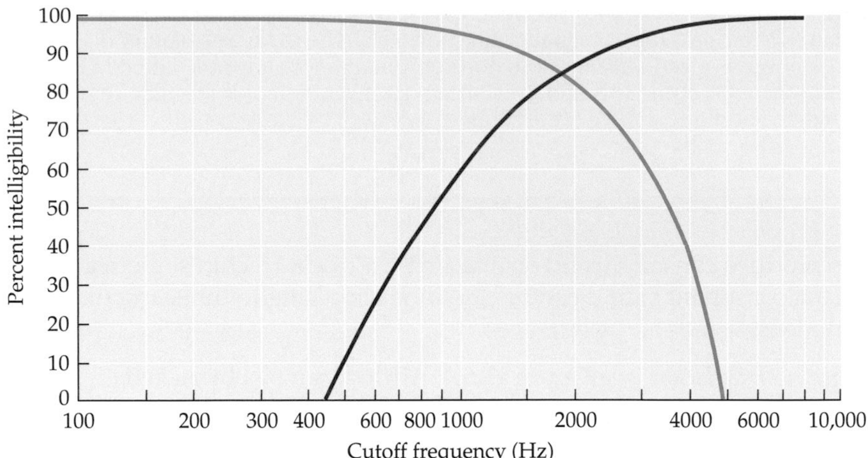

FIGURE 11.11 Because the speech signal has so many redundant acoustic characteristics, listeners can understand speech when all energy either below or above 1800 Hz is removed. The green line shows performance when energy above different frequencies (high pass) is available to listeners, and the red line shows performance when energy below different frequencies (low pass) is present. The red curve shows intelligibility when the cutoff is above the given *x* value, and the green curve shows intelligibility when the cutoff is below the given *x* value. Notice that intelligibility is excellent when all energy is removed below 500, 1000, and even 1500 Hz (green), and intelligibility is excellent when all energy is removed above 6000, 4000, and 2000 Hz (red). (After Fletcher and Galt, 1950.)

However, articulators can move only so fast, and forces of mass and inertia keep articulators from getting all the way to the position for the next consonant or vowel. Experienced talkers also adjust their production in anticipation of where articulators need to be next. In these ways, production of one speech sound overlaps production of the next. This overlap of articulation in space and time is called **coarticulation**. As we turn from speech production to speech perception, we will find that although coarticulation does not cause much trouble for listeners understanding speech, it has made understanding speech perception harder for researchers.

COARTICULATION AND LACK OF INVARIANCE To get a better sense of what coarticulation means, say the word *moody* a few times, and note the activity of your tongue as you form the 'd' sound. You will find that it starts in the back of your mouth, where it must be to form the 'oo' vowel sound, then touches the alveolar ridge just behind the teeth to form the 'd,' then ends up toward the front of the mouth to form the 'ee.' Now say the nonsense word *eedoom*. Reversing the vowel sounds means sending the tongue on the opposite journey, from front to alveolar ridge to back. As a result of the very different path taken by the tongue in these two utterances, the acoustic qualities of the 'd' in the two utterances are quite different.

This context sensitivity is a signature property of speech. One might expect context sensitivity to cause a significant problem for speech perceivers, because it means there are no "invariants" that we can count on to uniquely identify different speech sounds. For the earlier examples 'b,' 'd,' and 'g' (see Figure 11.10*a*), notice that the shape of the first formant (F_1) is pretty much the same for all three consonants when they precede the same vowel. F_1 is helpful in telling 'b,' 'd,' and 'g' apart from other speech sounds, but it does not help much in telling these sounds apart from one another. An F_1 like that shown in **Figure 11.12** is necessary for a sound to be 'b,' but it is not sufficient to inform the listener that the sound is 'b,' and not 'd' or 'g.' F_2 is very important for telling 'b' from 'd' from 'g,' but what F_2 tells the listeners depends on the quality of F_3 and the nature of the following vowel.

Explaining how listeners understand speech despite all this variation has been one of the most significant challenges for speech researchers. Context sensitivity due to coarticulation also presents one of the greatest difficulties in developing computer recognition of speech. We cannot program or train a computer to recognize a speech sound—consonant or vowel—without also taking into consideration which speech sounds precede and follow that

coarticulation The phenomenon in speech whereby attributes of successive speech units overlap in articulatory or acoustic patterns.

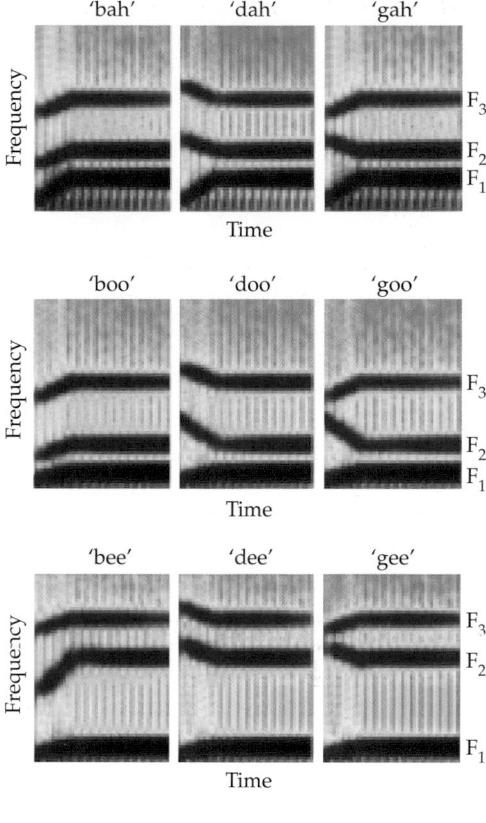

FIGURE 11.12 Spectrograms of 'd' sounds (center column), along with stop-consonant cousins 'b' (left) and 'g' (right). Changes in formants across time (formant transitions) for these sounds differ dramatically depending on the following vowels: 'ah' (top row), 'oo' (middle), and 'ee' (bottom).

sound. And we cannot identify those preceding and following sounds without also taking into consideration which sounds precede and follow them, and so on. You can see that the problem quickly becomes very difficult, and it may not surprise you that the most advanced computer speech recognition systems cannot recognize speech much better than a 2-year-old child can.

CATEGORICAL PERCEPTION How do the 2-year-olds do it? *Something* in the acoustic signal must lead them to perceive the 'd' in *deem, doom,* and *dam* as the same consonant. Almost 50 years ago, researchers invented machines that could produce speechlike sounds and started testing listeners to try to determine exactly what the acoustic cues were that enabled them to distinguish different speech sounds. They found, for example, that by varying the transitions of F_2 and F_3, they could produce sounds that listeners reliably reported hearing as 'bah,' 'dah,' or 'gah' (**Figure 11.13**). (See Web Activity 11.2: Categorical Perception.)

These researchers knew that making small, incremental changes to simple acoustic stimuli such as pure tones leads to gradual changes in people's perception of these stimuli. For example, tones would sound just a little higher in pitch with each small step in frequency. Surprisingly, speech sounds were not perceived in this way. When researchers started with a synthesized 'bah' and gradually varied the formant transitions moving toward 'dah' and then 'gah,' listeners' responses did not gradually change from 'bah,' to 'bah'-ish 'dah,' to 'dah,' to 'dah'-ish 'gah,' to 'gah.' Instead, listeners identified these sounds as changing abruptly from one consonant to another.

Furthermore, listeners appeared incapable of hearing that anything was different when two sounds were labeled as the same consonant. In this second part of the experiments, researchers played pairs of synthesized speech sounds and asked listeners whether the sounds were identical. Listeners

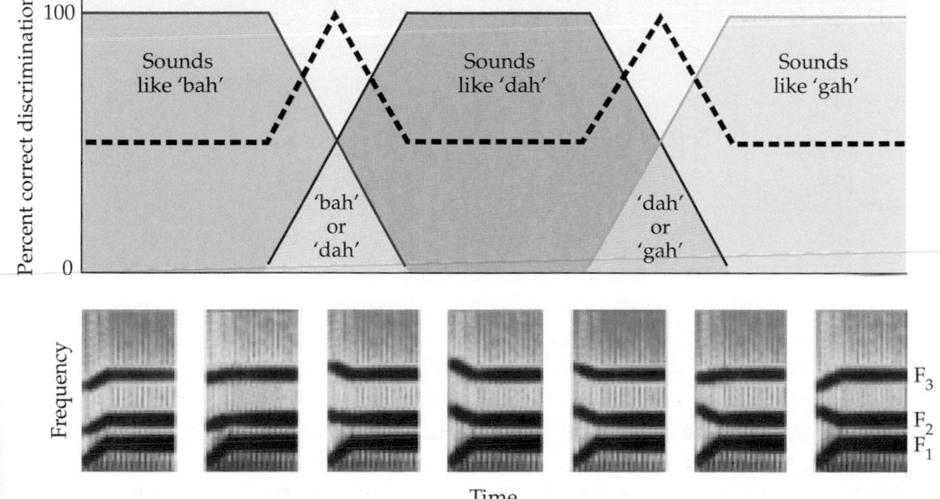

FIGURE 11.13 The sound spectrograms at the bottom of this figure indicate auditory stimuli that change smoothly from a clear 'bah' on the left through 'dah' to a clear 'gah' on the right. Perception does not change smoothly. All the sounds on the left sound like a 'bah' (blue curve) until we reach a sharp 'bah'–'dah' border. Listeners are much better at discriminating a 'bah' from a 'dah' than at discriminating two 'bah's or two 'gah's. The dashed black line indicates discrimination performance. The same is true for 'dah' (red curve) and 'gah' (green curve).

performed almost perfectly when detecting small differences between two sounds if one was 'bah' and the other was 'dah.' But if both sounds were 'bah' or both were 'dah,' performance dropped to chance levels (dashed line in Figure 11.13), even though the differences in formant transitions in the first and second pairs of stimuli were equally large.

This pattern of results has come to be called "categorical perception." As illustrated in Figure 11.13, three qualities define categorical perception. The first two were just described: a sharp labeling (identification) function and discontinuous discrimination performance. The third definitional quality of categorical perception follows from the first two: researchers can predict discrimination performance on the basis of labeling data. In short, listeners report hearing differences between sounds only when those differences would change the label of the sound, so the ability to discriminate sounds can be predicted by how listeners label the sounds.

HOW SPECIAL IS SPEECH? Categorical perception of speech sounds is not limited to the 'bah'/'dah'/'gah' dimension; it has been shown for many different contrasts between sounds in English, as well as other languages. These findings, along with the failure to find invariants that distinguish speech sounds from each other, led many speech researchers to suspect that humans had evolved special mechanisms just for perceiving speech. One very influential version of the "speech is special" idea, called the "motor theory" of speech perception (Liberman and Mattingly, 1985; Liberman et al., 1967), holds that processes used to produce speech sounds can somehow be run in reverse to understand the acoustic speech signal. Attempts have even been made to develop computer speech recognition by calculating back from the speech signal to articulations (**Figure 11.14**).

Over time, however, a number of problems with the motor theory have cropped up. First, it turns out that speech production is at least as complex as speech perception, if not more so. Every aspect of the acoustic signal relates to a particular aspect of the vocal tract. So if the acoustic signal is complex, this complexity must be the result of complexity in production.

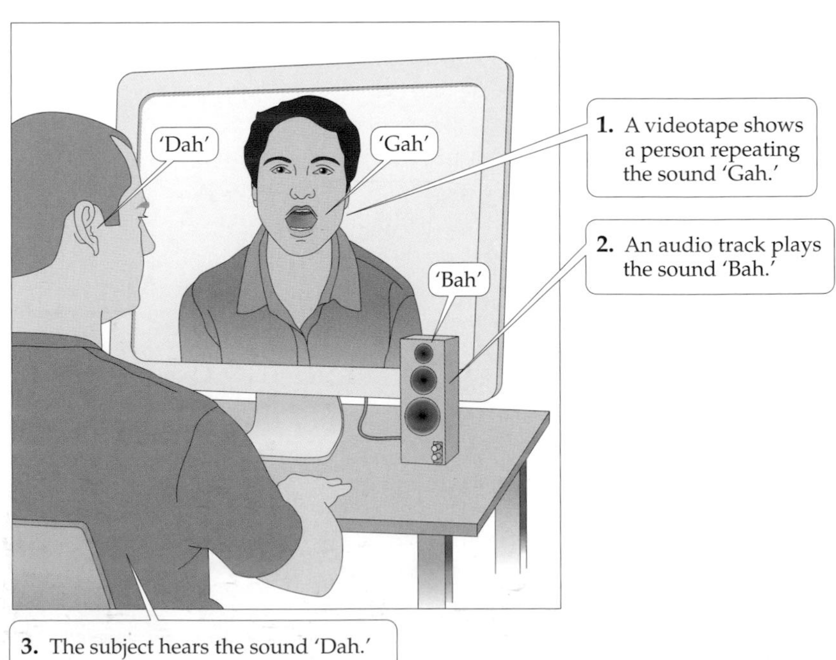

FIGURE 11.14 The motor theory was bolstered by, among other things, a somewhat peculiar finding by McGurk and MacDonald (1976). Experimental subjects were shown a video of a person saying the syllable 'gah' over and over. The audio track, however, was playing the sound 'bah' repeatedly. Incredibly, subjects consistently reported hearing a third syllable, 'dah,' even if they knew how they were being fooled because they heard 'bah' when they closed their eyes. (This effect really has to be experienced to be believed; try it in **Web Activity 11.3: The McGurk Effect** now.) According to motor theory advocates, the McGurk effect (as it came to be called) is caused by speech perception mechanisms fusing the visual cues to the positions of the articulators, as calculated from the acoustics.

(a)

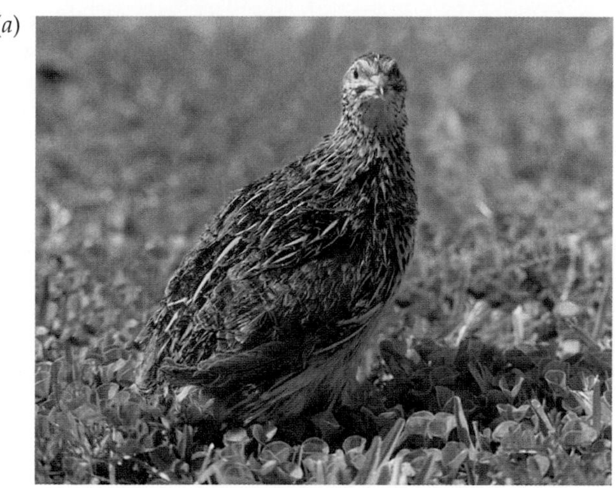

(b)

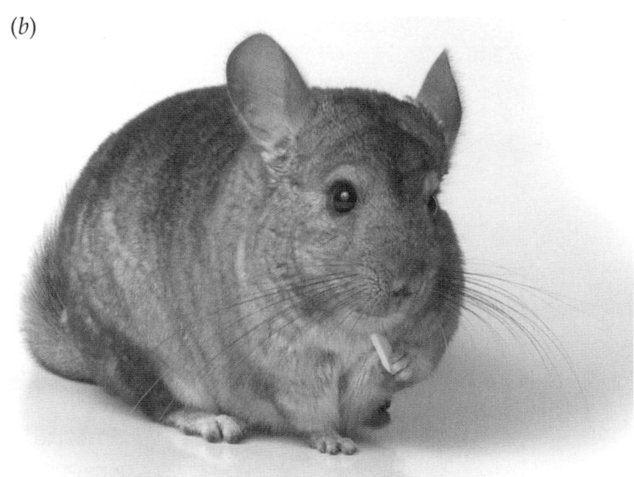

FIGURE 11.15 Speech perception by nonhumans. (*a*) Japanese quail can learn to tell 'd' from 'b' and 'g' preceding different vowels just as humans do. (*b*) Chinchillas have shown categorical perception of sounds varying from 'dah' to 'tah.' (*a* courtesy of Keith R. Kluender; *b* courtesy of Annie Huyler, Pioneer Valley Chinchillas.)

Trying to explain speech perception by reference to production is at least as difficult as explaining speech perception on the basis of acoustics alone.

A second reason to doubt that processes for perceiving speech are unique to humans is that numerous demonstrations have shown that nonhuman animals can learn to respond to speech signals in much the same way that human listeners do (Kluender, Lotto, and Holt, 2005; Kluender et al., 1998). For example, Japanese quail (**Figure 11.15***a*) can be taught to tell 'd' from 'b' and 'g' across the same sort of acoustic variation depicted in Figure 11.12 (Kluender, Diehl, and Killeen, 1987). Chinchillas (Figure 11.15*b*) have also shown classic categorical-perception effects (Kuhl, 1981; Kuhl and Miller, 1978).

Furthermore, we now know that categorical perception, one of the definitional characteristics of speech that was thought to be so unusual as to require a special processing mechanism, is not at all limited to speech sounds. Other types of auditory stimuli, such as musical intervals (Smith et al., 1994), are also perceived categorically, as are visual stimuli such as human faces (Beale and Keele, 1995) and facial expressions (Calder et al., 1996; De Gelder, Teunisse, and Benson, 1997; Etcoff and Magee, 1992). People even perceive differences between familiar animals categorically (R. Campbell et al., 1997) (**Figure 11.16**), and monkeys perceive images of cats versus dogs categorically (Freedman et al., 2001).

COARTICULATION AND SPECTRAL CONTRAST Contemporary research has turned increasingly to investigating how speech perception is explained by general ways that hearing, and perception more broadly, works. For example, perception of coarticulated speech appears to be at least partially explained

FIGURE 11.16 People categorically perceive changes between images of familiar animals such as monkeys and cows. The labels that observers use shift abruptly between "monkey" and "cow" when they identify such images. Observers also are better at discriminating two images when they label one as "monkey" and one as "cow." (After R. Campbell et al., 1997.)

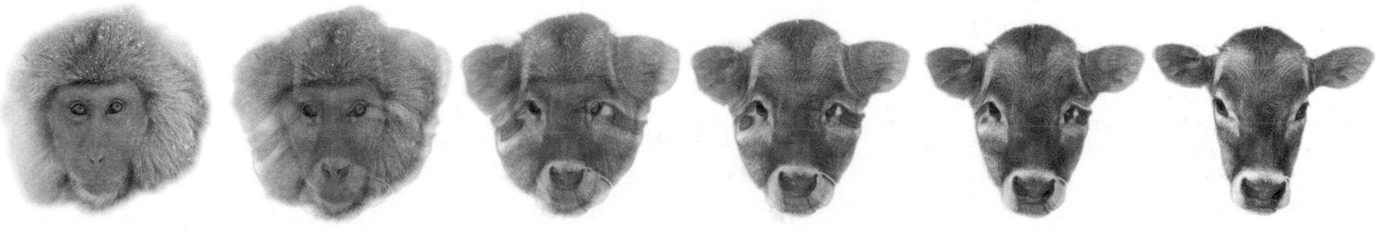

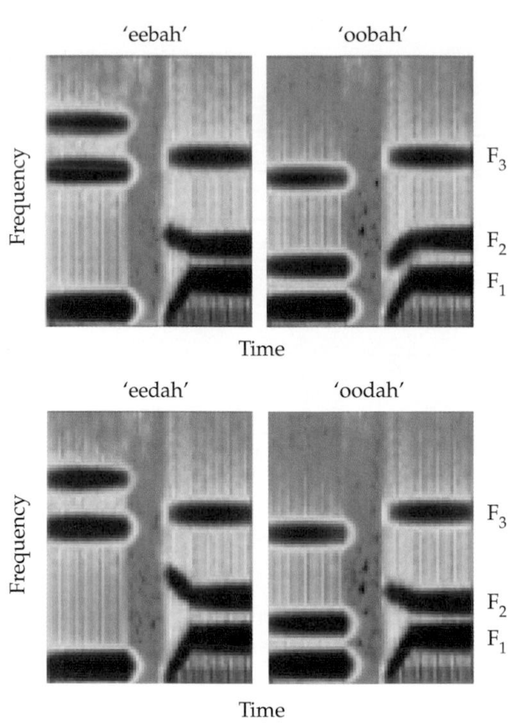

FIGURE 11.17 Because of coarticulation, consonant sounds such as 'bah' and 'dah' are acoustically very different, depending on the preceding vowel. Here, 'bah' is shown following 'ee' (top left) and 'oo' (top right), and 'dah' is shown following the same vowels (bottom). Note that F_2 in 'eebah' (top left) is acoustically identical to F_2 in 'oodah' (bottom right). Listeners hear the same consonant sound as 'b' following 'ee' and as 'd' following 'oo' because of the contrast between the spectrum of 'ee' and 'oo' and the spectrum of the following consonant.

by some fundamental ways that auditory systems work. Let's turn again to our example of stop consonants such as 'b' and 'd.' Two of the acoustic features that contribute to the perception of 'b,' as contrasted with the perception of 'd,' are the onset frequency and trajectory of the second formant (F_2). Because of coarticulation, the production of one speech sound always affects the production of the next sound; formants for one sound always are more like (assimilate to) the sounds that precede and follow. The onset of F_2 varies depending on whether the 'bah' or 'dah' follows vowels such as 'ee' (higher) or 'oo' (lower).

Perception of the syllables 'bah' and 'dah' works in a way that nicely fits the facts of coarticulation. The very same F_2 onset is heard as 'dah' following 'oo' and as 'bah' following 'ee' (**Figure 11.17**). Why does perception work this way? One idea is that listeners somehow "know" about how production works, perhaps through experience with speech. However, we know that perception by 4- to 5-month-old infants who cannot talk (Fowler, Best, and McRoberts, 1990), and even by birds (Lotto, Kluender, and Holt, 1997), is sensitive to the spectrum of preceding sounds when they hear syllables such as 'dah.' The reason is that auditory systems naturally work in a way to make it easier to understand coarticulated speech.

Because coarticulation always causes a speech sound to become more like the previous speech sound, auditory processes that enhance the contrast between successive sounds undo this assimilation. Listeners are more likely to perceive 'bah' (low F_2) when preceded by the vowel sound 'ee' (high F_2), and to perceive 'dah' (high F_2) when preceded by 'oo' (low F_2). Preceding sounds do not even have to be speech sounds. If, instead of playing 'ee' and 'oo' before syllables varying from 'bah' to 'dah,' we present only a single small band of energy at the frequencies where F_2 would be in 'ee' or 'oo,' perception of the following syllable changes just as it does with the full 'ee' or 'oo' vowel sound (Coady, Kluender, and Rhode, 2003). The onset of F_2 for 'bah' and 'dah' is perceived relative to whether the preceding energy is lower or higher in frequency. We perceive syllables such as 'bah' and 'dah' on the basis of the relative change in the spectrum: how the onsets contrast with the energy that precedes them.

You have encountered contrast effects several times before in this book. Remember that melodies are defined by changes between adjacent notes, and not by the exact notes in particular. While learning about vision, you saw many examples of contrast. Contrast plays a large role in the perception of lightness, color, and size, as well as line orientation, position, curvature, depth, and spatial frequency. Here, spectral contrast helps listeners perceive speech despite the lack of acoustic invariance due to coarticulation.

USING MULTIPLE ACOUSTIC CUES What do speech sounds, musical intervals, and faces all have in common? They are all stimuli that people have a great deal of experience perceiving. We spend a large chunk of our waking lives listening to speech and identifying people by their faces. Another thing that makes distinguishing between individual speech sounds and individual faces similar is that many small differences must be used together in order to discriminate different speech sounds and different faces (e.g., small changes in formant transitions and small changes in nose shape). At the same time, other stimulus differences must be ignored so that multiple instances of the same speech sound or multiple images of the same face can be classified properly (e.g., acoustic variation introduced when different speakers utter the same speech sound, or image variation introduced when a face is viewed from different angles).

To the extent that perception depends heavily on experience, speech is special only in that (1) humans have evolved unique anatomical machinery for producing it and (2) we spend a great deal of time practicing the perception of speech. The fact that there are no acoustic invariants for distinguishing speech sounds is really no different from many comparable situations in visual perception. For example, we saw in Chapter 6 that one particular cue for depth perception may fail us, but by taking multiple cues into account, we rarely make large mistakes when calculating distance relations.

The comparison with face recognition may be even more apt. Bob's nose may be quite similar to Ken's nose, Bob's eyes may be exactly as far apart as Paul's eyes, and Bob's mouth may be shaped just like Tom's mouth. But given enough experience with all three faces (and enough experience with face recognition in general), we can use the pattern of facial features to pick Bob out from a lineup every time—even if he is covering his mouth with his hand. Turning to speech perception, utterances of the syllables 'aba' and 'apa' can be distinguished from each other by at least 16 different characteristics of the acoustic signal (**Figure 11.18**) (Lisker, 1978). Listeners can make use of their experience with the co-occurrence of these multiple acoustic differences to understand speech.

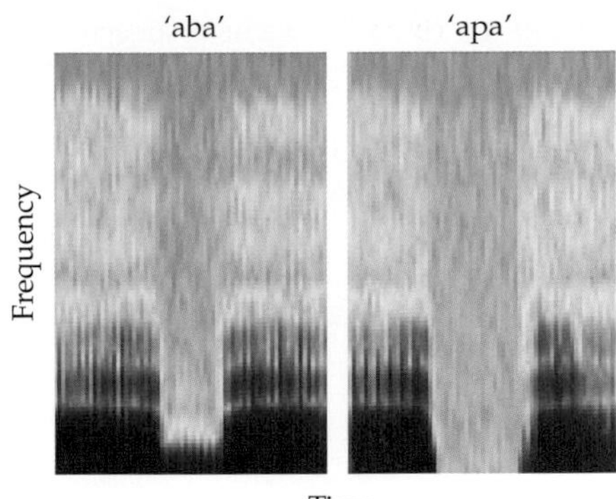

FIGURE 11.18 The simple distinction between 'aba' (left) and 'apa' (right) includes at least 16 acoustic differences. Some differences that are easy to see include duration of the first vowel, duration of the interval between syllables, and the presence of low-frequency energy in the middle of 'aba.'

To sum up, we don't need individual acoustic invariants to distinguish speech sounds; we just need to be as good at pattern recognition for sounds as we are for visual images. And one of the things that the billions of neurons in the brain do best is integrating multiple sources of information to recognize patterns (Kluender and Alexander, 2008). Computer simulations of neural connectivity (neural network models) designed to mimic the use of multiple attributes and associations between attributes are among the most successful artificial pattern recognizers yet invented by humankind. Interestingly, many neural network models (e.g., those developed by J. A. Anderson et al., 1977, or by Damper and Harnad, 2000) also show categorical-perception effects when the models are trained on enough examples.

Learning to Listen

In our discussion of vision earlier in the book, we saw that experience is incredibly important for visual perception, particularly the higher-level perception of objects and events in the world. Experience is every bit as important for auditory perception. This is especially true for the perception of speech; and unlike vision, experience with speech begins very early in development. In fact, babies gain significant experience with speech even before they're born!

Measurements of heart rate as an indicator of the ability to notice change between speech sounds have revealed that late-term fetuses can discriminate between different vowel sounds (Lecanuet et al., 1986). Prenatal experience with speech sounds appears to have considerable influence on subsequent perception. For one thing, newborns prefer hearing their mother's voice over other women's voices (DeCasper and Fifer, 1980). When 4-day-old infants in Paris were tested, they preferred hearing French instead of Russian (Mehler et al., 1988). Perhaps most amazingly, newborns prefer hearing particular children's stories that were read aloud by their mothers during the third trimester of pregnancy (DeCasper and Spence, 1986).

BECOMING A NATIVE LISTENER As we have seen, speech sounds can differ in many ways. Acoustic differences that matter critically for one language may be irrelevant or even distracting in another language. For example, the English language makes use of the distinction between the sounds 'r' and 'l,'

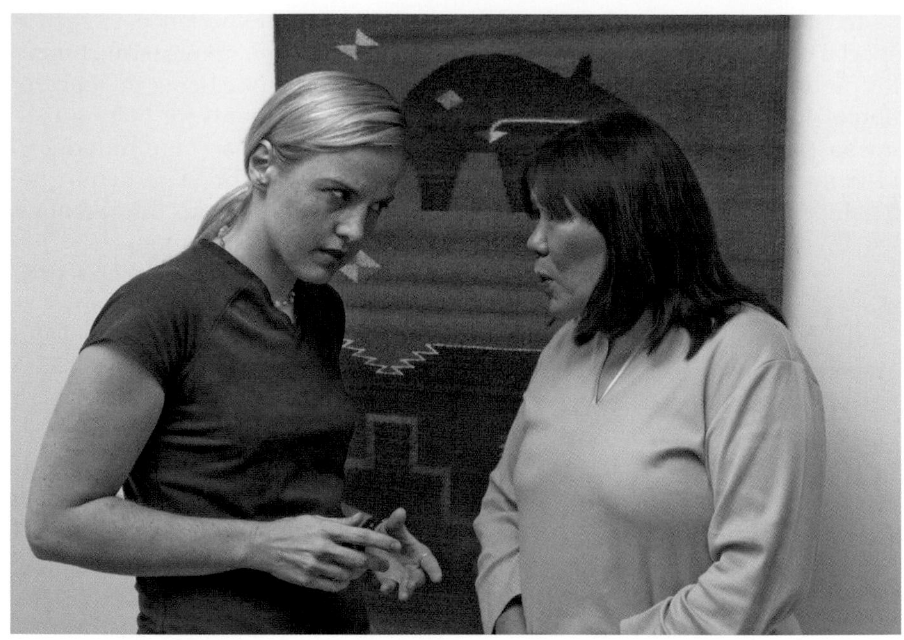

FIGURE 11.19 How we hear speech sounds depends on our experience with the speech sounds of our first language. Because of experience with one language, it is often difficult to perceive and produce distinctions in a new language. For example, most Japanese people learning English as a second language have trouble distinguishing between 'l' and 'r.'

whereas these two sounds are both very similar to only one sound (called a "flap") in Japanese. As another example, Spanish is one of many languages that uses only the five vowel sounds 'ee' (as in *beet*), 'oo' (as in *boot*), 'ah' (as in *bomb*), 'ay' (as in *bake*), and 'oh' (as in *boat*), whereas English employs numerous other vowel sounds.

As anyone who has spoken to a native Japanese speaker in English knows, the 'r'/'l' distinction is very difficult for Japanese people to pick up when they learn English as a second language (**Figure 11.19**). Because the difference between 'l' and 'r' is irrelevant to native Japanese speakers when they are learning their native language, it is adaptive for them to learn to ignore it, thus allowing them to focus on speech sound distinctions that are important in Japanese. When people have spent most of their lives listening to Japanese and not hearing the difference between 'r' and 'l,' we are not surprised that they have difficulty learning to produce the 'r' and 'l,' because the two sound much the same to a Japanese person. By the same token, a native Spanish speaker who complains that your dog just "beat him" is probably not claiming that Rover threw a punch; rather, the difference between 'ee' and 'ih' is less perceptible to the Spanish speaker because both of these English sounds are similar to the Spanish 'ee.'

Interestingly, studies show that infants begin filtering out irrelevant acoustic differences long before they begin to utter speech sounds (even before their babbling stage). One study found that by 6 months of age, infants from Seattle were more likely to notice acoustic differences that distinguish two English vowels than to notice equivalent differences between Swedish vowels, and infants from Stockholm were more likely to notice the difference between two Swedish vowels than between two English vowels (Kuhl et al., 1992). Tuning of perception for consonants appears to take a bit longer to develop, but by the time infants are 1 year old, they have also begun to ignore, just as their parents do, consonant distinctions not used in their native language (**Figure 11.20**).

Of course, it is possible, with much training, to learn to perceive and produce speech sound distinctions that you've spent most of your life ignoring. As you might expect, the longer a person uses only her first language, the

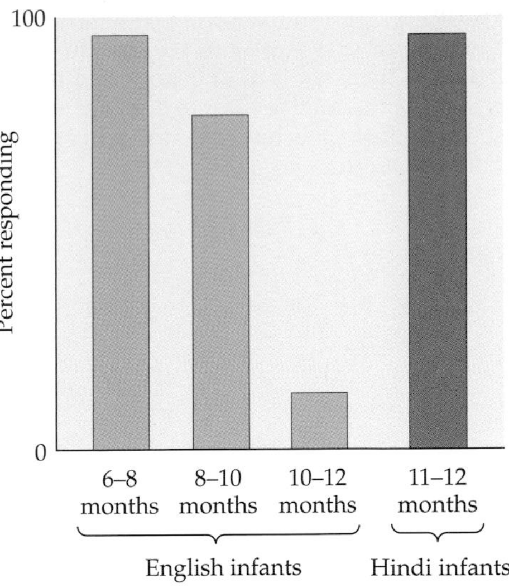

FIGURE 11.20 Hindi has a dental stop consonant produced with the tongue tip touching the teeth and a retroflex stop consonant that requires the tongue to bend up and back in the mouth. Adult speakers of English hear both of these sounds as 't' because they are similar to the English 't.' When Werker and Tees (1984) tested infants from English-speaking families in Vancouver, the youngest (6–8 months old) reliably responded to the difference between these two Hindi sounds. By age 1 year, however, the infants were mimicking their parents' behavior by ignoring the distinction between the two sounds.

longer it takes to learn to produce and perceive sounds from a second language (Flege, Bohn, and Jang, 1997; Imai, Flege, and Wayland, 2002). Many studies have been aimed at determining what makes new distinctions hard or easy for second-language learners to pick up. Learning is most difficult when both of the sounds in the second language are similar to a single sound in the first language (e.g., 'r' and 'l' for Japanese speakers learning English). Learning is easier if the two new sounds are both unlike any sound in the native language. For example, native English listeners have no problems distinguishing click sounds from Zulu because Zulu clicks are so unlike any English sounds. Learning also is easier if two new sounds from a new language are different in the same way as two sounds from the first language.

Picking up the distinctions in a second language is easiest if the second language is learned at the same time as the first. This is why language immersion programs are becoming popular in preschool and elementary curriculums of multicultural countries such as the United States. The downside to this strategy is that kids learning multiple languages at the same time usually take longer to master each of the languages individually than children exposed to only a single language take to master that one language (Bialystok and Hakuta, 1994). This is a natural consequence of having to learn not one but two sets of rules about when to ignore and when to pay attention to speech sound differences (as well as learning two vocabularies, two sets of grammatical rules, and so on).

LEARNING WORDS Thus far in this chapter, we have learned many things about the nature and complexity of speech sounds, and about how listeners perceive consonants and vowels. But the whole point of producing and perceiving these speech sounds is to put them together to form words, which are the units of language that convey meaning. How do novice language learners (infants) make the leap from streams of meaningless speech sounds to the meaningful groups of speech sounds that we call words?

First, let's state the obvious. Just like strings of musical notes, no string of speech sounds is inherently meaningful. The string 'd'–'aw'–'g' becomes meaningful to English-speaking infants, but to French-speaking, Spanish-speaking, and German-speaking infants this string remains completely meaningless because their parents refer to their furry house companion as *chien*, *perro*, and *Hund*, respectively. Infants in different places in the world must learn the words that are specific to their native language.

We have already seen how a series of consonants and vowels within a single word tend to "run into" one another because of coarticulation. It turns out the situation is not much better for a series of words forming a sentence. This fact is easily seen in **Figure 11.21**: without the letters at the bottom of the figure, you would have no idea where the word *where* ends and the word *are* begins.

Interestingly, our perception usually seems at odds with this acoustic reality. When we listen to someone talk to us in our native language, individual

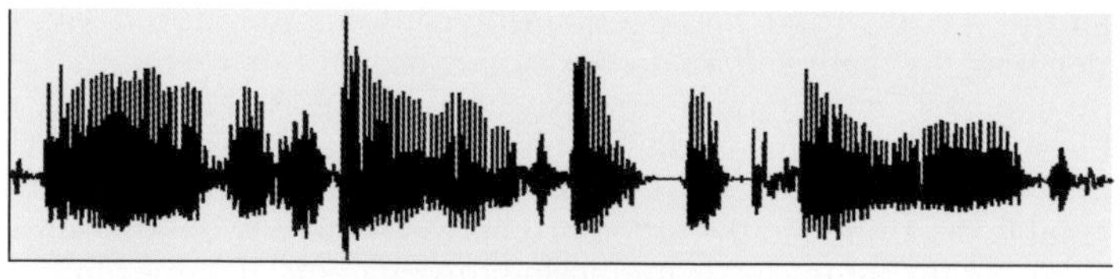

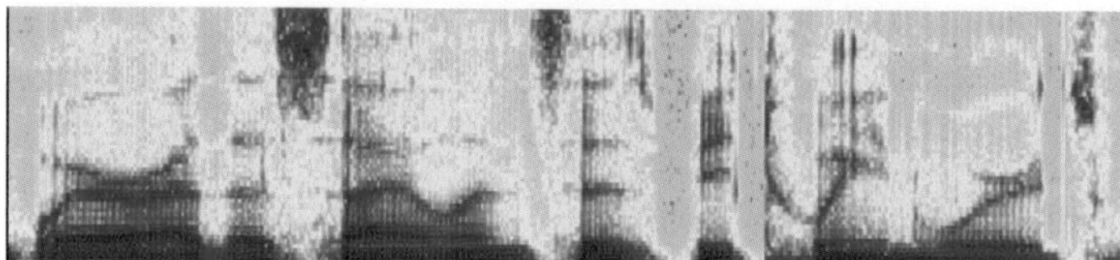

FIGURE 11.21 In this sentence—"Where are the silences between words?"—we can see that there are no breaks between the sounds of one word and the sounds of the next. Infants can use their experience with particular sequences of speech sounds to learn about boundaries between words.

words seem to stand out quite clearly as separate entities. But listening to someone speak in a different language is often a very different experience. Listen to the Chinese and Arabic speakers in **Web Activity 11.4: Word Breaks**. Unless you have experience with these languages, it probably sounds as if they include lots of really long words—some as long as whole English sentences. It may also seem as if people in these cultures speak much faster than English speakers do. Native Chinese and Arabic speakers probably say the same things about the English language and English speakers. This is the situation faced by infants the world over.

To study how infants learn words from the continuous streams of speech that they encounter in their environment, Saffran, Aslin, and Newport (1996) invented a novel language. The words of this new language all had three syllables—for example, *tupiro*, *golabu*, *dapiku*, and *tilado*. Next they created randomized sequences of these novel words, with words running together just as they do in fluently produced sentences. A sample sequence would be "tupirogolabudapikutiladogolabutupirotiladodapiku." Eight-month-old infants listened to a 2-minute sequence such as this while sitting on a parent's lap. After this brief period of learning, infants heard either "tupiro" (one of the novel words) or "pabiku" (a new combination of the same syllables used to produce the "real" novel words). The infants listened longer to the nonwords than to the words, indicating that after just 2 minutes of exposure, they had already begun to learn the words in this new "language." How did they do it?

Saffran and her colleagues suggest that the infants in their study learned the words by being sensitive to the statistics of the sequences of sounds that they had heard in the first part of the experiment. In the real world of language, words are simply sequences of speech sounds that tend to occur together. Other sequences occur together less often. For example, think about the sequence 'p'–'r'–'ih'–'t'–'ee'–'b'–'ay'–'b'–'ee.' An infant will hear the sounds making up the word *pretty* in many different contexts ("pretty dress," "pretty good," and so on) and the sounds making up the word *baby* in other contexts (e.g., "good baby," "baby doll"). In contrast, the sequence 'tyba' will almost never be heard in any other context, because no English words have this sequence of syllables. Saffran (2001, 2002) suggests that infants learn to pick words out of the speech stream by accumulating experience with sounds that tend to occur together; these are words (at least to babies). For example, infants eventually split the "word" *allgone* into two as they acquire more linguistic experience. When sounds that are rarely heard together occur in combination, that's a sign that there is a break between two words.

Speech in the Brain

Our earliest understanding of the role of cerebral cortex in the perception of speech and music was gained through unfortunate "natural" experiments in which people had lost their ability to understand speech following stroke or other brain injuries. However, it is difficult to draw strong conclusions about brain processes from brain injuries. Brain damage from stroke follows patterns of blood vessels, not brain function. Damage from stroke might cover just part of a particular brain function, leaving some of the function undamaged; or damage could cover a wide region that includes some or all of a particular brain function, as well as all or part of other functions. Performance following brain damage, along with later experimental findings, has taught us that different hemispheres of the brain are better at doing some types of tasks. For most people, the left hemisphere is dominant for language processing. The development of techniques for brain imaging, such as positron emission tomography (PET) and functional magnetic resonance imaging (fMRI), has made it possible for us to learn more about how speech is processed in the brain.

As we would expect on the basis of what we learned in Chapter 9, hearing sounds of any kind activates primary auditory cortex (A1). Further, we learned that the processing of complex sounds relies on additional areas of cortex adjacent to A1. These nearby areas of auditory cortex, called belt and parabelt regions, often are referred to as "secondary" or "association" areas. As one might expect, we see these areas activated when listeners hear speech and music. In addition, at these relatively early levels of cortical processing, activity in response to music, speech, and other complex sounds is relatively balanced across the two hemispheres (Binder, 2000).

When we listen to speech, additional areas of both left and right superior temporal lobes activate more strongly in response to speech than to nonspeech sounds, such as isolated tones and noise (**Figure 11.22**). Although we know that language is typically lateralized to one hemisphere, this activity in response to speech has been observed to be relatively balanced across both sides of the brain when researchers have been very careful to avoid higher-level effects of language (Zatorre and Binder, 2000).

At some point, however, processing of speech should become more lateralized to one temporal lobe because perceiving speech is part of understanding language. One challenge for researchers has been to create control stimuli

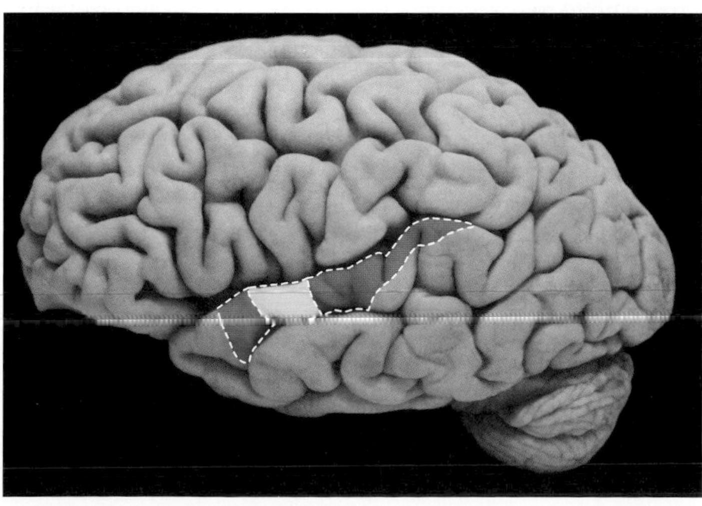

FIGURE 11.22 Listening to speech and similarly complex sounds results in the activation of cortical areas (blue) in both the left and the right superior temporal lobes (only the left is shown here). However, when listeners categorize sounds such as 'bah' and 'dah,' there is activation (yellow) a little farther anterior (forward) and ventral (lower), mostly on the left superior temporal lobe. When speech forms intelligible sentences, there is activation (green) even farther anterior and ventral only on the left side of the brain. (Courtesy of S. Mark Williams and Dale Purves, Duke University Medical Center.)

that have all the complex properties of speech without being heard as speech. We already learned that listeners are very good at understanding even severely distorted speech, so this makes it pretty difficult to construct stimuli that are complex like speech without being heard as speech.

Liebenthal et al. (2005) adopted a creative way to control for acoustic complexity while varying whether sounds would be heard as speech. They synthesized syllables varying incrementally from 'bah' to 'dah,' much like those in Figure 11.13, as their speech stimuli. Nonspeech control stimuli were the same series of syllables, except characteristics of F_1 transitions were flipped upside down. It is impossible for a human vocal tract to create such sounds, and listeners could not identify them as consonants.

While having their brains scanned, listeners participated in a categorical-perception task, discriminating pairs of stimuli from one or the other series of stimuli. For the 'bah'/'dah' speech series, performance was just like what we always find in studies of categorical perception: the discrimination of stimuli that would be labeled differently (e.g., 'bah' versus 'dah') was almost perfect, but the discrimination of other stimulus pairs was rather poor. For the nonspeech sounds, the accuracy of discrimination was similar for all pairs of stimuli. Hearing both series of stimuli resulted in increased activation in superior temporal cortex in both temporal lobes. When the sounds were speech ('bah' and 'dah'), however, the superior temporal cortex showed increased activation a bit anterior (forward) and ventral (lower) from the activation for control stimuli and mostly in the left hemisphere.

As with perception in general, cortical organization depends critically on experience, and the perception of speech sounds is tremendously experience-dependent. Because we know that English and Hindi speakers hear sounds like 'd' differently, we know that the way listeners discriminate 'bah' and 'dah' depends on experience. Liebenthal et al. (2005) may have revealed a place in the left temporal lobe where experience with English 'b' and 'd' shapes neural activity.

Another study demonstrated how these results might suggest the next step of the processing of speech into language. Scott et al. (2000) controlled for acoustic complexity while changing whether sentences were intelligible. They created "spectrally rotated" sentences that could not be understood by listeners. Rotated speech signals were spectrographically upside down. They could not be understood by listeners, but they were as complex acoustically as right-side-up sentences. Rotated stimuli activated superior temporal lobes comparably to intact, nonrotated sentences, suggesting that auditory processing in these areas is related more to complexity than to being speech per se. The essential difference between cortical responses to these two types of stimuli was that, in the left temporal lobe, activation in response to intact sentences continued farther forward of (anterior to) and lower than (ventral to) the region activated by rotated sentences. This activation was a little anterior and ventral to the 'b' and 'd' area activated in the categorical-perception task.

A great deal of research is being conducted to further our understanding of how speech is processed in the brain on its way to becoming part of words and sentences. For now, the evidence suggests that as sounds become more complex, they are processed in more anterior and ventral regions of superior temporal cortex farther away from A1 (Patterson and Johnsrude, 2008; Uppenkamp et al., 2006). When speech sounds become more clearly a part of language, they are processed farther forward in the left temporal lobe in areas that are more anterior and more ventral too.

Cortical processes related to speech perception could be distinguished from brain processes that contribute to the perception of other complex sounds in two other ways. Listeners have a wealth of experience simultaneously hearing speech and viewing talkers' faces, and the McGurk effect (see Figure 11.14) is evidence of the profound effects that visual cues can have on the way speech sounds are perceived. Some evidence suggests which brain areas are related to these audiovisual perceptual effects. For example, in studying participants silently lip-reading the face of a person saying the digits 1 through 10, Calvert et al. (1997) observed bilateral activation of superior temporal lobes like that found when listeners hear speech (e.g., Binder et al., 1994). Zatorre (2001) provided complementary findings in a study of people with cochlear implants who previously had been deaf. These listeners had increased brain activity in visual cortex when listening to speech. Zatorre hypothesized that this activation of visual areas of the brain is the result of increased experience and ability with lip-reading for these previously deaf individuals.

Finally, whenever people talk, they both hear the sounds they're producing and experience the movements of speech production in their own vocal tracts. One thing to learn from future studies of brain activity is how these processes of hearing and speaking interact. People have a lot of experience with the simultaneous activities of producing and perceiving our own speech, so one might expect to find brain regions where these related activities combine. (See Web Essay 11.1: Studying Brain Areas for Language Processing.)

Summary

1. Musical pitch has two dimensions: tone height and tone chroma. Musical notes are combined to form chords. Notes and chords vary in duration and are combined to form melodies.
2. Melodies are learned psychological entities defined by patterns of rising and falling musical pitches, with different durations and rhythms.
3. Rhythm is important to music, and to auditory perception more broadly. The process of perceiving sound sequences is biased to hear rhythm.
4. Humans evolved to be able to produce an extremely wide variety of sounds that can be used by languages. The production of speech sounds has three basic components: respiration, phonation, and articulation. Speech sounds vary in many dimensions, including intensity, duration, periodicity, and noisiness.
5. In terms of articulation and acoustics, speech sounds vary according to other speech sounds that precede and follow (coarticulation). Because of coarticulation, listeners cannot use any single acoustic feature to identify a vowel or consonant. Instead, listeners must use multiple properties of the speech signal.
6. In general, listeners discriminate speech sounds only as well as they can label them. This is categorical perception, which also has been shown for the perception of many other complex familiar auditory and visual stimuli.
7. How people perceive speech depends very much on their experience with speech sounds within a language. This experience includes learning which of the many acoustic features in speech tend to co-occur. Because of the role of experience in how we hear speech, it is often difficult to perceive and produce new speech sounds from a second language following experience with a first language.
8. One of the ways that infants learn words is to use their experience with the co-occurrence of speech sounds.
9. Speech sounds are processed in both hemispheres of the brain much like other complex sounds, until they become part of the linguistic message. Then, speech is further processed in anterior and ventral regions, mostly in the left superior temporal cortex.

Refer to the **Sensation and Perception** website **(www.sinauer.com/wolfe2e)** for activities, essays, study questions, and other study aids.

CHAPTER 12

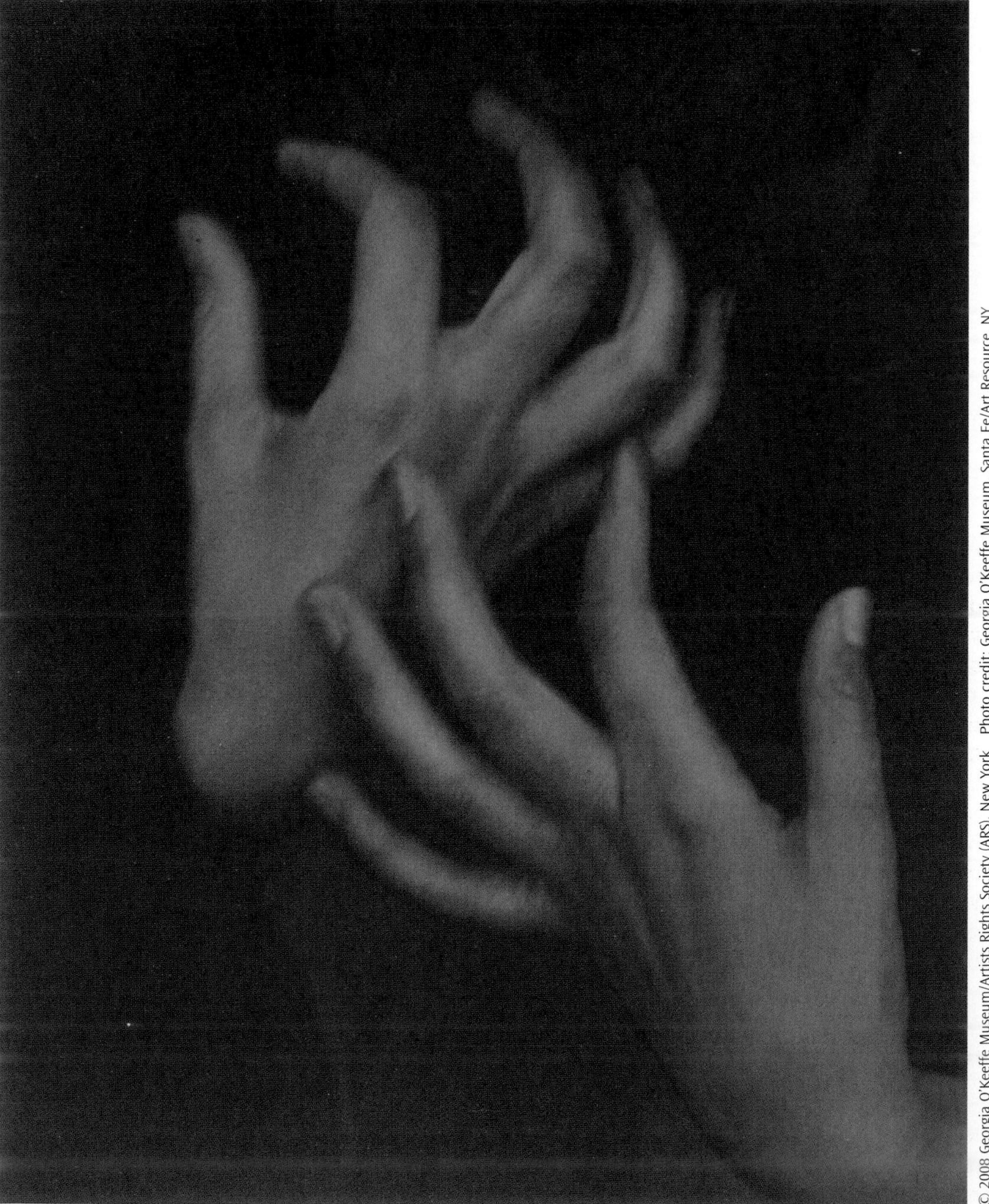

Alfred Stieglitz, *Hands*, 1919

Touch

Having studied the perceptual systems for vision and hearing, you should recognize a number of questions that curious minds want asked and answered about any sense. In this chapter we consider the following questions regarding the sense of touch:

- What are the physical stimuli for touch? More precisely, what forms of energy lead to the sensation of being touched?
- What is touch good for? What might the evolutionary "niche" of this sensory modality be?
- What is the sensory apparatus for touch, and how do these structures change touch stimuli into neural signals?
- Which neurophysiological pathways connect touch receptors to higher-order perception and cognition in the brain?
- How do we use touch input to determine the identity ("what" tasks) and location ("where" tasks) of objects in the world?
- How does the sense of touch compare with and interact with other sensory modalities?

Let's start with the first two of these questions. By its most narrow definition, the term *touch* is used to refer to the sensations caused by mechanical displacements of the skin. These displacements occur when you are poked by your 4-year-old nephew, licked by your dog, or kissed by your significant other. They occur any time you grasp, wield, or otherwise make contact with an object. We will use the term *tactile* (the adjective form of touch) to refer to these mechanical interactions and will expand the definition of *touch* to include the perception of temperature changes (thermal sensation), the sensation of pain, which occurs when our body tissues are damaged (or potentially damaged) in some way, itchiness, and the internal sensations that inform us of the positions and movements of our limbs in space. Collectively, these internal sensations are known as **kinesthesis** when they arise from muscles, tendons, and joints, and they are part of a broader system known as **proprioception**, which includes the vestibular system as well (see Chapter 15). The technical term for all these senses put together is **somatosensation**.

It is difficult to conceive of our species surviving without a sense of touch. Pain serves as a sophisticated warning system that tells us when something might be internally wrong or when an external stimulus may be dangerous, enabling us to defend our bodies as quickly as possible (e.g., by rapidly moving away from the noxious stimulus). Temperature sensations enable us to seek or create a thermally safe environment. Mechanical sensations play an important role in our intimate sexual and reproductive activities, and they provide a powerful means of communicating our thoughts and emotions nonverbally.

kinesthesis The perception of the position and movement of our limbs in space.

proprioception Perception mediated by kinesthetic and vestibular receptors.

somatosensation A collective term for sensory signals from the body.

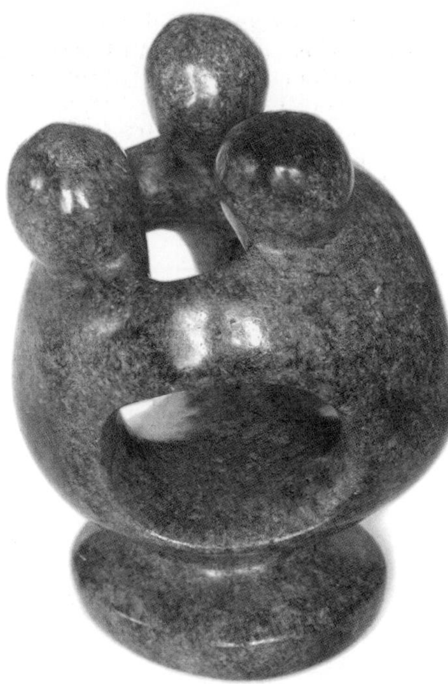

FIGURE 12.1 Soapstone sculpture from Zimbabwe.

On a more fundamental level, touch is important because we can use it to identify and manipulate objects that cannot be seen or heard. Blindfold yourself for at least 10 minutes and try doing some routine tasks, like making a sandwich, getting dressed, or taking a shower. The first thing you will notice while doing this exercise is just how much our species normally relies on vision to inform us about the world around us. But you should also discover that touch can substitute for vision to a surprising degree: You probably won't have as much trouble distinguishing the peanut butter jar from the jelly jar as you think you might. And if you pay attention, you will find that you don't actually use vision, or any sense other than touch, very much at all for some tasks (e.g., buttoning your shirt, brushing your teeth, opening that jar of peanut butter).

There is one more thing you may become acutely aware of during your experiment with the blindfold. Our eyes and ears can perceive signals from objects that are far from the body, but we must almost always be in direct contact with an object to perceive it by touch (exceptions to this rule include a jackhammer, whose vibrations on the street outside we can feel; and the sun, from which we feel warmth even though it is millions of miles away). Therefore, to use touch to learn about the world, we must act. If we want to know the weight of a beautiful soapstone sculpture like the one in **Figure 12.1**, we pick it up. We might also stroke it to feel its exquisite smoothness or press it to our forehead to feel its coolness. In sum, touch involves action, arguably to a greater degree than any of our other senses do.

Touch Physiology

The Sense Organ and Receptor Units for Touch

The sites of our sensing equipment for vision, audition, olfaction, and gustation are all located in organs (the eyes, ears, nose, and mouth, respectively) that are more or less dedicated to sensory processing. Some other animals have analogous appendages: antennae. You might think that, for touch, humans do not have a readily apparent sense organ. In fact, the human sense of touch is housed in what is actually the largest and heaviest of the sense organs, the skin, which covers an area of approximately 1.8 square meters and weighs about 4 kilograms. Touch receptors are embedded all over the body, in both hairless and hairy skin, as well as within our mouths and our muscles, tendons, and joints.

Although the external quality of the skin varies across different parts of the body (it is thicker in some parts and thinner in others, smoother in some regions and coarser in others, and so on), most skin includes the basic substructures shown in **Figure 12.2**. The receptor units for touch are embedded in both the outer layer, called the **epidermis**, and the underlying layer, known as the **dermis**. As Figure 12.2 illustrates, just as the eye has its rods and three types of cones, the skin has multiple types of touch receptors. These receptors form the basis for multiple "channels," specialized information-processing subsystems that each contribute to the overall sense of touch. For example, if we wrap our fingers around a cube of ice, different channels convey information about its temperature, its shape, and its texture.

We will discuss the receptors for these various channels in detail in the sections that follow (see **Web Activity 12.1: Somatosensory Receptors**). In general, however, each type of receptor can be characterized by three attributes:

1. *Type of stimulation to which the receptor responds*. Receptors respond to different stimulus events—for example, to pressure, vibration, or temperature changes.

epidermis The outer of two major layers of skin.

dermis The inner of two major layers of skin, consisting of nutritive and connective tissues, within which lie the mechanoreceptors.

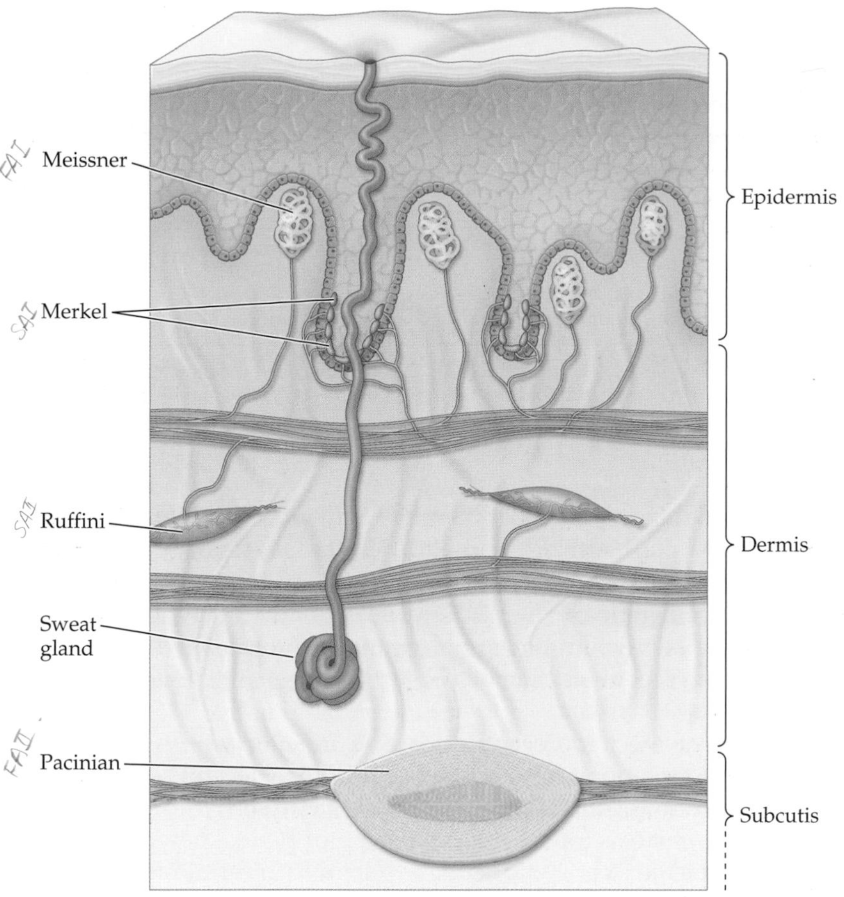

FIGURE 12.2 A cross section of hairless skin of the human hand, schematically demonstrating the locations of the four types of mechanoreceptors—Meissner corpuscles, Merkel cell neurite complexes, Ruffini endings, and Pacinian corpuscles—and illustrating the two major layers of human skin. The subcutis, which underlies these outer two layers as shown here, is not usually included in the formal definition of "skin." (After R. S. Johansson and Vallbo, 1983.)

2. *Size of the receptive field.* Receptors are activated when stimulation is applied to a particular area of the body, which constitutes the receptors' "receptive field" (recall that the same term is used for the receptors of other sensory systems). The size of the receptive field refers to the extent of the body area that elicits a receptor response.
3. *Rate of adaptation (fast versus slow).* A fast-adapting (FA) receptor responds with bursts of action potentials, first when its preferred stimulus is applied and then again when it is removed. It does not respond during the steady state between stimulus onset and offset. In contrast, a slow-adapting (SA) receptor remains active throughout the period during which the stimulus is in contact with its receptive field.

TACTILE RECEPTORS Tactile receptors are called **mechanoreceptors** because they respond to mechanical stimulation or pressure. A tactile receptor consists of a "nerve fiber" and an associated expanded ending. All tactile nerve fibers fall into a class called A-beta fibers, which have relatively wide diameters that permit very fast neural conduction. The four populations of tactile receptors that are found in the hairless skin on the palms are shown in Figure 12.2. (Note that there are also five major types of A-beta tactile receptors located in regions covered with hairy skin, such as the forearm. These mechanoreceptors and their associated afferent fibers have properties similar to those in hairless skin: two types are slowly adapting and three are fast adapting.) The tactile nerve fibers for the various types are assumed to terminate in different expanded endings. You may be surprised to learn that the specific kind of expanded ending for each type of nerve fiber has provoked considerable controversy among tactile scientists for over a century now, because it has proved extremely difficult to observe the physical connections directly.

mechanoreceptors Sensory receptors that are responsive to mechanical stimulation (pressure, vibration, and movement).

Meissner corpuscle A specialized nerve ending associated with fast-adapting (FA I) fibers that have small receptive fields.

Merkel cell neurite complex A specialized nerve ending associated with slow-adapting (SA I) fibers that have small receptive fields.

Pacinian corpuscle A specialized nerve ending associated with fast-adapting (FA II) fibers that have large receptive fields.

Ruffini ending A specialized nerve ending associated with slow-adapting (SA II) fibers that have large receptive fields.

TABLE 12.1 Response characteristics of the four mechanoreceptor populations

	Size of receptive field	
Adaptation rate	**Small**	**Large**
Slow	SA I (Merkel)	SA II (Ruffini)
Fast	FA I (Meissner)	FA II (Pacinian)

Note: FA I = fast-adapting type I; FA II = fast-adapting type II; SA I = slow-adapting type I; SA II = slow-adapting type II. The terminal ending associated with each type of tactile nerve fiber is shown in parentheses.

The expanded endings of the four different populations of tactile fibers in the hairless skin of the hand are named after the anatomists who first described them: **Meissner corpuscles**, **Merkel cell neurite complexes**, **Pacinian corpuscles**, and **Ruffini endings**. The endings of Meissner and Merkel receptors are located at the junction of the epidermis and dermis, whereas the Pacinian and Ruffini receptors are embedded more deeply in the dermis and underlying subcutaneous tissue.

The four types of mechanoreceptors can be independently classified according to their adaptation rates and the sizes of their receptive fields, as measured from activity of the tactile nerve fibers. These two dimensions lead to a second set of labels for the mechanoreceptor types, shown in **Table 12.1**. Each type of tactile fiber is particularly sensitive to certain features of mechanical stimulation, rendering it suitable for particular types of functions, as shown in **Table 12.2**.

- SA I fibers respond best to steady downward pressure, fine spatial details, and very low frequency vibrations of less than about 5 Hz. They are especially important for texture and pattern perception. Some activities particularly dependent on this touch channel include reading Braille and determining the location and orientation of the slot on the head of a screw that we can feel but not see. When a single SA I fiber is stimulated, people report feeling "pressure." These fibers are assumed to terminate in Merkel cell neurite complexes.

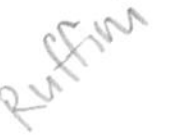

- SA II fibers in the skin (as well as in all fibrous tissues in the body) respond to sustained downward pressure, and particularly to lateral skin stretch, which occurs, for example, when we grasp an object. When you reach out for your coffee cup, the SA II fibers help determine when your fingers are shaped properly for picking up the cup. (Note that recent research has questioned whether the expanded terminals of the SA II

TABLE 12.2 Mechanoreceptors: Feature sensitivity and associated function

Mechanoreceptor population	Maximum feature sensitivity	Primary functions
SA I	Sustained pressure, very low frequency (< ~5 Hz) Spatial deformation	Texture perception Pattern/form detection
FA I	Temporal changes in skin deformation (~5–50 Hz)	Low-frequency vibration detection
FA II	Temporal changes in skin deformation (~50–700 Hz)	High-frequency vibration detection
SA II	Sustained downward pressure, lateral skin stretch, skin slip (low sensitivity to vibration across frequencies)	Finger position, stable grasp

fibers in the skin, the Ruffini endings, are as numerous as traditionally assumed.) When a single SA II fiber is stimulated, people do not experience any tactile sensation at all. Scientists have shown that in order to detect a stimulus, more than a single SA II fiber must be stimulated. These fibers are assumed to terminate in Ruffini endings.

- FA I fibers respond best to low-frequency vibrations from about 5 to 50 Hz. If your coffee cup is heavier than you expected and begins to slip across your fingers, this motion across the skin will cause just such vibrations, and your FA I fibers will help you correct your grip before your coffee spills all over you. When a lone SA I fiber is stimulated, people report a very localized sensation that they describe as "wobble" or "flutter." These fibers are assumed to terminate in Meissner corpuscles.
- FA II fibers respond best to high-frequency vibrations from about 50 to 700 Hz (the highest frequency tested to date). Such vibrations occur whenever an object first makes contact with the skin, as, for example, when a mosquito lands on your arm. Such vibrations are also generated when an object that you're holding contacts another object, so FA II fibers help you determine how hard you're tapping your pencil on your desk as you try to cram all this information into your brain. When a single FA II fiber is stimulated, people report a more diffuse sensation in the skin that corresponds to a "buzz." These fibers have been shown to terminate in Pacinian corpuscles.

Just as both rods and cones contribute to our perception of every individual visual stimulus, the four types of mechanoreceptors are always working together to inform us about every individual object we touch. Johnson (2002) gives the example of opening a door with a key. Feeling the shape of your key in your pocket requires the SA I (and maybe also the FA I) channel. Shaping your fingers to grasp the key involves the SA II channel. As you insert the key into the lock, your grip force increases so that the key does not slip, thanks to your FA I channel. Finally, your FA II channel tells you when the key has hit the end of the keyhole.

KINESTHETIC RECEPTORS In addition to the tactile mechanoreceptors in the skin, yet other types of mechanoreceptors lie within muscles, tendons, and joints. These are collectively referred to as **kinesthetic** receptors, and they play an important role in sensing where our limbs are and what kinds of movements we're making (Clark and Horch, 1986; L. A. Jones, 1999). The angle formed by a limb at a joint is perceived primarily through muscle receptors called **muscle spindles** (**Figure 12.3**), which convey the rate at which

kinesthetic Referring to perception involving sensory mechanoreceptors in muscles, tendons, and joints.

muscle spindle A sensory receptor located in a muscle that senses its tension.

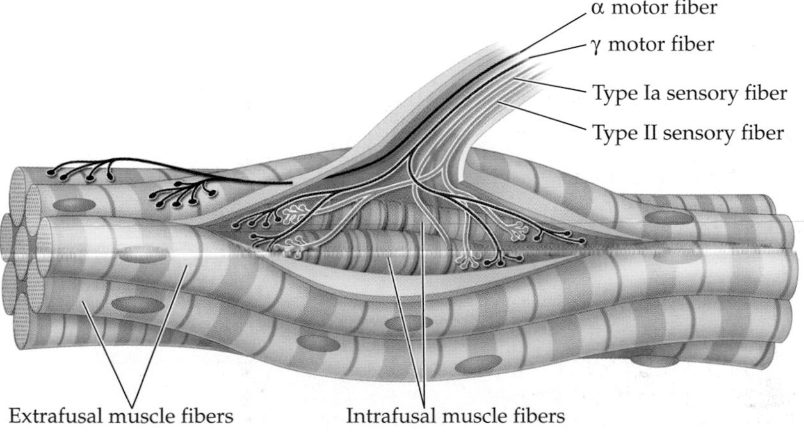

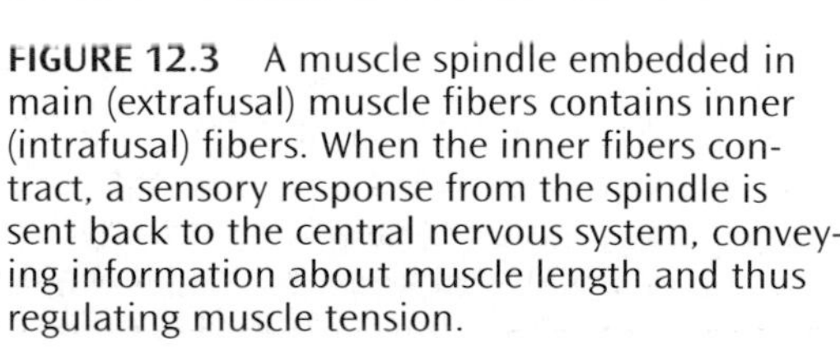
FIGURE 12.3 A muscle spindle embedded in main (extrafusal) muscle fibers contains inner (intrafusal) fibers. When the inner fibers contract, a sensory response from the spindle is sent back to the central nervous system, conveying information about muscle length and thus regulating muscle tension.

thermoreceptors Sensory receptors that signal information about changes in skin temperature.

warmth fiber A sensory nerve fiber that fires when skin temperature increases.

cold fiber A sensory nerve fiber that fires when skin temperature decreases.

the muscle fibers are changing in length. Receptors in the tendons provide signals about the tension in muscles attached to the tendons, and receptors directly in the joints themselves come into play particularly when a joint is bent to an extreme angle.

The importance of kinesthetic receptors is graphically illustrated by the strange case of a neurological patient named Ian Waterman (read *Pride and a Daily Marathon* [1991] by Jonathan Cole for more about this interesting individual). The cutaneous nerves that connected Waterman's kinesthetic and other mechanoreceptors to his brain were destroyed by a viral infection when he was 19 years old. Lacking kinesthetic senses, Waterman is now completely dependent on vision to tell him about the positions of his limbs in space. If the lights are turned off, Waterman cannot tie his shoes, walk up or down stairs, or even clap his hands, because he has no idea where his hands and feet are! Caught in an elevator when the lights went out, he was unable to remain standing and could not rise again until the illumination returned. (For additional details about Waterman's troubles, and the amazing degree to which he has compensated for his lack of kinesthetic receptors, see **Web Essay 12.1: Living without Kinesthesis**.)

THERMORECEPTORS **Thermoreceptors**, located in both the epidermal and dermal layers of the skin (see Figure 12.2), inform us about changes in skin temperature. There are two distinct populations of thermoreceptors (**Figure 12.4**): **warmth fibers** fire when the temperature of the skin surrounding the fibers rises; **cold fibers** (which outnumber warmth fibers by a ratio of about 30:1) fire in response to decreases in skin temperature.

Our bodies are constantly working to regulate their internal temperature, so under normal conditions the skin is kept between 30°C and 36°C (86°F and 96°F), and neither cold nor warmth fibers respond much while skin temperature remains within this range. If you bundle up in your long underwear and snowsuit but then sit inside in front of the fire, your skin temperature will probably rise above 36°C, and your warmth fibers will begin to fire. If you then take the snowsuit off and walk out into the snow, your skin temperature will rapidly begin to fall, and as soon as it goes below 30°C, your cold receptors will start firing.

Thermoreceptors also kick into gear when we make contact with an object that is warmer or colder than the skin. Objects in the environment are typically cooler than 30°C, so it is usually the cold fibers that tell us about the object. For example, steel conducts heat more efficiently than stone. Your cold fibers will thus fire less rapidly and for a shorter period of time when you touch a steel object than when you touch a stone object (because the steel object will warm more quickly to match your skin temperature). If

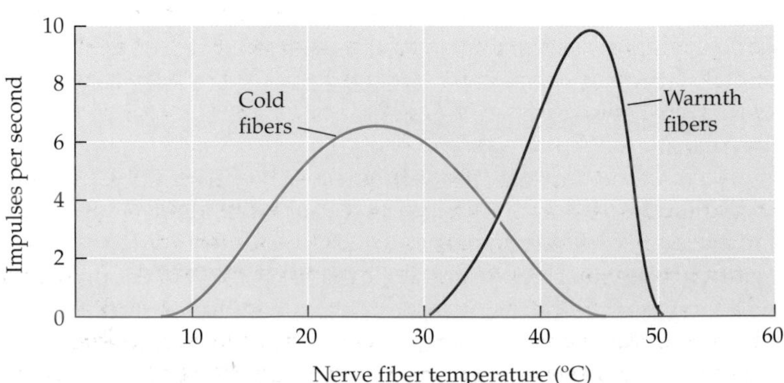

FIGURE 12.4 Thermal receptivity functions, showing the response of warmth and cold fibers to different temperatures. (After Guyton, 1991.)

you've had prior experience with steel and stone, you can interpret the thermoreceptor responses to make this distinction.

NOCICEPTORS Pain is the realm of touch that has the dubious honor of being home to the sensations we like the least. We may find some visual stimuli revolting and some olfactory or gustatory stimuli disgusting, but of all the sensations, it is pain that we take the most drastic actions to avoid. Pain begins with signals from **nociceptors**, touch receptors that have bare nerve endings and that respond to various forms of tissue damage or to stimuli that have the potential to damage tissue (including extreme skin temperatures lower than 15°C or higher than 45°C).

Nociceptors can be divided into two types by the nerve fibers, for which no specialized endings have been found. **A-delta fibers** respond primarily to strong pressure or heat and are myelinated, which enables them to conduct signals very rapidly. **C fibers** are unmyelinated and respond to intense stimulation of various sorts: pressure, heat or cold, or noxious chemicals. Both types of pain fibers are smaller in diameter than those coming from nonnociceptive mechanoreceptors in the skin—the wider-diameter fibers known as type "A-beta." Many painful events seem to occur in two stages: a quick sharp burst of pain followed by a throbbing sensation. These two stages may reflect the onset of signals first from the A-delta fibers and then from the C fibers (Price et al., 1977).

It might seem that pain perception has no upside, but consider what would happen if we had no nociceptors. We wouldn't be able to sense dangerously sharp or hot objects. Lacking alarms, we might soon lack fingers! Some diseases, such as Hansen's disease (leprosy) and diabetes, are characterized by the loss of pain sensation and provide real-life examples of the consequences. The case of "Miss C," reported by Melzack and Wall (1973), shows what can happen to people born with insensitivity to pain. Not only did Miss C lack pain sensation, but she did not sneeze, cough, gag, or protect her eyes reflexively. She suffered childhood injuries from burning herself on a radiator and biting her tongue while chewing food. As an adult, she developed problems in her joints that were attributed to lack of discomfort, for example, from standing too long in the same position. She died at age 29 from infections that could probably have been prevented in someone who was alerted to injury by painful sensations.

nociceptors Sensory receptors that transmit information about noxious (painful) stimulation that causes damage or potential damage to the skin.

A-delta fiber An intermediate-sized, myelinated sensory nerve fiber that transmits pain and temperature signals.

C fiber A narrow-diameter, unmyelinated sensory nerve fiber that transmits pain and temperature signals.

From Skin to Brain

Because the receptors for sights, sounds, tastes, and smells are all located in the skull, the pathways that deliver information from these receptors to the brain are fairly short. Touch messages, on the other hand, must travel as far as 2 meters to get from the skin and muscles of the feet to the brain. To cross this distance, the information must move up through the spinal cord. Initially the axons of various tactile receptors are combined into single nerve trunks, in much the same way that retinal ganglion axons converge in the optic nerve (see Chapter 2) and that cochlear hair cells converge in the auditory nerve (see Chapter 9).

Right from the start, though, we see two major differences between the visual and auditory pathways and the pathways for touch. First, whereas there are only two optic nerves and two auditory nerves, there are a number of somatosensory nerve trunks, arising in the hands, arms, feet, legs, and other areas of the skin. Second, axons in the optic and auditory nerves go directly to the brain, whereas axons in the older nerve trunks, which we discuss next, synapse first in the spinal cord. Once in the spinal cord, touch

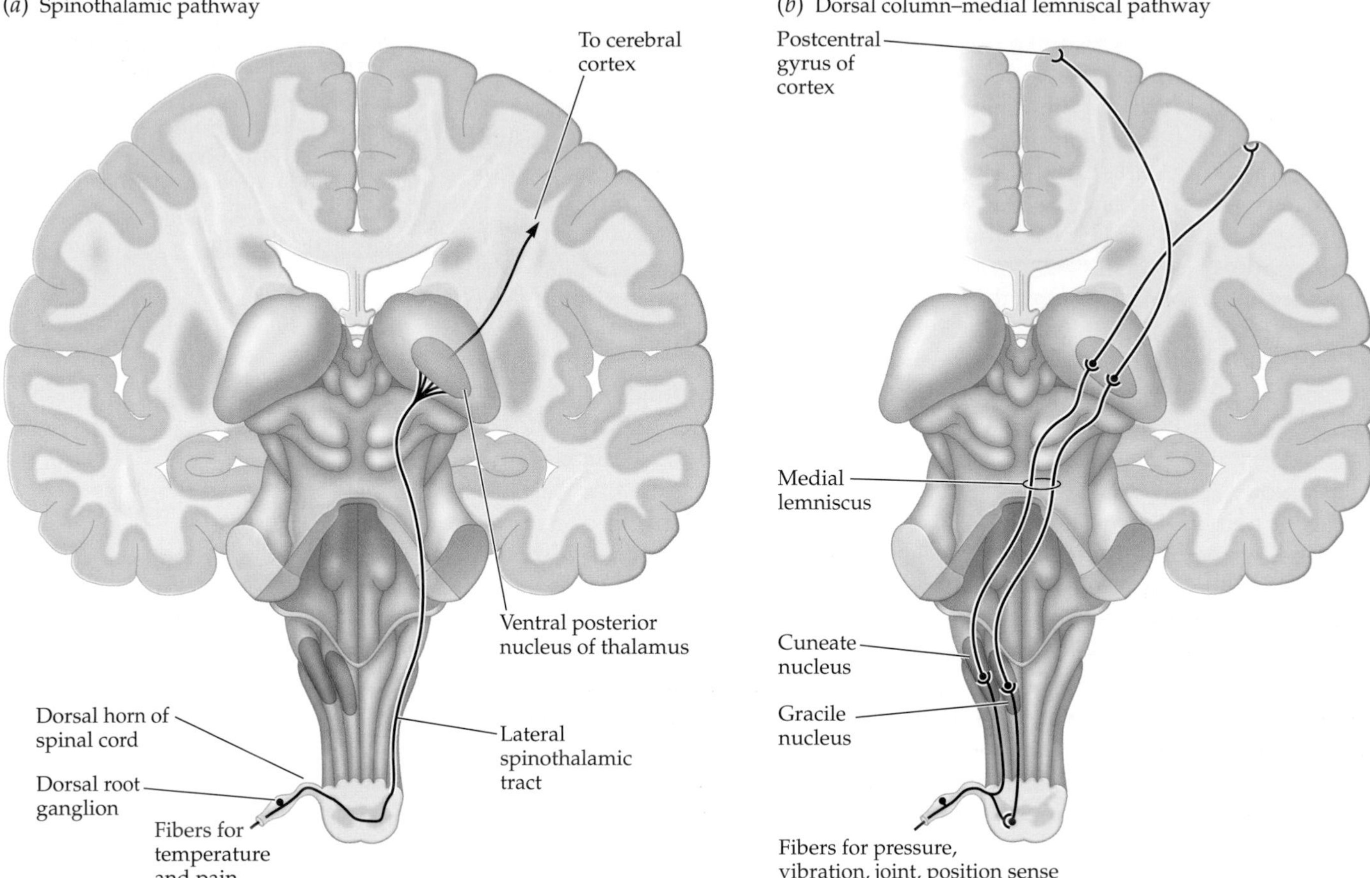

FIGURE 12.5 Pathways from skin to cortex. (*a*) Spinothalamic pathway. (*b*) Dorsal column–medial lemniscal pathway. (After Levine, 2000.)

information proceeds upward toward the brain via two major pathways, as shown in **Figure 12.5**. The evolutionarily older **spinothalamic pathway** (Figure 12.5*a*) is the slower of the two and carries most of the information from thermoreceptors and nociceptors. This pathway includes a number of synapses within the spinal cord, thus slowing conduction while providing a mechanism for inhibiting pain perception when necessary, as will be discussed shortly. The **dorsal column–medial lemniscal (DCML) pathway** (Figure 12.5*b*) includes wider-diameter axons and fewer synapses and therefore conveys information more quickly to the brain. Tactile and kinesthetic information carried along this pathway is used for planning and executing rapid movements, where quick feedback is a must.

Neurons in the DCML pathway first synapse in the cuneate and gracile nuclei, near the base of the brain (see Figure 12.5*b*). Activity is then passed on to neurons that synapse in the ventral posterior nucleus of the thalamus. Recall from Chapters 3 and 9 that the visual and auditory pathways also pass through the thalamus, each synapsing in its own modality-specific nucleus. Because this portion of the brain is largely shut down when we are asleep, the brain does not register (and therefore does not attempt to respond to) the relatively gentle touch sensations that occur, for example, when we roll over in our sleep.

From the thalamus, much of the touch information is carried up to the cortex (**Figure 12.6**) into **somatosensory area 1 (S1)**, located in the parietal lobe just behind the postcentral gyrus. S1 is analogous to V1 in vision (see Chapter 3). Neurons in S1 communicate with **somatosensory area 2 (S2)**, which lies in the upper bank of the lateral sulcus, and with other cortical areas. The

spinothalamic pathway The route from the spinal cord to the brain that carries most of the information about skin temperature and pain.

dorsal column–medial lemniscal (DCML) pathway The route from the spinal cord to the brain that carries signals from skin, muscles, tendons, and joints.

somatosensory area 1 (S1) The primary receiving area for touch in the cortex.

somatosensory area 2 (S2) The secondary receiving area for touch in the cortex.

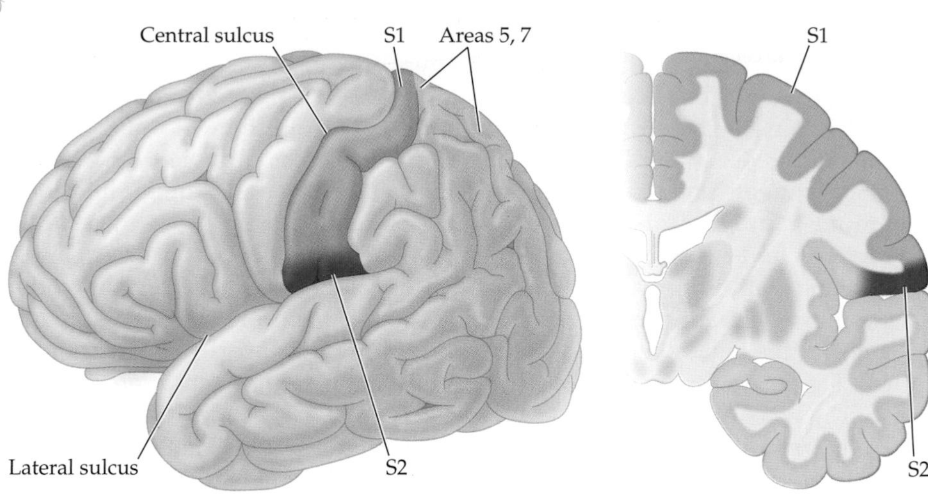

FIGURE 12.6 Primary somatosensory receiving areas in the brain. S1 includes Brodmann areas 1, 2, 3a, and 3b. Areas 5 and 7 are immediately posterior to S1. S2 lies within the lateral sulcus.

motor areas of the cortex, which control movements of body parts, are located just in front of the central sulcus. This adjacency enhances communication between the somatosensory and motor control systems.

Touch sensations that result from the skin being stimulated are spatially represented in area S1, and to some extent beyond, **somatotopically**. Somatotopy is analogous to the topographic spatial representation of events on the retina found in vision (see Chapter 3); adjacent areas on the skin are ultimately connected to adjacent areas in the brain (**Figure 12.7***a*). As a result, the somatosensory cortex is organized into a spatial map of the layout of the skin,

somatotopic Spatially mapped in the somatosensory cortex in correspondence to spatial events on the skin.

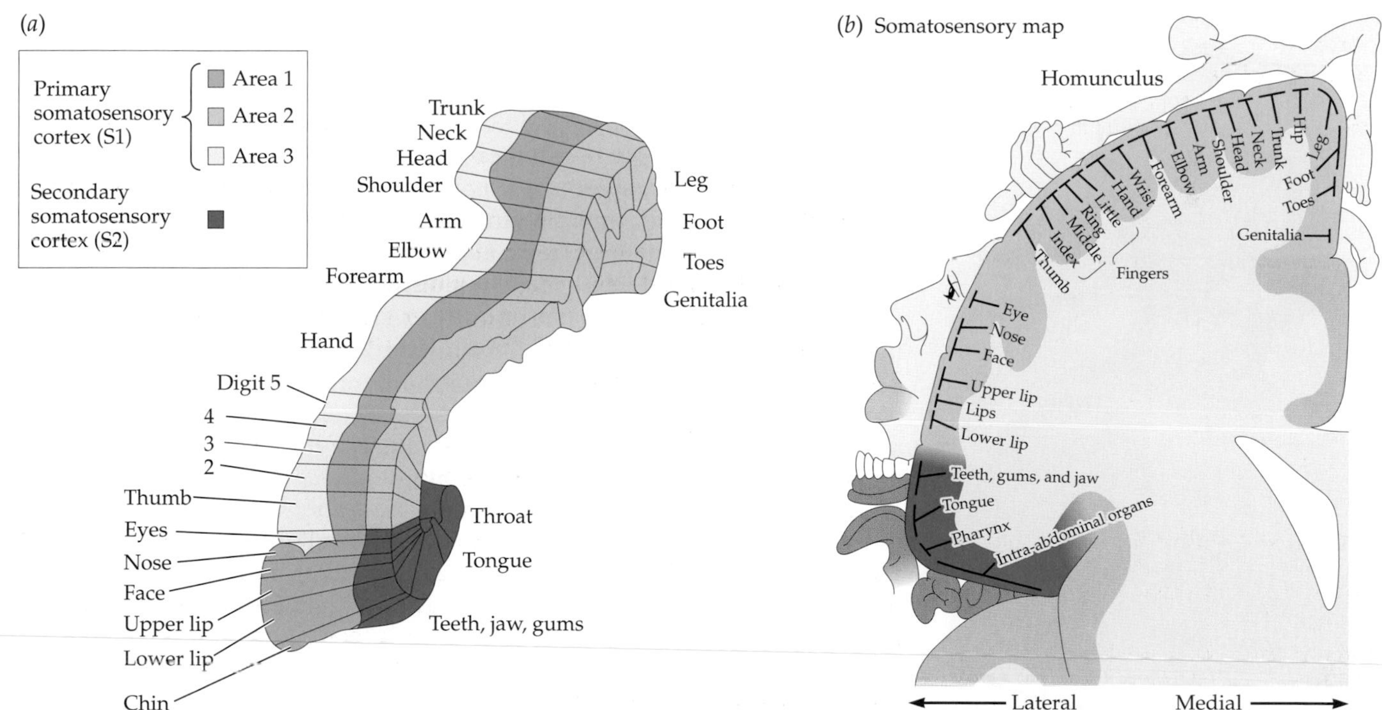

FIGURE 12.7 The sensory homunculus, showing brain regions that respond to stimulation of different parts of the body. (*a*) Multiple maps exist in primary and secondary somatosensory areas, three of which are shown within S1 and one within S2. (*b*) A schematic of the relative distribution of body parts in S1, as originally derived by Penfield and Rasmussen (1950).

homunculus A maplike representation of regions of the body in the brain.

phantom limb Sensation perceived from a physically amputated limb of the body.

often called the sensory **homunculus** (plural *homunculi*) (Figure 12.7*b*). We all have twin homunculi, one in each hemisphere of the brain. The left-hemisphere S1 receives information from the right side of the body and vice versa.

The sensory homunculus is derived largely from the work of Canadian neurosurgeon Wilder Penfield, who charted the somatotopic map with the aid of patients undergoing brain surgery to alleviate epilepsy. Because there are no pain receptors in the brain, the patients did not need to be anesthetized and could remain responsive. During the operation, Dr. Penfield systematically stimulated different parts of a patient's somatosensory cortex with an electrode. As the probe was moved from one location in S1 to another, the patient reported feeling sensations in the arms, legs, face, and so on. The correspondence between the stimulation and the sensation gave rise to a map of the body in the brain (see **Web Activity 12.2: The Sensory Homunculus**). In fact, the brain contains multiple sensory maps of the body. Separate maps are now known to exist in the different subareas of S1, and additional maps exist in secondary areas, as shown in Figure 12.7*a*.

Like the retinotopic map in area V1, Penfield's somatotopic map in S1 is distorted. The thumb, for example, grabs a big piece of real estate relative to its size. In contrast, sensations from the leg are processed in a relatively small portion of S1. In the visual system, the foveal area is overrepresented in V1 (cortical magnification; see Chapter 3) because there are many more photoreceptors in the fovea than in peripheral parts of the retina. Similarly, a larger chunk of S1 is dedicated to processing information from the lips and the fingers than from the neck because tactile receptors are much more heavily concentrated in the lips than they are in the neck. The relatively tight correspondence between body parts and areas of S1 can have unfortunate side effects in cases of limb amputation. If an amputee's left arm is missing, obviously no mechanoreceptors are sending touch signals from that arm. However, sporadic activity can continue in the area of the amputee's right S1 corresponding to the arm, leading to the perception of a **phantom limb**. At times, patients may perceive their phantom limbs to be in uncomfortable positions, leading to persistent (and very real) pain.

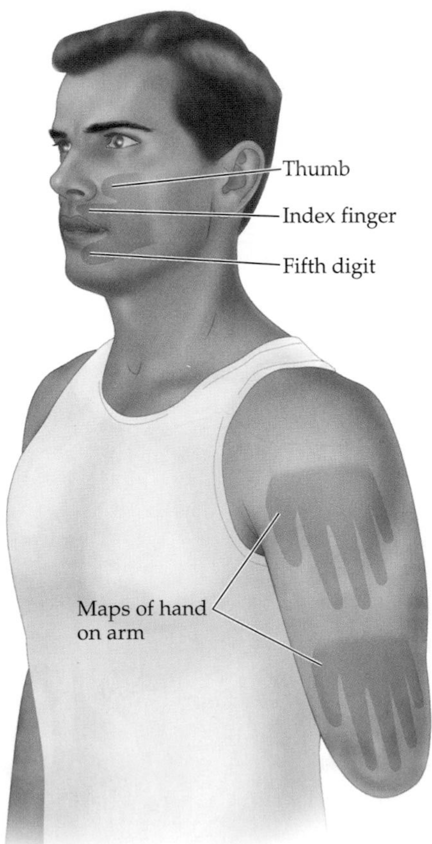

FIGURE 12.8 Phantom limbs may appear on the face and stump subsequent to amputation. Amputees report feeling the amputated hand when their face or remaining limbs are stimulated. (After Ramachandran, 1993.)

The psychologist Vilayanur Ramachandran recently made the astonishing observation that amputees often report feeling sensations in their phantom arms and hands when their faces or remaining limbs are touched (**Figure 12.8**). The source of this somatosensory confusion can be traced to an idiosyncrasy in the homunculus. Note in Figure 12.7 that the area responding to the face is located (somewhat arbitrarily) adjacent to the area responding to the hand and arm. Apparently the hand and arm areas of S1 are, to some extent, "invaded" by neurons carrying information from touch receptors in the face. However, other parts of the brain listening to the hand and arm areas are not fully aware of these altered connections, and therefore they attribute activity in these areas to stimulation from the missing limb. (You can read more about Ramachandran's fascinating studies on phantom limbs in **Web Essay 12.2: Phantom Limbs**.)

Projections from S1 form the basis for further analysis of objects and surfaces by the cortex of the brain. The results of some recent studies suggest that analogously to vision, the sense of touch may show a division between *what* and *where* systems in higher cortical centers. A patient studied by Reed, Caselli, and Farah (1996) showed an impairment in her ability to recognize objects by touch (*what*), but she showed no deficit in her spatial ability (*where*). Another patient could locate and manipulate objects by touch without recognizing them (Rossetti, Rode, and Boisson, 1995). Activation of the brain, observed with fMRI imaging, has been found in different areas, depending on whether the task is to locate an object or to recognize it tactually. And, as in vision, there is relatively more dorsal activation for locating objects and more ventral activation for recognizing objects (Reed, Klatzky, and Halgren, 2005; Reed, Shoham, and Halgren, 2004). You can learn more about the *what* versus *where* systems for touch by tapping into a lively debate on this topic among scientists interested in the neural circuitry that contributes to object processing (see Dijkerman and de Haan, 2007).

Lest you conclude that the neural organization of our brains for touch is permanent and unchanging, consider an experiment performed by Pascual-Leone and Hamilton (2001). These neuroscientists deprived normal, sighted volunteers of visual stimulation by having them wear a blindfold for 5 days. On each of the 5 days, they participated in an fMRI study during which pairs of Braille patterns were presented to the right index finger. Subjects were required to judge whether the two patterns within each pair were the same or different. Brain imaging found that on the first day, the Braille task activated only area S1 on the left side of the brain (which, you will recall, is activated by touching the right side of the body). But as the days progressed, the amount of activation in S1 declined while increasing in V1. Apparently area V1, which we think of as dedicated to vision, took over processing the spatial patterns introduced through the sense of touch. This change in V1 was transient: removing the blindfold led to a full return to what had been neurally observed before blindfolding. Such results reveal the remarkable **neural plasticity** of the somatosensory system. Plasticity is a recurring theme in sensory systems. We saw something very similar at the end of Chapter 3 in the discussion of visual development and strabismus, in which abnormal experience alters the wiring of the visual system. Note that the example we are discussing here shows that plasticity is a property of the adult brain and is not limited to the immature nervous system.

The pathways from the skin to the brain tell just one part of the story of the transmission of signals in touch. Downward pathways from the brain can alter the sensations produced by stimulating the periphery. Some of the most surprising effects of these downward pathways relate to the feeling of pain, which we discuss next.

neural plasticity The ability of neural circuits to undergo changes in function or organization as a result of previous activity.

substantia gelatinosa A jellylike region of interconnecting neurons in the dorsal horn of the spinal cord.

dorsal horn A region at the rear of the spinal cord that receives inputs from receptors in the skin.

gate control theory A description of the system that transmits pain that incorporates modulating signals from the brain.

- dorsal activation: locating
- ventral activation: recognizing

Pain

We tend to think of pain as an inevitable consequence of stress on or damage to our bodies, flowing from sensory levels to the conscious feeling of "ouch." The scientific study of pain, however, reveals it to be a highly subjective state with distinguishable components. What we think of as pain arises at multiple levels—sensory, emotional, and cognitive (Price, 2000)—which interact to create a conscious experience.

MULTIPLE LEVELS OF PAIN Pain sensations are triggered by the nociceptors, which were described earlier in this chapter. Neurons carrying nociceptive signals arrive at the spinal cord in an area called the **substantia gelatinosa** of the **dorsal horn**. Neurons there receive information *from* the brain as well as forming synapses with the neurons that are conveying sensory information from nociceptors *to* the brain (see Figure 12.5). According to the very influential **gate control theory** (Melzack and Wall, 1988) (**Figure 12.9**), the bottom-up pain signals from the nociceptors can be blocked via a feedback circuit located in the dorsal horn. When these gate neurons send excitatory signals, the sensory information is allowed to go through, but inhibitory signals from the gate neurons cancel transmission to the brain. The results of these interactions at the spinal cord are transmitted to somatosensory areas S1 and S2.

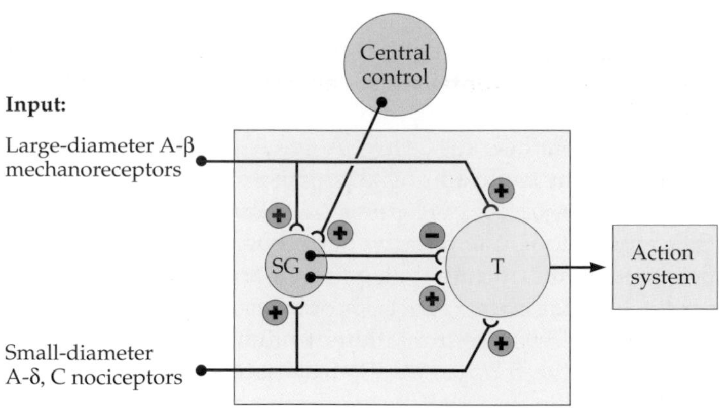

FIGURE 12.9 Gate control theory of Melzack and Wall (1988). Pain signals transmitted to the brain are moderated by activity in the substantia gelatinosa (SG) located in the dorsal horn of the spinal cord. The orange and green circles represent SG signals that decrease and increase pain, respectively, by their inhibitory and excitatory connections with transmission (T) cells. The transmission cells combine pain signals from the small-diameter fibers with signals inhibiting pain produced by stimulation of the large-diameter fibers. Direct excitatory pathways from both types of fibers are also found outside of the SG. As with the large-diameter fibers, the central control excites mechanisms in the SG that inhibit activation of transmission cells, thus decreasing the pain response.

The signals arising at S1 and S2 don't tell the whole story, however. We have known for some time that these areas are responsible for the sensory aspects of pain, but researchers recently used new methods to identify other areas of the brain that correspond to the emotional aspects of painful experiences. In one study (Rainville et al., 1997) (**Figure 12.10**), participants were hypnotized and their hands were placed in lukewarm or very hot water (which activated thermal nociceptors). The participants were sometimes told that the unpleasantness from the water was increasing or decreasing, and their brains were imaged during these periods by positron emission tomography (PET). The primary sensory areas of the cortex, S1 and S2, were activated by the hot water, but the suggestion of greater unpleasantness did not increase their response relative to the suggestion of decreased unpleasantness. In contrast, another area, the **anterior cingulate cortex (ACC)**, did respond differentially to the two hypnotic suggestions, by increasing or decreasing its activity according to the suggestion of increased or decreased unpleasantness. The researchers concluded that the ACC processes the raw sensory data from S1 and S2 in such a way as to produce an emotional response.

At a higher level still, pain can produce what Price (2000) called "secondary pain affect," which reflects the influence of cognition. Secondary affect is the emotional response associated with long-term suffering that occurs when painful events are imagined or remembered. For example, cancer patients who face a second round of chemotherapy may remember

anterior cingulate cortex (ACC) A region of the brain associated with the perceived unpleasantness of a pain sensation.

(*a*)

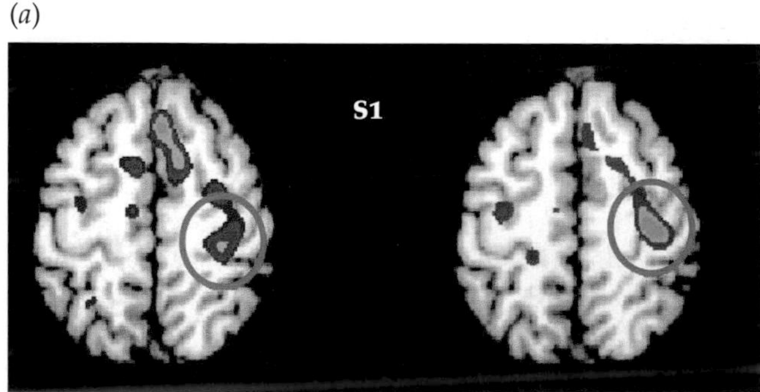

(*b*)

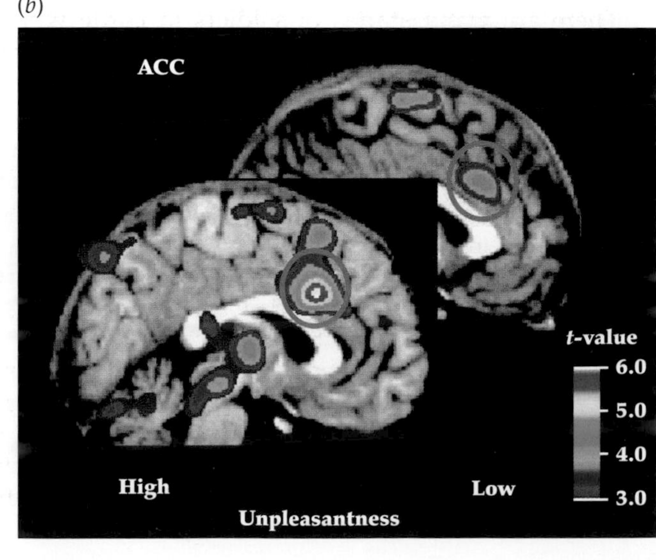

FIGURE 12.10 PET signals showing the effect of hypnosis on the brain, as observed by Rainville et al. (1997). (*a*) Primary somatosensory cortex (S1) was not affected by the suggested unpleasantness of pain (high on the left, low on the right). (*b*) The anterior cingulate cortex (ACC, circled), however, showed significantly different activation, depending on suggested unpleasantness.

the first and dread what is forthcoming. This component of pain is associated with the **prefrontal cortex**, an area concerned with cognition and executive control.

It may seem odd to associate pain with laughter, but at least some of the response people have to tickling seems to depend on nociceptors (Zotterman, 1939). And, just as signals from the brain can control pain perception, they appear to come into play when we try to tickle ourselves. Self-induced tickling not only produces less laughter; it also produces less activity in the somatosensory cortex, because of canceling signals (probably mediated by endogenous opiates) from other brain areas that know where the tickling stimulation came from (S.-J. Blakemore, Wolpert, and Frith, 1998).

As for itchiness, although research by Schmelz et al. (1997) suggests that pain and itch may be mediated by separate neural systems, researchers still understand relatively little about how itch works or how to relieve these nasty sensations. So, we will not discuss itch any further.

MODERATING PAIN Pain experiences are the complex result of sensory signals interacting with many other factors that have moderating effects. Damping of pain sensations (without losing consciousness) is called **analgesia**. Responses to noxious stimulation can be affected by analgesic drugs, of course, but perhaps more surprising are the attenuating effects of anticipation, religious belief, prior experience, or excitement. Studies also highlight the importance of interpersonal and broader social influences on the emotional component of pain.

At the level of the spinal cord, the gate neurons that attenuate pain can be activated by "counter-irritation" or "diffuse noxious inhibitory control"—extreme pressure, cold, or other noxious stimulation applied to another site distant from the source of the pain. For example, pain from electrically stimulating a tooth can be reduced by noxious stimulation of the hand (Motohashi and Umino, 2001). It appears that ascending signals from the counter-irritation reach the brain stem and initiate a new set of signals that are sent back down to the pain-blocking gate in the spinal cord (Rollman, 1991).

A different, and certainly more pleasant, way of modulating pain is to use relatively benign counterstimulation. Thus, although your mother may have told you not to scratch a mosquito bite, gate control theory says that rubbing the skin near the bite can, in fact, provide some relief. This effect results from the stimulation of fibers other than the nociceptors and can be produced by interactions between neurons within the spinal cord.

There are many stories of soldiers in battle who did not feel painful wounds until the stress was over. The analgesic effect was probably caused by **endogenous opiates**, chemicals released by the body that block the release or uptake of neurotransmitters necessary to transmit pain sensations to the brain. Differences between individuals with respect to pain responsiveness (that is, pain "thresholds") may reflect differences in their baseline levels of these substances. Externally produced substances such as morphine, heroin, and codeine are similar in chemical structure to these endogenous opiates, and thus they have similar analgesic effects. Other drugs, such as acetaminophen and ibuprofen, alleviate pain at its source, by counteracting chemicals that would otherwise start the nociceptors firing.

Research has shown that contact with those we love reduces brain activation in areas that regulate our emotions and bodily arousal responses to the threat of painful stimulation. In an fMRI study by Coan, Schaefer, and Davidson (2006), women experienced the threat of electric shock while holding their husband's hand, the hand of a male with whom they were unacquainted, or no hand at all. The magnitude of the neural response was

prefrontal cortex A region of the brain concerned with cognition and executive control.

analgesia Decreasing pain sensation during conscious experience.

endogenous opiates Chemicals released by the body that block the release or uptake of neurotransmitters necessary to transmit pain sensations to the brain.

hyperalgesia An increased or heightened response to a normally painful stimulus.

reduced when either the hand of the husband or an unknown male was touched, as compared to no hand contact. But the reduced neural response was greater when women touched their husband's hand, and was most effective for those in marital relationships deemed to be of the highest quality. Women who touched their husbands' hands also subjectively rated the threatening task experience as being less unpleasant.

Broader social influences on pain have also been found. For example, reports of painful strains of the arm from tasks requiring repetitive motion spread rapidly in Australia during the 1980s—like a contagious disease—but they were communicated by workers who did nothing more than talk to one another about their experiences. The cross talk could have multiple effects here, both heightening people's sensitivity to their suffering and providing a name for it.

PAIN SENSITIZATION Nociceptors provide a signal when there is impending or ongoing damage to the body's tissue. This is called "nociceptive" pain. Once damage has occurred, the site can become more sensitive, triggering the feeling of pain more readily than before. This experience is **hyperalgesia** and reflects an increased or heightened response to a normally painful stimulus. The resulting pain is called "inflammatory," and the heightened pain sensitivity usually goes away once the tissue heals. Pain can also arise in the absence of immediate trauma, because of damage to or dysfunction of the nervous system. The resulting pain is called "neuropathic." Some neuropathic pain reflects changes in the sensory fibers at the skin that do not normally produce pain but now become pain inducers (a phenomenon known as "allodynia"); other neuropathic pain arises from changes in the dorsal horn of the spinal cord. The changes at the level of the skin are called "peripheral," and those at the level of the spinal cord are called "central." The mechanisms by which neuropathic pain arises are increasingly understood at the cellular and molecular levels (Scholz and Woolf, 2002).

An important implication of sensitization research is that no single medication will alleviate all types of pain. Different underlying mechanisms for nociceptive, inflammatory, and neuropathic pain (peripheral or central) call for different analgesics.

Pleasant Touch

The traditional way of classifying different bodily sensations, introduced at the beginning of this chapter, is in terms of tactile, thermal, pain, and itch experiences. Collectively, these classic sensations are known as "discriminative touch." In just the last few years, however, scientists have uncovered a previously unknown fifth component that they named "pleasant" or "emotional" touch (McGlone et al., 2007). They have argued that the emotional properties of nonpainful bodily touch are mediated in large part by a class of unmyelinated (and thus, slower) peripheral C fibers known as "C tactile afferents" (or "CT afferents," for short) that are not related to either pain or itch. This type of C fiber, which differs from the C fiber associated with pain, seems to prefer mechanical stimulation in the form of slowly moving, lightly applied forces (like petting!).

Researchers have begun to think that CT afferents are located only in hairy skin, because a number of studies that have looked for them in hairless skin (e.g., palms and soles of the feet) have been unable to find any. It has been suggested, therefore, that these mechanical units form part of a neural subsystem that provides or supports emotional, hormonal, and behavioral responses to skin-to-skin contact with conspecifics, such as being stroked on the back of the hand, arm, or face by a girlfriend or boyfriend.

Pleasant touch is also processed in a different part of the brain than discriminative touch (Francis et al., 1999). Whereas primary somatosensory cortex is activated by the physical aspects of the stimulus (e.g., by the pressure it produces on the skin or a change in skin temperature), an area of the frontal lobes known to be involved in emotion, the orbitofrontal cortex, is activated by the pleasant qualities of the mechanical stimulation. The orbitofrontal cortex is activated by both painful and pleasant touch, suggesting that this region of the brain represents the emotional features of cutaneous stimulation, both rewarding and punitive (Rolls et al., 2003). There are indications that pleasant bodily contacts promote endorphin and oxytocin responses, which contribute to the feelings of well-being, confidence, and calmness.

Tactile Sensitivity and Acuity

Now that we've covered the physiological substrate of the touch system, we can turn to the psychological and psychophysical aspects. How sensitive are we to mechanical stimulation? What are the limits on tactile acuity in space and time? Put a bit differently, what are the smallest details that we can feel?

How Sensitive Are We to Mechanical Pressure?

To measure the minimum pressure that can be reliably sensed by a particular region of skin, we need a way to present well-defined amounts of pressure over and over again. In the nineteenth century, Max von Frey (1852–1932) developed an elegant and simple way to do this, using carefully calibrated stimuli, including horse and human hairs. Modern researchers typically use nylon monofilaments (e.g., fishing lines) of varying diameters. The smaller the diameter, the less force the line applies to the skin before it buckles.

To replicate von Frey's method yourself, touch different parts of your skin with a hair from your head and a bristle from a hairbrush to reveal the relative skin sensitivity to these two different forces. With the thinner hair, you will probably find that you can feel it on the more sensitive areas, such as your lips and perhaps some parts of your hand. You probably will not feel it pushing into your thigh or upper arm. With the bristle, however, you should discover that your skin is sensitive to mechanical pressure all over, but not uniformly so. For example, if you explore the skin on the back of your hand, you should be able to convince yourself that there are spots of greater and lesser sensitivity (Geldard, 1972).

Data from a more controlled pressure sensitivity study reveal that for both men and women, thresholds vary across different sites of the body (a high threshold means that that part of the body is less sensitive). In general, tactile pressure sensitivity is highest on the face, followed by the trunk and upper extremities (arms and fingers) and then the lower extremities (thigh, calf, and foot) (Weinstein, 1968). The pattern for males and females is very similar, except that women tend to be more sensitive to pressure than men. Sensitivity to temperature changes, as well as to pain, also varies markedly as a function of body site.

Another approach to measuring sensitivity is to ask, What is the smallest raised element we can feel as an otherwise completely smooth surface is passed over our skin? Like the storied princess who detected a pea under a pile of mattresses, we appear to be very sensitive to the pressure difference caused by a raised dot on a smooth surface. At a criterion of 75% detection, people can detect a dot only 1 micrometer high—that's a millionth of a meter, or 39 millionths of an inch! The dot seems to trigger detection by the FA I receptors, which also help us detect and correct for an object slipping

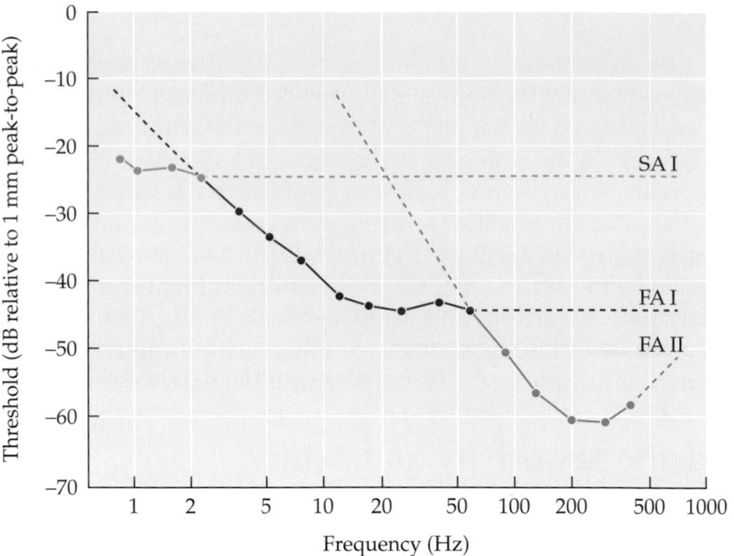

FIGURE 12.11 Minimally detectable displacement (threshold) of a vibrating stimulus applied to the human fingertip as a function of frequency. The y-axis measures vibratory intensity in decibels (relative to 1 millimeter of peak-to-peak displacement). Each of the three differently colored limbs of the overall vibrotactile sensitivity function (solid line) is believed to be mediated by the mechanoreceptor population most sensitive to that frequency range. The full vibratory response sensitivities of SA I, FA I, and FA II mechanoreceptor populations across the entire range of frequencies tested are revealed by the addition of dashed lines based on the results of corresponding neurophysiological studies of single-unit mechanoreceptor response. Researchers have proposed that SA I units mediate our threshold for vibrations below about 5 Hz; FA I fibers, for frequencies from about 5 to 50 Hz; and FA II units, for frequencies above about 50 Hz. (After Löfvenberg and Johansson, 1984.)

within our grasp. Even more impressive, when a texture that is made of many raised dots only a very small fraction of a micrometer high moves across the skin, the resulting vibrations trigger the FA II receptors deep within the skin, enabling us to distinguish the dot from a perfectly smooth surface (LaMotte and Srinivasan, 1991).

People are also sensitive to changes in pressure over time—that is, to tactile vibration. **Figure 12.11** shows absolute vibratory threshold (the minimum amount that a vibrating stimulus displaces the skin in order to be detected) as a function of the frequency presented to the fingertip (Löfvenberg and Johansson, 1984). In this study, people could detect the presence of vibrations from below about 5 hertz (Hz; 5 cycles in 1 second) up to about 400 Hz, the highest frequency that was tested. Other studies have confirmed that people can detect vibrations up to 700 Hz (Verrillo, 1963), the highest frequency tested to date.

Although people can detect vibrations over a wide frequency range, they are not equally sensitive to all frequencies, as Figure 12.11 clearly shows. Scientists now believe that the measurement of the threshold at a particular frequency of vibration depends only on the mechanoreceptor population that is most sensitive to that frequency. Since the various mechanoreceptor populations are sensitive to different frequencies, the overall psychophysical function for the detection of vibration (see Figure 12.11) reflects the contributions of different mechanoreceptor populations at different regions along it. Take a look at the corresponding vibration sensitivities of SA I, FA I, and FA II mechanoreceptor populations from less than 5 to 400 Hz, also shown in Figure 12.11. The SA I units would seem to mediate our absolute vibratory thresholds for frequencies below about 5 Hz; the FA I fibers, for frequencies from about 5 to 50 Hz; and the FA II units, for frequencies above about 50 Hz.

How Finely Can We Resolve Spatial Details?

Pressure detection is the tactile equivalent of detecting a spot of light, where the basic question is, Can you see or feel anything at all? For the tactile equivalent of visual acuity ("Can you make out the pattern of what you see or feel?"), try measuring your **two-point touch threshold**. As the name suggests, this is the smallest separation at which we can tell that we are being touched by two points and not just one. This experiment is best done with a partner, although it will work to some degree if you test yourself. A compass

two-point touch threshold The minimum distance at which two stimuli (e.g., two simultaneous touches) are just perceptible as separate.

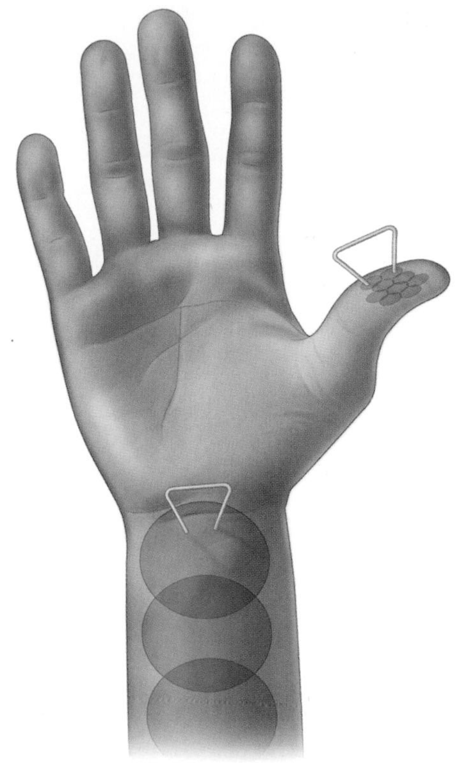

FIGURE 12.12 Two-point touch thresholds are determined primarily by the concentration and receptive-field sizes of touch receptors in an area of the skin. The triangles represent point stimulators, and the circles represent the areas of skin that would respond to a single stimulation.

(the kind that draws circles) is a useful stimulator, but you can use anything that enables you to vary the separation between two points, such as a bent paper clip. Pick one of your own or your partner's body regions and see if you can distinguish between a single point and both points. Then repeat the procedure with different separations of the two points (e.g., 0.5, 2, and 4 centimeters) and at different places on the skin (**Figure 12.12**).

Like sensitivity to pressure, spatial acuity varies across the body, but the extremities (fingertips, face, and toes) show the highest acuity. Results from a systematic study of two-point touch thresholds in females as a function of body site (**Figure 12.13**) demonstrate this finding quite clearly, and the pattern for males is very similar. More sensitive psychophysical methods show that on the fingertips we are capable of resolving a separation of only about 1 mm (Loomis, 1981). These results place tactile acuity somewhere between vision and audition: it is worse than visual acuity, but better than auditory spatial resolution.

Note the correspondence between the pattern of two-point thresholds across the body in Figure 12.13 and the relative distortion of different body

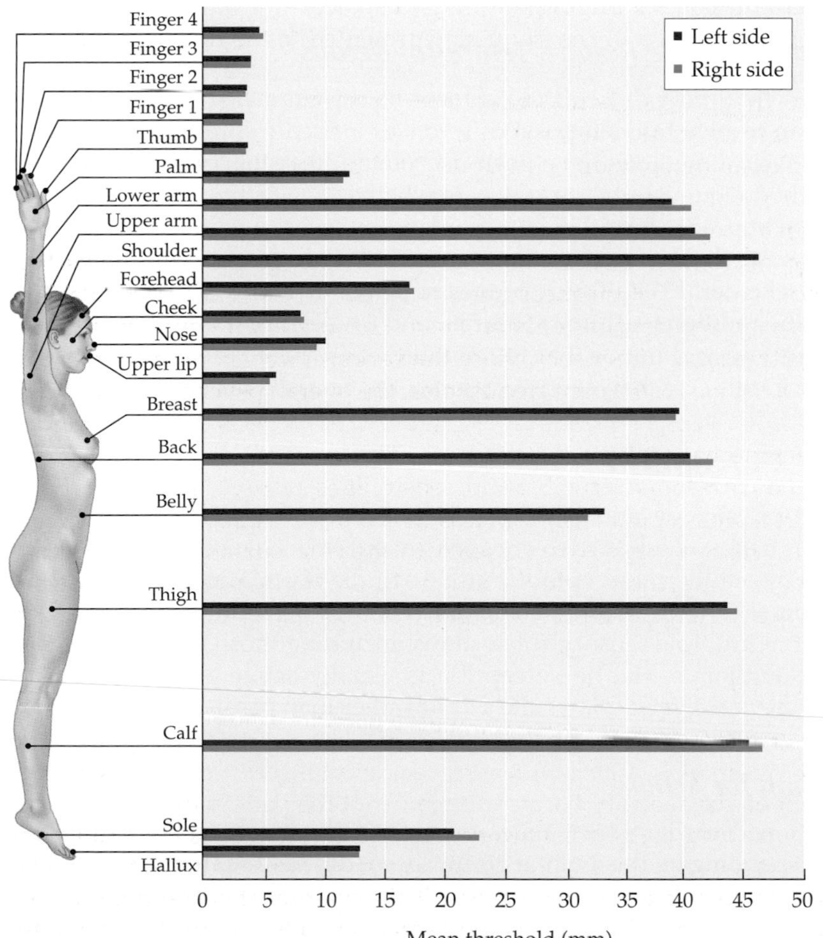

FIGURE 12.13 The minimal separation between two points needed to perceive them as separate (two-point threshold), when the points are applied at different sites on the body. (After Weinstein, 1968.)

parts in the sensory homunculus of Figure 12.7. This is not coincidental. The determination that two closely spaced points instead of just one are touching your skin—that is, a low two-point touch threshold—requires that your brain receive two separate signals. This means that at the skin, there must be a sufficient concentration of receptors, each with a small enough receptive field that the two contact points will elicit different responses. An additional constraint is that as the signals are sent to the cortex, they must not converge. A large enough chunk of cortical real estate is necessary to receive them separately. In short, the two-point touch threshold is low only when the density of receptors is relatively high, the receptive fields are small, and cortical convergence does not occur. (See **Web Activity 12.3: Two-Point Touch Thresholds.**)

Although useful, the traditional two-point touch test has some drawbacks, as you may see when you try your own experiment. Even if the two stimulated points feel like one, it is not quite the same as stimulating the skin with a single continuous contact. Therefore, asking people whether they are really being touched by one point or two will yield quite a different answer than asking them if it *feels like* one point or two, especially in sensitive areas like the fingertip. Alternatives that are more objective have been suggested, including judging whether an edge has a gap or indicating how a grating (a surface with alternating grooves and ridges) that is applied to the skin is oriented—along versus across the finger (Craig and Johnson, 2000). Tactile spatial acuity thresholds are mediated by the SA I (and possibly FA I) units, which have relatively small receptive fields and high receptor densities.

How Finely Can We Resolve Temporal Details?

It is somewhat more difficult to perform your own measures of how well people can resolve fine temporal differences in tactile stimulation. Various psychophysical methods have been used to address this question. A common method requires subjects to decide whether two tactile pulses delivered to the skin appear to be either simultaneous or successive in time. With this method, subjects can resolve a temporal difference of only 5 milliseconds (ms) (Gescheider, 1974). Touch proves to be better than vision (25 ms), but worse than audition (0.01 ms) (Sherrick and Cholewiak, 1986). As with spatial acuity, you will notice that touch falls somewhere between vision and audition; in this case, however, audition is the best and vision the worst.

Haptic Perception

With the physiology and basic psychophysics of the touch system now under our belts, we can turn to questions about how we use the information gathered by our thermoreceptors, muscle spindle fibers, Pacinian corpuscles, and so on. The term **haptic perception** refers to perceptual processing of inputs from multiple sensory subsystems, including those in skin, muscles, tendons, and joints. Haptic perception is usually active and information-seeking: the perceiver explores the world rather than passively receiving it.

Perception for Action

haptic perception Knowledge of the world that is derived from sensory receptors in skin, muscles, tendons, and joints, usually involving active exploration.

As mentioned earlier, touch relies on action to get information from the world. Expanding on this point a bit more, we can say that touch is active in two complementary ways. Using our hands to actively explore the world of surfaces and objects outside our bodies is *action for perception*. Using

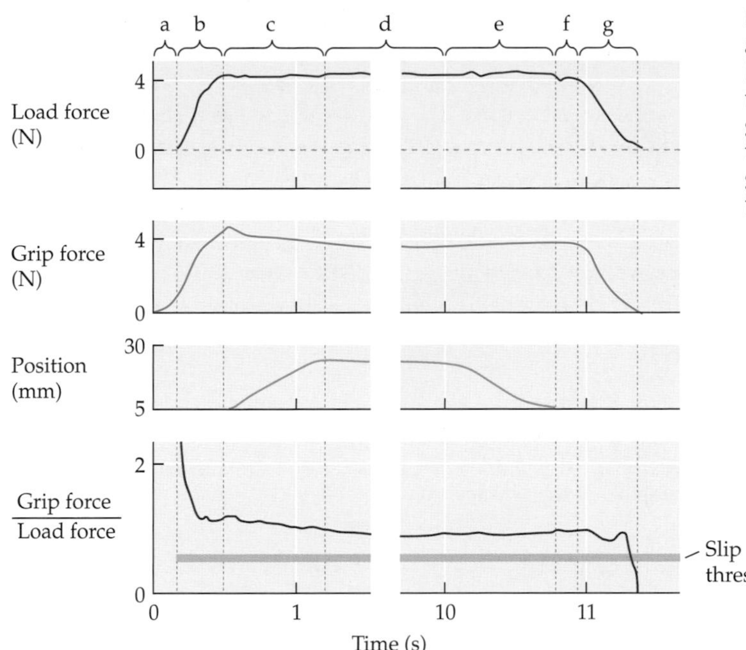

FIGURE 12.14 Force and position during lifting, grasping, and replacing a cube. Region a = grasp; b and c = lift; d = hold; e = lower; f and g = release. The load force (in newtons, abbreviated N) is in the gravitational direction, the grip force is imposed by the fingers pinching the cube, and the position is the height relative to the table. The ratio of grip force to load force is set so as to just prevent the cube from slipping. (After Westling and Johansson, 1984.)

somatosensation to control our impressive ability to grasp and manipulate objects in a stable and highly coordinated manner and to maintain proper posture and balance is *perception for action*.

In the section on kinesthetic receptors, we discussed how the loss of these internal touch receptors leads to a devastating inability to know (without looking) where our limbs are positioned. Westling and Johansson (1984) showed that mechanoreceptors in the skin also play critical roles when we are interacting with objects (**Figure 12.14**). These investigators anesthetized the skin on volunteers' hands so that activity in the mechanoreceptors was no longer available for processing. Even though their kinesthetic receptors were still active and they could still see what they were doing, the participants could no longer maintain a stable grasp of the objects they were required to lift, hold, and then replace on a supporting surface. Feedback from the mechanoreceptor populations in the skin appears to provide crucial information about when an object is about to slip on the skin. You may know this yourself from trying to unlock a door when your fingers are very cold!

Action for Perception

Let's now consider the "action for perception" side of haptic processing. Lederman and Klatzky (1987) coined the term **exploratory procedure** for a particular way of feeling an object in order to learn about one or more of its properties (**Figure 12.15**). Each exploratory procedure is optimal for obtaining precise details about one or two specific properties. For example, to find out how rough an object is, the best exploratory procedure is *lateral motion*—moving the fingers back and forth across the surface. This is the exploratory procedure that people freely choose when they wish to learn about roughness, and research indicates that it is also the one that works best.

To explain why each exploratory procedure is linked to a specific object property, we must consider both the neural structures that transduce information and the processes that operate on that information. For example, it has been shown that we adopt two different processes when judging the

exploratory procedure A stereotyped hand movement pattern used to contact objects in order to perceive their properties; each exploratory procedure is best for determining one (or more) object properties.

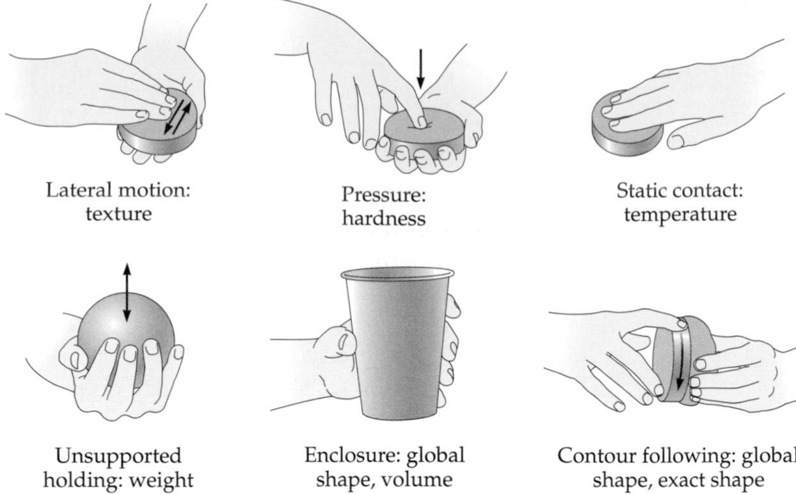

FIGURE 12.15 Exploratory procedures described by Lederman and Klatzky, and the object properties with which each is associated. (After Lederman and Klatzky, 1987.)

roughness of coarse as opposed to fine surfaces. Johnson and his colleagues (Johnson, 2002) have shown that the activity of slow-adapting mechanoreceptors (the SA I fibers) is a principal basis for the perception of surfaces that are at least moderately rough. These units are ten times as responsive when there is relative motion between the skin and the surface as when the fingers statically rest against the surface without motion. As your finger sweeps across a surface, the pattern of force across the receptors varies with the hills and troughs on the object's surface, providing a kind of spatial map of the variations in skin deformation that is sensed by the SA I fibers (and for the coarser surfaces possibly also by the FA I fibers). This map is passed on to higher-level neural structures, which integrate the lower-level information into an overall measure of the amount of variation. The brain then uses this neural measure to estimate the roughness of the surface. However, recent work further showed that when surfaces are very fine, the mechanoreceptors responsive to high-frequency vibrations, the FA II fibers, appear to encode surface roughness, although stroking with the fingers is still needed to set up the vibration (see Hollins, 2002). Hollins has suggested that scientific results obtained from the study of both coarse and fine surfaces support a dual-coding theory (as opposed to a single type of coding) for human roughness perception.

Hollins, Bensmaïa, and Washburn (2001) used a very clever psychophysical method known as selective adaptation to obtain scientific support for this dual-coding theory. They reasoned that if the high-frequency (FA II) mechanoreceptors are responsible for encoding the perceived roughness of fine surfaces, then if the fingertip is first selectively "adapted" (fatigued) to a very intense high-frequency vibration (e.g., 250 Hz), fine surfaces should subsequently not feel as rough as they do with the unadapted finger. In contrast, selectively adapting the fingertip to a high-intensity, low-frequency vibration (e.g., 10 Hz) should not affect how rough these same fine surfaces subsequently feel, because the mechanoreceptors that are most sensitive to such low-frequency vibration (SA I fibers, and possibly FA I fibers) do not encode the roughness of fine surfaces.

The results of this experiment nicely confirm the predictions, thus offering evidence in favor of dual-coding mechanisms for roughness. Selective adaptation has been more generally described as the "psychophysicist's microelectrode," in that this method offers a noninvasive complement to recording directly from neural fibers when studying a sensory system—in this case, somatosensation (for additional discussion of selective adaptation in spatial vision, see Chapter 3).

The What *System of Touch: Perceiving Objects and Their Properties*

Chapter 4 described the processes that underlie visual object recognition. We need somatosensation to control simple actions such as standing or grasping and to warn of danger through pain, but how much value does somatosensation have as an object recognition system? You know the answer if you have ever gotten out of bed in the dark to use the bathroom. The designers of coins know that it is imperative to be able to identify change while it is still in your pocket—hence the failure of the Susan B. Anthony dollar, which felt too similar to the quarter. And the next time you get dressed, try to keep your gaze constantly focused on your hands as you button your shirt and zip your zipper. This simple exercise should convince you that even when you can use vision, you sometimes rely on touch to recognize objects and their parts.

PERCEIVING MATERIAL VERSUS GEOMETRIC PROPERTIES People can perform haptic object recognition very well. Klatzky, Lederman, and Metzger (1985) asked people to identify each of 100 common objects (e.g., a fork, a brush, and a paper clip) placed in their hands. Not only did people perform almost perfectly without looking at the objects, but they also generally responded in less than about 2 seconds. However, the information used in haptic object recognition is quite different from that used in visual object recognition. Consider the difference between material properties—those that do not depend on the structure of a particular object, like its surface roughness—and geometric properties like size and shape. In haptic perception, the observer is in contact with the object being observed, so material properties of the object (is it soft? cold? fuzzy?) are easy to perceive and play a crucial role in the recognition process. In vision there is no physical contact, so thermal and textural properties of objects are much more difficult to perceive.

Therefore, the geometric properties of objects are the most important for visual recognition. Indeed, sparse line drawings may be quite easy to recognize visually, but they are hard to recognize when presented haptically as raised contours (**Figure 12.16**). To determine the overall shape of an object haptically, we usually must explore the object by tracing along its contours with our fingers. Integrating tactile information over time is possible but not very efficient, which is why the instantly recognizable material properties tend to be much more important in haptic recognition. (For more on this topic, see **Web Activity 12.4: Haptic Object Recognition.**)

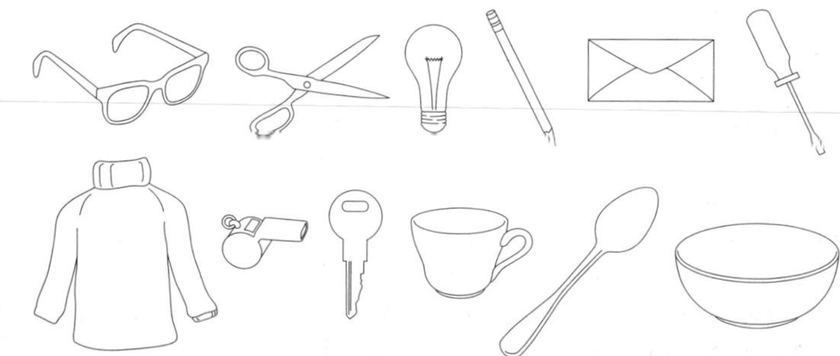

FIGURE 12.16 Examples of common objects that, in two-dimensional form, are easy to recognize visually but, when raised for haptic presentation, are not easily recognized by touch. (After Lederman et al., 1990.)

HAPTIC SEARCH As we saw in Chapter 8, a number of so-called preattentive features in the visual domain are presumed to be critical in the visual object recognition process. These features can be identified by the extent to which they "pop out" in a visual search task. For example, if you are searching for a red object, you will be equally fast at finding it regardless of how many green objects are presented along with it. This result implies that the "redness" of an object is available to recognition processes before attentional mechanisms examine the objects in the display and integrate the various features of each one.

Does the sense of touch also support preattentive feature detection? To find out, Lederman and Klatzky (1997) constructed a set of surfaces somewhat like a tactile slot machine with one key for each of six fingers. The subject's right hand is shown in **Figure 12.17***a*. Stimulus patches were mounted around the planar edges of each of six stimulus wheels. On each trial, the wheels were rotated until the desired stimulus patches were facing upward to form the haptic display. The entire display was then moved up to contact different combinations of the middle three fingertips of each hand. Using this apparatus, Lederman and Klatzky found that a number of haptic features do indeed pop out. As Figure 12.17*b* shows, participants in these experiments were just as fast at detecting a rough surface when there was no smooth surface in the tactile "display" as when there were as many as five smooth surfaces. Similarly, a hard surface popped out of a group of soft surfaces, a cool surface popped out of warm surfaces, and a surface with an edge popped out of perfectly flat surfaces.

However, not every haptic difference supports efficient search. For example, response times increased with the number of distractors when the task was to find a target with a horizontally oriented edge among distractors having vertical edges. Note that horizontal targets do pop out of vertical distractors in visual search tasks. This distinction fits nicely with the previous observation that haptic recognition relies extensively on material properties, but that the tactile system does not appear to be set up to efficiently process object contours.

FIGURE 12.17 An experiment investigating whether touch supports preattentive feature detection. (*a*) The apparatus used to display targets to the fingertips. The rotating drums bring either a stimulus patch or a cutout (no stimulus) to the upper surface, then rise as a whole to contact the middle three fingers of both hands (only one hand is shown). (*b*) The amount of time required to detect a rough target among smooth distractors as a function of the number of fingers stimulated. (After Lederman and Klatzky, 1997.)

(*a*)

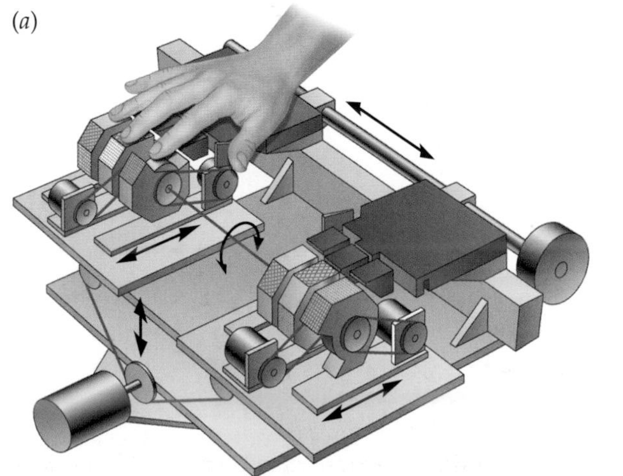

(*b*)

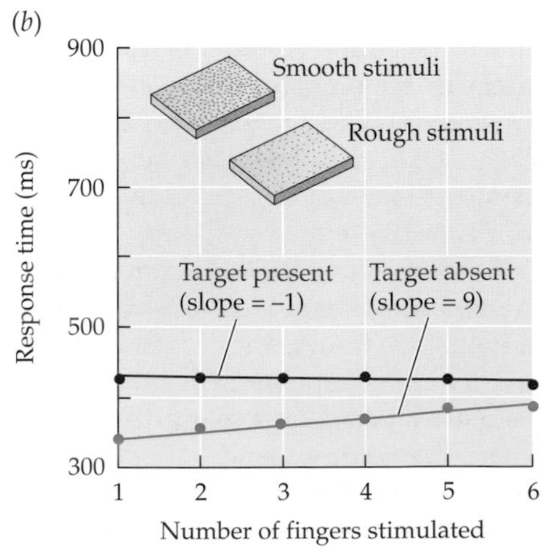

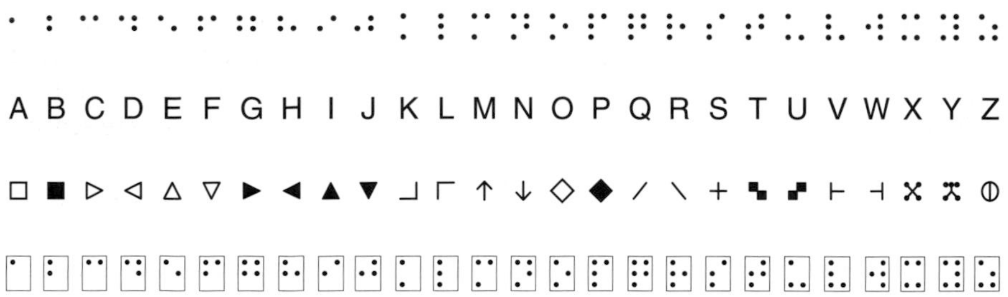

A B C D E F G H I J K L M N O P Q R S T U V W X Y Z

FIGURE 12.18 Selected character recognition sets used by Loomis, including Braille. (After Loomis, 1990.)

PERCEIVING PATTERNS WITH THE SKIN Even if pattern perception by touch is not terribly efficient, it can be done, especially if the patterns are small enough to be perceived by a single fingertip. Loomis (1990) has suggested that, to some extent, touch acts like blurred vision when the fingertip explores a raised pattern. He tested people's ability to identify a set of patterns including Braille symbols, English and Japanese letters, and geometric forms—a few of which are shown in **Figure 12.18**. Sometimes the patterns were presented to the fingertips as raised elements. Other times they were presented visually behind a blurring screen that matched the resolution of the eye with the more limited acuity of fingertip skin. Interestingly, Loomis found very similar patterns of visual and tactile confusion errors—that is, responses in which one pattern was confused for another. This finding suggests that a common, amodal decision process operates on both haptically and visually perceived patterns.

In the Braille alphabet, shown in the first row of Figure 12.18, each letter is formed by raising some of the dots in a 2 × 3 array. For the letter *A*, for example, a single dot is raised in the top left position; and for the letter *Q*, all dots except for the one in the lower right position are raised. This design reflects a compromise between the skin's acuity and its "field of view," the area of skin that we can take in all at once. It would be nice to include more than six dots in the array, but because of the spatial blurring imposed by the skin, denser patterns would be difficult to resolve and discriminate (remember that two-point thresholds on the fingertips are about 1 millimeter). Spreading a greater number of dots across a larger contact area would not work either, because then the pattern would extend beyond the fingertip. Unfortunately, people are unable to "read" more than one finger at a time, suggesting that our tactile field of view is very narrow.

TACTILE AGNOSIA Just as lesions in the temporal lobe can produce visual agnosia (see Chapter 5), lesions of the parietal lobe can produce **tactile agnosia**, an inability to identify objects by touch. In making a diagnosis of tactile agnosia, the neurologist needs to be able to eliminate other possibilities. Is the problem impaired motor control, which would prevent the exploratory procedures needed to effectively learn about an object's properties? Or might the problem be a higher-level cognitive dysfunction, such as a loss of access to object names?

We already described a patient who could not recognize objects by touch but could locate them. She had tactile agnosia with her right hand, due to a lesion in the left inferior parietal region of her brain, but the deficit did not extend to her left hand. Reed and Caselli (1994) documented that, although the patient could not recognize objects such as a key chain or a combination lock with her right hand, she could easily recognize these objects visually or with her left hand, ruling out a general loss of knowledge about objects. Other capabilities were normal in both hands, including sensory threshold

tactile agnosia The inability to identify objects by touch.

levels and the movements with which objects were explored. The patient could also discriminate between objects with different levels of weight and roughness using either hand. And she could answer questions about the haptic properties of named objects, such as whether an orange was harder than an apple, indicating that she had the ability to remember and imagine how objects felt.

Thus, the patient could acquire information with her impaired hand about an object's properties (e.g., its weight and roughness), and she had intact haptic knowledge about objects she had encountered in the past. What she lacked was a connection between these two components of object identification. That is, either she was unable to integrate the perceived properties into a coherent object representation, or she was unable to match perceived representations to stored representations in memory.

The Where *System of Touch: Locating Objects*

As in other sensory modalities, knowing *what* a haptic stimulus might be is only part of the perceptual problem. We also need to know *where* that stimulus is located because we often want to do something with it. If you are already touching an object, you obviously know where it is (a tree limb that you bump your head on is in the air; one that you stumble over has fallen to the ground). If you are not yet touching the object but can see it, your sense of vision can work out where the object is and guide your reaching behavior. But what about groping for the snooze button on your alarm clock when your eyes have not yet opened for the day? As mentioned already, there is evidence that touch, like vision, has a specialized neural pathway for dealing with questions of where objects are located, as compared to knowing what they are like.

HAPTIC OBJECT LOCALIZATION Like visual and auditory localization, haptic object localization first requires that we establish a **frame of reference**. For vision, the center of the reference frame—the **egocenter**—is located near the bridge of the nose, between the two eyes; the auditory egocenter is a point smack in the middle of the head (between the two ears). One way to get at your haptic egocenter is to place your left index finger on top of the edge of a desk or table, close your eyes, and try to match this location by placing your right index finger on the bottom of the desk (**Figure 12.19**). If you do this many times, you may find that you consistently err to the left. Conversely, if you try to match the location of your right index finger with your left, you will be more likely to err to the right. A careful analysis of errors in a task of this type led Haggard et al. (2000) to conclude that there is, in fact, no single fixed frame of reference for the haptic perception of locations. In the case of the index-finger reaching task, the egocenter appears to be located at the shoulder of the arm doing the reaching. In other tasks, the egocenter may move to other positions on the body.

Although you might think you're pretty accurate at determining how external objects are oriented in haptic space, research has shown that people make surprisingly large and systematic errors. Try the following task, which is illustrated in **Figure 12.20**. Have a friend place two pencils in front of you within reach, one far off to your left and the other far off to your right. Position your hands in a natural way on both rods. The orientation of the left pencil should be fixed so that its length lies crosswise to the fingers of your left hand. The right pencil should be set in a random position beneath your right hand. Rotate the right pencil until it feels parallel to the left pencil. Now have a look at how the two pencils are aligned with respect to each

frame of reference The coordinate system used to define locations in space.

egocenter The center of a reference frame used to represent locations relative to the body.

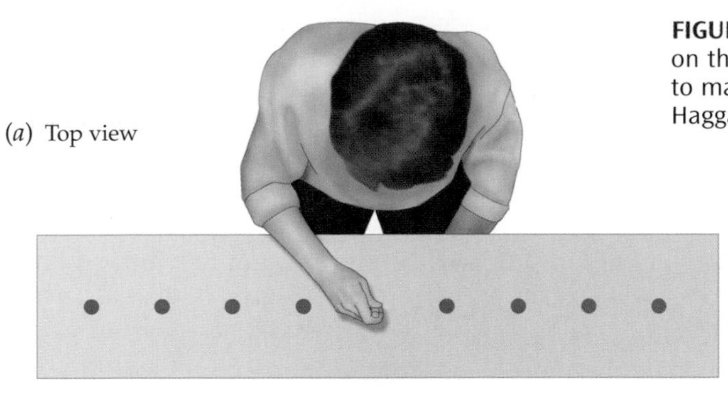

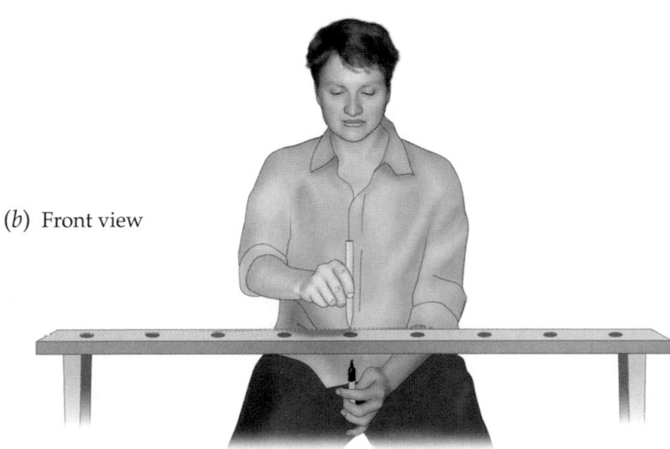

FIGURE 12.19 Locating the haptic egocenter. One hand places a stylus on the target on the upper table surface, and the other hand attempts to match up underneath the table in the corresponding location. (After Haggard et al., 2000.)

other. Are they physically parallel? Figure 12.20 illustrates a task in which people try to orient rods to appear "parallel" within tabletop space.

Kappers (2007) showed that, on average, the orientation of the two rods consistently differed by 40 degrees! Across individuals, the deviation ranged from 8 to as much as 91 degrees! Although spatial errors made in this haptic parallelism task were typically very large, the average trends were quite consistent. Subjects tended to judge what was parallel by weighting their orien-

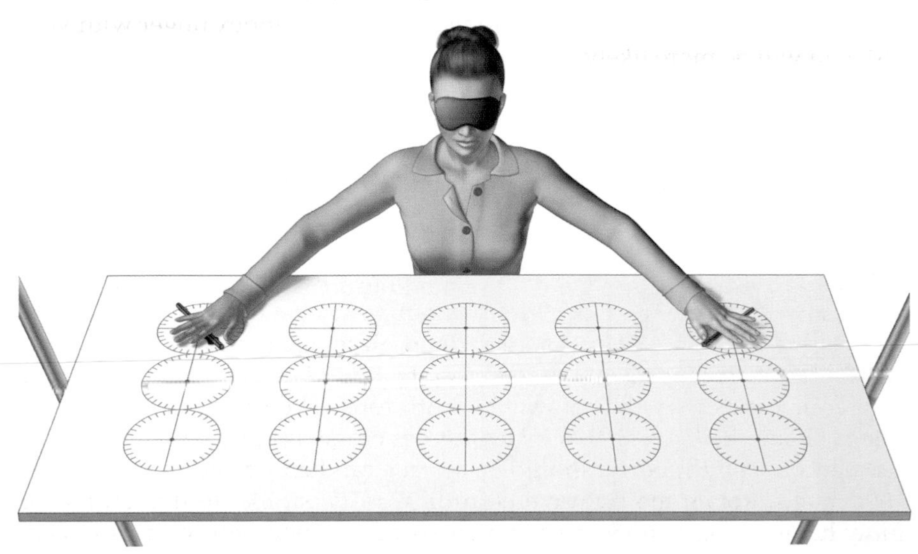

FIGURE 12.20 Haptic perception of tabletop space. The two bars in this figure are arranged to represent how a hypothetical subject would orient them in the actual experiment to appear close to "parallel." (After Kappers, 2007.)

body image The impression of our bodies in space.

tation judgments with respect to two different spatial frames of reference: one that was egocentric (with reference to the body, and commonly centered on the hand); the other, allocentric (with reference to external space).

BODY IMAGE Understanding how we haptically perceive space becomes even more fascinating when we find that the impression we have of our bodies in space (called the **body image**) is highly changeable. We have all heard of clinical reports of individuals with abnormal brain function who report "out-of-body" experiences in which the conscious sense of self lies outside the physical body. It is as if the observer were looking at his or her body, but from someone else's point of view. A study by Ehrsson (2007) showed just how easy it is to induce an illusory "out-of-body" experience in healthy subjects. Here is how he did it.

As depicted in **Figure 12.21**, the participant (let's call him "Frank") sat in front of two cameras placed beside each other. Frank wore virtual-reality goggles connected to the cameras for a stereo view. The experimenter stood at Frank's side and used a plastic rod to stroke his physical chest (unseen by the cameras). Being very careful to use exactly the same timing, the experimenter used a second rod to simultaneously "stroke" Frank's "phantom chest," an area in front of and just below the cameras (see figure). Frank could see the back of his body sitting in the chair and the experimenter's hand moving down toward a point below the two cameras. When subjects were asked what they experienced, they reported viewing their own body from behind, with their heads located at the site of the cameras (like the phantom's head in Figure 12.21). In addition they reported feeling the tap on the phantom's chest just below the cameras. (Ehrsson was careful to address other control questions to ensure that the out-of-body experience could not be attributed to suggestibility or to the subjects' compliance to the task.) (See **Web Activity 12.5: The Rubber Hand Illusion** for another way to elicit an out-of-body experience.)

Note also that we are not the only primates who can modify their body schemas. Iriki, Tanaka, and Iwamura (1996) showed how quickly the body images of regular tool-using Japanese monkeys could be modified. The monkeys practiced using a handheld tool, as they would a rake, to retrieve distant food objects. After this task was repeated for only 5 minutes, the visual receptive fields of bimodal cells that received converging inputs from both vision and touch actually grew in size to include the complete length of the tool in addition to the hand. The neuroscientists proposed that such neural modifications represent how the monkey brain incorporated the tool into the body image as an extension of the monkey's own hand.

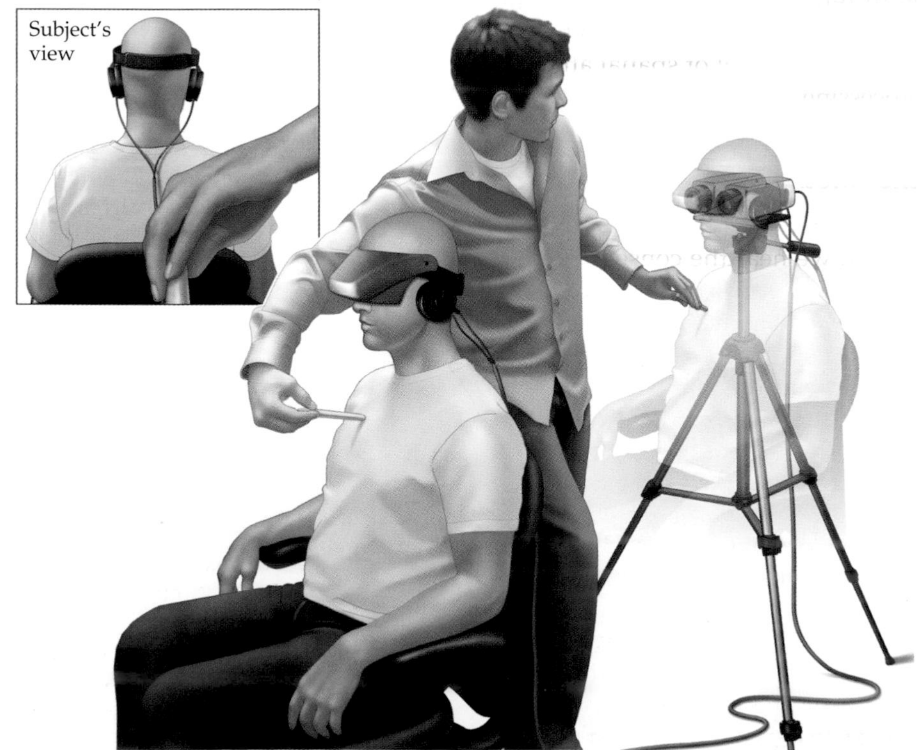

FIGURE 12.21 The experimental setup used to induce an out-of-body experience. (After Ehrsson, 2007.)

Tactile Spatial Attention

Although the last 50 years or so have produced a considerable amount of research on visual and auditory attention (see Chapter 8), only in the last decade have scientists begun to investigate the nature of the processes that underlie tactile attention. In this section we focus on tactile spatial (as opposed to nonspatial) attention.

When people anticipate being touched in a particular location, they can voluntarily direct their attention to that location. Attention that is directed to the tactile modality in this way is known as **endogenous** (or top-down) control. In one study (Spence, Pavani, and Driver, 2000), participants were asked to indicate whether a sustained force or a series of pulses was delivered to a fingertip (**Figure 12.22**). The stimulated fingertip could be on the left or the right hand. A visual precue, in the form of an arrow, predicted which hand would receive the stimulation. If people could make use of this precue to direct attention to the predicted hand, it was expected that they would be faster at deciding whether the stimulus was sustained or pulsed. And indeed, this was the case: the precue sped up responses relative to a no-cue control. Occasionally, however, the precue directed the participant's attention to the wrong hand, and on such trials, people responded more slowly than in the no-cue condition.

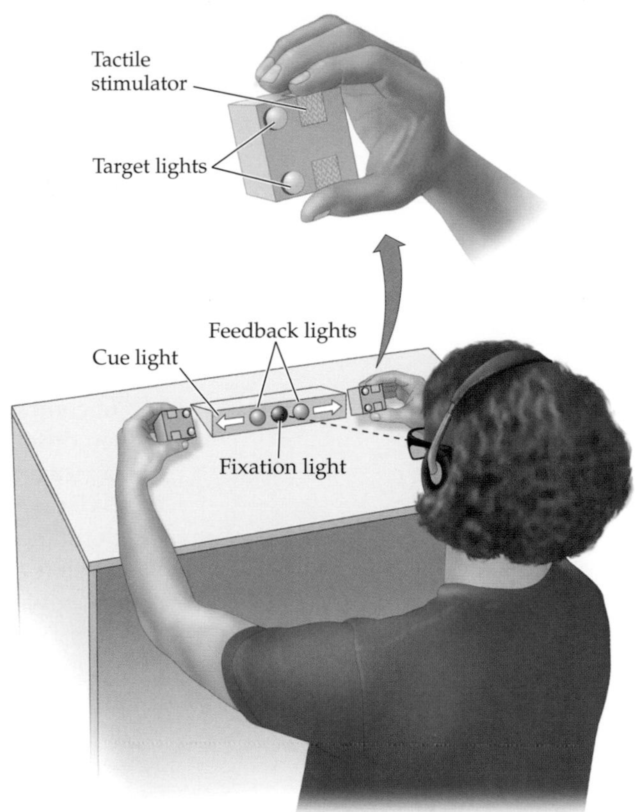

FIGURE 12.22 Studying competition between sensory modalities. In each hand the subject holds a cube that has a vibrotactile stimulator and a light, either of which can signal the required response. The arrows at fixation are used to direct attention. (After Spence, Pavani, and Driver, 2000.)

These effects are exactly analogous to attentional cueing effects in vision and audition. Thus, we see that tactile attention, like visual and auditory attention, is a limited resource that must be allocated in one way or another. You will probably have realized that directing one's attention endogenously or voluntarily to a stimulus event is not the only way in which people control spatial attention. It is also possible to reflexively direct one's spatial attention to an abruptly occurring tactile stimulus that takes place at a particular location or part of the body. Such reactive control of spatial attention is known as **exogenous** (or bottom-up) processing.

Interactions between Touch and Other Modalities

Touch does not occur only in the absence of other sensory input, of course. We commonly touch objects that we see, and we hear the consequences of contact. How does the perceptual system as a whole deal with signals from multiple modalities? Sometimes they compete, and sometimes the whole is an integrated combination of the different inputs.

Competition can arise when resources are limited—that is, when attention comes into play in a particular task. Do the different modalities compete with each other for attentional resources as well? Consider the fact that the pressure stimulus of your posterior on your seat seems to have lost out to this visual text in the current competition for your attention (until now, that is). In the lab, Spence, Nicholls, and Driver (2001) did a cross-modal version of the same sort of cueing experiment that was described in the previous paragraph: they led participants to expect a stimulus to be presented via one modality and then sometimes presented it in a different modality. The participants were instructed to indicate with a foot pedal whether a target stimulus appeared on their left or right side. The stimulus could be noise from a loudspeaker (audition), a red circle at the location of the loudspeaker (vision),

endogenous spatial attention A form of top-down (knowledge-driven) control of spatial attention in which attention is voluntarily directed toward the site where the observer anticipates a stimulus will occur.

exogenous spatial attention A form of bottom-up (stimulus-driven) spatial attention in which attention is reflexively directed toward the site at which a stimulus has abruptly appeared.

or a rod pressing the finger while it touched the loudspeaker (touch), and a cue could direct attention toward any of the three modalities.

Again, responses were faster when the cue was valid and slower when it was invalid. Interestingly, the greatest cost for an invalid cue occurred when observers expected a tactile stimulus but a visual or auditory stimulus was presented instead. This result may imply that the sense of touch has a particularly restricted attentional channel—that once attention is focused on the touch modality, it is relatively difficult to reallocate it. Or it may be that visual attention and auditory attention are shared to some extent, because expectancies in those modalities could be directed to a common location in external space, whereas the expectancy for touch was directed to a location on the body.

In contrast to attentional competition, intersensory integration can occur when different modalities receive information about the same object. Suppose, for example, that you're touching sandpaper. The roughness you feel also depends on the roughness you see. Participants in an experiment by Lederman, Thorne, and Jones (1986) saw and felt different sandpaper surfaces that they believed were one and the same. When they were asked about how closely packed the elements in the surface were, they were more strongly influenced by vision. When asked about the roughness of the surface, however, touch became more important and vision less important.

In some circumstances, one modality may appear to dominate. In a classic study pitting vision against touch, Rock and Victor (1964) had people grasp a square while looking at it through a distorting lens. What these participants felt was pretty much what they saw: a rectangle. But dominance by one modality over the other is not the rule. A more general model is that people integrate the signals from two modalities, producing a weighted average. That is, they use x percent of the information from one modality and (100 – x) percent from the other. The relative weighting reflects the quality of the signal from each modality.

Ernst and Banks (2002) demonstrated such integration with an apparatus that simultaneously created touch and sight of the same virtual display. The display consisted of a plane with a raised bar across the middle (**Figure 12.23**). The virtual visual display was produced with stereo glasses and an appropriate pair of random dot stereograms, one presented to each eye (see Chapter 6, "Random Dot Stereograms," Figure 6.32), creating the visual illusion of a bar stepping up from a plane. The corresponding virtual touch display was created with a device that generated forces that pushed back on the hand whenever contact was made with the simulated surface. When the bar heights presented to the two modalities were discrepant (the touched bar higher than the viewed bar or vice versa), the perceived height of the bar was a weighted compromise between them, with vision more strongly weighted than touch. When the

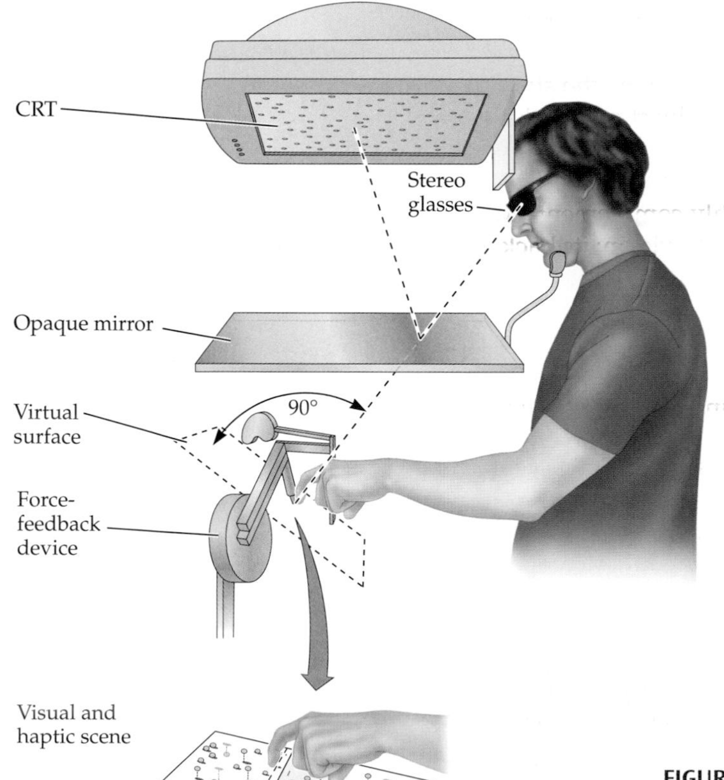

FIGURE 12.23 Testing the integration of sensory modalities. The observer could see a virtual surface of dots through stereo goggles, which gave the appearance of a raised bar across the surface, and could touch the virtual surface and receive resisting forces consistent with the surface height. (After Ernst and Banks, 2002.)

investigators made the information from vision less reliable by randomly changing the apparent height of some of the surface dots, the weight assigned to touch increased, and it played a greater role in determining the perceived height of the bar.

Multiple modalities may collaborate by signaling different, but complementary, sources of information about an object. The discussion of object perception emphasized that vision and touch are intrinsically complementary: one well suited to convey an object's geometry; and the other, its material. For a quite different example of intermodal cooperation, consider an intriguing study about the perception of object shape by Fiona Newell et al. (2001).

In the learning phase of the experiment, observers studied a set of Lego shapes, each fixed in a particular orientation, using vision or touch (**Figure 12.24**). In the recognition phase, previously studied shapes were presented, oriented either as they had been during the study phase or reversed 180 degrees, along with unstudied shapes. Again using vision or touch, the subjects were required to indicate whether each tested shape was old (previously studied) or new. People who studied and were tested in the same modality, whether vision or touch, recognized old shapes better when they were presented in the same orientation as during the study phase, indicating that memory for the shapes was orientation-sensitive. But now for the surprise: for people who studied and were tested in different modalities—vision changed to touch, or vice versa—recognition was actually better when the studied shapes were reversed in orientation during the recognition phase! Why should this be?

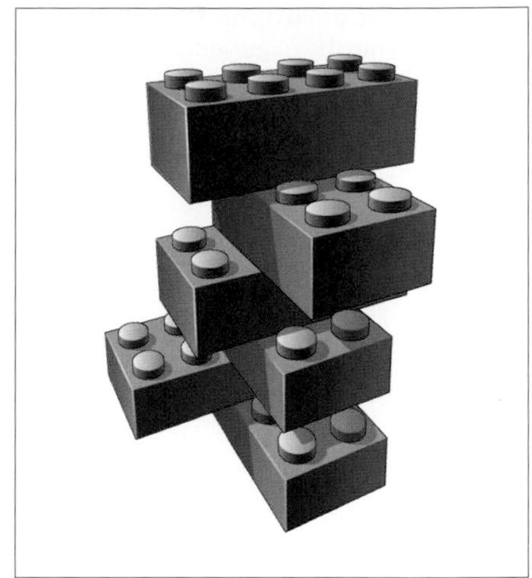

FIGURE 12.24 An example of the unfamiliar object shapes used in Newell's experiment. (After Newell et al., 2001.)

The authors noticed that when haptically exploring the shapes, subjects placed their thumbs on the front surface and their other fingers around the back surface, suggesting that they learned more about the back of the object. For people who studied with vision and were tested with touch, reversing the object meant that the previously visible (front) surface was then the one that was more accessible to manual exploration (back). For people who studied with touch and were tested with vision, reversing the object meant that the more effectively explored back surface was then what was accessible to vision. Thus, it would appear that two modalities might most efficiently process an object's shape by using two different, but highly complementary, sources of information: the object's front processed best with vision; its back, with haptics.

Virtual Haptic Environments

One form of low-tech tactual interface that has been around for some time is derived from **Tadoma**, a method used by deaf and blind people to track speech in real time, and named after its first known American practitioners, Tad Chapman and Oma Simpson. In this method, the haptic listener spreads the fingers of one hand across the speaker's lips, jaw, and throat. Movements and vibrations of the speaker's speech apparatus provide inputs to the cutaneous and kinesthetic components of the recipient's haptic system, and these signals can be translated by a skilled recipient into spoken words.

The existence of Tadoma has inspired researchers to develop a virtual display that can transmit information analogous to that from the speaker's vibrating bone and moving jaw delivered to the perceiver's hand. This device is called the Tactuator (Tan et al., 1999). Eventually such devices might translate recorded speech to the hand of a deaf-blind user, an outcome made possible by understanding the capabilities and limitations of touch.

Tadoma A method by which those who are both deaf and blind can perceive speech in real time using their hands.

The experiment by Ernst and Banks described earlier used a virtual haptic environment. Anyone who has played a video game has been in a virtual

virtual haptic environment A synthetic world that may be experienced haptically by operation of an electromechanical device that delivers forces to the hand of the user.

environment. The actions of the player (e.g., button presses or joystick movements) are sensed by the machine and filtered through a program that creates a simulated world, causing new events and outcomes that are fed back to the user through vision and audition. Although some joysticks employ crude vibration, what is missing from most of these environments at present is haptic feedback. However, interfaces have recently been developed that provide such feedback in the form of vibration or sustained forces to the hand.

Imagine yourself, for example, exploring the inside of a box in a **virtual haptic environment**. The environment has been programmed so that some locations within it are assigned to walls of the box. These locations simulate rigid surfaces with material properties such as coefficients of friction. You grasp a handle and move your hand, which causes motion of a probe in the simulated environment. When the probe reaches the location that has been assigned to a wall, you encounter resisting forces on the handle, which depend on variables such as your angle and speed of approach to the wall. This example is very simple; devices in use today are also capable of creating diverse objects varying in shape, size, surface texture, and softness.

Haptic virtual environments would be useful in many applications other than video games. One such application is training physicians for minimally invasive surgery, in which the surgeon manipulates an implement inserted into the body through a small incision while viewing the surgical site on a video display. In a virtual haptic training environment, the patient's body is replaced by a dummy, and the surgical tool connects to a computer that tracks the trainee's movements. The computer contains a simulation of the patient that describes body structures and their properties, such as slipperiness and softness. As the computer tracks the surgeon's actions with the tool, it determines the effect they would have on the simulated patient, and it generates high-precision graphics and forces to feed back to the surgeon. Such systems are currently under development (**Figure 12.25**). Commerce on the Internet is another potential domain for force-feedback devices that could allow products to be felt as well as seen.

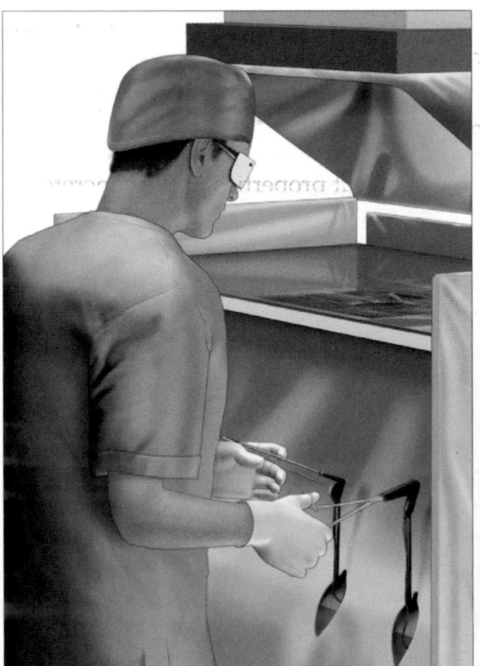
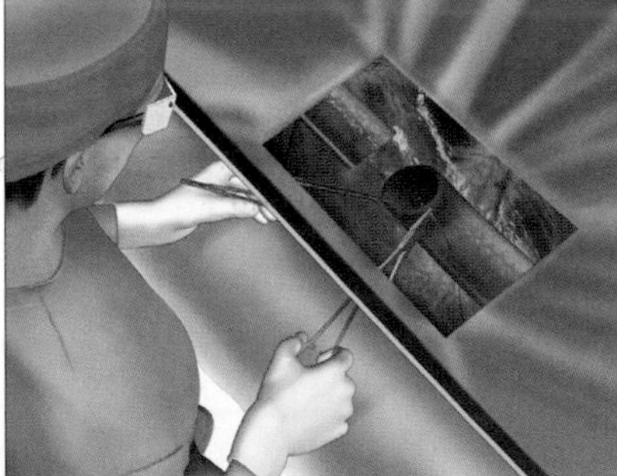
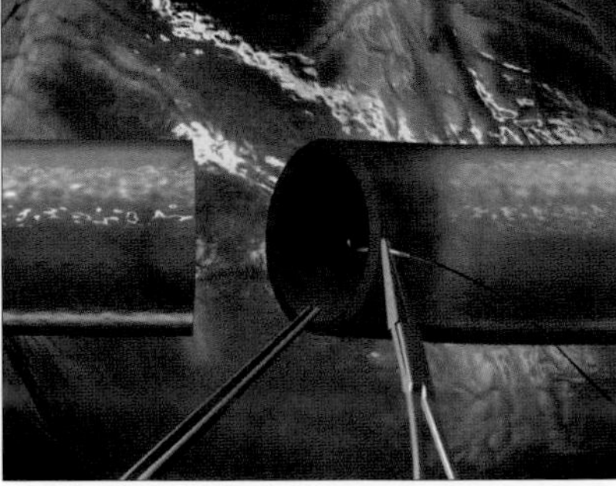

FIGURE 12.25 A virtual surgical trainer. A novice surgeon receives high-precision graphics and force feedback about a blood vessel that is being repaired. (After photographs from Boston Dynamics.)

Summary

1. The sense of touch produces a number of distinct sensory experiences, most recently including pleasant or emotional touch. Each type of experience is mediated by its own sensory receptor system(s). Touch sensors are responsive not only to pressure, but also to vibration, changes in temperature, and noxious stimulation. The kinesthetic system, which also contributes to our sense of touch, is further involved in sensing limb position and the movement of our limbs in space.
2. Four classes of pressure-sensitive (mechano-) receptors have been found within hairless skin, and another five classes within hairy skin. The organs used to sense limb position and movement (namely, our muscles, tendons, and joints) are more deeply situated within the body. Thermoreceptors respond to changes in skin temperature that occur, for example, when we contact objects that are warmer or cooler than our bodies. Nociceptors signal tissue damage (or its potential) and give rise to sensations of pain.
3. The pathways from touch receptors to the brain are complex. Two major pathways have been identified: a fast pathway that carries information from mechanoreceptors, and a slower one that carries thermal and nociceptive information. Only the second pathway synapses when it first enters the spinal cord. These pathways project to the thalamus and from there to the primary somatosensory area, located in the parietal lobe just behind the central sulcus. This area contains several somatotopically organized subregions, in which adjacent areas of the body project to adjacent areas of the brain. The neural organization of the brain for touch has been shown to be remarkably plastic, even in adults.
4. Downward pathways from the brain play an important role in the perception of pain. According to the gate control theory, signals along these pathways interact at the spinal cord with those from the periphery of the body. Such interactions can block the pain signals that would otherwise be sent forward to the brain. The sensation of pain is further moderated by areas in the cortex.
5. Investigators have measured sensitivity to mechanical force by applying nylon hairs of different diameters to the skin. They determine spatial acuity of the skin by measuring the two-point touch threshold, and more precisely by discriminating the orientation of gratings applied to the skin. Tactile pressure sensitivity and spatial acuity vary with body site because of varying concentrations of different types of mechanoreceptors. The minimum depression of the skin needed to feel a stimulus vibrating at a particular rate (frequency) provides a measure of vibration sensitivity.
6. The sense of touch is intimately related to our ability to perform actions. Signals from the mechanoreceptors are necessary for simple actions such as grasping and lifting an object. Conversely, our own movements determine how touch receptors respond and, hence, what properties of the concrete world we can feel. Touch is better adapted to feeling the material properties of objects than it is to feeling their geometric features (e.g., shape), particularly when an object is large enough to extend beyond the fingertip.
7. Like other sensory modalities, touch gives rise to internal representations of the world, which convey the positions of objects using the body as a spatial reference system. Touch-derived representations are inputs to higher-level functions like allocation of attention and integration with information from other modalities.
8. The psychological study of touch is useful for a number of applications. Virtual touch environments that transmit forces to the touch receptors can provide a basis for training people to perform remote operations like surgery and perhaps, in the future, will convey the illusion of touched objects over the Internet.

Refer to the
Sensation and Perception
website
(www.sinauer.com/wolfe2e)
for activities, essays, study questions, and other study aids.

CHAPTER 13

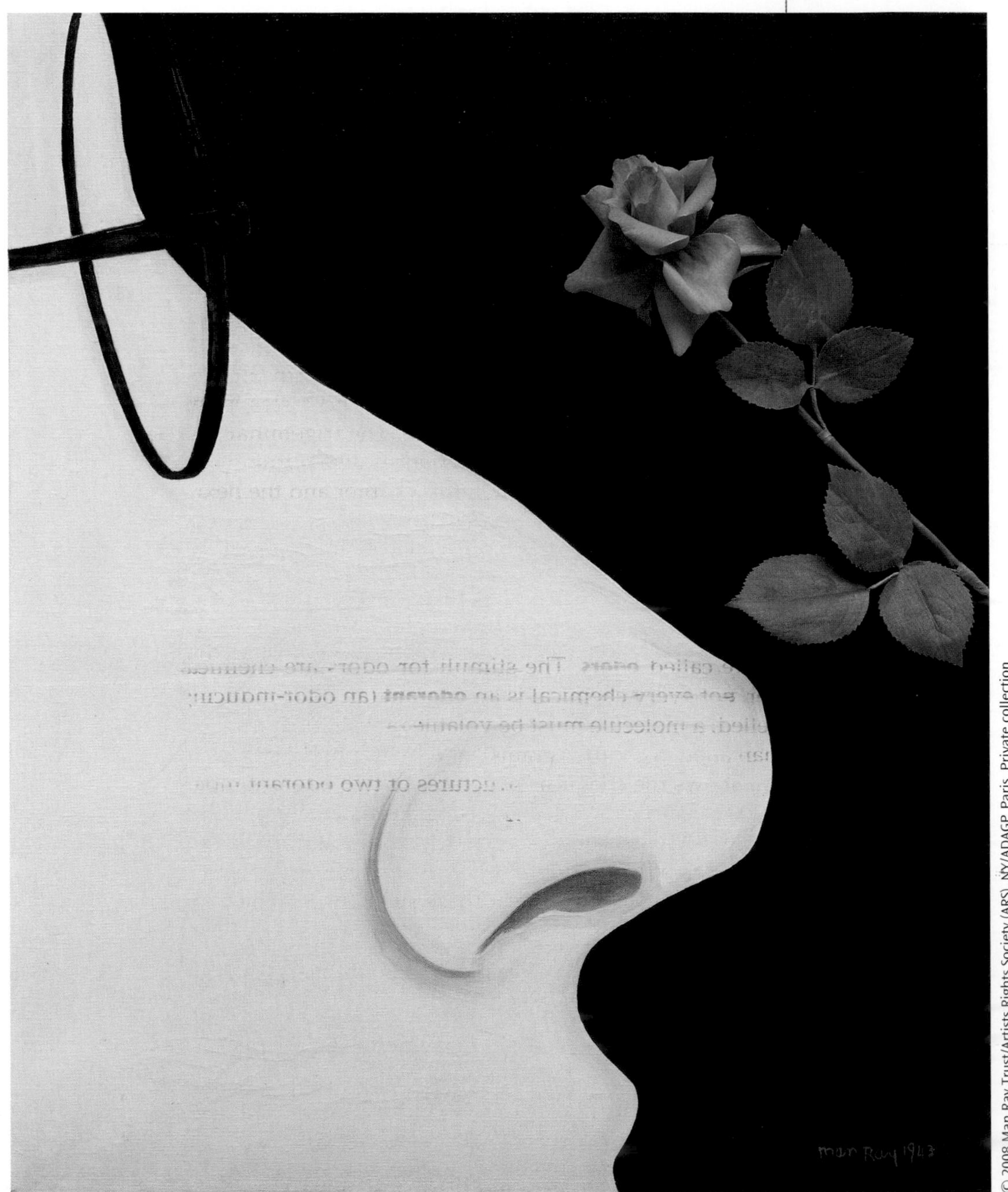

Man Ray, *The Artificial Florist*, 1943

Olfaction

The story of the next two chapters begins at the dawn of life itself. When single-cell organisms first appeared on Earth, their basic purpose in life was to take in some substances (food) and avoid others (toxins). As these organisms evolved into multicellular creatures, detecting chemicals in the environment continued to be crucial for survival. Systems to detect and analyze environmental molecules were thus the first senses to evolve.

Humans have two main chemical detection systems: one for molecules floating in the air, and another for molecules that we put in our mouths. The technical names for these two systems are **olfaction** and **gustation**, respectively. The former, more commonly known as "smell," is the subject of this chapter. Gustation, which you probably know as "taste," will be explored in the next chapter (although, as you'll see, the distinction between tastes and smells is not as clear as you probably think). Another chemical sensing system that is important for both our experiences of smell and tastes is the trigeminal system, innervated by the trigeminal nerve. The trigeminal system enables us to *feel* gustatory and olfactory experiences, like burning and cooling. You will learn more about this system in this chapter and the next.

Olfactory Physiology

Odors and Odorants

Olfactory sensations are called **odors**. The stimuli for odors are chemical compounds. However, not every chemical is an **odorant** (an odor-inducing substance). To be smelled, a molecule must be volatile (able to float through the air), small (less than about 5.8×10^{-22} grams), and hydrophobic (repellent to water). **Figure 13.1***a* shows the chemical structures of two odorant molecules. However, many molecules that would seem to meet the basic requirements still don't smell to us. Two examples are natural gas (methane) and a by-product of methane, carbon monoxide (Figure 13.1*b*). Our evolutionary ancestors would have had no reason to detect these substances, which are not dangerous in the concentrations found in nature. But because carbon monoxide buildups in enclosed spaces such as homes with gas furnaces can be fatal, gas companies add a compound (tertiary-butyl mercaptan) that we smell as rotten eggs, to act as a warning signal when a stove's pilot light goes out. We also can't smell the molecules that make up the air we breathe, such as oxygen and nitrogen.

The Human Olfactory Apparatus

Unlike vision and audition, but like touch and taste, the human olfactory system is tacked onto an organ that serves another purpose. The primary

olfaction The sense of smell.

gustation The sense of taste.

odor A general smell sensation of a particular quality. For example, "The cake had a chocolate *odor*." By contrast, when referring to a specific chemical entity, the term *odorant* should be used.

odorant Any specific aromatic chemical. For example, "You were given the *odorant* menthol to smell."

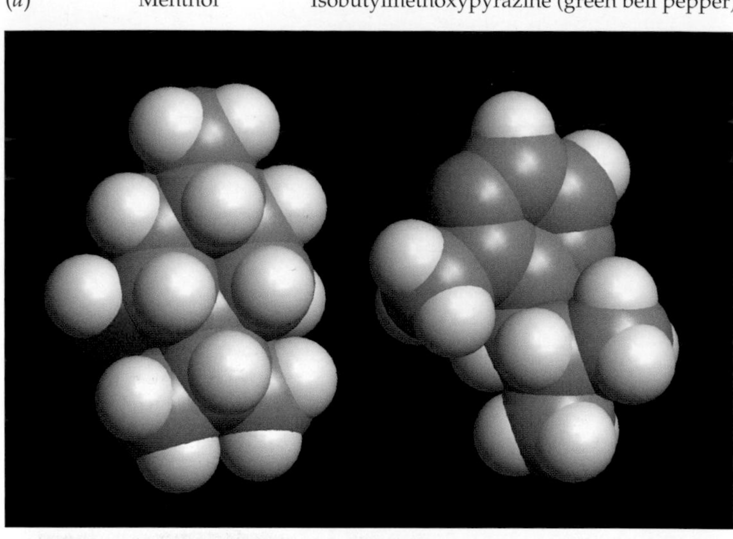

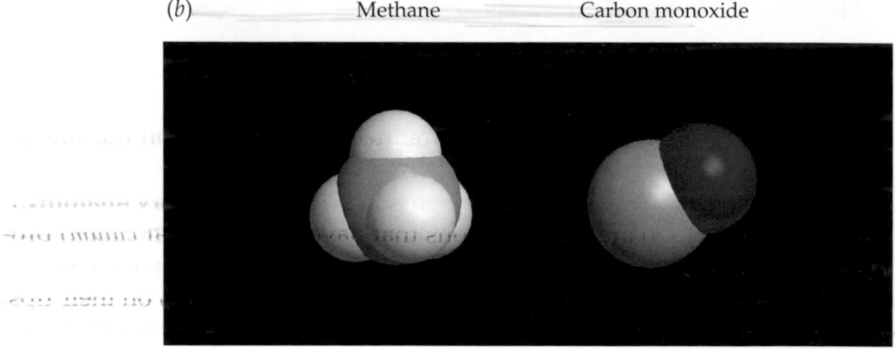

FIGURE 13.1 Odorants. Most small, volatile, and hydrophobic molecules activate the sense of smell (*a*), but there are notable exceptions to the rule, such as methane and carbon monoxide (*b*).

olfactory cleft A narrow space at the back of the nose into which air flows, where the main olfactory epithelium is located.

olfactory epithelium A secretory mucosa in the human nose whose primary function is to detect odorants in the inspired air. Located on both sides of the upper portion of the nasal cavity and the olfactory clefts, the olfactory epithelium contains three types of cells: olfactory sensory neurons, basal cells, and supporting cells.

function of the nose (**Figure 13.2**) is to filter, warm, and humidify the air that we breathe. But the inside of the nose has small ridges called turbinates that add turbulence to incoming air, causing a small puff of each breath to rise upward, pass through a narrow space called the **olfactory cleft**, and settle on a yellowish patch of mucous membrane called the **olfactory epithelium** (**Figure 13.3**). This is the "retina of the nose." We have an olfactory epithelium at the back of each nasal passage, about 2.75 inches up from the nostril. Each

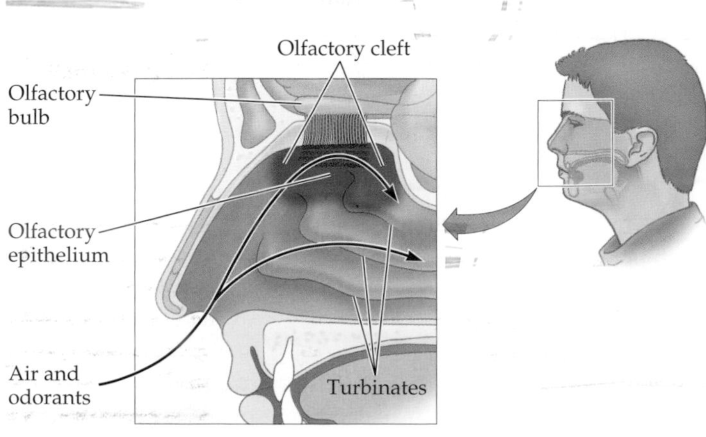

FIGURE 13.2 The nose. Although the primary function of the nose is to warm and humidify the air that we breathe, the nose also directs odorants onto the olfactory epithelium.

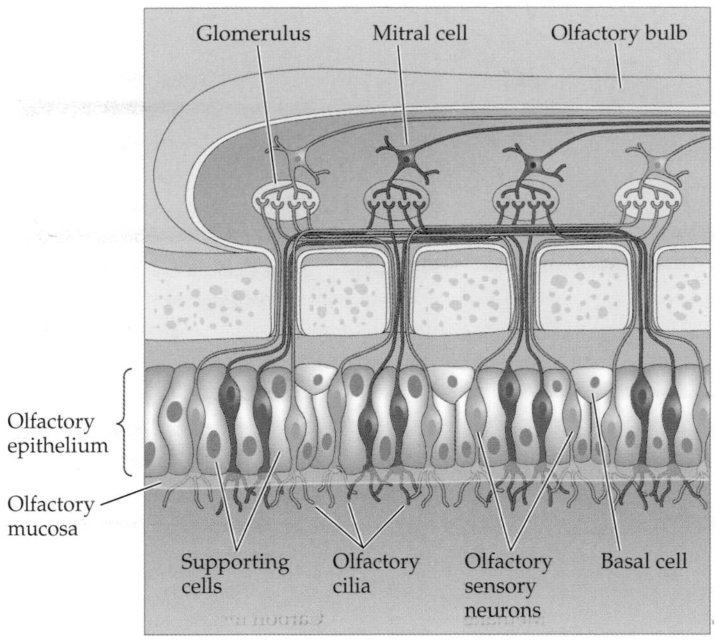

FIGURE 13.3 The retina of the nose. The olfactory epithelium contains three types of cells: olfactory sensory neurons (OSNs), basal cells, and supporting cells. The OSNs are located beneath a watery mucous layer on the epithelium; the hairlike olfactory cilia of the OSN dendrites project through the mucus and are the receptor sites for odorant molecules. The different colors of the OSNs represent the glomeruli onto which they will converge. All blue OSNs go to blue glomeruli, all purple to purple, and so on. This schematic illustrates the fact that different OSNs expressing the same receptors converge on the same glomeruli no matter where they are in the olfactory epithelium.

epithelium measures about 1 to 2 square inches (depending on the size of the nose) and contains three types of cells: **supporting cells**, **basal cells**, and **olfactory sensory neurons** (**OSNs**). (See Web Activity 13.1: Olfactory Anatomy.)

OSNs (**Figure 13.4**) are small neurons that have **cilia** (singular *cilium*) protruding into the mucus covering the olfactory epithelium. These cilia, which are actually the OSN's dendrites, have **olfactory receptors** (**ORs**) on their tips. The interaction between an odorant and the OR stimulates a cascade of bio-

supporting cells One of the three types of cells in the olfactory epithelium. This cell type provides metabolic and physical support for the OSNs.

basal cells One of the three types of cells in the olfactory epithelium. The basal cells are precursor cells to olfactory sensory neurons.

olfactory sensory neurons (OSNs) The main cell type in the olfactory epithelium. OSNs are small neurons located beneath a watery mucous layer in the epithelium. The cilia on the OSN dendrites contain the receptor sites for odorant molecules.

cilia Hairlike protrusions on the dendrites of olfactory sensory neurons. The receptor sites for odorant molecules are on the cilia, which are the first structures involved in olfactory signal transduction.

olfactory receptor (OR) The region on the cilia of olfactory sensory neurons where odorant molecules bind.

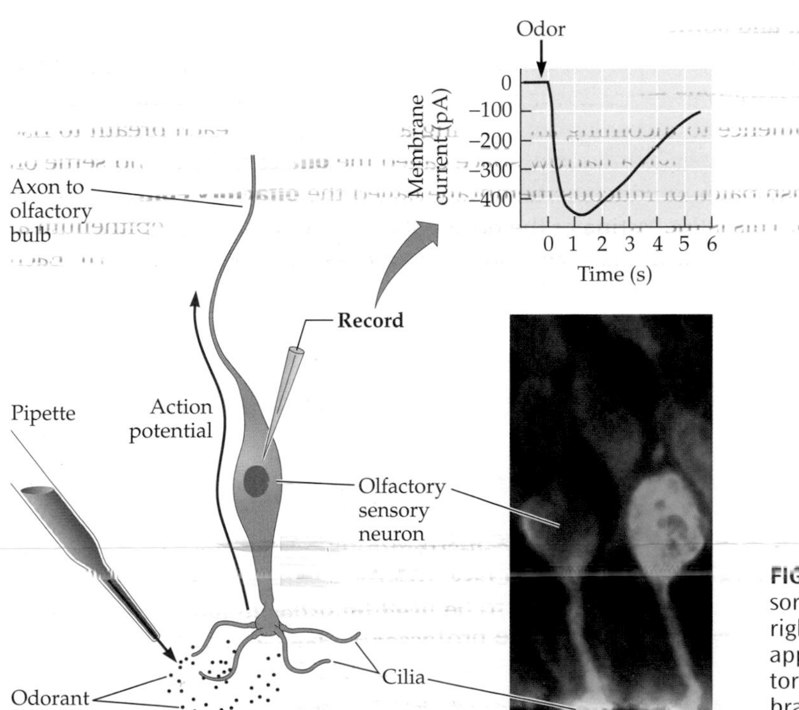

FIGURE 13.4 A fluorescence image of an olfactory sensory neuron (lower right), with a schematic graph (upper right) of an action potential sequence following odorant application. The OSN collects odorant molecules via receptors on its dendrites and sends action potentials to the brain through its axons. (Scan courtesy of C. Balmer and A. LaMantia.)

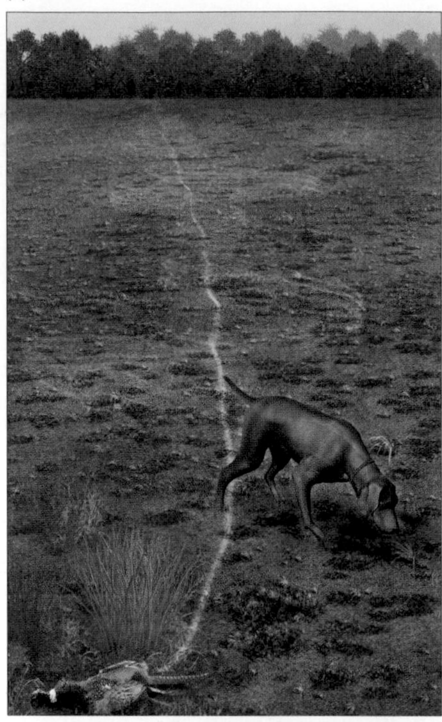
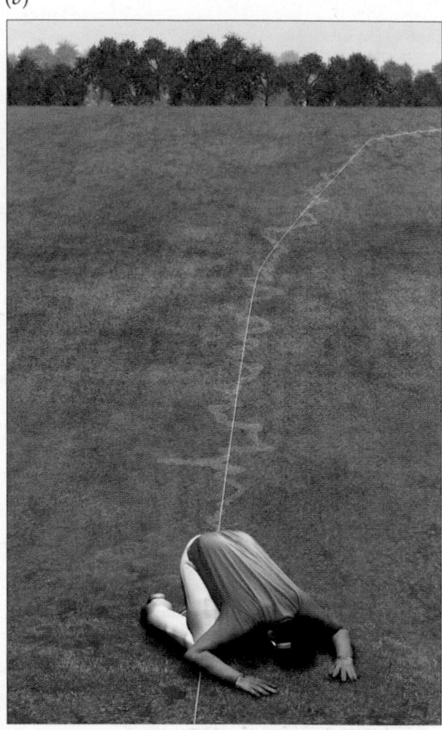

FIGURE 13.5 Tracking scents. (*a*) The path (red) of a dog following the scent trail (yellow) of a pheasant dragged through a field. (*b*) The path (red) of a human following a scent trail (yellow) of chocolate essential oil through a field. (After Porter et al., 2007.)

chemical events, ultimately producing an action potential that is transmitted along the axon of the OSN to the olfactory bulb (Schild and Restrepo, 1998). To initiate an action potential, about seven or eight odor molecules must bind to a receptor, and it takes about 40 of these nerve impulses for a smell sensation to be reported.

We have approximately 20 million OSNs, split between the epithelia of our right and left nostrils. This is more receptors than we have in any other sensory system except vision, and these receptors enable us to distinguish thousands of different odors. However, the number of receptors we have is paltry compared to a bloodhound's 220 million OSNs. In addition, a much higher proportion of a dog's brain is dedicated to olfaction: about 5%, compared to 0.1% for humans. Researchers suspect that humans can smell about the same number of scents as dogs (the bloodhounds aren't talking, so we can't be sure), but dogs can sense odors at concentrations nearly 100 million times lower than the concentrations that humans can detect (Krestel et al., 1984; Willis et al., 2004). Nevertheless, in a recent study humans were able to follow a 10-meter-long scent track of chocolate aroma while on all fours in an open grass field (Porter et al., 2007), and the tracking pattern that the participants used was strikingly similar to that of a dog (**Figure 13.5**). Other amazing smellers include pigs, which can smell the scent of truffles (the mushroom, not the chocolate) under 6 inches of soil; and salmon, which use smell to find the waters of their birth from hundreds of miles away (Dittman and Quinn, 1996).

cribriform plate A bony structure riddled with tiny holes, at the level of the eyebrows, that separates the nose from the brain. The axons from the olfactory sensory neurons pass through the tiny holes of the cribriform plate to enter the brain.

anosmia The total inability to smell, most often resulting from sinus illness or head trauma.

The axons on the ends of OSNs opposite the cilia (dendrites) pass through the tiny sievelike holes of the **cribriform plate**, a bony structure at the level of the eyebrows that separates the nose from the brain (**Figure 13.6**). A hard blow to the front of the head can cause the cribriform plate to be jarred back or fractured, slicing off the fragile olfactory axons, and consequently inducing **anosmia** ("smell blindness"), the total absence of a sense of smell. Stem cells in the olfactory epithelium can form new OSNs; indeed, all

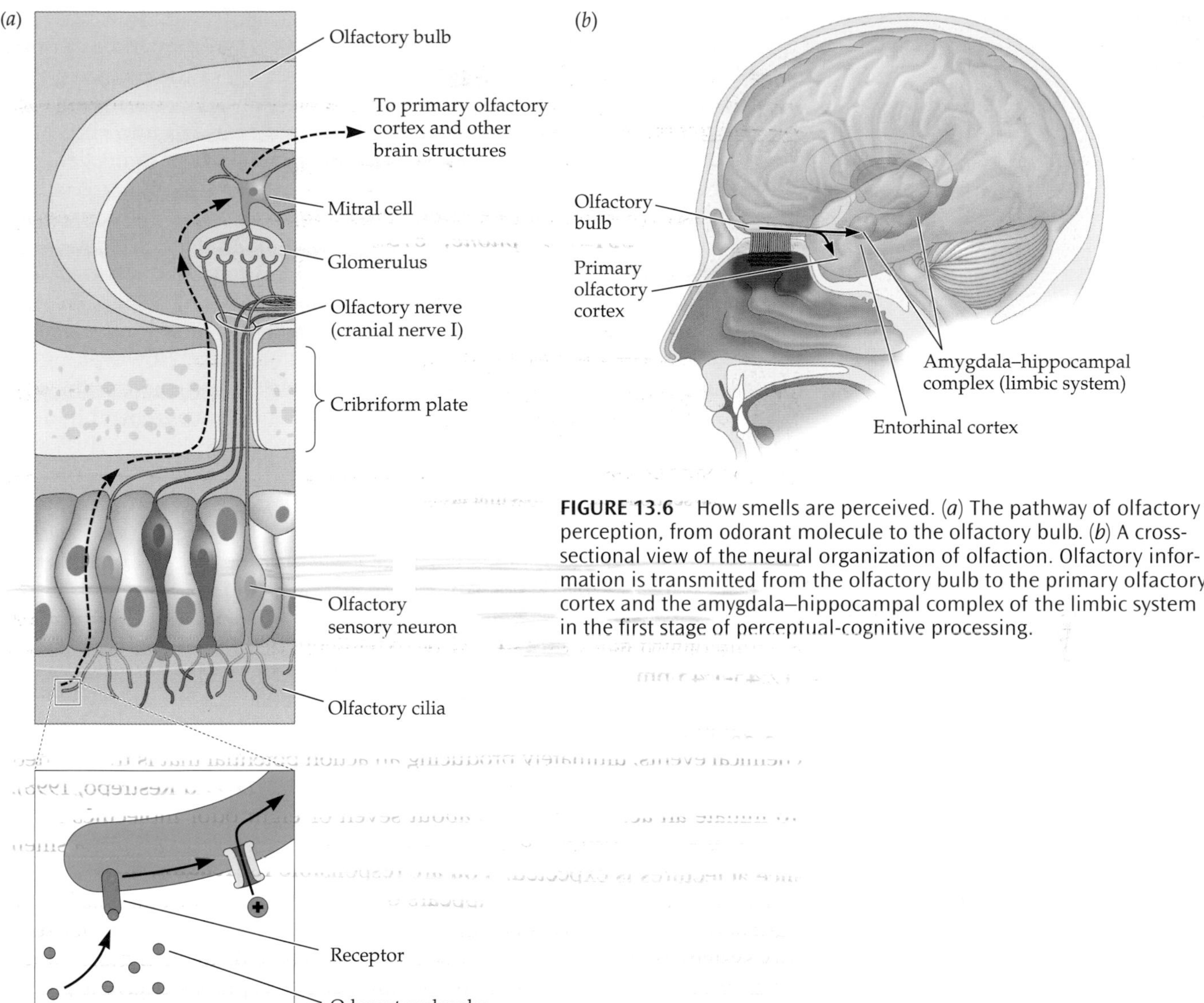

FIGURE 13.6 How smells are perceived. (*a*) The pathway of olfactory perception, from odorant molecule to the olfactory bulb. (*b*) A cross-sectional view of the neural organization of olfaction. Olfactory information is transmitted from the olfactory bulb to the primary olfactory cortex and the amygdala–hippocampal complex of the limbic system in the first stage of perceptual-cognitive processing.

of our OSNs die and regenerate about once every 28 days. However, fractured cribriform plates typically scar over, preventing the new OSN axons from passing through to the brain and crippling the sense of smell for life.

Head trauma is not the only way to produce anosmia. The most common cause of olfactory loss is upper respiratory tract infection (e.g., sinus infection); the second most common cause is sinonasal disease (such as polyps), followed by head trauma; only 30% of anosmias are caused by head trauma. Certain medications can also cause smell loss or disturbance, particularly those used for treating high blood pressure or elevated cholesterol levels. The rarest form of anosmia is congenital; only 3% of people with anosmia are born anosmic. The likelihood of recovery is best when anosmia is caused by infection or disease, because often when the underlying illness is treated, normal smell function returns.

It is worth commenting here that compared to loss of vision or hearing, olfactory loss is paid little attention by both the medical and the general community. In a questionnaire administered to students at the University of Pennsylvania, loss of the sense of smell was ranked equal to losing one's big toe (Wrzesniewski, McCauley, and Rozin, 1999). However, anosmia can cause great suffering, because it affects many aspects of our lives, most noticeably our experience of taste, as we will discover in the next chapter. There is also a profound connection between psychiatric depression and our sense of smell. People who lose their sense of smell can fall into clinically serious depressive states, and people who are diagnosed with depression often concomitantly complain of a weakened sense of smell (Pause et al., 2001). The neurobiological connection between olfactory and emotional processing enables a bidirectional interaction between them (Herz, 2007).

Given the impact of anosmia on quality of life, treatment and attention are critical, especially since the incidence of anosmia is surprisingly high. From a survey by the National Institutes of Health in 1994, it was conservatively estimated that one of every 100 people suffers from anosmia. However, more recent estimates indicate that as many as 14 million Americans over the age of 55 have a severely compromised sense of smell. Including younger adults, it appears that about one in 20 Americans may have some olfactory dysfunction. Olfactory loss can also be the first symptom of neurological disorders such as Alzheimer's and Parkinson's diseases. It is therefore very important to investigate olfactory loss when it occurs. Many smell and taste clinics throughout the country administer simple tests to determine the causes and treatment possibilities for olfactory loss and dysfunction.

In someone with a healthily functioning sense of smell, the OSN axons pass through the cribriform plate, bundle together to form the **olfactory nerve** (cranial nerve I), and enter a blueberry-sized extension of the brain just above the nose, called the **olfactory bulb** (see Figure 13.6). We have two olfactory bulbs, one in each brain hemisphere. Unlike the other senses we've studied so far, olfaction is **ipsilateral**, meaning that the right olfactory bulb gets information from the right nostril and the left olfactory bulb gets information from the left nostril.

Within the olfactory bulb are globular tangles of axons from the OSNs that are synapsed with dendrites from **mitral cells** and **tufted cells**. These spherical bundles are called **glomeruli** (singular *glomerulus*). Molecular genetic studies in mice have shown that all neurons expressing a particular OR type, *no matter where they are on the nasal epithelium*, converge onto one glomerulus pair (consisting of one medial and one lateral glomerulus) in the olfactory bulb (Mombaerts et al., 1996). Thus, all the ORs detecting methyl salicylate, for example, a synthetic chemical that smells like wintergreen mint, send their axons to a single glomerulus pair. Higher brain structures receiving information from the olfactory bulbs therefore know that a signal coming from this glomerulus pair is consistent with sniffing wintergreen. However, this relatively simple picture is complicated by the fact that each glomerulus may receive axons from several different receptor types.

Though they number in the millions, OSNs converge onto a relatively small number of glomeruli. The mouse, whose brain and OR physiology are much more devoted to olfaction than are those of humans, has 2000 glomeruli. It was therefore speculated that humans with far fewer functioning ORs would have about 700 glomeruli (see the next section for more details). However, very recent immunohistochemistry research from Charles Greer's laboratory at Yale University revealed that humans have as many as 6000 glomeruli; three times as many as the mouse for only a third the number of receptors (Maresh et al., 2008). This discovery is quite a surprise and suggests that using the mouse olfactory system as a model for humans, which has traditionally been the case, may be inaccurate. Stay tuned!

Central brain structures that process olfactory information from the olfactory bulb include the **primary olfactory cortex**, **amygdala–hippocampal complex**,

olfactory (I) nerves The first pair of cranial nerves. The axons of the olfactory sensory neurons bundle together after passing through the cribriform plate to form the olfactory nerve.

olfactory bulb The blueberry-sized extension of the brain just above the nose, where olfactory information is first processed. There are two olfactory bulbs, one in each brain hemisphere, corresponding to the right and left nostrils.

ipsilateral Referring to the same side of the body (or brain).

mitral cells The main projective output neurons in the olfactory bulbs.

tufted cells A secondary class of output neurons in the olfactory bulbs.

glomeruli Spherical conglomerates containing the incoming axons of the olfactory sensory neurons. Each OSN converges onto two glomeruli (one medial, one lateral).

primary olfactory cortex The neural area where olfactory information is first processed, which includes the amygdala–hippocampal complex and the entorhinal cortex.

amygdala–hippocampal complex The conjoined regions of the amygdala and hippocampus, which are key structures in the limbic system. This complex is critical for the unique emotional and associative properties of olfactory cognition.

and **entorhinal cortex** (see Figure 13.6). These are all part of a network of brain structures known as the **limbic system**, which is involved in many aspects of emotion and memory. As we will see later, these connections are the key to the unique associative learning and emotional properties of olfaction.

entorhinal cortex A phylogenetically old cortical region that provides the major sensory association input into the hippocampus. The entorhinal cortex also receives direct projections from olfactory regions.

limbic system The encompassing group of neural structures that includes the olfactory cortex, the amygdala, the hippocampus, the piriform cortex, and the entorhinal cortex. The limbic system is involved in many aspects of emotion and memory. Olfaction is unique among the senses for its direct and intimate connection to the limbic system.

Olfactory receptor cells are different from all other sensory receptor cells in that they are not mediated by a protective barrier and instead make direct contact with the brain. By contrast, visual receptors are protected by the cornea, receptors for hearing are protected by the eardrum, and taste buds are buried in papillae. One consequence of the fact that the olfactory sensory neurons are direct conduits into the brain is that many drugs can be inhaled. In spite of their direct linkage into the brain, OSN axons are among the thinnest and slowest in the body. Therefore, even though the nose connects directly to the brain, the time it takes to perceive an odor is long compared to our other sensory experiences. The lag time between sniffing and the brain's registering a smell varies, averaging approximately 400 milliseconds (ms) (almost half a second); compare this to the 45 ms it takes for the visual cortex to register an image presented to the retina. This half-second duration for odorant registration does not take into account the time it takes to react to a scent, which effectively doubles the perceptual time, making olfaction a particularly slow sense. You yourself have probably observed that smells seem to *emerge* gradually, rather than flashing into your awareness.

These distinctions bring up the subtle differences between sensation and perception in olfaction. Sensation occurs when a scent is neurally registered; perception occurs when we become aware of detecting the scent. Similarly, odors tend to linger—because of both ambient airflow and receptor clearance speed. The relatively slow speed and lingering features of olfaction have been the central obstacles for developing effective "smell-o-vision" and smell virtual-reality technologies.

The Genetic Basis of Olfactory Receptors

In 1991, molecular biologists Linda Buck and Richard Axel (who were rewarded with a Nobel Prize for their efforts) showed that the genome contains about 1000 different olfactory receptor genes, each of which codes for a single type of OR. All mammals appear to have pretty much this same set of 1000 genes, but interestingly, some of the OR genes in each species are nonfunctional "pseudogenes": the genes are present on the chromosomes, but the proteins coded for by the genes never get produced. In dogs and mice, about 20% of the OR genes are pseudogenes; in humans, the proportion is much higher, between 60% and 70%.

We don't have a precise percentage for humans because researchers have found individual variability in the number of receptors expressed. One person may express 348 ORs while another expresses 388, but both have a "normal" sense of smell. The differences between the two, however, will likely manifest in sensitivity to certain odorants. That is, certain specific chemicals will smell stronger to one person than they do to another, and thus the *perception* of certain odors may be different. In olfaction, there may truly be different noses for different people (Menashe et al., 2003).

In general, the more receptors that are expressed, the more sensitive one is to odorants. A highly intense odor tends to be perceived as less pleasant than the same scent at a lower intensity (see also the "Olfactory Hedonics" section of this chapter). We see this relationship with intensity in all our senses. Very bright lights and loud sounds are inherently more unpleasant than moderate-intensity lights and sounds, and our relative acuity in vision and hearing will individually affect how much we can tolerate (see Chapter

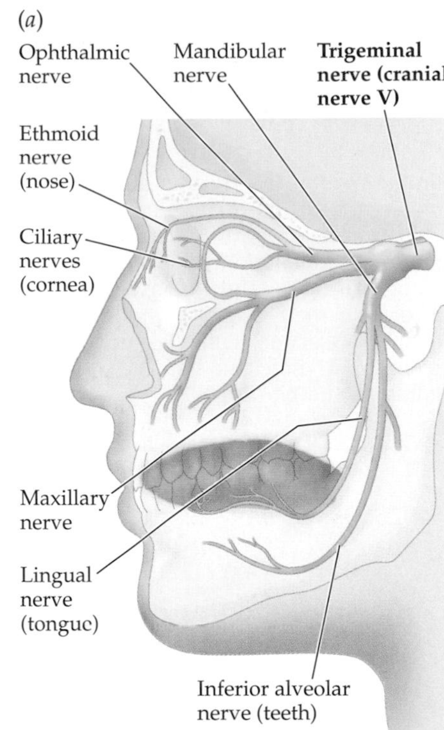

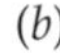

(b)

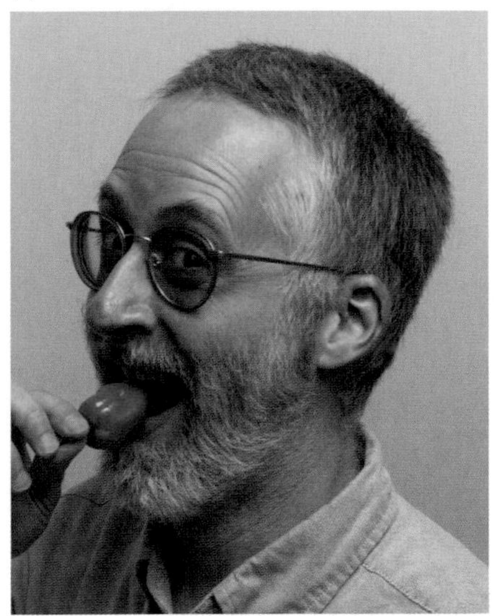

FIGURE 13.7 The trigeminal nerve's role in the perception of odors. (*a*) The trigeminal nerve carries information from somatosensory receptors in the nose and face to the thalamus and then on to the somatosensory cortex. (*b*) The irritation or excitement (depending on your culinary preferences) caused by eating chili peppers is due to trigeminal nerve stimulation.

9 for more detail). Genetic variation in receptor expression may be the one innate factor in the modulation of our odor likes and dislikes.

Some researchers have recently suggested that the high proportion of OR pseudogenes in humans is the result of an evolutionary trade-off between vision and olfaction. Yoav Gilad and his colleagues (2004) observed that Old World primate species such as gorillas and rhesus monkeys have about 30% OR pseudogenes, but most New World species (e.g., squirrel monkeys) have a lower proportion (about 18%). The one New World exception is the howler monkey, which also has about 30% OR pseudogenes. It turns out that the howler monkey has something in common with Old World primates that other New World monkeys do not: trichromatic color vision. Brains can get only so big, so to free up the brain space necessary to house human ancestors' evolving visual analysis tools (including trichromatic vision), we may have dropped the ability to analyze the odorants detected by certain OR genes, and they then became pseudogenes. The payoff from superior visual detection must have been better for our ancestors' survival than the disadvantages from diminished olfactory acuity.

The Feel of Scent

As mentioned at the start of this chapter, our experience of odors often has a *feel* to it as well as a smell. This is because most odorants stimulate the somatosensory system to some degree through polymodal nociceptors (touch, pain, and temperature receptors) inside the nose. For example, menthol feels cool and ammonia feels burning. These sensations are mediated by the **trigeminal nerve** (cranial nerve V) (**Figure 13.7***a*). In many cases it is impossible to distinguish between the sensations traveling up cranial nerve I from olfactory receptors and those traveling up cranial nerve V from somatosensory receptors. For example, the nasal cooling (cranial nerve V) and specific scent (cranial nerve I) associated with the smell of peppermint fuse to produce a holistic sensory experience. Trigeminal stimulation accounts for why our eyes tear when we chop onions and why we sneeze when we sniff pepper. High levels of trigeminal stimulation (e.g., munching habanero peppers; Figure 13.7*b*) can produce a severe burning sensation, and trigeminal activity has been linked to the facial–head pain felt in migraine headaches. "Smelling salts" (made from ammonia combined with eucalyptus oil) revive us because of their trigeminal activation.

trigeminal (V) nerves The fifth pair of cranial nerves, which transmit information about the 'feel' of an odorant (e.g., menthol feels cool, and cinnamon feels warm), as well as pain and irritation sensations (e.g., ammonia feels burning).

From Chemicals to Smells

Now that we know something about the physiological basis of olfaction, we can ask the following crucial question: How does the biochemical interaction between an odorant and an OR, and subsequent neurological processing in the olfactory bulbs and later brain structures, result in the psychological perception of a scent such as lemon? Buck and Axel's seminal discovery of olfactory receptor genes has produced an explosion of research surrounding this question over the past decade, but a fully comprehensive theory of how we perceive scents has still not been developed.

Theories of Olfactory Perception

At present, the best-accepted biochemical theory (first proposed in its modern form in the 1950s by the British scientist John Amoore) is based on the match between the shapes of odorants and odor receptors. It was dubbed "shape theory" but is better denoted as "shape-pattern theory." In a nutshell, **shape-pattern theory** contends that odorant molecules have different shapes and olfactory receptors have different shapes, and an odorant will be detected by a specific OR to the extent that the odorant's molecules fit into the OR (**Figure 13.8**). Gordon Shepherd and his students pioneered the idea that when a given odorant is sniffed, a particular pattern is generated across the glomeruli. Differences in those spatial patterns provide the basis for the array of odors that we perceive.

The most recent molecular research suggests that scents are detected by means of a combinatorial code. Different scents activate different arrays of olfactory receptors in the olfactory epithelia, producing specific firing patterns of neurons in the olfactory bulb. The specific pattern of electrical activity in the olfactory bulb then determines the particular scent we perceive. That is, different patterns are elicited for the perception of vanilla, orange, urine, and skunk (for example), and the various patterns for specific scents turn out to be highly consistent across individuals (Zou, Li, and Buck, 2005).

However, there are also alternative explanations of how olfaction works. The strongest alternative to shape-pattern theory is **vibration theory**, championed most recently by Luca Turin (Turin, 1996). In essence, vibration theory proposes that, because of atomic structure, every smell molecule has a different vibrational frequency, and molecules that produce the same vibrational frequencies have the same smell. Turin reported that various chemicals that have predictably similar vibrations because of their molecular composition also have similar smells. For example, all citrus odors fall into the same class

shape-pattern theory The current dominant biochemical theory for how chemicals come to be perceived as specific odorants. Shape-pattern theory contends that different scents—as a function of odorant-shape to OR-shape fit—activate different arrays of olfactory receptors in the olfactory epithelia. These various arrays produce specific firing patterns of neurons in the olfactory bulb, which then determine the particular scent we perceive.

vibration theory An alternative to *shape-pattern theory*, describing how olfaction works; most recently championed by Luca Turin. Vibration theory proposes that every perceived smell has a different vibrational frequency, and that molecules that produce the same vibrational frequencies will smell the same.

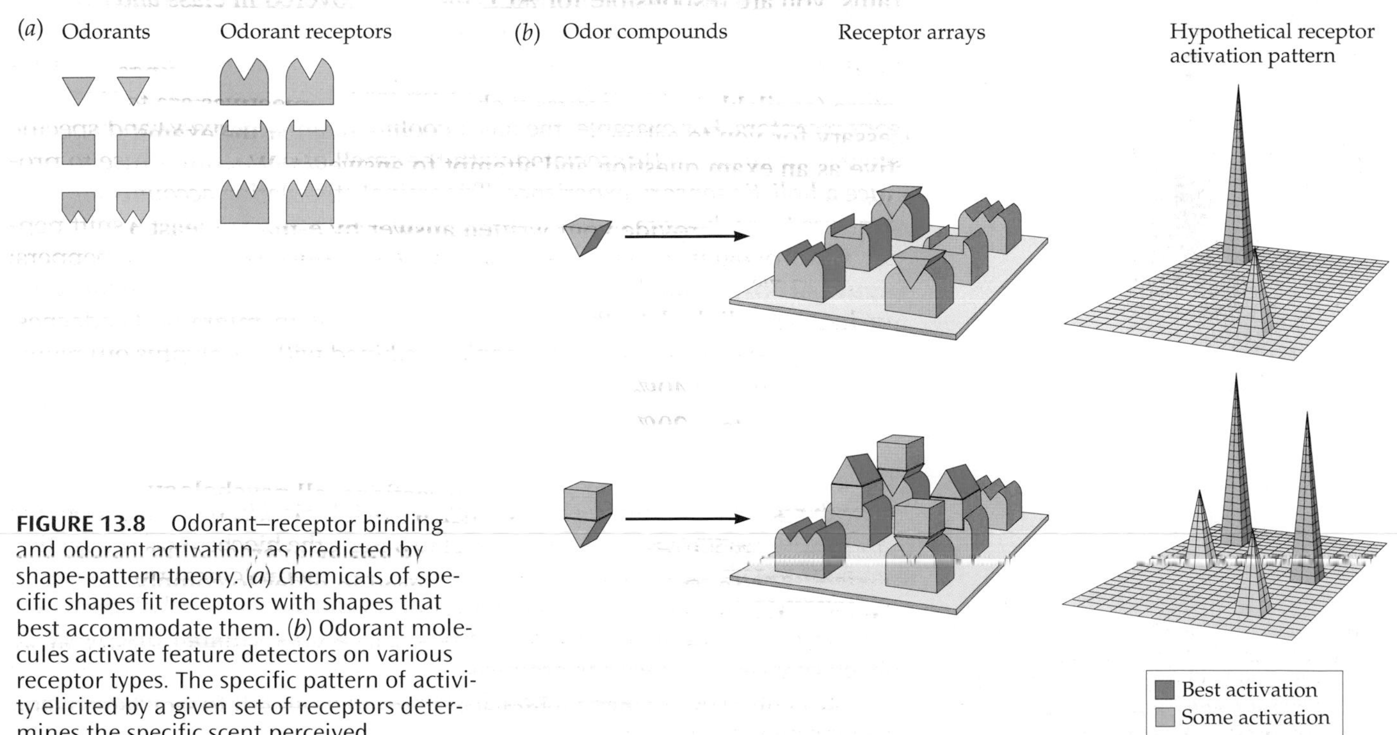

FIGURE 13.8 Odorant–receptor binding and odorant activation, as predicted by shape-pattern theory. (*a*) Chemicals of specific shapes fit receptors with shapes that best accommodate them. (*b*) Odorant molecules activate feature detectors on various receptor types. The specific pattern of activity elicited by a given set of receptors determines the specific scent perceived.

of vibrational frequency. But other independent researchers have not validated Turin's claims (Keller and Vosshall, 2004).

Much less research has focused on the vibration theory than on the shape-pattern theory, so current advances may unfairly bias our understanding. Nevertheless, vibration theory cannot explain several conundrums of olfactory perception, such as specific anosmias and the different scents produced by stereoisomers, which shape-pattern theory can explain.

A **specific anosmia** is the inability to smell one specific compound amid otherwise normal smell perception. Most specific anosmias are to steroidal musk compounds, and the condition appears to be genetic. The most studied specific anosmia is an inability to smell the compound androstenone, which is found in armpit sweat and pork. Fifty percent of the population has a specific anosmia to androstenone. Interestingly, of the remaining 50% who can smell it, about half describe the smell as a "sweet musky-floral" scent, while the other half describe it as an unpleasant "urinous" odor. A recent cloning study of human olfactory receptors showed that the variability in detection of the odorant androstenone, as well as its perceived pleasantness, is due to genetic differences in OR expression between individuals (Keller et al., 2007).

Serendipitous observation also revealed that through repeated testing, sensitivity to androstenone could be induced in about half of the people who were initially unable to detect it (Wysocki, Dorries, and Beauchamp, 1989). That is, a proportion of the people who were anosmic to this particular chemical developed an ability to smell androstenone through repeated exposure. This change in detection ability to a specific chemical cannot be explained by vibration theory. Nor can vibration theory explain why some people perceive the scent as sweet-floral and others as urinous. However, shape-pattern theory can account for these observations.

It is presumed that the specific anosmia and the various perceptions of the chemical androstenone are genetically determined. That is, in individuals with the specific anosmia, the receptors that detect androstenone are nonfunctional (coded by pseudogenes), and different receptors detect the compound in those who perceive a floral scent than those who perceive a urinous odor. From other areas of biology, we know that genes can be "turned on" by environmental factors, and because each olfactory receptor is coded for by a specific gene, it is conceivable that the receptors for detecting androstenone can be activated through repeated presentation of the chemical. Other studies have shown that increased sensitivity to some common odorants, such as benzaldehyde (cherry–almond aroma) and citralva (lemon–orange scent) can be induced through repeated exposure to these chemicals, particularly for females (Dalton, Doolittle, and Breslin, 2002; Diamond et al., 2005). Furthermore, recent studies in fruit flies have shown that genetically hardwired OSNs can be altered by exposure to specific chemicals (Sachse et al., 2007). Plasticity and modulation through environmental influences appear to be basic principles in olfaction.

Another mark in favor of shape-pattern theory comes from the study of **stereoisomers**. Stereoisomers are molecules that are mirror-image rotations of one another; and although they contain all the same atoms, they can smell completely different. For example, *d*-carvone (the right-handed isomer) smells like caraway (**Figure 13.9***a*), and *l*-carvone (the left-handed isomer) smells like spearmint (Figure 13.9*b*). According to shape-pattern theory, this difference arises because the rotated molecules do not fit the same receptors (as if you were trying to put your right hand into your left-hand glove); thus, different receptors are activated for these two molecules, causing dif-

specific anosmia The inability to smell one specific compound amid otherwise normal smell perception.

stereoisomers Isomers (molecules that can exist in different structural forms) in which the spatial arrangement of the atoms are mirror-image rotations of one another, like a right and left hand. Also called *optical isomers*.

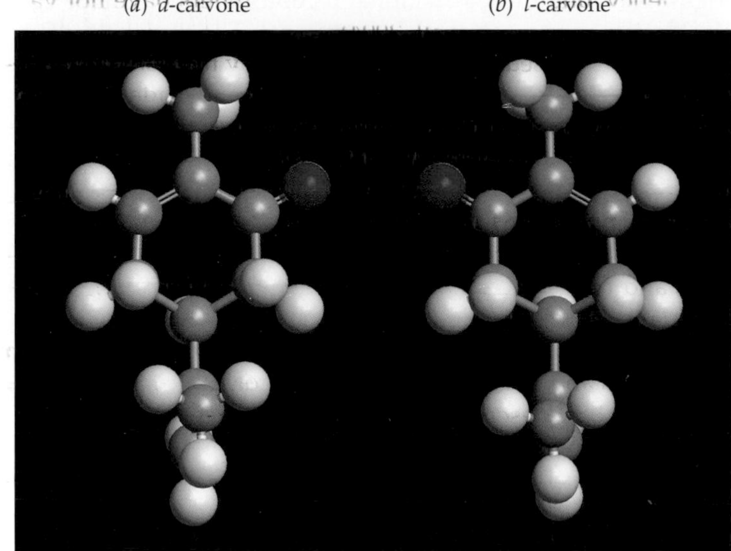

FIGURE 13.9 The stereoisomers *d*-carvone (*a*) and *l*-carvone (*b*) contain the same atoms yet smell completely different: *d*-carvone smells like caraway, *l*-carvone like spearmint. Shape-pattern theory can account for this fact.

ferent scents to be perceived. Vibration theory cannot explain why stereoisomers smell different, because the vibration of stereoisomers is the same. More recent, and more direct, evidence for shape-pattern theory comes from experiments using cloned olfactory receptors, which have revealed chemical–receptor interactions in vitro that show specific odorants binding with specific receptors.

Like so many debates in psychology, it may be that neither shape-pattern nor vibration theory is a complete theory of smell (recall the initial conflicts between the trichromatic and opponent-process theories of color vision, for example). Shape-pattern theory currently has better general explanatory value, but it is also true that all molecules vibrate and all receptors are made of atoms that vibrate. This leaves room for vibrational interactions between odor molecules and receptors to play a role.

The Importance of Patterns

You may have noticed a potential discrepancy in how we have accounted for odorant perception. As we've seen, we can discriminate many thousands of odors, yet our genes code for only about 1000 olfactory receptors, and 600 to 700 of them are nonfunctional. How can we detect so many different scents? To start to see the way out of this conundrum, recall that, in vision, we can tell the difference between thousands of different colors, even though we have only *three* types of cones. Each type of olfactory receptor responds to the structure of certain molecules only. However, a molecule may have features that stimulate several different receptors. Moreover, each receptor appears to have various "feature detectors" that contribute to further specificity in OR activation. Thus, a different *set* of feature detectors is activated when we smell chocolate compared to when we smell a rose (see Figure 13.8*b*).

As with detecting colors, we detect odors by considering the *pattern* of activity across various different receptor types. The intensity of an odorant also changes which receptors (and hence patterns) will be activated, which is why weak and strong concentrations of an odorant do not smell quite the same. The fact that receptor activation is affected by odor intensity likely

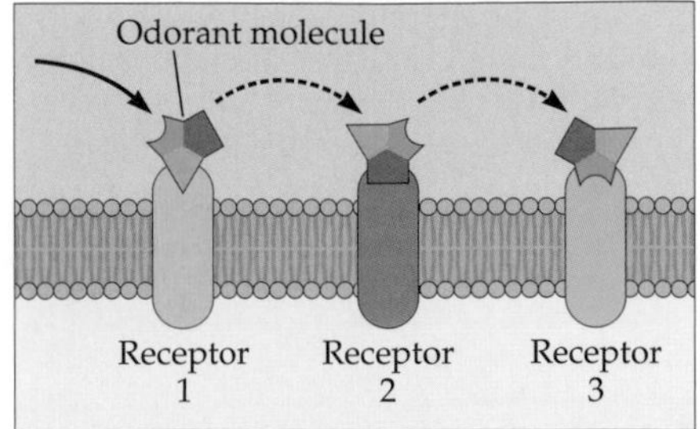

FIGURE 13.10 The hypothetical role of OR receptor activation timing and order. A single molecule binds first to receptor type 1, then a split second later to receptor type 2, then to receptor type 3. Brains are especially well suited to recognize patterns of responses such as this, so the number of odorants we can recognize greatly exceeds the number of receptor types available.

explains why dogs with many more functional receptors than we have can perceive considerably lower concentrations of odorants. The timing of olfactory receptor activation is probably also important; an odorant that activates several receptors will also stimulate them in a specific time order. Another odorant might stimulate the same receptors in a different order, and the difference might lead to the perception of a different smell (**Figure 13.10**). Thus, different odor perceptions can be due to different OR firing patterns or to firing of the same receptors at a different rate or sequence.

The flip side of the pattern perception mechanism is that if two molecules, or combinations of molecules, activate the same receptors in the same order, we end up smelling the same thing. For example, the feature detectors for the single molecule phenyl ethyl alcohol and a real live rose in the garden, whose scent is composed of more than 1000 different molecules, might both result in the same basic pattern of activation and hence the same perception of "rose" (this phenomenon should be reminiscent of metamers in color vision).

Odor Mixtures

Just as we rarely hear pure tones outside of auditory perception experiments, we rarely smell "pure odorants" outside of an olfactory perception lab. Almost all of the olfactory stimuli that we encounter in the real world are mixtures, like the thousand-molecule rose scent emanating from a flower bed that we discussed in the previous section. How do we process the components in an odorant mixture? There are two broad possibilities: *analysis* and *synthesis*. Auditory mixtures provide the classic example of analysis. A high note and low note played simultaneously on a piano each can be analyzed out of the mix and perceived separately (**Figure 13.11*a***). Color mixtures provide the classic example of synthesis. If we mix red and green lights, the resulting color that we see is yellow (Figure 13.11*b*). Red and green cannot be analyzed out, because the two lights have been synthesized into something else. Is olfaction (Figure 13.11*c*) an analytical or a synthetic sense?

Although we are capable of discriminating thousands of different odorants, intuition tells us that most mixtures are perceived as unitary wholes. For example, the smell of bacon is very distinctive, and most people would perceive it to be a unitary sensation. But there is no "bacon" odorant; the sensation we recognize as bacon is made up of a combination of many different volatile chemicals. To test the synthetic/analytical nature of olfactory perception, Laing and his colleagues (Laing and Francis, 1989; Laing and Glemarec, 1992) conducted a series of experiments in which they asked

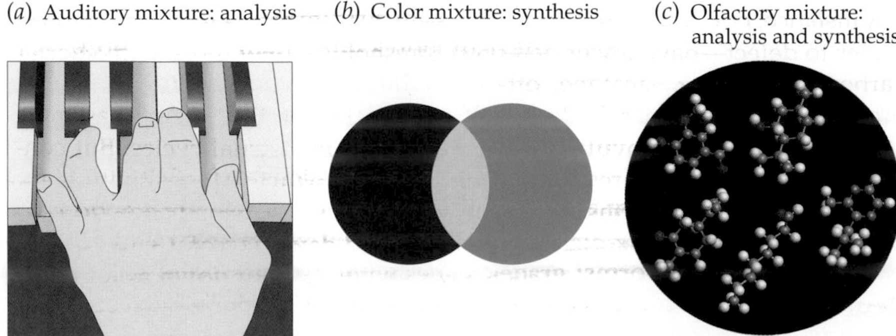

FIGURE 13.11 The roles of analysis and synthesis in sensory perception. We can break the three tones out of the musical chord being played in (*a*), but we cannot separately perceive the high- and medium-wavelength light rays mixing in the center of (*b*). When we mix odorants (*c*), we perceive the mixture primarily synthetically, but some degree of analytical perception is possible. Analytical ability varies with prior training and with the odorants that comprise a mixture.

untrained participants, participants who received preliminary "odor training," and experienced perfumers and flavorists to identify the constituents of mixtures containing between one and five common odorants. The average discrimination rate from all the participants combined was no more than three components in a five-component mixture. However, the more training the participant had the better they did. Thus, it appears that olfaction is primarily a synthetic sense, but that a certain amount of analytical ability can be developed with training.

Odor Imagery

Though visual and auditory imagery is possible, humans appear to have little or no ability to conjure odor "images." For example, you can probably easily generate a visual image of a Hershey's chocolate kiss right now (you might even start salivating). But can you really reproduce the smell of chocolate in your "mind's nose"? Brain-imaging studies (e.g., Kosslyn et al., 1995) have shown that many of the same parts of the brain that would be involved in actually seeing the kiss are also involved in visually imaging it; with olfaction, however, similar studies suggest that the degree of overlap between smelling an odor and "imaging" it is much weaker. Dreams with olfactory sensations are also very rare (Carskadon et al., 1989; Zadra, Nielsen, and Donderi, 1998). Other animals, such as rodents, which rely predominantly on smell as the sense to negotiate the world, may well think and dream in smell. Because we do not think in smell, it is not necessary to have stored representations of olfactory experiences. Nevertheless, since the olfactory system appears to be highly flexible and modulated by learning and environmental experiences throughout life, one might be able to develop the capacity to create sensory representations of smells with training. Many perfumers and chefs insist that they can image olfactorily.

Olfactory Psychophysics, Identification, and Adaptation

The subfield of psychology called **psychophysics** was introduced in Chapter 1. The goal of the psychophysicist is to quantify the psychological experience of our sensory world. In this section we will briefly discuss some of the nuts-and-bolts questions addressed by olfactory psychophysics; then we'll go on to consider the related and more interesting questions of how we identify and adapt to odors.

Detection, Discrimination, and Recognition

Perhaps the most basic question we can ask for any sense is, How much stimulation is required before we perceive something to be there? As with other senses, our olfactory *detection thresholds* depend on a number of factors. For instance, odorant molecules with longer carbon chains (e.g., vanillin) are easier to detect—have lower detection thresholds—than those with shorter carbon chains (e.g., acetone, otherwise known as nail polish remover). Women also have generally lower olfactory detection thresholds than men, especially during the ovulatory period of their menstrual cycles. But contrary to popular belief, research has shown that olfactory sensitivity is *not* heightened during pregnancy (Cameron, 2007; Hummel et al., 2002; Laska et al., 1996). Taste is another story, as we'll see in the next chapter.

Our ability to detect odors also declines with age, because of a change in the proportion of OR cell regeneration to cell death. The outcome is that as we get older the number of odor receptors that die off continues to rise

psychophysics The science of defining quantitative relationships between physical and psychological (subjective) events.

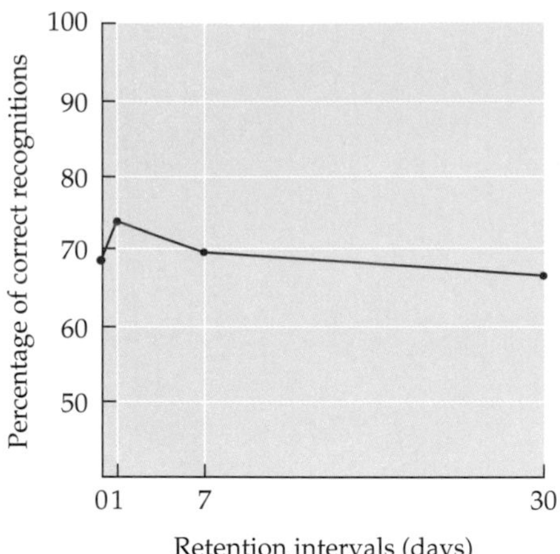

FIGURE 13.12 The first point on this graph at 70% indicates odor recognition accuracy with only a 30-second delay from learning. Note, however, that this accuracy level is the same after a week and has dropped only about 3% after a retention interval of a month. This retention rate remains relatively constant over intervals at least as long as a year. (From Engen and Ross, 1973.)

beyond the number that are regenerated (Kern et al., 2004). This ratio continues to worsen in favor of cell death as we grow older, such that after the age of 85 it is estimated that about 50% of the population has effectively become anosmic (Hummel et al., 2007; J. C. Stevens and Cain, 1987). Taste and trigeminal perception, however, have not been shown to decline in sensitivity with age, which explains why the elderly favor foods that are spicy (trigeminal) and salty (taste) (Stevens, Plantinga, and Cain, 1982).

As already noted, a healthy person can *discriminate* thousands of odors. The more "nose" training we have (e.g., professional perfumers and wine tasters), the more odors we can discriminate; some claims suggest that professionals can distinguish up to 100,000 odors (Dobb, 1989). Note, however, that discrimination is not the same thing as *recognition*, the ability to remember whether or not we've smelled an odor before. It takes as much as three times as many odorant molecules floating through the nose to recognize an odor than it does to simply detect that the odor is there. You've probably experienced this phenomenon yourself: you register that you smell something before you realize that you know the smell.

Another interesting feature of odor recognition is its durability. In controlled experiments, a 30-second delay between odor presentation and testing produces a precipitous drop in recognition accuracy, but what we remember after 30 seconds is very close to what we remember after 3 days, a month, or even a year (**Figure 13.12**) (Engen, Kuisma, and Eimas, 1973; Engen and Ross, 1973; Murphy et al., 1991; Rabin and Cain, 1984). Again, you probably recognize this phenomenon from your own life. If you smelled a certain flower only once when you were a child, and you came upon that flower again 20 years later, you might very well know that the odor was familiar. Our memory for odors is especially potent if emotion is experienced during initial exposure (Herz, 1997).

Psychophysical Methods for Detection and Discrimination

Researchers wanting to measure how sensitive people are to an odorant or whether they can discriminate one odor from another use various psychophysical methods. A common technique for determining someone's odor detection threshold is called the **staircase method** (or "reverse staircase method"). There are various versions of the staircase method. In a typical procedure, an odor is presented in ever-increasing concentration increments until the participant reports being able to "smell something" for several increments. Then the odor concentration is decreased incrementally until the participant reports no detection.

staircase method A psychophysical method for determining the concentration of a stimulus required for detection at the threshold level. A stimulus (e.g., odorant) is presented in an ascending concentration sequence until detection is indicated, and then the concentration is shifted to a descending sequence until the response changes to "no detection." This ascending and descending sequence is typically repeated several times, and the concentrations at which reversals occur are averaged to determine the threshold detection level of that odorant for a given individual. Also called *reverse staircase method*.

triangle test A test in which a participant is given three odors to smell, of which two are the same and one is different. The participant is required to state which is the odd odor out. The order of the three odors given (e.g., same, same, different; different, same, same; same, different, same) is typically manipulated and the test repeated several times for greater accuracy.

These reversals are repeated a number of times, and the odorant concentrations at the point where reversals occur are averaged to determine the approximate concentration needed for that person to detect the odorant. As a reversal point is reached, the increments by which an odorant's concentration is raised and lowered can be fine-tuned for precision. Staircase methods can be used to determine a general benchmark for olfactory sensitivity. They can also be used to determine detection thresholds across a range of different odors for specific and individualistic testing.

To determine whether someone can discriminate between two odors, the most common psychophysical test used is called the **triangle test**. In a triangle test, a participant is given three odors to smell, of which two are the same and one is different. The participant is required to state which is the odd odor out. The order of the three odors given (e.g., same, same, different; different, same, same; same, different, same) is typically manipulated and the test repeated several times to establish accuracy.

Identification

Attaching a verbal label to a smell is yet another step beyond odor recognition. Olfaction has been called "the mute sense" because we are often so lost for verbal descriptors for our olfactory experiences (Ackerman, 1990). All of us have had the experience of not being able to come up with the name of something that we know; for example, what was the name of your fourth-grade teacher? This experience is known as the "tip-of-the-tongue" phenomenon. In the olfactory domain, suppose you take a sniff of something from a bottle that provides no visual clues to what it contains and you immediately know that the scent is extremely familiar, but you just can't come up with the name for it. Borrowing from the verbal scenario, we call this experience the **tip-of-the-nose phenomenon** (Lawless and Engen, 1977), and it can be very frustrating.

There are some important differences between the tip-of-the-nose state and the tip-of-the-tongue state. For one, in the tip-of-the-tongue state we might not know the exact word we're looking for, but we might know its first letter, its general word configuration, the number of syllables in the word, and so on ("Starts with a *K*, two syllables, sounds like a German word … Aha, my fourth-grade teacher was Mrs. Kaiser!"). In the tip-of-the-nose state, we typically know nothing about the label we're searching for. But even though we are clueless about the odor's name, we do usually know how to respond to it appropriately. If you smelled maple syrup, even if you couldn't name it you would know it was something that you liked to eat; whereas if you smelled shoe polish, you would know that it wasn't something you'd want to put in your mouth. (These examples might remind you of brain damage patients with visual agnosia, who often know how to use an object even if they don't know what it's called.)

Anthropologists have found that in all known languages, there are fewer words that refer exclusively to our experience of smells than there are for any other sensation (Classen, Howes, and Synnott, 1994). In English, *aromatic, fragrant, pungent, redolent*, and *stinky* pretty much exhaust the list of adjectives that specifically describe olfactory stimuli and nothing else. More common terms used to describe odors, like *floral* or *fruity*, are references to the odor-producing objects (flowers and fruits), not the odors themselves. We also borrow terms from other senses (chocolate smells *sweet*, grass smells *green*, and so on).

Various possibilities explain why our sense of smell and language are so disconnected. First, unlike what happens in other sensory systems, olfactory information is not integrated in the thalamus prior to processing in the cortex, and it is argued that the thalamus has relevance for language. Second, a large body of evidence indicates that the majority of olfactory processing occurs in the right hemisphere of the brain, whereas language processing is known to be dominated by the left hemisphere (see Royet and Plailly, 2004, for review). It has even been suggested that odors are hard to name because of competition between odor and language processing for cognitive resources that share the same neural substrates (Lorig, 1999). This latter theory is supported by a recent study using brain-imaging techniques, which showed that the presence of an odor altered the semantic processing of words and degraded word encoding, but did not influence nonsemantic processing (Walla et al., 2003). (See also **Web Essays 13.1: Olfactory Lateralization** and **13.2: Verbal–Olfactory Interactions**.)

When odor identification is measured in a way that can trigger the tip-of-the-nose state, it is equivalent to a free-recall memory test; you have to come up with the name for the odor yourself without any clues. Another way that odor identification is measured is by recognition, where, like a

tip-of-the-nose phenomenon The inability to name an odorant, even though it is very familiar. Contrary to the tip-of-the-tongue phenomenon, one has no lexical access to the name of the odorant, such as first letter, rhyme, number of syllables, and so on, when in the tip-of-the-nose state. This is one example of how language and olfactory perception are deeply disconnected.

multiple-choice exam question, various alternates are given and the person must pick the correct name to go with that odor. Scratch-and-sniff odor recognition tests like this are very important in clinical situations; particularly for detecting the early stages of neurological disorders like Alzheimer's disease. Prior to forgetting people's names or where the car keys are, people in the first stages of Alzheimer's are unable to correctly identify odors. This is because Alzheimer's is foremost a disease of semantic loss, and because language and smell are so weakly connected in the first place, this system is most vulnerable to the first signs of semantic deterioration. The sooner people are correctly diagnosed with Alzheimer's disease and treated, the better their quality and duration of life will be.

Adaptation

Have you ever had the experience of noticing coworkers or classmates who seem to be pouring a bottle of cologne over their head every morning, leaving you choking on the overpowering aroma? Can't they smell anything? Or perhaps you've noticed that, after having a bottle of perfume for a few months, you can't smell the fragrance in it anymore. Or you've gone away on vacation and returned home to find that your house seems to have a "funny" smell that it didn't have when you left. What's going on? The answer has two parts: the first involves the nose, and the second the mind.

The sense of smell is a change detector system. When a new chemical comes along, your olfactory receptors fire in response to it, and you perceive a scent. For example, when you first enter a bakery, you notice the mouthwatering aromas of the cakes, cookies, pies, and breads. But if you stand inside inspecting the sweet baked goods for a while, you may find that by the time you've picked out what cake you want for dessert, you can no longer smell it. What has happened here is that the odorant molecules that make up the bakery aroma have bound to the corresponding olfactory sensory neurons in your nose. When this happens the ORs retreat into the cell body (Firestein, 2001). The receptors are therefore no longer physically available to respond to the bakery scent molecules. This response is a process in "receptor recycling." Specifically, odorant binding to an OR causes the OR to be internalized into its cell body, where it becomes unbound from the odorant and is then recycled through the cell and emerges again in a number of minutes. Receptor recycling is a mechanism common to all receptors in the class to which ORs belong: **G protein–coupled receptors (GPCRs)**.

This process is called **receptor adaptation**. The precise length of time for adaptation to occur varies as a function of both the individual (Dalton, 2002) and the odorant (Pierce et al., 1996). On average it takes about 15 to 20 minutes of continuous exposure to an odorant for the molecules to stop eliciting an olfactory response, but adaptation can also occur in less than a minute. Receptor adaptation can also be undone relatively quickly. Stepping outside the bakery for a few minutes gives unbound olfactory receptors a chance to accumulate on the cell surface again, so when you walk back in you can enjoy the appetizing scents once more. The magnitude of adaptation is also affected by odor intensity (Kadohisa and Wilson, 2006). As odor concentration increases, the degree of adaptation decreases. For example, it takes longer to adapt to the odor wafting from an apple pie baking in the oven than to the scent emanating from a cool slice of pie on the kitchen counter.

One way to prolong the effect of smelling a scent before adaptation kicks in is to dispense an odor intermittently. For example, bursts of air freshener alternated with no scent will draw out the time before your receptors are smothered by the air freshener molecules and duck for cover. Dalton (1996)

G protein–coupled receptors (GPCRs) The class of receptors that are present on the surface of olfactory sensory neurons. All GPCRs are characterized by a common structural feature of seven membrane-spanning α-helices.

receptor adaptation The biochemical phenomenon that occurs after continuous exposure to an odorant, whereby the receptors stop responding to the odorant and detection ceases.

also showed that psychological processes can have an effect on adaptation rates. In one experiment, half the participants were told that an odorant they were being exposed to was "healthful," while the other participants were told the odorant was "hazardous." Twenty minutes after initial exposure, the participants smelling the supposedly healthful odorant had adapted to it, whereas the participants who thought they were smelling a hazardous chemical actually became sensitized—they reported the smell as even more intense after 20 minutes than at the start of the experiment. These different reactions from the two sets of participants occurred even though all of them had been smelling *the very same odorant*, isobornyl acetate, which has a balsam woody odor and is completely harmless.

cross-adaptation The reduction in detection of an odorant following exposure to another odorant. Cross-adaptation is presumed to occur because the two odorants share one or more olfactory receptors for their transduction, but the order of odorant presentation also plays a role.

One of the benefits of olfactory adaptation is that it enables us to filter out stable background odors, and this filtering ability can be enhanced through active sniffing—that is, taking deliberate quick inhalations (Kepecs, Uchida, and Mainen, 2007). Active sniffing makes OR neurons less responsive to stable odors and more responsive to new odors (Verhagen et al., 2007). For example, if we are at a car dealership and think we smell something burning, we typically engage in active sniffing to (1) see if we are right and (2) determine which Ferrari is smoldering. In vision and hearing, perceptual stimuli in the foreground can be segregated from stimuli in the background through spatial analysis of the scene. In olfaction, spatial analysis is compromised because background and foreground odors merge in the air. However, provided that background and foreground odors are at least briefly separated in time (new car smell first and then burning odor), active sniffing enables us to separate components of an olfactory scene.

In some cases, exposure to one odorant can raise the odor detection threshold for a second, completely different odorant. For example, when you're picking out a perfume in a department store, your nose may become fairly useless at differentiating the fragrances after several samples, despite the salesperson's insistence that the perfumes are quite different from each other (**Figure 13.13**). This phenomenon is called **cross-adaptation**, and it is presumed to occur when the odorants in question rely on similar sets of olfactory receptors. However, this simple explanation is complicated by the fact that most cross-adaptation relationships are nonreciprocal. For example, smelling pentanol (a chemical used in some paints) seems to have a strong cross-adapting effect on next smelling propanol (used as an antiseptic and solvent), whereas smelling propanol first has only a small cross-adapting effect on next smelling pentanol (Cain and Engen, 1969). Furthermore, exposure to the first odorant can sometimes *enhance* sensitivity to the second odorant. (See **Web Activity 13.2: Odor Adaptation and Habituation.**)

Regardless of why they occur, cross-adaptation effects, like self-adaptation effects, usually go away after a couple of minutes. Professional perfumers, who may have to smell hundreds of scents per day and thus don't have a couple of minutes to spare, use a trick of sniffing their bare arm or cotton shirt sleeve between smelling odorants; doing this effectively clears the nose even at a fast pace of odorant presentation. Nobody knows why this works, but it does. The next time you find yourself suffering from numb nose in a department store, try it.

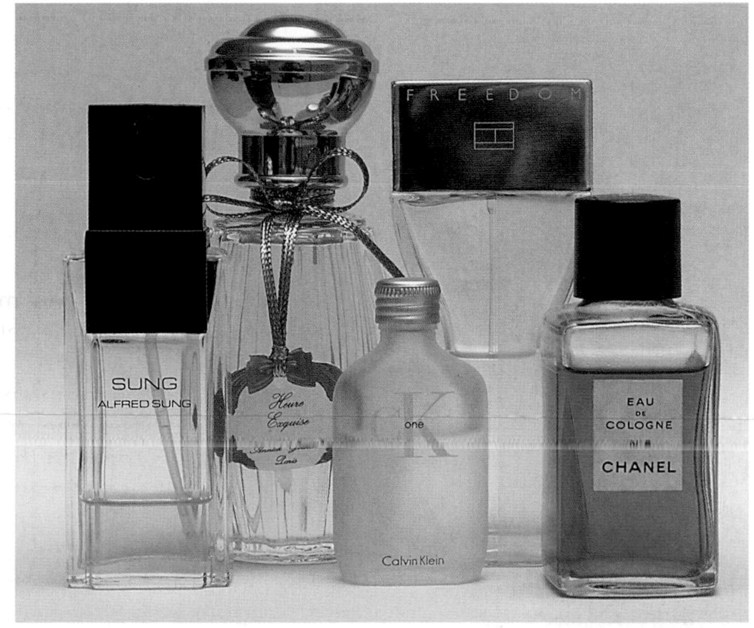

FIGURE 13.13 Do these five fragrances smell the same? No, but because of olfactory cross-adaptation, if you've smelled four of them in succession, the subtleties of the fifth one may be lost to your nose.

Cognitive Habituation

Receptor adaptation explains why you lose the delicious aroma of the bakery after you've been in the store for awhile, but can smell it again after a short break outside. If you took a job at a bakery, however, a different process would take place. This is the phenomenon that your friend who can't smell his cologne is experiencing, and it's the reason why you don't smell your house unless you go out of town for a couple of weeks. It is a psychological effect called **cognitive habituation**.

In short, when we live with an odor, we cognitively habituate to it and no longer react to it, or we show a very diminished response to it. For example, textile workers exposed daily to acetone exhibited acetone detection thresholds that were eight times higher than those of a comparable group of control subjects. However, their thresholds to another chemical (butanol), to which neither group had been regularly exposed, were no different from each other (Wysocki et al., 1997). We habituate to some degree to stimuli presented to all our senses (you will eventually learn to sleep through your roommate's snoring, for example), but attention can bring us out of habituation with every sense except smell. Unlike receptor adaptation, which can be undone in a few minutes, cognitive habituation requires weeks to reverse, even for pungent trigeminal stimulants like acetone (Dalton et al., 1997; Wysocki et al., 1997). For example, if you stopped wearing your cologne for 5 days, you would still *not* be able to smell it well once you put it back on. But if you abstained for 2 weeks or more, you would.

Dalton (2002) suggested that at least three mechanisms could be involved—either singularly or in interaction—in producing olfactory habituation. First, the olfactory receptors that are internalized into their cell bodies during odor adaptation may be more hindered after continuous exposure and take much longer to recycle than they normally would. Second, from continuous exposure, odorant molecules may be absorbed into the bloodstream, then transported to the olfactory receptors via nasal capillaries when we breathe out through the nose. As long as the odorant chemicals remain in the bloodstream, we will be constantly adapted (Maruniak, Silver, and Moulton, 1983). Finally, cognitive-emotional factors, such as the process observed in the experiment in which participants were told that odors were harmful and then did not adapt, may be involved (but in the reverse direction) in cognitive habituation.

Another feature of odor perception that highlights the importance of attention is that we cannot smell while we're asleep (Carskadon and Herz, 2004). Unlike responses to auditory stimuli, presenting participants who were in deep sleep—known as slow-wave sleep (SWS) or dreaming (REM) sleep—with trigeminally activating odors such as peppermint and pyridine, even at high concentrations, did not awaken them or elicit EEG (electroencephalogram) sleep pattern changes. Nevertheless, a recent functional neuroimaging (fMRI) study reported that presenting an odor during SWS that had previously been present during an awake learning task produced hippocampal changes consistent with those observed in memory consolidation (B. Rasch et al., 2007). However, the odor had no effect if it was presented during other sleep stages or REM sleep. This finding suggests that odors may be detected by the brain during SWS. However, other neuroimaging research on awake subjects during smell tasks indicates that attention to odors alters brain activity and odor detection ability (Zelano et al., 2005; Plailly et al., 2008). It may be that, because attention is effectively cut off during sleep, so is our ability to respond to odors. Note again the issue of sensation versus perception. Although odors may be registered by the brain without conscious awareness, olfactory perception depends on attention.

cognitive habituation The psychological process by which, after long-term exposure to an odorant, one is no longer able to detect that odorant or has very diminished detection ability.

Olfactory Hedonics

The most immediate and basic response we have to an odor is whether we like it or not. Such affective evaluations are known as **odor hedonics.** In tests of odor hedonic evaluation, ratings for how pleasant, familiar, and intense a person finds a given odorant are typically taken. These measures are then used to determine the hedonic value of a specific smell. It is obvious that perceived pleasantness is related to our liking for an odor. But how are familiarity and intensity related?

odor hedonics The liking dimension of odor perception, typically measured with scales pertaining to an odorant's perceived pleasantness, familiarity, and intensity.

Familiarity and Intensity

As in many other life situations, we tend to like odors that we've smelled many times before. That is, we tend to like familiar odors better than unfamiliar odors. Moreover, we often perceive pleasant odors as familiar, even if we haven't smelled them before (Moskowitz, Dravnieks, and Klarman, 1976; Sulmont, Issanchou, and Koster, 2002). Thus, ratings of odor pleasantness and familiarity show a linear relationship with odor liking.

Intensity has a more complex relationship to odor liking and often shows an inverted-*U* function, but this depends on the odorant. A rose scent may be evaluated as more positive with increasing intensity, up to a point—then the function reverses, and as the scent becomes stronger it is judged to be more disagreeable (**Figure 13.14***a*). By contrast, a weak fishy odor may be acceptable, but as intensity increases, its perception becomes steadily more negative (Figure 13.14*b*). Note also that individual differences in the number and type of receptors expressed may influence one's sensitivity (intensity perception) and hence the predisposition to experience specific odorants along a pleasantness continuum.

Nature or Nurture?

A long-standing debate in olfaction centers around whether hedonic responses to odors are innate or learned. Researchers on the *innate* side of the debate claim that we are born with a predisposition to like or dislike various smells. In other words, rose is inherently a good smell and skunk is inherently a bad smell, the way bitter taste is inherently unpleasant to us and sweet inherently pleasant (see Chapter 14). In contrast, researchers taking the *learned* view hold that we are born merely with a predisposition to learn to like or dislike smells, and that whether a smell is liked or not is determined by the emotional value (good or bad) of the experiences that have been associated with it. That is, if we like rose and dislike skunk, the reason is that we have a good and a bad association, respectively, with these two scents. We need not have direct contact with a skunk to form such an association, though, because cultural learning provides meaning to many unencountered stimuli.

If asked to take a position yourself, on the sole basis of your own personal experiences, it's pretty likely you would come down on the innate side of the debate. After all, who could like the smell of skunk, and who wouldn't like the smell of a rose? In fact, however, a great deal of evidence suggests

(*a*)

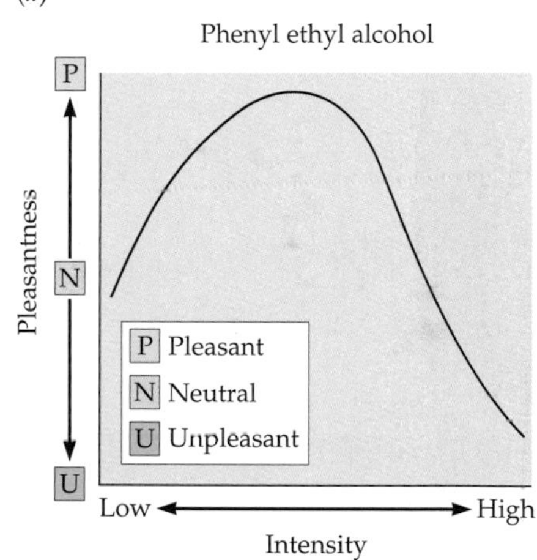

(*b*)

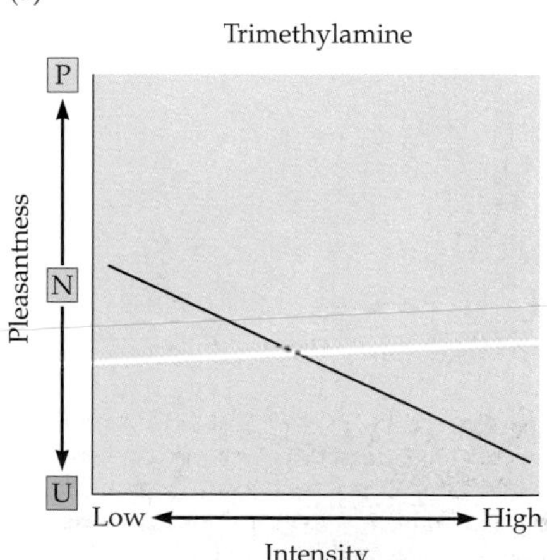

FIGURE 13.14 Pleasantness ratings of odorants plotted against intensity. (*a*) The relationship between odor intensity and pleasantness is often described by an inverted-*U* function, if the odorant is initially considered pleasant, as the synthetic rose scent (phenyl ethyl alcohol) usually is. (*b*) For an odorant that is initially considered tolerable (but not necessarily pleasant), such as fishy smelling trimethylamine, the relationship may more aptly be described by a linear graph like this.

gestation Fetal development during pregnancy.

that odor hedonics are almost exclusively learned. A good place to start looking for such evidence is with infants. If odor preferences are innate, then newborns should display them. However, researchers have repeatedly found that when presented with odorants that they have probably never encountered before, infants and children often display very different preferences from those of adults. For instance, infants do not find the smells of sweat and feces unpleasant (Engen, 1982; M. Stein, Ottenberg, and Roulet, 1958), and toddlers often do not hedonically differentiate between odorants that adults find either very unpleasant (e.g., butyric acid, found in rancid foods) or pleasant (e.g., amyl acetate, which smells like banana).

One difficulty in doing these types of studies is that the olfactory system is fully functional by the third month of **gestation** (6 months before the baby is born) (Schaal, Marlier, and Soussignan, 1995, 1998; Winberg and Porter, 1998), and odorant molecules do find their way into the womb. So it is difficult to know exactly how much exposure even a newborn infant has had to an odorant. But exposure to odorants in utero has led to yet another line of evidence in support of the learned view of hedonics: Mennella and colleagues found that mothers who consumed distinctive-smelling volatiles (e.g., garlic, alcohol, and cigarette smoke) during pregnancy or breast-feeding had infants who showed greater preferences for these smells than did infants who had not been exposed to these scents (Mennella and Beauchamp, 1991, 1993; Mennella, Johnson, and Beauchamp, 1995). What we learn about odors prenatally and during infancy and early childhood can also go on to influence our food and flavor preferences in adulthood (Haller et al., 1999). This correlation suggests that it might be a good idea for women to eat lots of spinach and liver and other healthful foods during pregnancy and lactation.

Cross-cultural data provide further support that associative learning, rather than hardwired responses, is responsible for olfactory preferences. No scientific studies to date have found cross-cultural agreement for hedonic responses to common everyday smells, either "good" or "bad" (Ayabe-Kanamura et al., 1998; Schleidt, Hold, and Attila, 1981). And many anecdotal and observational examples illustrate the culturally polarized responses that we have to specific odors. For example, many Asians consider the smell of cheese to be disgusting, yet most Westerners consider it anything from comfort food to an extravagant indulgence. In contrast, the Japanese often enjoy a meal for breakfast called *nattō* (a fermented soybean dish) (**Figure 13.15**) that most Westerners wouldn't bring near their mouths (some say it smells like burning rubber). Both cheese and *nattō* are high in protein and similarly nutritious; the reason they are preferred, or not, as foods has to do with our learned associations with their scents.

In case you're thinking that the examples of odors given so far aren't really *that* bad, and that there must be consensus on really horrid stenches, this also doesn't seem to be the case. Fecal smells are not high on most North Americans' "best smells list," but the Masai of Africa like to dress their hair with cow dung as a cosmetic color treatment. And in a recent study undertaken by the US military to create a stink bomb (to be

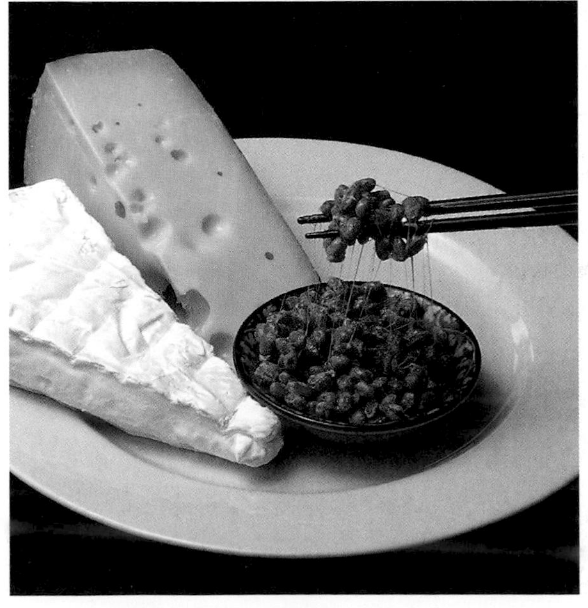

FIGURE 13.15 The Japanese regularly eat *nattō* (right) for breakfast, but Westerners do not equate the smell of this food with eating. In contrast, cheese, which most Westerners enjoy, is considered disgusting by most Japanese eaters.

used for crowd dispersal), it was impossible to find an odor (including "US Army issue latrine scent") that was unanimously considered repellent across ethnic groups (Dilks, Dalton, and Beauchamp, 1999). Recent laboratory studies directly aimed at testing the learning hypothesis have shown that a novel odorant can be made to be perceived as good or bad as a function of the associations (good or bad) made to it (Herz, Beland, and Hellerstein, 2004). Note, however, that from an experimental perspective it is much easier to demonstrate that odor preferences can be learned than to prove that no odors exist to which innate responses may be shown.

In an attempt to support the view that odor pleasantness has an innate basis, a recent study tested whether an odorant's physical and chemical structure could predict how pleasant or not it would be perceived to be (Khan et al., 2007). The researchers found that the molecular structure of odorants was able to account for 30% of the variance in participant's responses (70% was not accounted for this way) and therefore argued that a portion of odor pleasantness perception may be innate. Further research evaluating individual differences in OR expression and the perception of odorants with specific molecular structures is needed.

An Evolutionary Argument

The theory that odor preferences in humans are formed through associative learning rather than being innate can be defended on the basis of evolutionary principles (Herz, 2001). *Specialist* animal species live in very specific habitats and thus have a limited number of food sources and predators. For such species, hardwired responses to particular odors are adaptive. California ground squirrels, for example, exhibit an instinctive defensive response the first time they are exposed to the odor of their natural predator, the Pacific rattlesnake, but they don't show the same response to the scent of Pacific gopher snakes, which are not their natural predators (**Figure 13.16**) (Coss et al., 1993; Poran and Coss, 1990).

Generalist species (including humans, rats, and cockroaches), on the other hand, can exploit many different habitats. Their available resources and potential predators can vary widely across environments, so it is not adaptive for these species to have predetermined olfactory responses to any particular odor. Instead, generalists need to be especially prepared to learn and remember what to approach and what to avoid on the basis of experience.

(*a*)

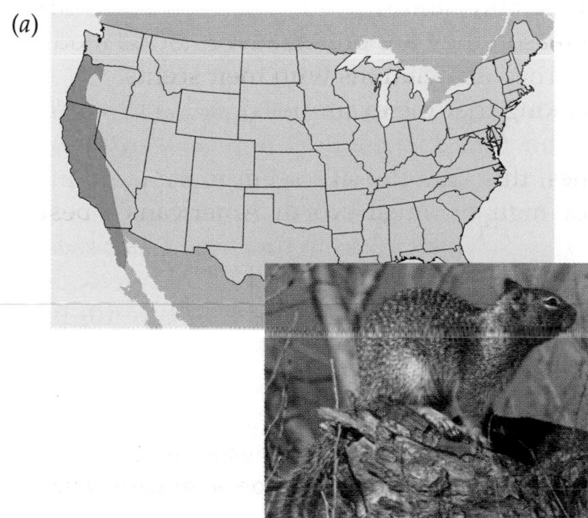

(*b*)

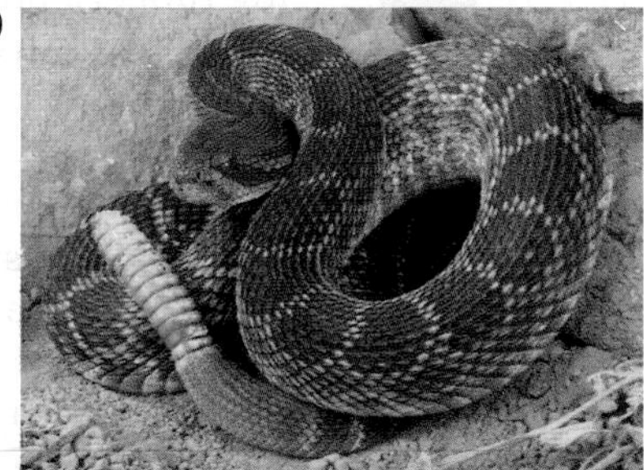

FIGURE 13.16 The California ground squirrel lives in a restricted habitat (*a*), so it has only a few natural predators, including the Pacific rattlesnake (*b*). Studies have shown that, unlike humans, specialist spec such as the California ground squirrel show innate odor responses this case to avoid the scent of the animal that will try to eat the

learned taste aversion The avoidance of a novel flavor after it has been paired with gastric illness. The smell, not the taste, of the substance is key for the learned aversion response in humans.

Clear evidence that learning is a critical mechanism by which generalists acquire odor responses is shown by **learned taste aversions**. Rats and humans can be made to avoid a flavor by being made sick after consumption. See Chapter 14 for an explanation of the critical role of olfaction in flavor perception. For example, presenting a rat with a sweet-tasting, banana-smelling drink and then injecting the rat with lithium causes nausea and creates a conditioned avoidance of this flavor in the future. Similarly, children who experienced chemotherapy after ingesting a novel flavor of ice cream (mapletoff) subsequently refused to eat mapletoff ice cream (Bernstein, 1978).

Researchers have shown that in humans the conditioned aversion is to the smell, not the taste, of the substance (Bartoshuk and Wolfe, 1990). In rats, it remains unclear whether there is a discrete role for taste in this type of aversion learning. The long-term effects of learned taste aversion for humans are clearly adaptive. If poison is ingested, it is best to learn to avoid it permanently, rather than having to repeat the mistake until it kills you. The key point is that for generalists, banana and mapletoff are not inherently meaningful smells in themselves; rather, it is their association to positive or negative experiences that makes us interpret them as good or bad.

Caveats

Although a great deal of evidence suggests that odor hedonics are learned, we must note two caveats. First, trigeminally irritating odors may elicit pain responses, and all humans have an innate drive to avoid pain (although even this drive can be overcome by cultural influences, as attested by the popularity of chili peppers in many ethnic cuisines). Second, as has been mentioned several times, the potential variability in the receptor genes and pseudogenes that are expressed across individuals may influence odor intensity perception and consequently pleasantness. For example, people who like the smell of skunk may exhibit this response in part because they are missing receptors for detecting some of the more pungent volatiles, whereas people who are particularly repulsed by this scent may be endowed with a greater number of receptors that are keenly attuned to the mercaptan and sulfide aspects of this bouquet. Therefore, the "perceived" intensity of a scent may be partly responsible for its perceived (un)pleasantness. Recall that for many odors, an inverted-*U* function exists between liking and intensity. Genetic differences in OR expression appear to extend to ethnicities as well (Menashe et al., 2003), which may help explain why it has been impossible to develop a universally effective stink bomb.

Olfaction, Memory, and Emotion

In the mid-1960s in Britain, Moncrieff (1966) asked adult respondents to provide hedonic ratings for a battery of common odors. A similar study was conducted in the United States in the late 1970s (Cain and Johnson, 1978). Included in both studies was the odorant methyl salicylate, a scent we call "wintergreen." In the British study, wintergreen was given one of the lowest pleasantness ratings; in the American study, it was rated the most pleasant of the scents tested in the study. There is a historical reason for this difference. In Britain, the smell of wintergreen is associated with medicine; in particular, wintergreen was added to analgesics used during World War II, a time that the adults in the 1966 study would not have remembered fondly. Conversely, in the United States the smell of wintergreen is exclusively a candy smell, so it has only sweet, positive connotations. As this example demonstrates, the key to olfactory associative learning is the experience that occurs when the odor is first encountered, and in particular, the emotional connotation of that experience (Bartoshuk, 1991; Engen, 1991; Herz, 2001).

When an odor is liked or disliked because of what it has been associated with in our past, we are also recalling a memory when we smell it. Many of our odor experiences, such as most Britons' and Americans' experiences with wintergreen, are too vague to conjure specific memories, and only the feelings of good or bad remain. However, one of the most distinctive features of olfaction is its ability to elicit our most emotional and evocative personal recollections.

Odors have earned the reputation of being the "best cues" to memory, but are they? To address this question, Herz (1998, 2004) compared recollections stimulated by a particular smell—for example, popcorn—with memories evoked by the sight of popcorn, the sound of popcorn popping, the feel of popcorn kernels, or simply the word *popcorn* (**Figure 13.17**). The take-home message from these studies is that, in terms of their vividness and accuracy, memories evoked by odors are as good as—but not any better than—memories evoked by sights, sounds, feel, or words. (See **Web Activity 13.3: Sensory Memory Cues**.)

As already noted, however, memories triggered by odor cues are distinctive in one important way: their emotionality. Across a wide range of experiments that assessed both laboratory-induced memories and naturalistic autobiographical memory, a consistent pattern of results emerged (Herz, 1998, 2004; Herz and Cupchik, 1995; Herz et al., 2003): when experiencing a recollection, participants list more emotions associated with olfactory cues than they do with other sensory modalities, they rate those emotions as having greater intensity, and they report particular memories as being more emotionally laden when they are elicited by odors compared to when they are cued by another sense. People also feel more transported to the original time and place when a scent is eliciting their recall than when that same memory is triggered via another sensory system.

Despite the conventional wisdom, then, odors appear to be no better than other sensory cues at eliciting an *accurate* recollection. Instead, the emotion and evocativeness of odor-elicited memories leads to the false impression that such memories are especially accurate. The confidence that one's recollections are true, which is so hard to resist when memories are colored by emotional experience, is quite similar to what often emerges during eyewitness testimony in the courtroom. Eyewitnesses recalling emotionally charged episodes are often extremely confident that their recollections are accurate, but research shows that these memories are often incorrect (Busey et al., 2000).

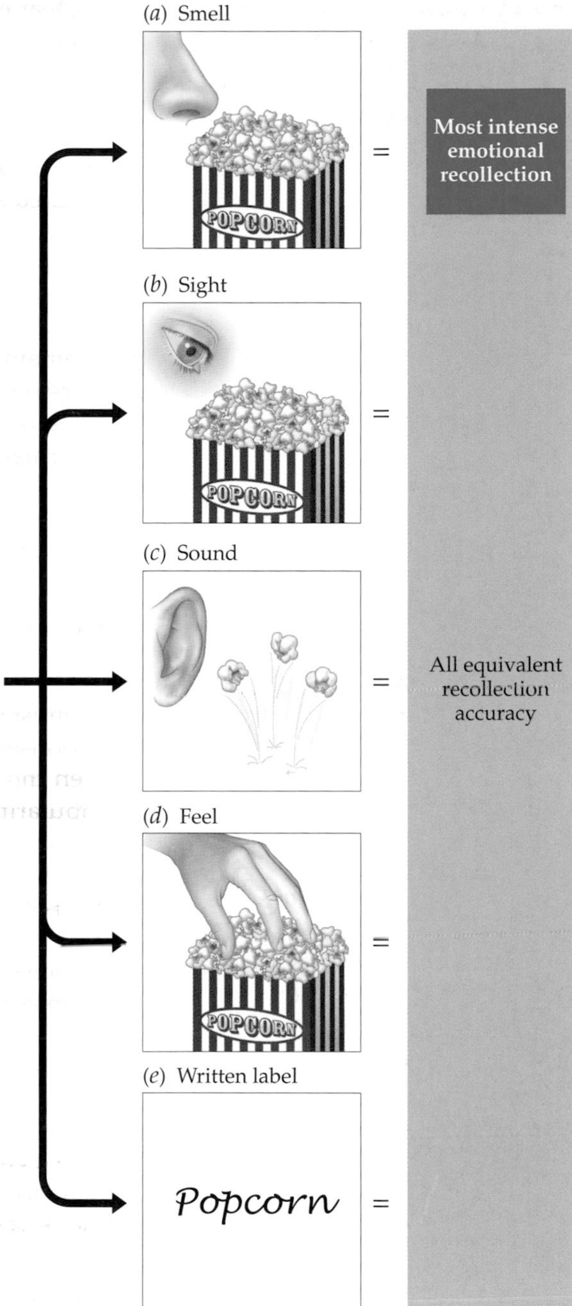

FIGURE 13.17 The smell (*a*), sight (*b*), sound (*c*), feel (*d*), and verbal label (*e*) of popcorn elicit memories that are equivalent in terms of their accuracy. However, odor-induced recollections are more intensely emotional, and this quality has earned odorants a reputation as particularly good cues for memory.

Neuroanatomical and Evolutionary Connections between Odor and Emotion

Neuroanatomy supports the proposition that our olfactory system is especially prepared to learn the affective significance of odors. The amygdala, which synapses directly with the olfactory nerve, is critical for emotional associative learning (M. Davis and Whalen, 2001). A recent neuroimaging study showed that when participants recalled a significant personal memory connected to the smell of a specific perfume, the amygdala was markedly more activated than when they recalled the same memory connected to the sight of the perfume bottle, or when they smelled or saw a nonmeaningful perfume (Herz et al., 2003).

The **orbitofrontal cortex**, where olfaction is processed, is also the cortical area responsible for assigning affective value—that is, our hedonic judgments in response to a wide range of stimuli (R. J. Davidson, Putnam, and Larson, 2000). Furthermore, the most ancient part of the brain, the rhinencephalon—literally, the "nose brain"—which comprises the olfactory cortex and limbic areas, developed first from olfactory structures. Only later in evolution did limbic structures such as the amygdala develop. It is interesting to consider that our hedonic and emotional reactions to stimuli in general may have their origin in our sense of smell.

Almost all species of animals use smell or chemical communication for the most basic behaviors necessary for survival: recognizing kin, finding reproductively available mates, locating food, and determining whether an animal or object is dangerous (see the next section). Only in humans have visual and auditory information mostly replaced smell for imparting this kind of crucial knowledge about the world. Yet our olfactory system has retained some of its basic functions. The most immediate responses we have to odors are simple binary opposites: like or dislike, approach or avoid. Emotions convey similar messages: approach what is good, safe, and joyful, and avoid what is bad, dangerous, or liable to cause grief. Thus, emotions and olfaction are functionally analogous. Both enable the organism to react appropriately to its environment, maximizing its chances for basic survival and reproductive success. Viewed in this context, the human emotional system can be seen as a highly evolved, abstract cognitive version of the basic behavioral motivations instigated by the olfactory system in animals (Herz, 2000, 2004).

orbitofrontal cortex The part of the frontal lobe of the cortex that lies above the bone (orbit) containing the eyes. The orbitofrontal cortex is responsible for processing olfaction. It is also the area of the brain critical for assigning affective value to stimuli—in other words, determining hedonic meaning.

main olfactory bulb (MOB) The olfactory bulb; the blueberry-sized extension of the brain just above the nose; the first region of the brain where smells are processed. In humans we simply refer to "olfactory bulb(s)," but in animals with accessory olfactory bulbs, we distinguish between "main" and "accessory."

accessory olfactory bulb (AOB) A smaller neural structure located behind the main olfactory bulb that receives input from the vomeronasal organ.

vomeronasal organ (VNO) A chemical sensing organ at the base of the nasal cavity with a curved tubular shape. The VNO evolved to detect chemicals that cannot be processed by the olfactory epithelium, such as large and/or aqueous molecules—the types of molecules that constitute pheromones.

The Vomeronasal Organ and the Question of Human Pheromones

In animals that rely on smell for survival, the olfactory system consists of two subdivisions: the **main olfactory bulb (MOB)** and the **accessory olfactory bulb (AOB) (Figure 13.18)**. The AOB is an add-on to the back of the MOB. Neurons from these two systems do not interconnect, and the two systems function separately in the integration of specific chemicals. In order for the AOB to be activated, a structure different from the nose needs to be engaged. This structure is called the **vomeronasal organ (VNO)**, sometimes also referred to as "Jacobson's organ" after the Danish anatomist who discovered it.

The VNO is found in some amphibians, most reptiles (but not birds), and many mammals, including New World primates. When snakes open their mouths and appear to be licking the air, they are actually moving chemicals from the air into their vomeronasal organ. In mammals, the VNO is cigar shaped and located at the top back of the nasal cavity. The VNO can respond to some olfactory stimuli, but it responds primarily to chemicals that are higher in molecular weight than can be detected by the olfactory sensory

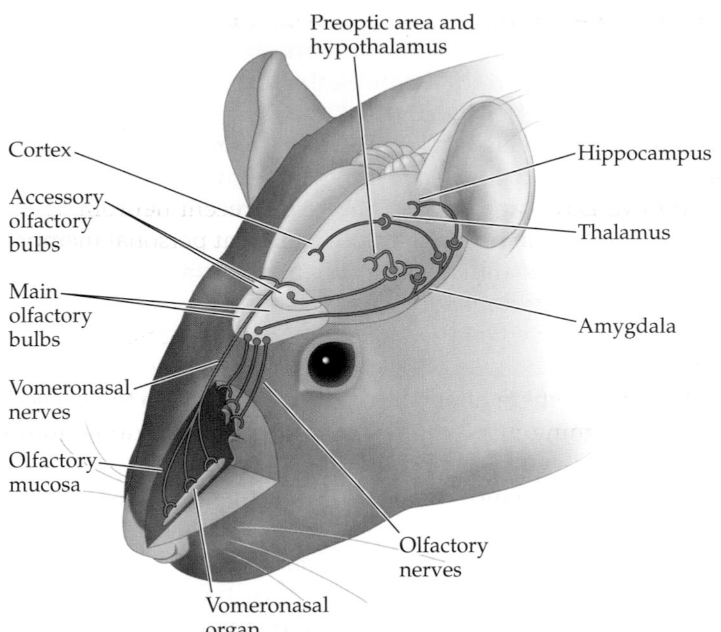

FIGURE 13.18 The olfactory system of a hamster, showing the location of the vomeronasal organ and accessory olfactory bulbs. Note that no functional vomeronasal organ or accessory olfactory bulbs have been found in humans. (Adapted from an illustration by Dr. Michael Meredith.)

neurons, as well as to chemicals that are nonvolatile. It also detects chemicals dissolved in water (as opposed to only in air). Whether humans possess a functioning VNO has been the focus of much recent debate, but it is now generally accepted that although human embryos may have a VNO, this tissue is not neurally connected and disappears shortly after birth. Moreover, we do not have an AOB for VNO neurons to connect to in the brain.

In animals that possess a VNO, its primary function is the detection of **pheromones**. Pheromones are not odors. They are chemicals that may *or may not* have a smell. The word *pheromone* is derived from the Greek *pherein*, meaning "to carry," and *hormon*, meaning "to stimulate." It was first coined in 1959 by Peter Karlson, a German biochemist, and Martin Lüscher, a Swiss entomologist, to describe a chemical substance that carries a message about the physiological or behavioral state of one insect to another, and which in turn leads to a specific reaction in the receiver insect. That is, pheromones are chemical communication. Today, the more generalized definition of a pheromone is *a chemical compound produced by one animal that elicits a specific behavioral or physiological response in another animal of the same species.*

Pheromones are most important for communication in the social insects, like ants, termites, and bees, but they also convey important information for many noninsect species, including primates. There are many examples of this form of chemical communication. Pheromones are used to identify territory. For example, a tiger will rub a tree with glands from its cheeks to claim it, just the same way that a cat rubs your leg with its eyebrow and rump glands to mark you as its territory! Pheromones also initiate alarm or defense reactions. When a honeybee stings us, the chemical released from the stinger (which happens to smell like banana) is a cue to other bees to join in—unfortunately for us! Most important, for many animals pheromones are critically involved in communication about reproductive behavior. They can provide signals to males about when a female is fertile and provide signals to females to initiate sexual behavior. For example, a male rhesus monkey will ignore a female rhesus in heat if his nose is blocked and a female sow will not go into **lordosis** (the position necessary for impregnation) if she isn't exposed to the male pig pheromone androstenone.

pheromone A chemical emitted by one member of a species that triggers a physiological or behavioral response in another member of the same species. Pheromones are signals for chemical communication and do not need to have any smell.

lordosis The position that a sow needs to assume in order to be impregnated. It involves the inward curving of the spinal column and exposure of the genitals.

releaser pheromone A pheromone that triggers an immediate behavioral response among conspecifics.

primer pheromone A pheromone that triggers a physiological (often hormonal) change among conspecifics. This effect usually involves prolonged pheromone exposure.

Pheromones produce two kinds of effects. The two types of pheromones that cause these effects are known as **releaser** and **primer pheromones**. Primer pheromone effects are slow and produce a physiological change in the recipient over time. For example, female rodents that are housed together will come into estrus at the same time after several cycles. Releaser pheromone effects are fast and always produce behavioral responses. The consequence of the banana aroma from a bee sting is one example. Sexual cues and behavioral responses to those cues, such as lordosis, are other examples of releaser pheromone effects. In contrast, primer pheromones may produce no behavioral consequences and may be noticeable only in terms of physiological changes.

There is one good example of a primer pheromone effect in humans. It is known as the "McClintock effect" after Martha McClintock, who identified this phenomenon in college while pursuing her undergraduate degree. The McClintock effect is shown when women who are in physical proximity (e.g., live together) over time start to have menstrual cycles that coincide. That is, women who move into college residence together at the beginning of the school term will likely be having their periods in sync with one another by the time Christmas break rolls around. It appears that one woman in the group becomes the "driving" female and the cycles of the other women in the group change to match hers. So far, we have not discovered what factors determine who the driving female is.

The McClintock effect is believed to be caused by chemicals present in human sweat that are capable of priming the hormonal systems of other individuals. An important feature of any pheromone effect is that all this takes place without any conscious awareness and no smell is detected. However, this human pheromone story is not without controversy. Some researchers have argued that the McClintock effect is a statistical artifact and not a real physiological phenomenon. Furthermore, we do not have a functioning VNO or AOB. Therefore, how is this effect happening, if indeed it truly is? Some have suggested that, presuming the effect is real, hormonal information may be transmitted from one woman to another through another system altogether, such as absorption through the skin (Herz, 2007).

Given that the sexual interactions of most animals seem to be affected by pheromones, it is no surprise that a human "aphrodisiac" pheromone has been the holy grail of the perfume industry. Although direct evidence for a human releaser pheromone has not been observed, several new findings suggest that we may transmit odors that affect our sexuality.

The chemical androstadienone is a steroid derivative of the male sex hormone testosterone (it is chemically related to androstenone, which was mentioned earlier), and its presence in male body fluids (e.g., sweat) is higher than in females. For these reasons, androstadienone has been studied as a potential human sexual pheromone. In several studies androstadienone has been observed to improve women's mood, *but* only when women are in the presence of men (Jacob, Hayreh, and McClintock, 2001; Lundstrom and Olsson, 2005). In the presence of a female experimenter, androstadienone had no impact on female participants' mood. Another study with a male experimenter found that androstadienone also increased self-rated sexual arousal and cortisol levels (Wyert et al., 2007). These results have led to the speculation that androstadienone is a "modulator" pheromone for women in certain social contexts (i.e., the presence of men). Note, however, that the levels of androstadienone that women were exposed to in these studies were a million times higher than the amount a normal male actually emits. Thus, the ecological validity of androstadienone as a human pheromone is questionable.

With respect to potential chemicals emitted by females, a recent study (G. Miller, Tybur, and Jordan, 2007) found that professional exotic lap dancers earned almost twice as much in tips (averaging $335 a night versus $185) when they performed during the ovulatory phase of their menstrual cycles compared to the menstrual phase of their cycles. Moreover, dancers who were taking birth control pills (and were thus hormonally infertile) showed *no* change in tip earnings over time and also earned less overall than did dancers who were not using hormonal contraception (average earnings $193 versus $276). Since the dancers all claimed they performed the same way every day and that their behavior to the patrons was consistent, the explanation offered is that the women were *perceived* as more attractive to the male patrons when they were most fertile through some mechanism other than behavioral or visual cues. This other mechanism is proposed to be chemical. The degree to which conscious smelling by the male patrons was involved, however, was not tested. Another study found that odors emitted by breast-feeding women increased sexual desire among other women by 24% if they had a partner and 17% if they were single (Spencer et al., 2004).

Thus, female body odors that vary with hormonal status appear to influence human sexual arousal. In addition to illustrating a biological basis for olfactory influences on behavior, these findings are consistent with the view that when odors acquire meaning they are able to elicit emotional and behavioral responses consistent with that meaning. The scent of ovulating women may be arousing to men because of their past sexual experiences, and the scent of lactating women may be an aphrodisiac to other women also because of its learned connotations. Whether perceptible odors and/or imperceptible chemical signals influence human sexuality currently remains unknown.

Summary

1. Olfaction is one of the two chemical senses; the other is taste (see Chapter 14). To be perceived as scent, a chemical must possess certain physical properties; however, even some molecules that possess these characteristics cannot be smelled. Olfaction has some unique physiological properties, one of which is that only about 35% of the genes that code for olfactory receptors in humans are functional. Another unusual feature is that most smells also stimulate the somatosensory system via the trigeminal nerve, and it is often impossible to distinguish the contribution of olfactory sensation from trigeminal stimulation.
2. The dominant biochemical theory of odor perception—shape-pattern theory—contends that the fit between a molecule and an olfactory receptor (OR) determines what molecules are detected as scents, and that specific odorant molecules activate arrays of ORs, producing specific patterns of neural activation for each perceived scent. However, this theory is not universally accepted, and alternate explanations exist (e.g., vibration theory).
3. Almost all odors that we encounter in the real world are mixtures, and we appear not to be very good at analyzing the discrete chemical components of scent mixtures. Olfaction is thus primarily a synthetic, as opposed to analytical, sense. However, analytical olfactory ability can be developed with training. True odor imagery is also weak (or nonexistent) for most people, but training may also facilitate this ability.
4. The psychophysical study of smell has shown that different odorant intensity levels and different cognitive functions are required for odor detection, discrimination, and recognition. Identification differs from odor recognition in that, in the former, one must come up with a name for the olfactory sensation. It is very difficult to name even very familiar odors—an experience known as the tip-of-the-nose phenomenon—one of several indications that linguistic processing is highly disconnected from olfactory experience.

Refer to the
Sensation and Perception
website
(www.sinauer.com/wolfe2e)
for activities, essays, study questions, and other study aids.

5. Another important discrepancy between the physical experience and the psychological experience of odors is the difference between receptor adaptation and cognitive habituation. Receptor adaptation occurs after continuous odorant exposure over a number of minutes, can be undone after a few minutes away from the odorant, and is explained by a basic biochemical mechanism. By contrast, cognitive habituation occurs after long-term exposure (e.g., in a living or work environment) to a particular odorant and takes weeks away from the odorant to undo. At present, the mechanisms responsible for the cognitive habituation effect are not fully understood.
6. The most immediate and basic response we have to an odor is whether we like it or not; this is hedonic evaluation. Odor hedonics are measured by pleasantness, familiarity, and intensity ratings. Pleasantness and familiarity are linearly related to odor liking; odor intensity has a more complex relationship to hedonic perception. Substantial evidence suggests that our hedonic responses to odors are learned and not innate, even for so-called stenches. That we have learned to like or dislike various odors rather than being born with hardwired responses is evolutionarily adaptive for generalist species like humans. The caveats to the learned proposition are odors that are highly trigeminally irritating (pain-inducing) and the potential genetic variability in the number and types of receptors expressed across individuals, which may influence olfactory sensitivity (intensity) and hence odor hedonic perception.
7. The key to olfactory associative learning is the emotional value of the context in which the odor is first encountered. If the emotional context is good, the odor will be liked; if it is bad, the odor will be disliked. Emotional associations with odors can also elicit full-blown episodic memories. Emotional potency distinguishes odor-evoked memories from memories triggered by other sensory cues. The neuroanatomy of the olfactory and limbic systems and their neuroevolutionary development illustrate how emotional processing and olfactory processing are uniquely and intimately interrelated.
8. Pheromones are chemicals emitted by individuals that affect the physiology and/or behavior or other members of the same species and may or may not have any smell. In all mammals that have been shown to use pheromones for communication, detection is mediated through the vomeronasal organ and processed by the accessory olfactory bulb. Humans do not possess a functional VNO or AOB, but some evidence suggests that human chemical signals can affect menstrual synchrony. Exposure to very high doses of androstadienone, a chemical in sweat, has also been suggested to act as a modulator pheromone for women in the presence of men. The mechanism by which these chemicals are perceived has not yet been determined. Perceptible female body odors that vary with hormonal status such as ovulation and lactation may also influence sexual arousal. The existence of true human pheromones, however, remains controversial.

CHAPTER 14

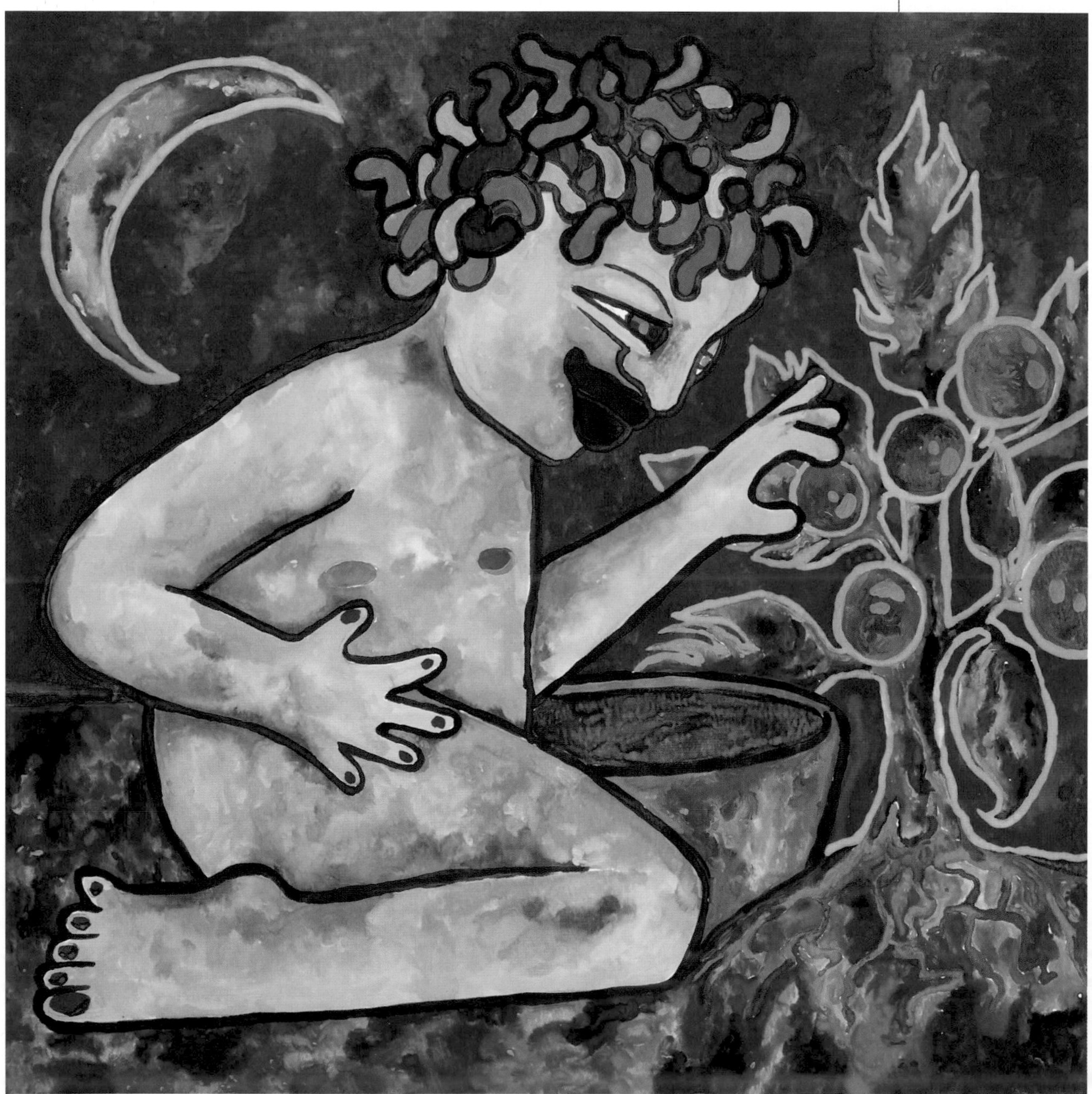

Photo credit: Stephen Petegorsky

Joanne Delphia, *Midnight Harvest*, 2004

Taste

Calvin Trillin, a writer who makes wonderful observations about the joys of eating, described his 4-year-old daughter's reaction to "polishing off a particularly satisfying dish of chocolate ice cream." She said, "My tongue is smiling."

What makes tongues smile? As with our noses, the basic answer to this question is molecules. Olfaction and gustation are often grouped together as the chemical senses, and in terms of physiology, these two sensory systems are in some ways quite similar. But the chemicals we taste have already entered our mouths and are about to move even farther into our bodies. Thus, taste serves the most specific function of any of the senses: discerning which chemicals we need to ingest because they are nutritious and which we need to spit out because they may be poisonous. Perhaps this is why something about our liking or disliking of tastes and flavors seems to be very different from the liking or disliking that one might associate with the color red or the sound of middle C on the piano. Nature has equipped us to care passionately about food because that passion holds the key to our survival.

Taste versus Flavor

Before delving any further into the gustatory system, we need to clear up a very old misunderstanding. According to the early Greeks, sensations perceived from foods and beverages in the mouth were tastes, and sensations perceived by sniffing were smells. In fact, however, food molecules are almost always perceived by both our gustatory and our olfactory systems. The molecules we taste are dissolved in our saliva and passed over the taste receptors on our taste buds, as we'll discuss in this chapter. But when we chew and swallow foods, other molecules are released into the air inside our mouths and forced up behind the palate into the nasal cavity, where they contact the olfactory epithelium and stimulate our olfactory receptors (**Figure 14.1**). The brain then knits these **retronasal olfactory sensations** together with our gustatory sensations into a kind of metasensation that goes by the name **flavor**.

It is quite easy to prevent the airflow that carries odorants through the retronasal passage. Children do it all the time when they hold their noses while eating spinach. Try the following experiment now—but use a piece of chocolate if you're still not crazy about spinach. Pinch your nose before putting the chocolate in your mouth, then chew it and note the sensation, which will be almost pure taste (sweet with a bit of bitter). Then, just before swallowing, release your nose. The volatile molecules responsible for the chocolate sensation will immediately be drawn up behind your palate and into the nasal cavity, and you will understand the difference between taste and flavor. You've probably noticed before that flavor is similarly impoverished

retronasal olfactory sensation The sensation of an odor that is perceived when chewing and swallowing force an odorant in the mouth up behind the palate into the nose. Such odor sensations are perceived as originating from the mouth, even though the actual contact of odorant and receptor occurs at the olfactory mucosa.

flavor The combination of true taste (sweet, salty, sour, bitter) and retronasal olfaction.

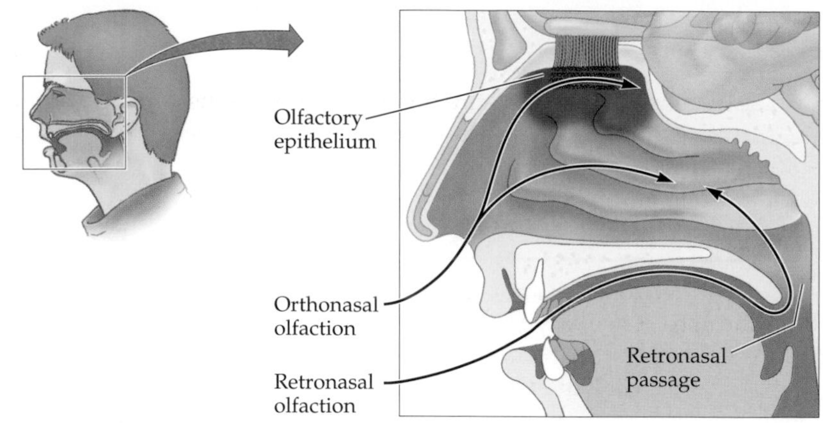

FIGURE 14.1 Molecules released into the air inside our mouths as we chew and swallow food travel up through the retronasal passage into the nose, where they then move upward and contact the olfactory epithelium.

when you have a stuffy nose. Web Activity 14.1: Taste without Smell asks you to test this phenomenon with other stimuli.

Foods are also perceived by the somatosensory system via touch, temperature, and pain receptors in the tongue and mouth. Some of these sensations have protective functions: the burn of acid (which might damage your stomach if swallowed), the heat pain from scalding coffee, the pain of biting the tongue, and so on. Somatosensations also provide information about the nature of foods and beverages. For example, we get information about the fat content of foods from tactile sensations such as oily, viscous, thick, and creamy.

Localizing Flavor Sensations

You should have realized something else when you performed the chocolate experiment described in the previous section: even though you now know that the chocolate sensation originates from the olfactory receptors in your nose, you probably still perceived the flavor as coming entirely from your mouth. This perception is due in part to the tactile sensations evoked by chewing and swallowing, and in part to taste. Because you taste and feel the food only in your mouth (not in your nose), your brain concludes that the sensations must have arisen entirely from the mouth. Exceptions include foods such as horseradish, wasabi, and spicy mustard, which give off volatile chemicals that activate pain receptors all the way up through the retronasal passage. But these exceptions prove the rule: when we eat these foods, we experience the sensations as coming from our noses as well as our mouths.

Now consider the following curious case. A patient with normal olfaction but damaged taste and oral touch reported that she could smell lasagna, but when she ate it, it had no flavor. A similar effect was produced in a laboratory using a small amount of lidocaine and a large amount of blueberry yogurt. Subjects in this study had their left **chorda tympani** (one of the **cranial nerves** that carries information from taste receptors to the brain) anesthetized with the lidocaine while they tasted the yogurt. In this situation, the subjects reported that the blueberry sensation—which is entirely due to retronasal olfaction—seemed to come only from the right side of the mouth. Moreover, the intensity of the blueberry sensation was reduced, and this intensity was reduced even further when both taste nerves were blocked (D. J. Snyder et al., 2001).

In both the patient and the experimental subjects, the pathway from the mouth to the nasal cavity was completely intact. Why, then, were their retronasal lasagna and blueberry sensations reduced? Recent brain-imaging research by Dana Small appears to answer this question: the brain processes odors differently, depending on whether they come from the mouth or

chorda tympani The branch of cranial nerve VII (the facial nerve) that carries taste information from the anterior, mobile tongue (the part that can be stuck out). The chorda tympani nerve leaves the tongue with the lingual branch of the trigeminal nerve (cranial nerve V) and then passes through the middle ear on its way to the brain.

cranial nerves Twelve pairs of nerves (one from each pair for each side of the body) that originate in the brain stem and reach sense organs and muscles through openings in the skull.

through the nostrils. This distinction makes good sense functionally because the significance of odors in the mouth is very different from that of odors sniffed from the outside world. Without the proper cues to tell us where an odorant is coming from, input from the olfactory receptors apparently cannot be routed to the proper brain area to connect the smell sensation with the food stimulus.

The connections between taste and smell have been understood by the food industry for many years (Noble, 1996). For example, if a company is marketing pear juice and wants to intensify the sensation of pear, it will add sugar. The increase in sweetness (a pure taste sensation) will increase the perceived olfactory sensation of pear. However, this will work only for pairs of taste and retronasal olfaction that are commonly experienced. If our pear juice company were to add salt, the pear sensation would not increase. Thus, learning plays a role in this phenomenon.

The pervasiveness of food additives such as carrageenan, guar gum, and other thickening agents shows that the food industry also has a good handle on the effects of somatosensation on food perception. And the ingredient lists of most processed foods include at least one artificial coloring, testifying to the importance of yet another sense, vision, in how we perceive foods.

taste buds Globular clusters of cells that have the function of creating the neural signals conveyed to the brain by taste nerves. Some of the cells in the taste bud have specialized sites on their apical projections that interact with taste stimuli. Some of the cells form synapses with taste nerve fibers.

papillae Structures that give the tongue its bumpy appearance. From smallest to largest, the papillae types that contain taste buds are fungiform, foliate, and circumvallate; filiform papillae, which do not contain taste buds, are the smallest and most numerous.

Anatomy and Physiology of the Gustatory System

Taste perception consists of the following sequence of events (the structures involved are illustrated in **Figure 14.2**): Chewing breaks down food substances into molecules, which are dissolved in saliva. The saliva-borne food molecules flow into a taste pore that leads to the **taste buds** embedded in structures called **papillae** (singular *papilla*) that cover the tongue (if the olfactory epithelium is the retina of the nose, the tongue is the retina of the

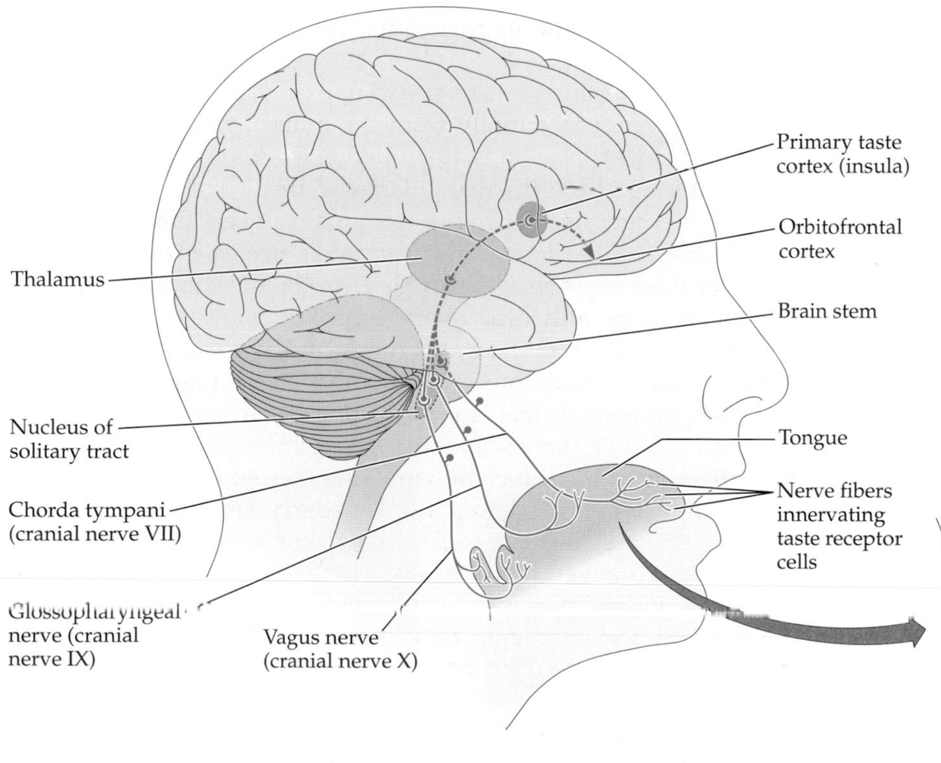

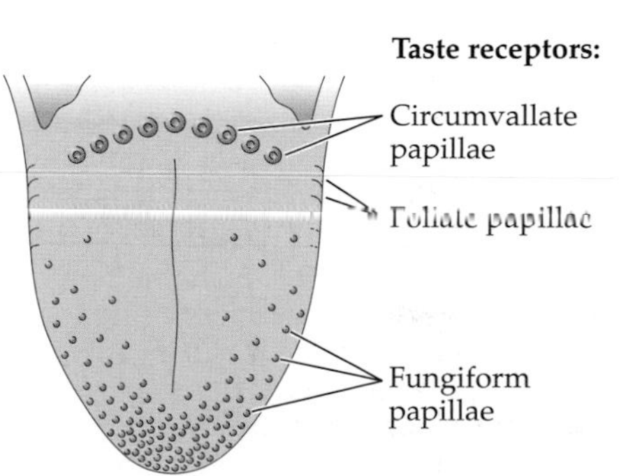

FIGURE 14.2 The locations of each type of taste papilla are identified in the diagram of the tongue shown here. Neural signals from the taste buds in those papillae are transmitted via cranial nerves VII, IX, and X to the brain.

mouth). Each taste bud, in turn, contains a number of **taste receptor cells.** Each taste receptor cell responds to a limited number of molecule types; when one of its preferred molecules makes contact with it, it produces action potentials that send information along one of the cranial nerves to the brain. See **Web Activity 14.2: Gustatory Anatomy** for an interactive overview of the system, which is described in greater detail in the sections that follow.

taste receptor cells Cells within the taste bud that contain sites on their apical projections that can interact with taste stimuli. These sites fall into two major categories: those interacting with charged particles (e.g., sodium and hydrogen ions), and those interacting with specific chemical structures.

filiform papillae Small structures on the tongue that provide most of the bumpy appearance. Filiform papillae have no taste function.

fungiform papillae Mushroom-shaped structures (maximum diameter 1 millimeter) that are distributed most densely on the edges of the tongue, especially the tip. Taste buds (an average of six per papilla) are buried in the surface.

foliate papillae Folds of tissue containing taste buds. Foliate papillae are located on the rear of the tongue lateral to the circumvallate papillae, where the tongue attaches to the mouth.

circumvallate papillae Circular structures that form an inverted *V* on the rear of the tongue (three to five on each side). Circumvallate papillae are moundlike structures surrounded by a trench (like a moat). These papillae are much larger than fungiform papillae.

Papillae

Papillae give the tongue its bumpy appearance and come in four major varieties, three of which contain taste buds.

Filiform papillae, the ones *without* any taste function, are located on the anterior portion of the tongue (the part we stick out when giving someone a raspberry) and come in different shapes in different species. In cats, they are shaped like tiny spoons with sharp edges. The filiform papillae on our tongues do not have these sharp edges, which is why you will find lapping milk from a bowl considerably more difficult than your cat does.

Fungiform papillae, so named because they resemble tiny button mushrooms, are also located on the anterior part of the tongue. They are visible to the naked eye, but blue food coloring swabbed onto the tongue makes them particularly easy to see (the blue food coloring stains the filiform papillae much better than the fungiform papillae, so the fungiform papillae appear as light circles against a darker blue background). Fungiform papillae vary in diameter, but the maximum is about 1 millimeter. On average, about six taste buds are buried in the surface of each fungiform papilla. If we stain the tongues of many individuals, we see a large amount of variation (**Figure 14.3**). Some tongues have so few fungiform papillae that their stained tongues appear to have polka dots on them. Other tongues have so many that the polka dots are wall-to-wall.

Foliate papillae are located on the sides of the tongue at the point where the tongue is attached. Under magnification, they look like a series of folds. Taste buds are buried in the folds.

Finally, **circumvallate papillae** are relatively large circular structures forming an inverted *V* on the rear of the tongue. These papillae look like tiny islands surrounded by moats. The taste buds are buried in the sides of the moats.

Although most people don't realize this, there are also taste buds on the roof of the mouth where the hard and soft palates meet. To demonstrate these, wet your finger and dip it into salt crystals. Touch the roof of your mouth and move your finger back until you feel the bone end (the margin between the hard and soft palates). You will experience a flash of saltiness as you move the salt crystals onto the taste buds arrayed on that margin.

(*a*) Nontaster

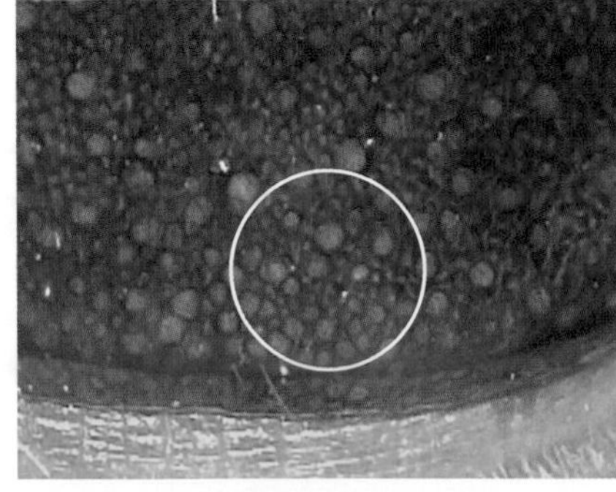

(*b*) Supertaster

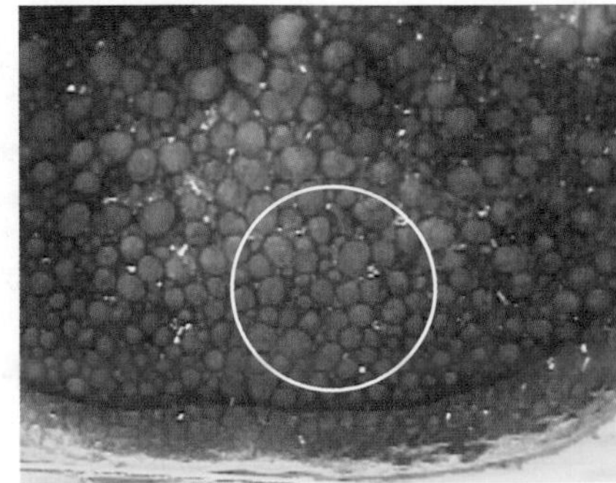

FIGURE 14.3 Examples showing typical variability in density of fungiform papillae from one individual to the next. The circles (6 mm diameter) show a template used to provide counts of the number of fungiform papillae, which can then be compared across individuals (the circle is about the size of a hole made by a paper punch). In extreme cases, normal individuals may have as few as 5 fungiform papillae in that area or as many as 60.

In sum, the taste buds are distributed in a line across the roof of the mouth and in papillae distributed in an oval on the tongue. Fungiform papillae make up the front of the oval, and foliate and circumvallate papillae make up its rear. Note that we have no subjective awareness of this distribution of taste buds. (For more on this topic, see **Web Essay 14.1: Scientific Urban Legend—The Bogus Tongue Map.**)

microvilli Slender projections on the tips of some taste bud cells that extend into the taste pore.

Taste Buds and Taste Receptor Cells

Each taste bud is a cluster of elongated cells, organized much like the segments of an orange (**Figure 14.4**). The tips of some of the cells—the taste receptor cells—end in slender **microvilli** (singular *microvillus*) containing the sites that bind to taste substances. In an earlier era, these microvilli were mistakenly thought to be tiny hairs; we now know that microvilli are extensions of the cell membrane.

Taste nerve fibers were once believed to be connected to receptors on one end and the brain at the other end. A considerably more complex series of events is now beginning to emerge. At least some receptors are on cells that do not synapse with taste nerve fibers; the information they convey must get to the nerve fibers in some other way (Herness et al., 2005; Roper, 2006).

In fungiform papillae, the taste nerve fibers that enter the taste buds branch so that an individual cell can be innervated by more than one taste fiber and an individual taste fiber can innervate more than one cell. Taste receptors have a limited life span. After about 10 days they die and are replaced by new cells. This constant renewal enables the taste system to recover from a variety of sources of damage, and it explains why our taste systems remain robust even into old age. Recordings from taste nerve fibers show that different receptor cells contacted by branches of a single fiber show similar specificities to taste stimuli. In other words, it appears that the nerve fibers are somehow able to select the cells with which they will synapse so that the message they convey remains stable, even though the receptor cells are continually replaced.

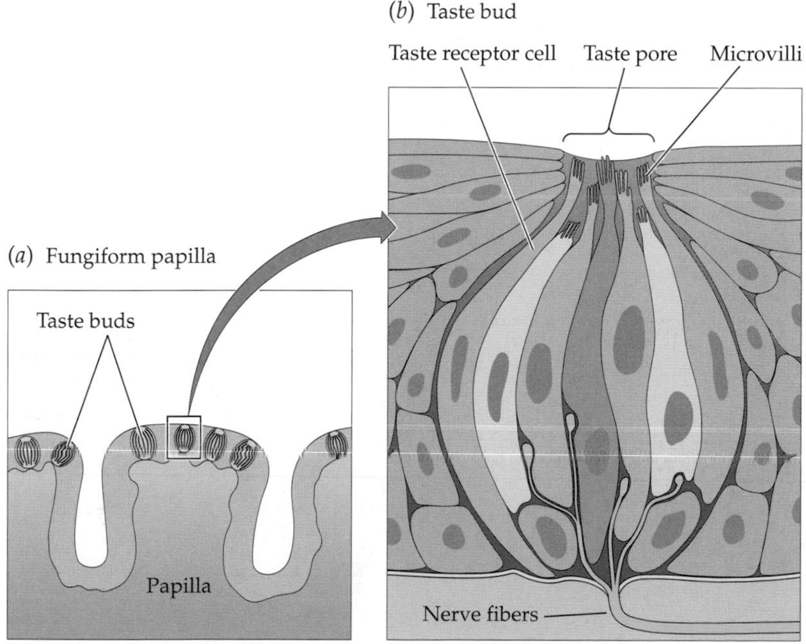

FIGURE 14.4 Taste buds. (*a*) The location of the taste buds buried in the tissue on the tops of the fungiform papillae. (*b*) Cross section of a taste bud.

tastant Any stimulus that can be tasted.

The mechanisms that permit a taste cell to recognize a taste stimulus, known as a **tastant**, contacting its microvilli can be divided into two large categories (**Figure 14.5**). One class of tastants is made up of small, charged molecules that taste salty or sour. Small openings, called "ion channels," in microvilli membranes allow some types of charged particles to enter cells but bar others. When the charged particles in salty and sour foods enter salty and sour receptor cells, these cells signal their respective tastes.

Tastants in the second class, which produce sensations that we label as sweet or bitter, are perceived via a mechanism similar to that in the olfactory system, using G protein–coupled receptors (GPCRs). The GPCRs wind back and forth across microvillus membranes, and when a particular tastant molecule "key" is fitted into the "lock" portion of a GPCR on the outside of the membrane, the portion of the GPCR inside the cell starts a cascade of molecular events that eventually causes an action potential to be sent to the brain.

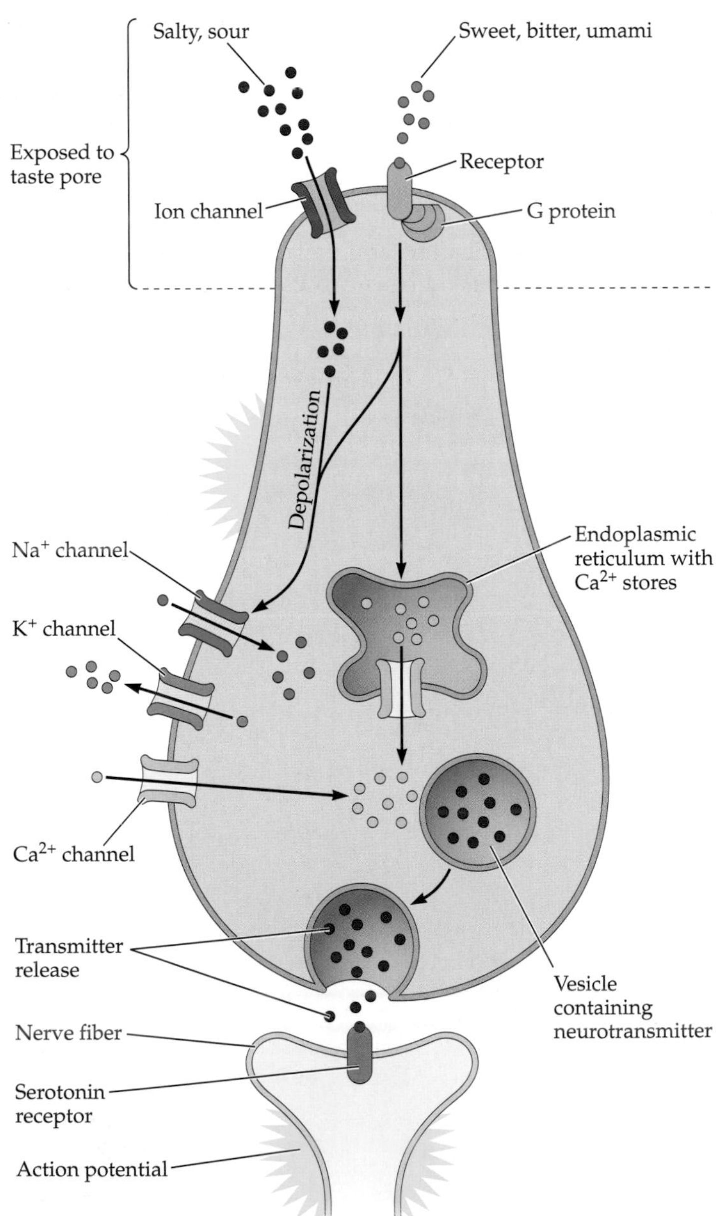

FIGURE 14.5 Diagram of a taste receptor cell illustrating the different receptor mechanisms for ionic stimuli (salty and sour), as well as those using a lock-and-key mechanism (sweet, bitter, umami).

Taste Processing in the Central Nervous System

After leaving the taste buds through the cranial nerves, gustatory information travels through way stations in the medulla and thalamus before reaching the cortex (**Figure 14.6**) (Pritchard and Norgren, 2004). The primary cortical processing area for taste—the part of the cortex that first receives taste information—is the **insular cortex**. The **orbitofrontal cortex** receives projections from the insular cortex. Some orbitofrontal neurons are multimodal. That is, they respond to temperature, touch, and smell, as well as to taste, suggesting that the orbitofrontal cortex may be an integration area.

insular cortex The primary cortical processing area for taste—the part of the cortex that first receives taste information.

orbitofrontal cortex The part of the frontal lobe of the cortex that lies above the bone (orbit) containing the eyes.

Inhibition plays an important role in the processing of taste information in the brain. One of the functions of this inhibition may be to protect our whole-mouth perception of taste in the face of injuries to the taste system. Our brains receive taste input from several nerves (see Figure 14.6). Damage to one of them diminishes its contribution to the whole; however, that damage also releases the inhibition that is normally produced by the damaged nerve. The result is that whole-mouth taste intensities are relatively unchanged. Unfortunately, this preserved whole-mouth perception comes with a cost in some cases. Localized taste damage is often accompanied by "phantom taste" sensations (recall the phantom limbs experienced by many limb amputees, described in Chapter 12), as if the release of inhibition permits even noise in the nervous system to be perceived as a taste.

Descending inhibition from the taste cortex to a variety of other structures (DiLorenzo and Monroe, 1995) may also serve other functions. For example, mouth injuries that lead to oral pain make it harder to eat. The inhibition of such pain perceptions by taste-processing parts of the brain would make eat-

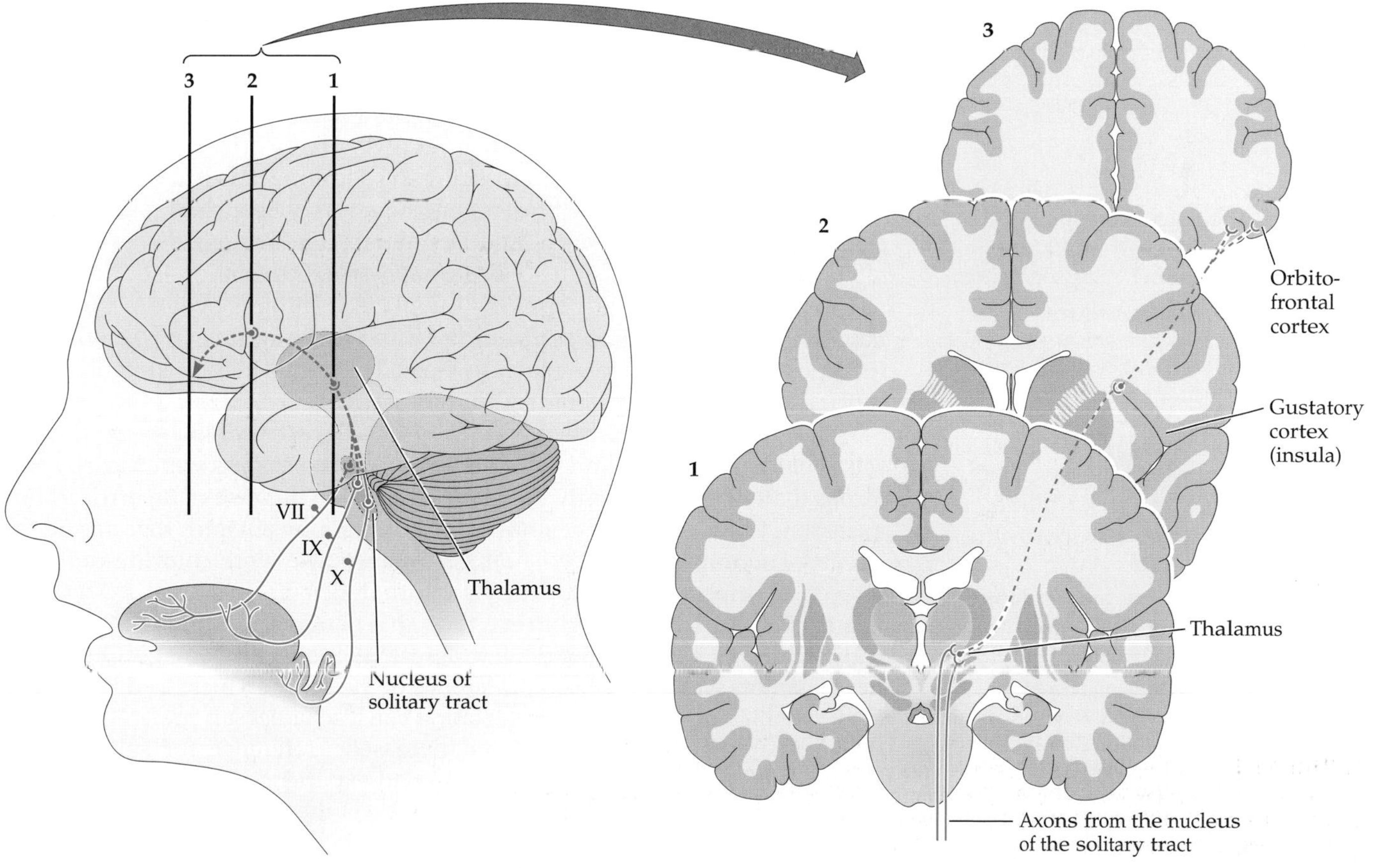

FIGURE 14.6 Taste information projects from the tongue to the medulla, then to the thalamus (shown in cross section 1 of the brain), then to the insula (cross section 2), and finally to the orbitofrontal cortex (cross section 3).

ing easier and thus increase the likelihood of survival (because no matter how much the mouth hurts, we still have to eat). Consistent with this principle, patients with a serious oral pain disorder (burning mouth syndrome) were shown to have localized taste damage as well (Grushka and Bartoshuk, 2000). Furthermore, women who have taste damage are more likely to suffer from severe nausea and vomiting during pregnancy (Sipiora et al., 2000), and cancer patients, whose chemotherapy and radiation therapy is known to damage the taste system, are more likely to experience coughing, gagging, and hiccups. In all these cases, inhibitory signals from the taste cortex that normally help prevent eating-disruptive symptoms (oral pain, vomiting, hiccuping, and so on) may have been turned off because of the damage to the taste system.

The Four Basic Tastes

We learned in the previous chapter that we are able to distinguish many different odorants. Already in this chapter, however, we have seen that when olfaction is taken out of the equation, much of the complexity of the sensations evoked by foods vanishes. Thus, we are led to believe that the number of basic taste qualities is quite small. In fact, the current universally accepted list includes only the four **basic tastes** previously mentioned in the section on taste buds and taste receptor cells: **salty**, **sour**, **bitter**, and **sweet**. As we discuss these in the sections that follow, note that one of the most important features of these basic tastes is that our liking (or disliking) for them is "hardwired" in the brain; that is, we are essentially born liking or disliking these tastes. This is very different from the way we learn to like or dislike odors.

Salty

Salts are made up of two charged particles: a cation (positively charged) and an anion (negatively charged). For example, common table salt is NaCl; the sodium is the cation (Na^+) and the chloride is the anion (Cl^-). Although all salts taste at least a little salty to humans, pure NaCl is the saltiest-tasting salt around. Sodium must be available in relatively large quantities to maintain nerve and muscle function, and loss of body sodium leads to a swift death.

Our ability to perceive saltiness is not static. Gary Beauchamp and his colleagues (Bertino, Beauchamp, and Engelman, 1982) showed that diet can affect the perception of saltiness. Fortunately for those on low-sodium diets, reduced sodium intake increases the intensity of saltiness over time. Individuals who are initially successful in reducing their sodium intake will find that foods they used to love may now taste too salty. This adjustment in perception helps them keep their sodium intake down.

Our liking for saltiness is not static either. Early experiences can modify salt preference. In 1978 and 1979, several hundred infants were fed soy formulas that were accidentally deficient in chloride because of an error in formulation. Chloride deficiency has effects on our physiologies that mimic the effects of sodium deficiency. Thus, the infants who were chloride-deficient offered an important way to study sodium deficiency in humans. The Centers for Disease Control and Prevention in Atlanta monitored these infants, and a variety of studies were done to assess any potential damage. One of the consequences was that the salt preference of the children increased (L. J. Stein et al., 1996). Experiences during gestation can also affect salt preference. Crystal and Bernstein (1995) found an increased preference for salty snacks among college students whose mothers had experienced moderate to severe morning sickness during pregnancy. The exact mechanisms by which these abnormal metabolic events enhance salt preference are still not understood.

basic tastes The four taste qualities that are generally agreed to describe human taste experience: sweet, salty, sour, bitter.

salty The taste quality produced by the cations of salts (e.g., the sodium in sodium chloride produces the salty taste). Some cations also produce other taste qualities (e.g., potassium tastes bitter as well as salty). The purest salty taste is produced by sodium chloride (NaCl), common table salt.

sour The taste quality produced by the hydrogen ion in acids.

bitter The taste quality, generally considered unpleasant, produced by substances like quinine or caffeine.

sweet The taste quality produced by some sugars, such as glucose, fructose, and sucrose. These three sugars are particularly biologically useful to us, and our sweet receptors are tuned to them. Some other compounds (e.g., saccharin, aspartame), are also sweet.

Sour

As you may remember from high school chemistry, a solution containing hydrogen ions (H^+) and hydroxide ions (OH^-) in equal proportions produces water (HOH, or H_2O). As the relative proportion of H^+ increases (decreasing the pH level), the solution becomes more *acidic*. Why do you need to be reminded of all this? Because sour is the taste of acids. Some individuals like the sourness of acids in relatively low concentrations. Many adults enjoy pickles and sauerkraut, both of which get their sour tastes from lactic acid, and the success of sour candies shows that many children like sour tastes that adults reject (Liem and Mennella, 2003). At high concentrations, however, acids will damage both external and internal body tissues.

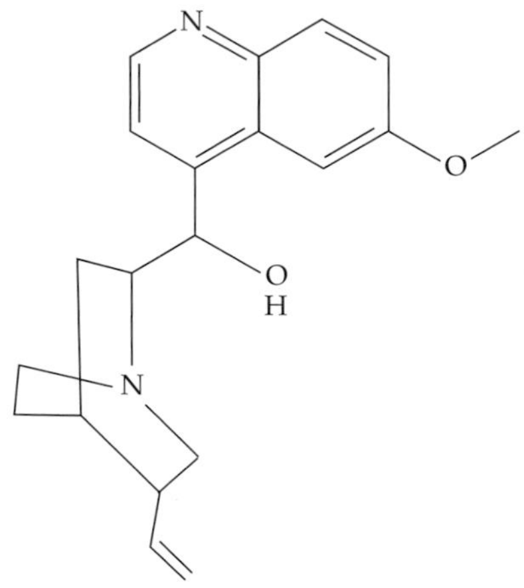

FIGURE 14.7 The molecular structure of quinine ($C_{20}H_{24}N_2O_2$), a prototypically bitter substance.

Bitter

The Human Genome Project revealed a multigene family responsible for about 25 different bitter receptors. The HUGO Gene Nomenclature Committee has established the rules for naming genes. (HUGO stands for Human Genome Organisation, an international organization of scientists involved in human genetic and genomic research.) The bitter gene family is *Tas2r* (*Tas#r* stands for taste, with the "2" indicating bitter—we will see below that a "1" indicates sweet); numbers following the *r* indicate the particular gene that is a member of that family. The bitter genes are located on three different chromosomes: 5, 7, and 12. Some of the bitter stimuli that excite each of the receptors expressed by these genes are now known. For example, a group of phytonutrients (compounds derived from edible plants) have been shown to stimulate taste receptors expressed by *Tas2r16*. One of these compounds, salicin, is an extract from willow bark that we know well as a compound related to aspirin (Bufe et al., 2002). But for most of the bitter stimuli we experience routinely, the receptors are still unknown.

Quinine (**Figure 14.7**), which is used to treat malaria, is one example of a bitter compound. Tonic water (which contains quinine), was originally formulated as a treatment for malaria (now, however, we know that unfortunately it does not contain enough quinine for that purpose). Tonic water does, however, contain enough quinine to taste very bitter, and for this reason lots of sugar was added to make the tonic water palatable. This approach works because sweet and bitter tastes inhibit one another; tonic water tastes much less bitter than the quinine content alone would and also tastes much less sweet than the sugar added alone would. Tonic water actually contains about the same amount of sugar as do other carbonated beverages.

Each bitter receptor does not project via a specific bitter neuron. What this means is that, although a great many different compounds taste bitter, we generally do not distinguish between the tastes of these compounds (Mueller et al., 2005); we simply avoid them all. The diversity of receptors for bitterness enables species or even individuals in a given species to have varying responses to an array of bitter compounds. One of the most famous of these is "taste blindness" to PTC (phenylthiocarbamide) found in humans—a phenomenon we will revisit later in this chapter.

Not coincidentally, compounds that taste bitter to us tend to be poisonous. However, some bitter stimuli are actually good for us. For example, bitter compounds in some vegetables help protect against cancer. We would like to be able to "turn off" these bitter sensations to make it easier for people to eat their vegetables. Along these lines, Robert Margolskee, a pioneer in studies of bitter transduction, used his understanding of the bitter system to identify a substance that can inhibit some bitter sensations: adenosine monophosphate

(AMP) (Ming, Ninomiya, and Margolskee, 1999). AMP may actually function as a natural bitter inhibitor in mother's milk. A number of compounds in milk, such as casein (milk protein) and calcium salts, taste bitter; and, as we will see later, aversions to bitter tastes are present at birth. The presence of AMP in mother's milk may suppress those bitter tastes enough to allow milk to be palatable to babies who are particularly responsive to them.

Bitter perception is also affected by hormone levels in women. Sensitivity to bitterness intensifies during pregnancy and diminishes after menopause (Duffy et al., 1998). These differences make sense in the context of the function of bitterness as a poison detection mechanism. Intensifying the perception of bitter early in pregnancy, when toxins exert their maximum effects, has clear biological value. Consistent with this correlation, some of the aversions during pregnancy occur with foods or beverages that have bitter tastes (e.g., coffee).

Sweet

Sweetness is evoked by sugars, simple carbohydrates that generally conform to the chemical formula $(CH_2O)_n$, where n is between 3 and 7. Glucose, one of the sweetest-tasting sugars, is the principal source of energy in humans (as well as nearly every other living thing on Earth). Common table sugar, sucrose (**Figure 14.8**)—which is a combination of glucose and yet another sugar, fructose—tastes even sweeter.

The biological function of sweet is different from that of bitter, and the way taste receptors are tuned supports that biological difference. Many different molecules taste bitter. Our biological task is not to distinguish among them but rather to avoid them all. Thus, we have multiple bitter receptors to encompass the chemical diversity of poisons, but they all feed into a common line leading to rejection. With regard to sweet, some biologically useless sugars have structures very similar to those of glucose, fructose, and sucrose. In this case, then, the task of the taste system is to tune receptors so specifically that the biologically important sugars stimulate sweet taste but the others do not.

Consistent with the biological purpose of sweet, the family of genes expressing sweet receptors is very small: *Tas1r2* and *Tas1r3*. (We will discuss a third member of this family, *Tas1r1*, later). These genes express three different G protein–coupled receptors: T1R1, T1R2, and T1R3.

Simple molecules (monomers) can form chains of varying length (polymers). When the chain has only two units, it is called a dimer; when the two units are different, it is called a heterodimer. Receptors T1R2 and T1R3 combine to form the heterodimer that is now thought to be the primary sweet receptor (**Figure 14.9**). The complex extracellular portion of this combination (which resembles the form of a Venus flytrap) provides a variety of positions at which sweeteners with very different chemical structures can bind. For example, sweet proteins are very large compared to smaller sweeteners like sucrose, and these sweet proteins can act like wedges that insert into the trap of the Venus flytrap domain and trigger the receptor. Smaller sweeteners (sugars, saccharin, aspartame, and so on) can interact with this same site or with other sites on the receptor.

The discovery that a single receptor is responsible for all sweet perception was very exciting to taste investigators, but it introduced a new sweetness puzzle. Different sweeteners stimulate different parts of the receptor, but whatever the source of stimulation is, the receptor produces the same signal. Therefore, all sweeteners—sugars and artificial sweeteners alike—would produce the same sweetness. However, artificial sweeteners like saccharin and aspartame do not taste exactly like sugar; if they did, there would be no need

FIGURE 14.8 The molecular structure of sucrose, common table sugar. This disaccharide is formed from a combination of a glucose molecule and a fructose molecule. Glucose, which is easily extracted from sucrose by the digestive system, is the main fuel that powers almost every biological engine (including the human brain currently reading this book).

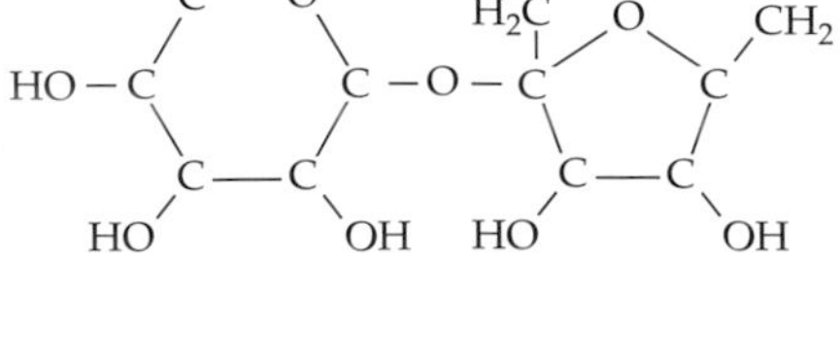

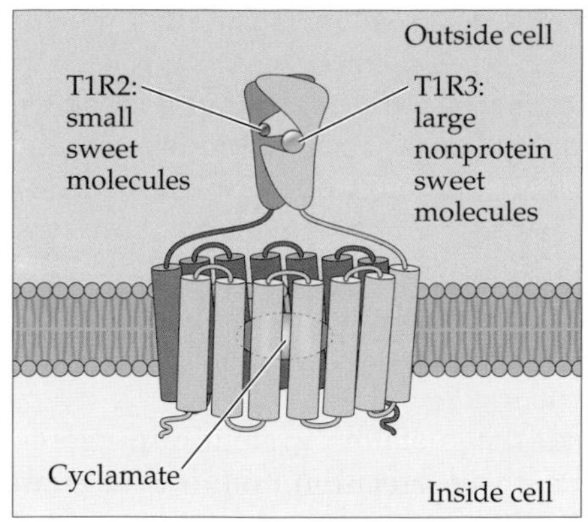

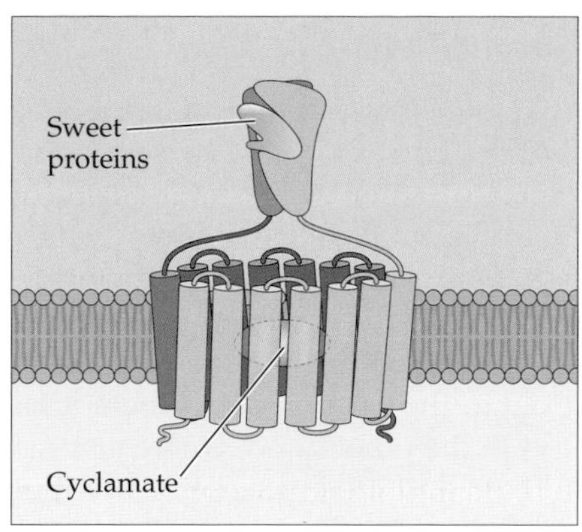

FIGURE 14.9 Structure of the T1R2–T1R3 heterodimer sweet receptor, showing binding sites for both large and small sweet molecules. (After Temussi, 2007.)

to continually search for better artificial sweeteners. Some claim that artificial sweeteners produce additional tastes that account for the difference. For example, saccharin tastes bitter as well as sweet to many. But some of us (the author included) do not taste the bitterness of saccharin at all; we are quite convinced that it is the nature of the sweetness that differs. Genetic studies may offer some help here. The receptor T1R3 appears to be able to function alone to respond only to high concentrations of sucrose (Zhao et al., 2003). This unique functionality could create the difference that many of us perceive between the sweetness of sucrose and that of artificial sweeteners.

Since our taste system can produce sweet receptors so precisely tuned to the biologically useful sugars, what is going on with artificial sweeteners? As far as we know, these sweeteners are biologically useful for only those interested in losing weight, but there is some doubt about whether even this is true.

Saccharin was discovered in 1879 when a research fellow working on coal tar derivatives failed to wash up before dinner and subsequently noticed that the tar residue on his hands tasted sweet. Another artificial sweetener was discovered in 1937, by a graduate student working in what must have been a messy lab. When he tasted sweet while smoking a cigarette, he realized that some compound in the lab must be responsible. In this way, cyclamate was discovered. Cyclamate was very popular for a few years, but suspicions were raised that it was carcinogenic. Although that suspicion was challenged and cyclamate remains legal in a number of other countries, the FDA (Food and Drug Administration) banned it in the United States. Artificial sweeteners are attractive to dieters because their sweet taste comes with essentially no calories. Countless dieters count on this property to help them watch their weight, but a 1986 epidemiological study showed that women who consumed artificial sweeteners actually gained weight (Stellman and Garfinkel, 1986).

That same year, John Blundell, an English expert on weight regulation, published a provocative article suggesting that aspartame (the artificial sweetener sold as NutraSweet) increases appetite (Blundell and Hill, 1986). Was the benefit of the reduced calories lost when individuals using aspartame actually increased their caloric intake in subsequent meals? T. L. Davidson and S. E. Swithers (2004) elaborated on this kind of thinking. They point to the fact that the "obesity epidemic" reflected in increasing weight in the American public occurred over the same years as the introduction of low-calorie foods into the American market. They argue that the uncoupling of the sensory properties of these diet foods from their metabolic consequences disrupts regulation, leading to weight gain.

Survival Value of Taste

Like olfactory receptors, taste receptors detect specific features of molecules. But the two associated senses evolved to serve quite different functions. The sense of smell helps us identify objects in our environment. Indeed, for many animals (e.g., rodents), olfaction is the primary means for knowing what surrounds them in the world. Consistent with this purpose, the olfactory system is capable of distinguishing a large number of different molecules, and an individual animal can learn about whatever olfactory stimuli exist in the environment where it happens to live.

On the other hand, we've just seen that the gustatory system responds to a fixed and much smaller set of molecules. This precise tuning is consistent with the role of taste as a system for detecting nutrients and "antinutrients" (substances that are either helpful or harmful, respectively, to our bodies) before we ingest them.

Each of the four basic tastes is responsible for a different nutrient or antinutrient, and has evolved according to its purpose. For example, the bitter taste subsystem is nature's poison detector. In terms of chemical structure, poisons are quite diverse. This diversity makes sense because any built-in poison detector must be able to recognize many different compounds. On the other hand, given that we don't really care if we can discriminate among poisons, since we just want to avoid them all, we could hook all of those receptors up to a few common lines to the brain. As we saw earlier, this is exactly how the bitter subsystem is set up.

Similarly, the sour subsystem is configured to reject any acidic solution without distinguishing exactly what is causing the acidity of the solution to be so high. The other two taste subsystems enable us to detect, and therefore selectively ingest, foods that our bodies need: sodium (salty) and sugars (sweet).

The Pleasures of Taste

Pfaffmann wrote a famous paper in 1960 entitled "The Pleasures of Sensation," in which he underlined unique features of the sense of taste with regard to affective experience. Taste provides not only sensory information about certain nutrients, but also pleasure (sweet, salty, and, for children, sour) and displeasure (bitter). The pleasure or displeasure that these tastes evoke is present at birth. That is, with no experience, an infant will like sweet and dislike bitter and strong sour. Salty receptors are not completely mature at birth, but when they do become functional, infants will like relatively dilute salts.

Some of the most impressive evidence for this hardwired affect with taste came from the work of Jacob Steiner on facial expressions in newborn infants (Steiner, 1973). Steiner found that infants responded with stereotyped facial expressions when sweet, salty, sour, and bitter solutions were applied to their tongues. Sweet evoked a "smilelike" expression followed by sucking (**Figure 14.10***a*). Sour produced pursing and protrusion of the lips (Figure 14.10*b*). Bitter produced gaping, movements of spitting, and in some cases, vomiting movements. Even infants born without cerebral hemispheres (a condition known as "anencephaly") showed the same facial expressions, suggesting that these expressions are mediated by very primitive parts of the brain.

This hardwired affect responds to body need. For example, craving for salt was demonstrated by a dramatic case described in 1940. A 3½-year-old boy with an intense craving for salt died when his salt intake was restricted during a hospital stay. An autopsy revealed a tumor of his adrenal gland

(a) 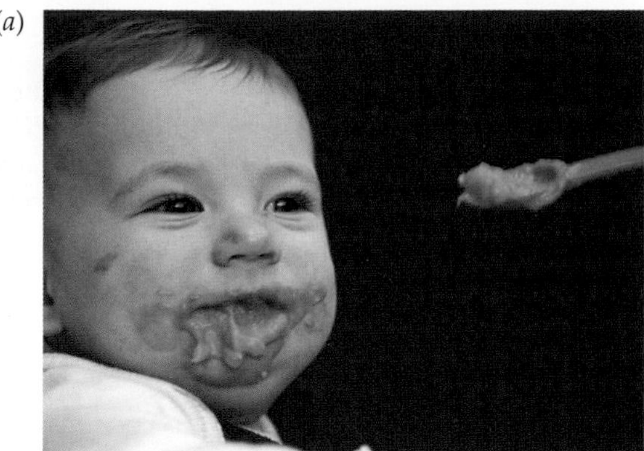

(b) 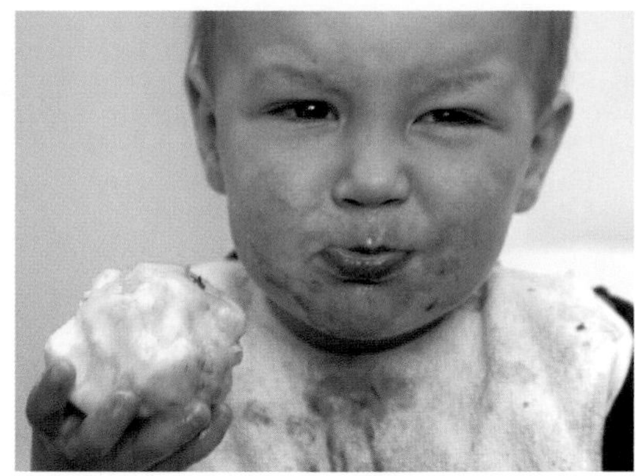

FIGURE 14.10 The two toddlers' facial expressions reveal the taste qualities that they are experiencing. (*a*) Sweet potato produces the typical smile associated with the acceptance of sweet. (*b*) Green apple produces the puckery face associated with sour.

that had caused his body to lose sodium. His salt craving had enabled his body to retain enough sodium to keep him alive (Wilkins and Richter, 1940).

The fact that the basic tastes provide both information and affective experience enables organisms to solve critical nutritional problems immediately, without having to learn (which takes time). The newborn baby can nurse because the sweet taste of mother's milk is pleasurable. The baby can also reject poisons because the bitter tastes they evoke are aversive. The athlete who sweats or the new mother who loses blood can replace lost sodium because of the pleasant taste of salt.

Specific Hungers

Early on, Curt Richter proposed a simple mechanism for the regulation of nutrients: the **specific hungers theory**. According to this view, the need for a nutrient causes the body to crave it. Ingestion of the nutrient reduces the craving and brings the body back into balance. The case of the boy with the salt craving described in the previous section provided support for this theory. Another source of support was a treatment for schizophrenia that was popular in the 1940s. At the time, some experts believed that the brain, which depends on glucose for fuel, could be forcibly rested if blood glucose were driven to very low values with insulin. Intense cravings for sweet were an unexpected by-product of the therapy. Later laboratory studies confirmed that insulin injections produce increased liking for sweet.

Even more support for the idea of specific hungers seemed to come from the work of a pediatrician, Clara Davis. She allowed a group of 6-month-old infants to eat whatever they liked, to see if they would choose wisely (C. M. Davis, 1928). The infants thrived, leading Davis to conclude that, when allowed to choose among a variety of healthy foods, infants had the ability to select a healthy diet.

The success of the specific hungers theory spurred further investigations that ultimately proved that the theory was limited only to sweet and salty. In one of the early studies, rats were fed a diet deficient in vitamin B_{12}, which made them sick. When the rats were offered a choice of remaining on the same diet or switching to a diet containing B_{12}, they immediately switched. But Paul Rozin conducted a crucial control. He gave the control rats the choice of the original diet or a different diet that was also deficient in B_{12}. These rats also immediately switched to the different diet. Thus, the rats in the original study were not specifically seeking B_{12}; they had simply learned to avoid the diet that made them ill (Rozin, 1967).

Rozin's work ended belief in specific hungers as an explanation of dietary regulation for anything beyond sugar and salt. In retrospect, we can see that

specific hungers theory The idea that deficiency of a given nutrient produces craving (a specific hunger) for that nutrient. Curt Richter first proposed this idea and demonstrated that cravings for salty or for sweet are associated with deficiencies in those substances. However, the idea proved wrong for other nutrients (e.g., vitamins).

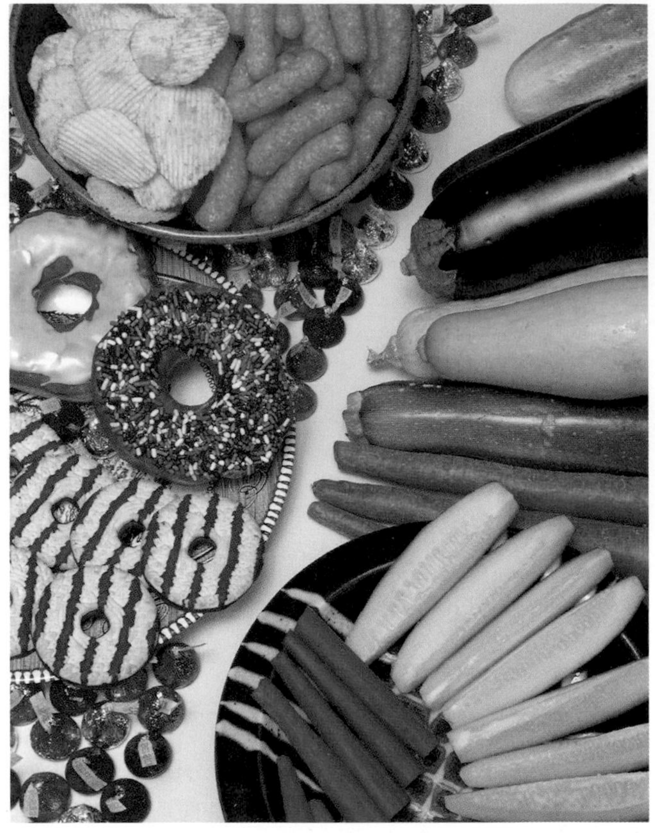

FIGURE 14.11 In our evolutionary past, when food was scarce and we had to expend considerable physical effort to get it, specific hungers for sugar and salt were adaptive. In the current era, in which foods are plentiful and easily obtained, these specific hungers (combined with the profit motive for the food industry) lead many to consume too much junk food. The nutrients in vegetables are, alas, largely undetectable, so we cannot develop specific hungers for them.

the theory lacked an important ingredient. For craving to cause an animal to seek out and take in a needed nutrient, a sensory cue would have to be unambiguously associated with the nutrient. The saltiness of salt and the sweetness of sugar could serve as such cues, but the B_{12} molecule does not produce a detectable cue in food (**Figure 14.11**).

We were left with a problem, though. How did Clara Davis's infants know how to select a healthy diet if specific hungers do not operate for all nutrients? It turned out that they were not selecting a healthy diet at all. They were simply eating a variety of the foods presented because they got bored eating single foods. Because all of the choices were healthy, all the infants needed to do was eat a variety. In the modern world, eating whatever we like will not produce good health, because too many of the available foods are not healthy. In fact, the specific hungers that are genuine can do us considerable harm; just think about our love for sweet and salty junk foods.

If specific hungers don't control all of what we eat, what does? Our likes and dislikes of food depend very much on our likes and dislikes of the retronasal olfactory sensations associated with foods. As we saw in the previous chapter, these olfactory likes and dislikes are not hardwired as those for taste are. Thus, our affect toward foods is made up of the hardwired affect contributed by taste, combined with the learned affect contributed by retronasal smell.

The gastrointestinal tract (commonly referred to as the gut) plays a crucial role in this learning. The macronutrients (nutrients that provide calories) are carbohydrates (long chains of sugar molecules), proteins (chains of amino acids), and fats (chains of fatty acids attached to glycerol). Except for the special case of sugar (a very short chain), these macronutrient molecules are too large to be sensed by taste or olfactory receptors. When foods containing these macronutrients enter the gut, however, the macronutrients are broken into their constituent pieces. These pieces stimulate chemoreceptors in the gut, and the brain makes us like the sensory properties (primarily the retronasal olfactory sensations) of the foods (conditioned food preferences). On the other hand, if we experience nausea after eating, the brain makes us dislike the sensory properties of the foods (conditioned food aversions). Thus, we regulate our intake through a combination of hardwired basic tastes and learned responses to food flavors.

umami The taste sensation evoked by monosodium glutamate.

monosodium glutamate (MSG) The sodium salt of glutamic acid (an amino acid).

The Special Case of Umami

Umami arose as a candidate for a fifth basic taste as part of advertising claims by manufacturers of **monosodium glutamate (MSG)**, the sodium salt of glutamic acid. Identified by Japanese chemists in the early 1900s, MSG was initially marketed as a flavor enhancer, said to suppress unpleasant tastes and enhance pleasant ones. When taste experts proved skeptical, MSG manufacturers went on to claim that MSG was a fifth basic taste, speculating that it signaled protein and thus played an important role in nutrition. However, the umami taste is not perceptible in many foods containing proteins. Another reason why umami is an unlikely candidate for a fifth basic taste is that some individuals like it but others do not. Basic tastes signal nutrients with hardwired affect, so if umami were a basic taste, the vast majority of people would react to it in the same way.

Because glutamate is an important neurotransmitter, receptors for the molecule are common throughout the body. The argument that such receptors might have been harnessed by the taste system to signal umami gained respectability when neuroscientists Nirupa Chaudhari and Steve Roper identified a version of a glutamate receptor in rat taste papillae (Chaudhari, Landin, and Roper, 2000). The glutamate receptor is linked to the sweet receptors. Sweet compounds stimulate the heterodimer made up of T1R2 and T1R3; umami stimulates another heterodimer, made up of T1R1 and T1R3.

Of special interest, Robert Margolskee (also a pioneer in the study of the sweet receptor) recently discovered that many taste receptors, including the glutamate receptor, are found in the gut. This exciting discovery suggests a different function for umami. Protein molecules are too large to be sensed by taste or smell, but proteins are made up of amino acids, including glutamic acid. When eaten, proteins are broken down into their constituent amino acids, providing stimuli for the glutamate receptors in the gut. These receptors can signal the brain that protein has been consumed. In this way, glutamate receptors can fulfill the function attributed to umami, but this is done in the gut, not the mouth. Consistent with this finding, John Prescott (a cognitive psychologist who studies the chemical senses) showed that consumption of a novel-flavored soup with MSG added to it produces a conditioned preference for the novel flavor. Simply holding the soup in the mouth does not (Prescott, 2004).

Because glutamate is a neurotransmitter, concerns have been raised about its safety in the human diet. MSG became particularly notorious in the 1960s. First it became associated with Chinese restaurant syndrome—a constellation of symptoms including numbness, headache, flushing, tingling, sweating, and tightness in the chest—that was reported by some individuals after consuming MSG (Kwok, 1968). Then Dr. John Olney, a toxicologist, suggested that MSG might induce brain lesions, particularly in infants (Olney and Sharpe, 1969). In response to these concerns, MSG was removed from baby foods in the 1970s. The final conclusion as of now (see Walker and Lupien, 2000) is that MSG in large doses may be a problem for some sensitive individuals, but apparently does not present a serious problem for the general population. For those who are sensitive, however, MSG can pose a serious risk.

The Special Case of Fat

Like protein, fat is a very important nutrient. Also like protein, fat molecules are too large to stimulate either taste or olfaction but are broken into their constituent parts by digestion in the gut. Fat molecules are made up of fatty acids attached to a support structure. Whole fat molecules stimulate the trigeminal nerve in the mouth, evoking tactile sensations like oily, viscous, creamy, and so on; but some fat molecules may be partially digested while still in the mouth, thus releasing fatty acids. Neurobiologist Tim Gilbertson's discovery of fatty acid receptors on the tongues of rats led to the idea that stimulation of these fatty acid receptors might play a hardwired role in our love of fat. Just as with glutamate, however, nature uses a more general method to ensure that we love fat-containing foods. Anthony Sclafani (a learning theorist who is an expert on conditioned food preferences) showed that fat in the gut produces conditioned preferences for the sensory properties of the food containing fat. Once we understand the role of conditioning in food preferences, we should have a healthy skepticism about the value of so-called diet foods. Mimicking the sensory properties of normal foods but reducing the caloric content disrupts normal regulatory mechanisms, as noted by Davidson and Swithers (see the discussion of sweet earlier in this chapter).

Coding of Taste Quality

A major source of historical controversy in the taste literature revolved around whether tastes are coded mainly via **labeled lines**, in which each taste neuron would unambiguously signal the presence of a certain basic taste, or via patterns of activity across many different taste neurons. We've seen examples of both types of coding in other senses. For example, color vision and olfaction use pattern coding. A single type of cone cannot tell us the wavelength of a light ray, but the pattern of activity across our three cone types can give us this information. Hearing, on the other hand, uses a mechanism more akin to the labeled-line approach: certain neurons always respond best to 5000-Hz tones, others always respond best to 5100-Hz tones, and so on. Which scheme is used in the gustatory system?

Given what we've already learned about the functions of the four basic tastes, it is easy to construct an evolutionary argument for labeled-line coding. Recall that in olfaction, which uses pattern coding, mixtures of two different compounds very often produce a third smell sensation that bears no resemblance to the smells of the mixture components. Such a coding system would be disastrous for the purpose of the taste system. For example, poisonous plants contain components with a variety of tastes. If bitterness were to synthesize with these other tastes, we would not be able to parse it out and thus avoid the poison. The functions of the four tastes are well served by their independence from each other. In addition, studies have shown that we are, in fact, very good at analyzing taste mixtures. For example, tonic water, which contains a combination of quinine and sugar, tastes bittersweet: we have no difficulty identifying its two components—bitter and sweet.

The historical controversy arose because initial research seemed to indicate that most neurons coming from taste buds respond to more than one of the four basic tastes. In Carl Pfaffmann's classic work recording from single cat chorda tympani fibers, these fibers were not specific to the four basic tastes. For example, some fibers responded to both acid and salt, and others responded to both acid and quinine (Pfaffmann, 1941). How could such a system code sour, salt, and bitter without confusion? Subsequent research showed that although "pure" labeled lines from individual receptor types

labeled lines A theory of taste coding in which each taste nerve fiber carries a particular taste quality. For example, the quality evoked from a sucrose-best fiber is sweet, that from an NaCl-best fiber is salty, and so on.

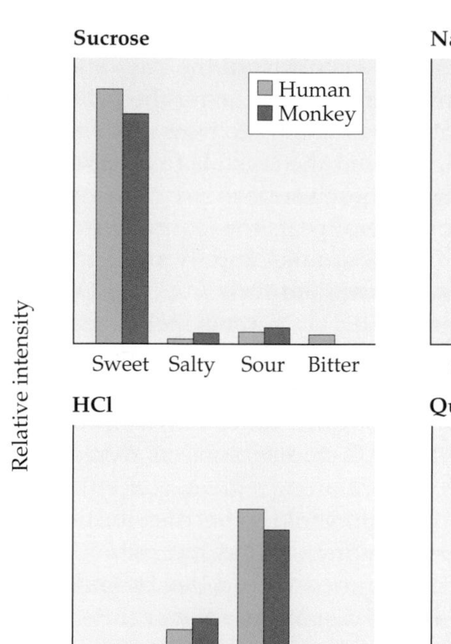

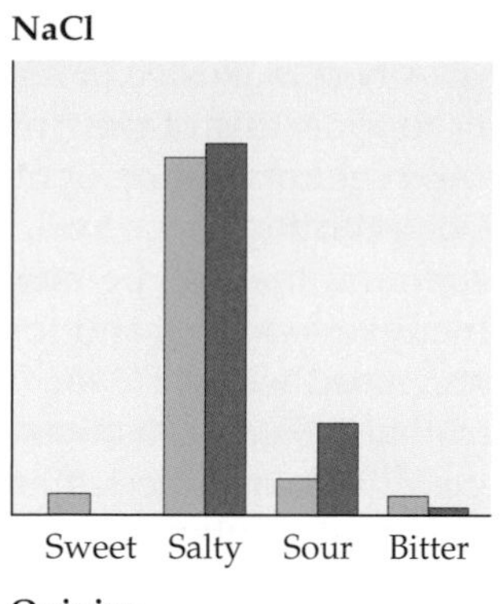

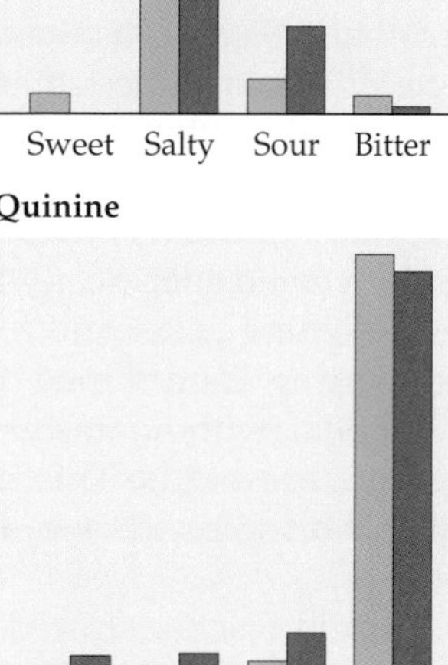

FIGURE 14.12 The tastes that human subjects perceive for each of four stimuli: sucrose, NaCl, HCl, and quinine. Also shown are the tastes that a monkey would perceive if the monkey's sweet-best fibers coded sweetness, NaCl-best fibers coded saltiness, HCl-best fibers coded sourness, and quinine-best fibers coded bitterness. (Monkey data from Sato, Ogawa, and Yamashita, 1975.)

are rare, most taste nerve fibers do have a clear "favorite" stimulus. Marion Frank (1973) named the fiber types "NaCl-best," "sucrose-best," and so on.

The fact that taste nerve fibers are not exclusively tuned to single basic tastes means that we rarely, if ever, experience "pure tastes." For example, sour tastes are perceived when acid-best fibers are activated, but acids also activate NaCl-best fibers (**Figure 14.12**). Thus, a solution of hydrochloric acid (HCl) will taste primarily sour, but also salty.

nontaster of PTC/PROP An individual born with two recessive alleles for the *Tas2r38* gene and unable to taste the compounds phenylthiocarbamide or propylthiouracil.

Taste Adaptation and Cross-Adaptation

As we've seen throughout this book, all sensory systems show adaptation effects, in which constant application of a certain stimulus temporarily weakens subsequent perception of that stimulus. In taste, our constant adaptation to the salt in saliva affects our ability to taste salt; in addition, adaptation to certain components in one food can change the perception of a second food. (See Web Essay 14.2: Water Tastes.)

You've experienced cross-adaptation yourself if you've ever noticed that a beverage like lemonade tastes too sour after you eat a sweet dessert. The sugar in the dessert adapts the sweet receptors so that the subsequent lemonade tastes less sweet and more sour than normal.

Genetic Variation in Taste Experience

In 1931 a chemist named Arthur Fox discovered that we do not all live in the same taste worlds (A. L. Fox, 1931). Fox was synthesizing the compound phenylthiocarbamide (PTC) (**Figure 14.13***a*), when some spilled and flew into the air. A colleague nearby noticed a bitter taste, but Fox tasted nothing. A test of additional colleagues revealed a few more **nontasters** like Fox who

(*a*) Phenylthiolcarbamide

(*b*) Propylthiouracil

FIGURE 14.13 The chemical structures of PTC (*a*) and PROP (*b*). The portions shaded in blue are those responsible for the bitter taste.

taster of PTC/PROP An individual born with one or both dominant alleles for the *Tas2r38* gene and able to taste the compounds phenylthiocarbamide and propylthiouracil. Tasters of PTC/PROP who also have a high density of fungiform papillae are supertasters.

tasted little bitterness in the compound, but most (**tasters**) perceived it as bitter. The next year Albert Blakeslee (a famous geneticist of the day) and Fox took PTC crystals to a meeting of the American Association for the Advancement of Science and set up a voting booth for attendees to register their perceptions. About one-third of those polled found the crystals to be tasteless, while two-thirds found them to be bitter. These proportions captured the imagination of many researchers, and for several years the *Journal of Heredity* sold papers impregnated with PTC for further studies. Family studies eventually confirmed that taster status was an inherited trait (e.g., the Dionne quintuplets were all found to be tasters in 1941). Nontasters carried two recessive alleles, whereas tasters had either one or both dominant alleles.

Initially, individuals were simply classified according to whether they could taste PTC, but eventually threshold studies came into vogue. In a threshold method invented specifically for PTC studies, subjects were given eight cups, four containing water and four containing a given concentration of PTC. Correct sorting determined the threshold. The distribution of thresholds was bimodal, with nontasters showing very high thresholds and tasters showing low thresholds. This distribution varied by sex and race: women had lower thresholds than men, and Asians had lower thresholds than Caucasians.

In the 1960s, Roland Fischer shifted tests to a chemical relative of PTC that was safer to test—propylthiouracil (PROP) (Figure 14.13*b*)—and focused on the nutritional implications of the genetic variation in taster status (Fischer and Griffin, 1964). Fischer suggested that tasters were more finicky eaters: because bitter tastes are more intense to these individuals, they tend to dislike foods high in bitter compounds, such as many vegetables, that nontasters find more palatable. Fischer also related taster status to body type (e.g., weight) and health. Alcoholics and smokers were found to contain a lower proportion of tasters than would be expected by chance, presumably because unpleasant sensations (e.g., bitterness) produced by alcoholic beverages and tobacco acted as deterrents. The effect of genetic variation in taste was even related to cancer risk, as will be described shortly.

In 2003, Dennis Drayna and his colleagues discovered the location of the gene that expresses PTC/PROP receptors (Kim et al., 2003). This gene is a member of the bitter family introduced earlier and is designated *Tas2r38*. Individuals with two recessive alleles are nontasters; those with either one or both dominant alleles are tasters.

Supertasters

By the 1970s, the "direct" psychophysical methods introduced by Harvard's S. S. Stevens led to a new look at genetic variation in taste. Instead of measuring thresholds—the dimmest sensations—investigators could look at suprathreshold taste and plot the psychophysical functions showing how perceived taste intensity varies with concentration. Stevens and his students showed that the same relation held for many different sensory modalities, including taste:

$$\psi = \phi^{\beta}$$

where ψ is perceived intensity, ϕ is concentration, and β takes on different values for different sensory modalities (S. S. Stevens and Galanter, 1957). Of special interest for the present purposes, β takes on different values for different taste qualities. For example, bitterness grows more slowly with concentration than sweet does (**Figure 14.14**). That is, the value of β for bitter is smaller than the value of β for sweet.

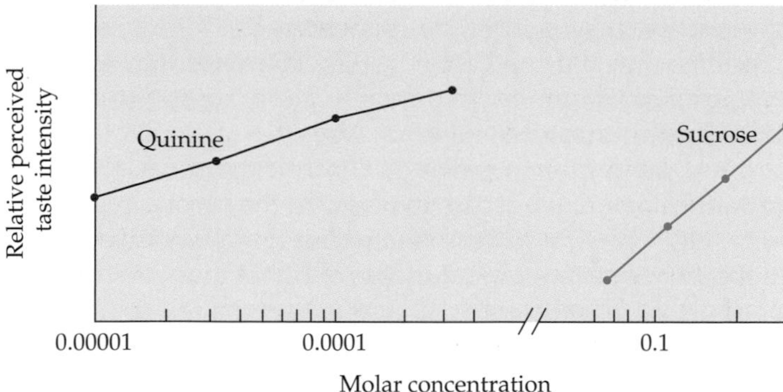

FIGURE 14.14 Psychophysical functions for quinine and sucrose. The logarithm of the perceived taste intensity is plotted against the logarithm of the concentration. In this plot, β is the slope of the function. The value of β for quinine is 0.3; for sucrose, 0.8. (Data from Bartoshuk, 1979.)

cross-modality matching The ability to match the intensities of sensations that come from different sensory modalities. This ability enables insight into sensory differences. To the average nontaster of PTC/PROP, for example, the bitterness of black coffee roughly matches the pain of a mild headache; for a supertaster, the bitterness of black coffee roughly matches the pain of a severe headache.

supertaster An individual who perceives the most intense taste sensations. A variety of factors may contribute to this heightened perception; among the most important is the density of fungiform papillae.

Two of S. S. Stevens's students—Joseph Stevens and Lawrence Marks—made another fundamental discovery in this era: humans are very good at **cross-modality matching** (J. C. Stevens, 1959). For example, we can match the loudness of a sound to the brightness of a light, and we can match both of these to the intensity of a taste. This finding led to yet another way to study variability in individuals' perceptions of the bitter taste of PTC and PROP (Marks et al., 1988): we could ask subjects to match the bitterness of PROP to other sensations completely unrelated to taste (**Figure 14.15**). For example, nontasters matched the taste of PROP to very weak sensations (the sound of a watch or a whisper). Tasters proved to be a heterogeneous lot. For some, PROP was likened to very intense sensations, such as the brightness of the sun or the most intense pain ever experienced. These individuals were labeled **supertasters**. "Medium tasters" matched PROP to weaker stimuli, such as the smell of frying bacon or the pain of a mild headache (Bartoshuk, Fast, and Snyder, 2005).

Armed with genotypes, ratings of the bitterness of PROP, and counts of fungiform papillae, Valerie Duffy (a pioneer in the modern movement among nutritionists to evaluate food behavior in terms of the sensory properties of foods instead of only their nutrient content), along with her student John Hayes and colleagues (Hayes et al., 2008), was able to show that a combination of PROP genotype and tongue anatomy divided individuals into the three groups already described: nontasters, tasters, and supertasters. This research showed that PROP status and number of fungiform papillae are independent. The

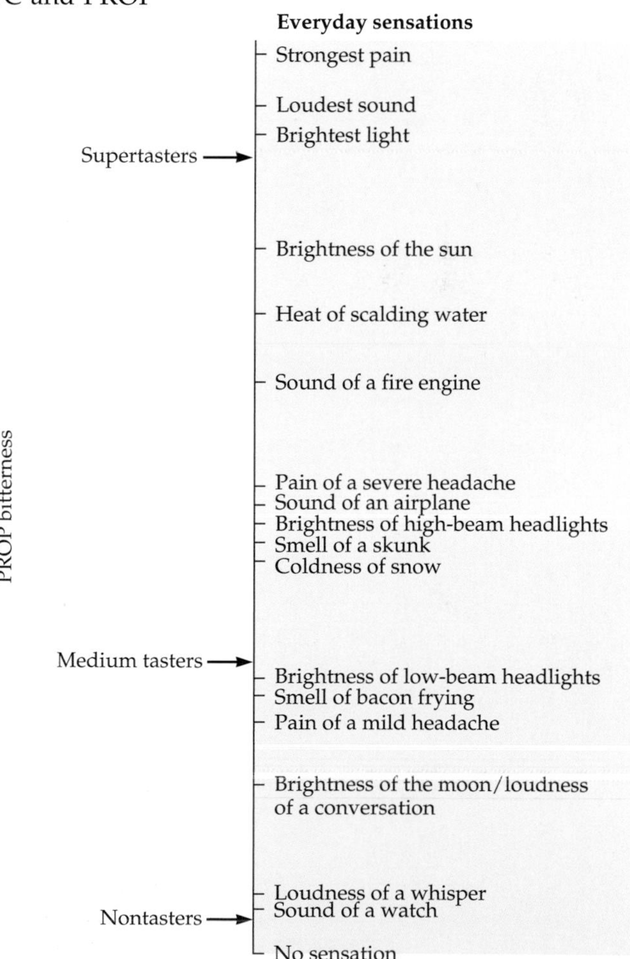

FIGURE 14.15 Cross-modality matching. The levels of bitterness of concentrated PROP perceived by nontasters, medium tasters, and supertasters of PROP are shown on the left. The perceived intensities of a variety of everyday sensations are shown on the right. (Data from Fast, 2004.)

combination of ability to taste PROP and possession of a very large number of fungiform papillae produces a PROP supertaster; PROP tasters with fewer fungiform papillae are medium PROP tasters. PROP nontasters show the whole range of number of fungiform papillae. Thus, a person can be a PROP nontaster but be a supertaster in all other ways.

Those with the most fungiform papillae not only experience the most intense taste sensations in general, but also experience the most intense sensations of oral burn (e.g., chilis) and oral touch (fats, thickeners in foods) because fungiform papillae are innervated by nerve fibers that convey burn and touch sensations, as well as those that convey taste sensations. In addition, because of central connections between taste and retronasal olfaction, those who experience the most intense taste sensations also perceive more intense retronasal olfaction and thus more intense flavor.

Pathology adds yet another source of variation in our oral sensations. Surprisingly, removing input from one of the taste nerves (by anesthesia or damage) can actually intensify taste sensations (e.g., Lehman et al., 1995). This intensification results because inputs from the different taste nerves inhibit one another in the brain. Loss of input from one nerve releases others from that inhibition. In some cases, the result is actual intensification of whole-mouth taste.

Although the concept of supertasters originated because of studies on PROP bitterness, we now understand that a variety of factors contribute to the intensities of oral sensations. Thus, supertasters are best defined simply as those who experience the most intense taste sensations, but we add a note of caution: given the many sources of variation, we find ourselves with different types of supertasters.

Health Consequences of Taste Sensation

With these new insights, the potential links between responsiveness to PROP and health have become the focus of renewed interest. The new psychophysical methods permitted Valerie Duffy to show that variation in the sensory properties of foods and beverages affects food preferences and thus diet. Because diet is a major risk factor for a variety of diseases, genetic variation in taste plays a role in these diseases. For instance, some vegetables produce unpleasant sensations (e.g., bitter) to medium tasters and supertasters, leading these individuals to eat fewer of them. Reduced vegetable intake is in turn a risk factor for colon cancer.

Sure enough, Duffy and her colleagues found that, in a sample of older men getting routine colonoscopies at a Department of Veterans Affairs hospital, those tasting PROP as most bitter had the most colon polyps, a precursor to colon cancer (Basson et al., 2005). On the other hand, fats can produce unpleasantly intense sensations to supertasters, leading them to eat fewer high-fat foods and thereby lowering their risk of cardiovascular disease (Duffy, Lucchina, and Bartoshuk, 2004). These sensory links to behavior that affects health are not limited to diet. Fischer's early suggestion that nontasters are more likely to smoke and consume alcohol has proved correct (Duffy et al., 2004; D. J. Snyder et al., 2005).

Pleasure and Retronasal versus Orthonasal Olfaction

There is still much that is not understood about the links between retronasal and orthonasal (through the nostrils) olfaction, including the pleasure or displeasure associated with these sensations. We know that we learn to like or dislike smells, but do we learn these preferences separately for retro- and orthonasal olfaction? David Laing, an Australian expert on the chemical senses, suggested that this may be the case. He noted that many of us like the smell of recently cut grass, but few would like such a sensation if it turned up in food. On the other hand, when an aversion is learned retronasally, it often shows up with orthonasal olfaction as well. Bartoshuk recounts getting carsick on a childhood vacation while simultaneously eating chocolate-covered cherries. She now not only avoids the cherries, but finds cherry-scented soaps disgusting as well.

Chili Peppers

The pleasure that some people experience from chili peppers deserves special attention. We are not born liking chili peppers. Rozin studied the acquisition of chili pepper preference in Mexico and found that the process depended on social influences. Chili is gradually added to the diet of young children beginning at about age 3, and the children observe their family members enjoying it. By age 5 or 6, children voluntarily add chili to their own food. At some point the chili is liked for its own sake.

A variety of arguments based on presumed health benefits have been introduced to account for our love of chili peppers. For example, some have argued that chilis kill microorganisms in food, thus acting as a preservative. Others have argued that chilis contain vitamins A and C, which give them adaptive value (in other words, the pain of the chili serves as a cue for the presence of the vitamins). The pleasure that some people experience from chilis has also been linked to the idea that the resulting burn leads to the release of endorphins, the brain's internal painkillers.

One of the most interesting features of the liking for the burn of chili peppers is its near total restriction to humans. Rozin has documented a few cases on record of animals showing a liking for chilis, but in all cases these were pets fed chili pepper by their human companions. When Rozin tried to produce liking for chilis in rats, he failed. But one of Rozin's students, Bennett Galef, who is famous for the study of social interactions among rats, was finally able to get rats to like a diet seasoned with a mild level of cayenne pepper by exposing the rats to a "demonstrator" rat that had just eaten the diet. It seems that growing to like chili peppers is a social phenomenon for rats as well.

The burn that we experience from chili peppers is highly variable across individuals (**Figure 14.16**). The variability comes from two sources. First, as noted earlier, individuals with the most fungiform papillae (supertasters) have the most fibers mediating pain, and thus they perceive the most intense oral burn from chilis. Second, capsaicin, the chemical that produces the burn in chilis, desensitizes pain receptors. This means that individuals who consume chilis quite often (once every 48 hours is sufficient) are chronically desensitized. Chili peppers produce considerably less burn to those who are desensitized.

Desensitization can come to your rescue if you accidentally order a meal that proves to be overspiced for your palate. After the first mouthful, wait until the burn has subsided. The mistake many diners make is to keep trying to eat. As long as the capsaicin continues to be applied, desensitization does not occur. Desensitization occurs during the decline of the burn (B. G. Green, 1993). Once the initial burn has faded, the rest of the meal can be consumed with relative comfort.

FIGURE 14.16 Do these images inspire fear or delight in your taste buds?

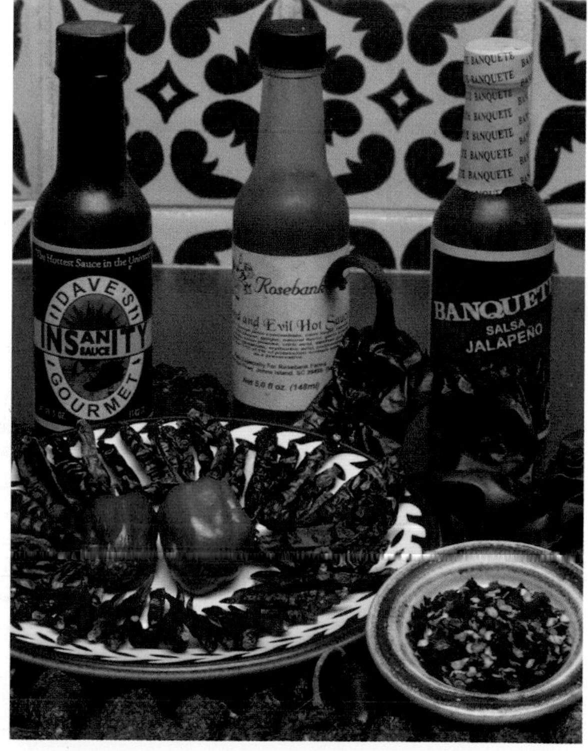

Capsaicin desensitization has important clinical value. The ancient Mayan Indians used a concoction made of chilis to treat the pain of mouth sores. Wolffe Nadoolman, then a medical student at Yale working in Bartoshuk's laboratory, created a similar remedy by adding cayenne pepper to a recipe for taffy. Cancer patients often develop painful mouth sores from chemotherapy and radiation therapy, and if these patients suck on the capsaicin candies, capsaicin is brought into contact with the pain receptors stimulated by the sores. The pain receptors are then desensitized and the pain is dramatically reduced (Berger et al., 1995). Although capsaicin can be used to reduce pain at any body site, the skin is a potent barrier that prevents capsaicin from contacting pain receptors. Thus, capsaicin remedies for disorders like arthritis are rarely very satisfactory. In the mouth, the mucous membrane permits capsaicin to easily contact pain receptors, so there, desensitization is fast and powerful.

Summary

Refer to the
Sensation and Perception
website
(www.sinauer.com/wolfe2e)
for activities, essays, study questions, and other study aids.

1. Flavor is produced by the combination of taste and retronasal olfaction (olfactory sensations produced when odorants in the mouth are forced up behind the palate into the nose). Flavor sensations are localized to the mouth, even though the retronasal olfactory sensations come from the olfactory receptors high in the nasal cavity.
2. Taste buds are globular clusters of cells (like the segments in an orange). The tips of some of the cells (microvilli) contain sites that interact with taste molecules. Those sites fall into two groups: ion channels that mediate responses to salts and acids, and G protein–coupled receptors that bind to sweet and bitter compounds.
3. The tongue has a bumpy appearance because of structures called papillae. The filiform papillae (most numerous) have no taste buds. Taste buds are found in the fungiform papillae (front of the tongue), foliate papillae (rear edges of the tongue) and circumvallate papillae (rear center of the tongue), as well as on the roof of the mouth.
4. Taste projects ipsilaterally from the tongue to the medulla, thalamus, and cortex. It projects first to the insula in the cortex, and from there to the orbitofrontal cortex, an area where taste can be integrated with other sensory input (e.g., retronasal olfaction).
5. Taste and olfaction play very different roles in the perception of foods and beverages. Taste is the true nutritional sense; taste receptors are tuned to molecules that function as important nutrients. Bitter taste is a poison detection system. Sweet taste enables us to respond to the sugars that are biologically useful to us: sucrose, glucose, and fructose. Salty taste enables us to identify sodium, a mineral crucial to survival because of its role in nerve conduction and muscle function. Sour taste permits us to avoid acids in concentrations that might injure tissue.
6. Umami, the taste produced by monosodium glutamate, has been suggested as a fifth basic taste that detects protein. However, umami lacks one of the most important properties of a basic taste: hardwired affect. Some individuals like umami, but others do not. The presence of glutamate receptors in the gut suggests that protein detection occurs there. Digestion breaks down proteins into their constituent amino acids, and the glutamate released stimulates gut glutamate receptors, leading to conditioned preferences for the sensory properties of the foods containing the protein.
7. The importance of taste to survival requires that we be able to recognize each of the taste qualities, even when it is present in a mixture. By coding taste quality with labeled lines in much the same way that frequencies are coded in hearing, nature has ensured that we have this important capability. These labeled lines are noisy. For example, acids are able to stimulate fibers mediating saltiness, as well as those mediating sourness. Thus, acids tend to taste both salty and sour.

8. Foods do not taste the same to everyone. The Human Genome Project revealed that we carry about 25 genes for bitter taste. The most studied bitter receptor responds to PROP and shows allelic variation in humans leading to the designations, "nontaster" for those who taste the least bitterness and "taster" for those who taste the most. In addition, humans vary in the number of fungiform papillae (and thus taste buds) they possess. Those with the most taste buds are called supertasters and live in a "neon" taste world; those with the fewest live in a "pastel" taste world. Psychologists discovered these differences by testing people's ability to match sensory intensities of stimuli from different modalities. For example, the bitterness of black coffee matches the pain of a mild headache to nontasters but resembles a severe headache to supertasters. The way foods taste affects palatability, which in turn affects diet. Poor diet contributes to diseases like cancer and cardiovascular disease.
9. For taste, unlike olfaction, liking and disliking are hardwired; for example, babies are born liking sweet and salty and disliking bitter. When we become deficient in salt or sucrose, liking for salty and sweet tastes, respectively, increases. Junk foods are constructed to appeal to these preferences. Liking the burn of chili peppers, on the other hand, is acquired and, with the exception of some pets, is essentially limited to humans. Because taste buds are surrounded by pain fibers, supertasters perceive much greater burn from chilis than do nontasters.

CHAPTER 15

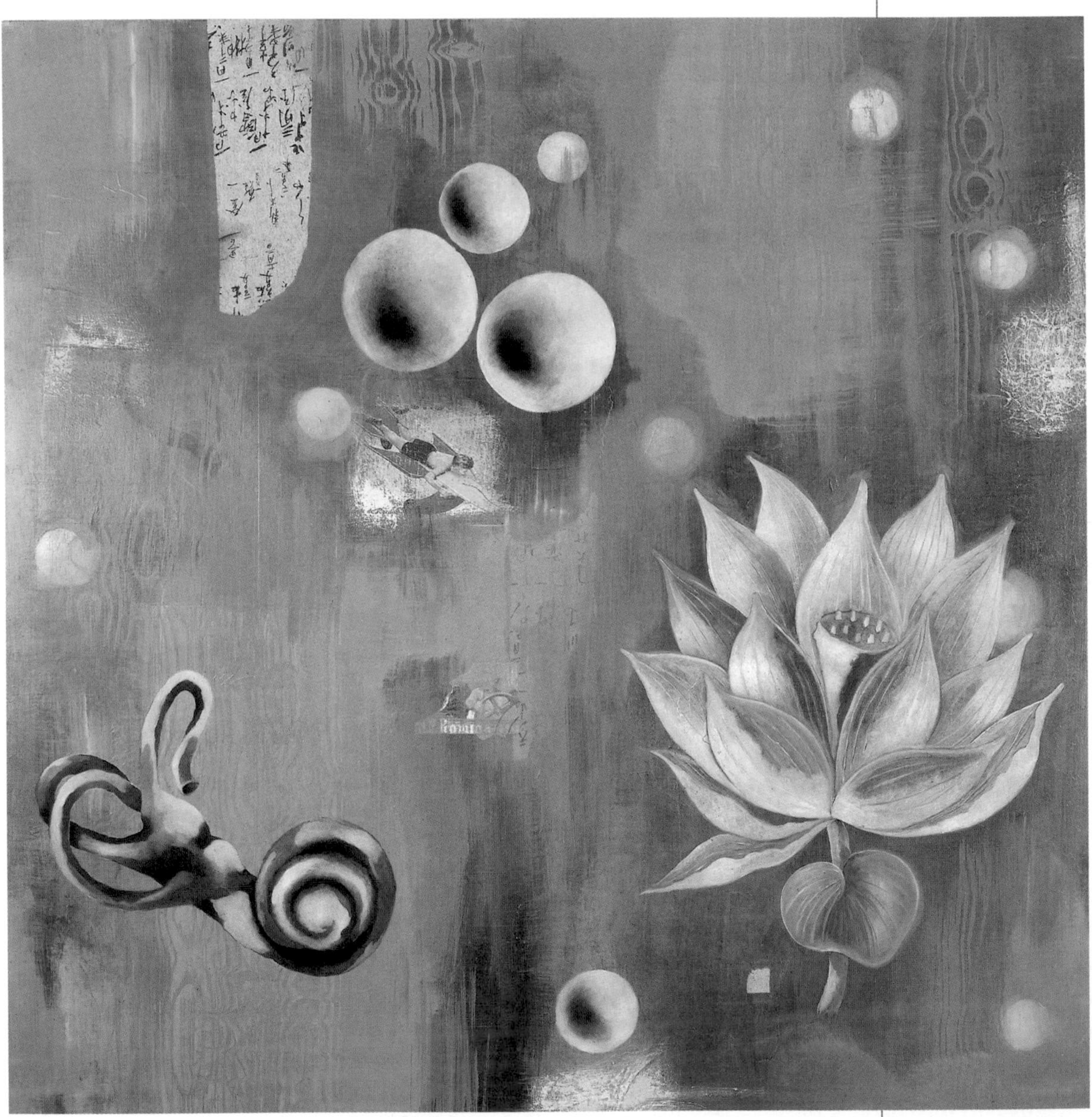

Jody Guralnick, *Organs of Hearing and Balance*, 2000

Spatial Orientation and the Vestibular System

Remember when you were a child and you used to spin around until you were dizzy and couldn't walk straight? Perhaps you even lost your balance and fell? Why were you dizzy? The sensations did not arise from one of the five senses that Aristotle recognized—vision, hearing, touch, taste, or smell. Your dizziness arose from contributions of the vestibular system to your sense of spatial orientation.

The **vestibular system**—sometimes called the vestibular labyrinth—is a set of specialized sense organs located in the inner ear right next to the cochlea (a hearing organ discussed in Chapter 9). These organs sense motion of the head, as well as the orientation of gravity, and make a predominant contribution to our sense of tilt and our sense of self-motion. Taken together, the senses of tilt and self-motion comprise our sense of **spatial orientation**.

You may be asking, "Wait a minute, why didn't I learn about the vestibular system and spatial orientation when I first learned about the five senses?" Good question. Perhaps you should have. The vestibular "sixth sense" provides fundamental contributions that are often overlooked. For example, the vestibular system contributes to clear vision when we move and helps us maintain balance when we stand. And it is so crucial that some patients even report cognitive deficits when it fails. Yet, despite these essential contributions, the vestibular system toils in anonymity. Much of the time, we remain unaware of it until it stops working properly.

The fundamental nature of the vestibular system is emphasized by the fact that the vestibular organs appeared very early in evolutionary history and have remained relatively unchanged. The fossil record shows the presence of distinct vestibular organs dating back 400 million years. The system is not only ancient but largely automatic. While you are aware of the normal function of your eyes and ears, a patient may only become acutely aware of their vestibular sensation—experiencing dizziness, spatial disorientation, imbalance, blurred vision, and/or illusory self-motion—when problems develop (see **Web Essay 15.1: Meniere's Syndrome**).

Obviously, we can no longer ask Aristotle—who is credited with first cataloging our sensory systems—why he did not include spatial orientation or our vestibular sense among the specialized sensory systems, but we can speculate. One explanation may be that it was not until the nineteenth century that scientists understood that the vestibular system is a specialized set of sense organs. Up to then, the vestibular system had been considered an entrance to the cochlea. In fact, the name *vestibular* records this error for posterity because *vestibule* means "entrance." But this explanation is not entirely satisfactory, since Aristotle had cataloged other senses without detailed anatomical or physiological knowledge.

Another explanation may be the inconspicuous nature of our vestibular sense. In fact, as we'll see, many responses evoked by the vestibular system

vestibular system The set of five organs—three semicircular canals and two otolith organs—located in each inner ear that sense head motion and head orientation with respect to gravity. Also called *vestibular labyrinth*.

spatial orientation A sense comprised of three interacting sensory modalities: our senses of linear motion, angular motion, and tilt.

(*a*)

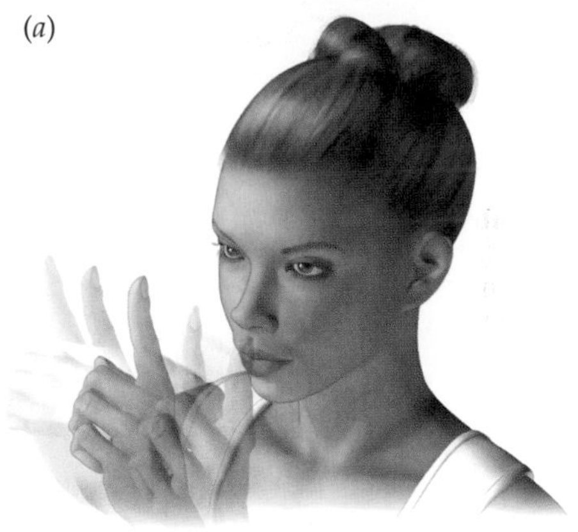

Subject's view

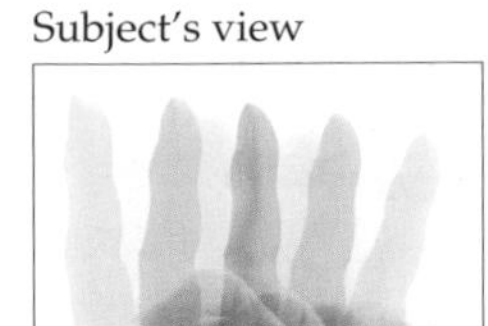

(*b*)

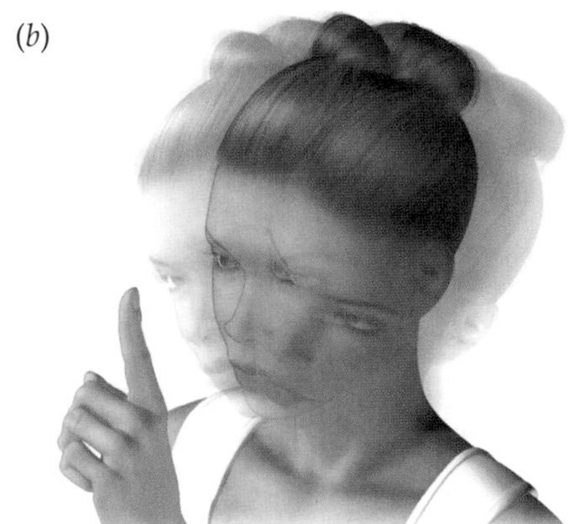

Subject's view

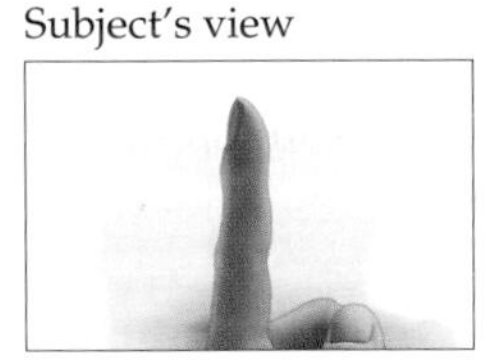

(*c*)

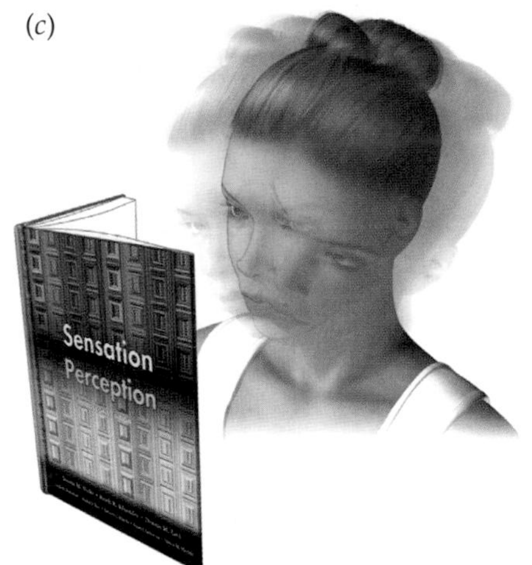

Subject's view

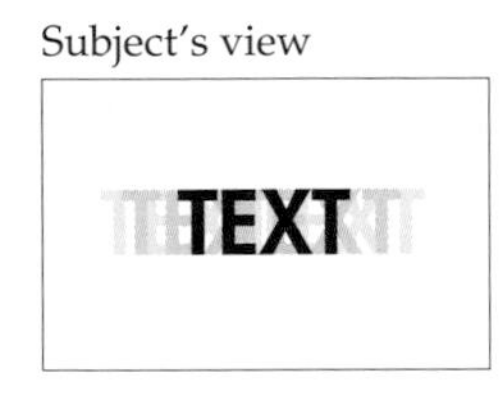

FIGURE 15.1 Demonstration of the vestibulo-ocular reflex. (*a*) As your fingertip moves faster and faster in front of your face, the fingertip begins to blur. (*b*) When you shake your head back and forth, the fingertip remains clearer. (*c*) Text also remains clearer during head shaking.

are reflexive and linked to the outputs of other sensory systems. For example, the vestibular system helps us see clearly by reflexively rotating the eyeballs in the sockets to compensate for head rotation—thereby helping to keep visual images stable on the retina. To demonstrate this to yourself, move your hand back and forth in front of your face (**Figure 15.1***a*). Start slowly and then move your hand faster and faster. Focus on a fingertip and notice that it starts to appear more and more blurry as your hand moves back and forth at a higher frequency. Now hold your hand in front of your face and shake your head from side to side as if to say "no" (Figure 15.1*b*). Again, start slowly and gradually increase the speed. At higher frequencies of motion, you should notice that each fingertip stays in focus more readily and at higher speeds when you move your head than when you move your hand. You can compensate for head movement more readily than hand movement because of a vestibulo-ocular reflex that we will discuss in more detail later.

Before we move on, there is one more lesson to draw from this example. Rotate your head back and forth while you read this text (Figure 15.1*c*). Until now, you probably didn't perceive any head motion. In fact, your head often moves around, but you do not typically perceive your head motion, because the vestibular system usually performs its job automatically—with little, if any, conscious awareness. But now that I've called your attention to it, as you continue to shake your head you can perceive your head rotating, can't you? Thus, it is not that you are unable to perceive vestibular stimulation but rather that under normal circumstances it is relegated to the attentional background.

Modalities and Qualities of Spatial Orientation

Our sense of spatial orientation is based on three *sensory modalities*: the senses of linear motion, angular motion, and tilt. Why do we call these "modalities," as though they were different senses? Vision and audition are different modalities, but we would say that color and depth perception are different qualities, not different modalities. The key lies in the energy transduced and the receptors. Color and depth are different interpretations of the same light collected by the same rods and cones in the retina—hence, *qualities*. Seeing and hearing involve different stimulation energy—light and pressure waves, respectively—and different types of receptors.

Sensing linear motion, angular motion, and tilt involves different receptors and/or different stimulation energy—hence, *modalities*. Specifically, the vestibular system transduces three distinct stimulation energies—gravity, angular acceleration, and linear acceleration—using two different types of sense organs. The force of gravity, pulling us toward the center of the Earth, is transduced by a set of vestibular organs called the **otolith organs**. The otolith organs provide a predominant contribution to our sense of the tilt of our heads. In addition to gravity, the otolith organs also sense linear acceleration, which is a change in linear velocity. This signal makes a predominant contribution to our sense of linear motion. Similarly, the **semicircular canals** sense angular acceleration, which is a change in angular velocity; this signal makes a predominant contribution to our sense of angular motion. The sensitivity of the vestibular system to acceleration—angular acceleration for the semicircular canals and linear acceleration for the otolith organs—demonstrates that the vestibular system is principally sensitive to *changes* in motion. Constant motion—whether angular or linear—does not result in vestibular signals that directly indicate motion.

Note that the otolith organs sense two stimuli with physically distinct causes: gravity and linear acceleration. This makes the signals from the otolith organs ambiguous, because the otolith organs transduce both linear acceleration and the relative orientation of gravity into a neural signal. As Einstein noted, the physics of the situation assures that no device can tell the difference between gravity and linear acceleration. Therefore, it will be up to the brain to figure out if you are accelerating or feeling the pull of gravity. See Web Essay 15.2: Gravity versus Linear Acceleration for more on the equivalence of these two forces.

Each of the three spatial orientation modalities includes two qualities: direction and **amplitude**. As an example of direction, perceived linear motion might be forward, up, and to the left. As an example of amplitude, the speed of our perceived motion can be large (as when we're flying in an airplane) or small (as with a baby crawling).

The Three Spatial Orientation Modalities: Angular Motion, Linear Motion, and Tilt

Our sense of orientation in space is made up of at least three interacting sensory modalities—a **sense of angular motion**, a **sense of linear motion**, and a **sense of tilt**. To experience your sense of angular motion, simply close your eyes and rotate your head from side to side as if to say "no." Primarily because of the contributions of the vestibular system, you should experience a perception of angular velocity that is roughly proportional to the actual angular velocity of your head.

Relatively pure linear motion is more difficult to achieve passively, but the experience of riding in a car, train, or bus provides an example. Try the following when you are a passenger in a car. With your eyes closed, pay attention to your sense of motion as the driver backs the car out of the garage, brings the car to a stop, and then begins to accelerate forward. Initially, you should perceive backward translation (i.e., backward linear motion). You should also perceive the cessation of translation as the car comes to a stop, and then forward translation as the car accelerates.

Finally, to experience your sense of tilt, simply close your eyes and nod your head as if to say "yes." Pitch your head forward and hold it there for several seconds; then pitch your head backward and hold it there. You should experience a perception of head tilt that represents your tilt sensory modality.

otolith organs The mechanical structures in the vestibular system that sense both linear acceleration and gravity.

semicircular canals The three toroidal tubes in the vestibular system that sense angular motion.

amplitude The magnitude of displacement (increase or decrease) of a head movement (e.g., angular velocity, linear acceleration, tilt).

sense of angular motion The spatial orientation modality that senses motion resulting from rotation.

sense of linear motion The spatial orientation modality that senses translation.

sense of tilt The spatial orientation modality that senses head inclination with respect to gravity.

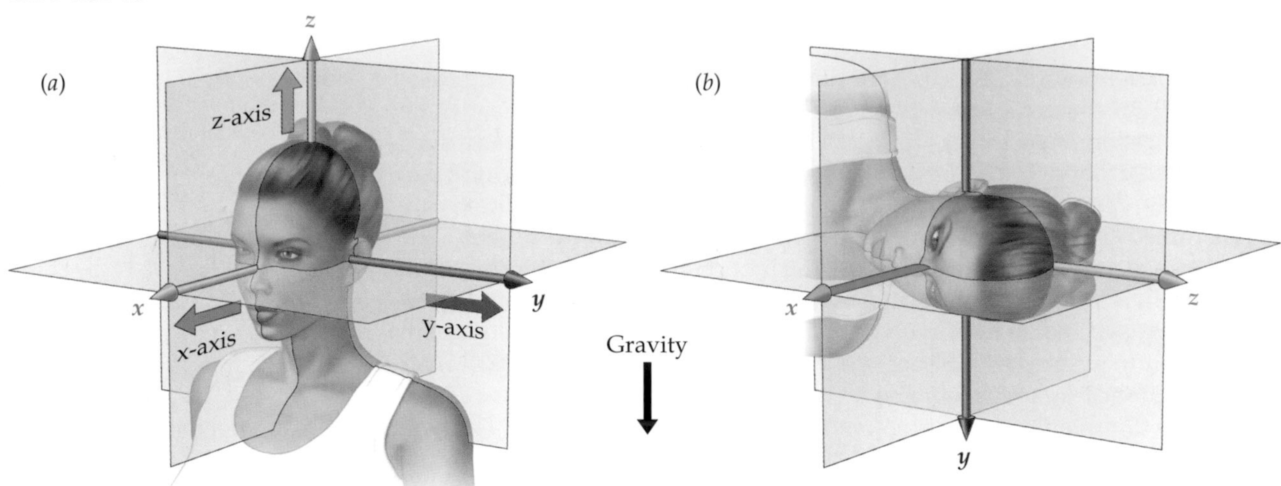

FIGURE 15.2 Movement of the head can be described in terms of a simple fixed coordinate system. The x-axis always points forward relative to the current orientation of the head, the y-axis always points out the left ear, and the z-axis always points out the top of the head. As part (*b*) illustrates, this coordinate system always moves with the head.

FIGURE 15.3 Bodies can turn (rotate) in three directions. The head can move with a pure roll velocity around the x-axis (*a*, *d*), a pure pitch velocity around the y-axis (*b*, *e*), or a pure yaw velocity around the z-axis (*c*, *f*). More generally, at any instant the head can rotate about any arbitrary rotation axis made up of varying roll, pitch, and yaw rotation velocity components.

Basic Qualities of Spatial Orientation: Direction and Amplitude

DIRECTION As mentioned earlier, direction is a quality for each of the spatial orientation modalities. To help clearly classify direction, we first define a simple coordinate system that moves with the head (**Figure 15.2**). The x-axis always points forward, the y-axis always points out the left ear, and the z-axis always points out the top of the head.

Let's consider the three directions for our sense of rotation. The head can rotate with a roll angular velocity (**Figure 15.3*a***), as when you tilt it left or right from upright. Or it can rotate with a pitch angular velocity, as when you nod "yes" (Figure 15.3*b*). Or the head can rotate with a yaw angular velocity, as when you shake your head "no" (Figure 15.3*c*). Roll, pitch, and yaw angular velocities are always defined with respect to the head. For example, even when you're lying on your side (see Figure

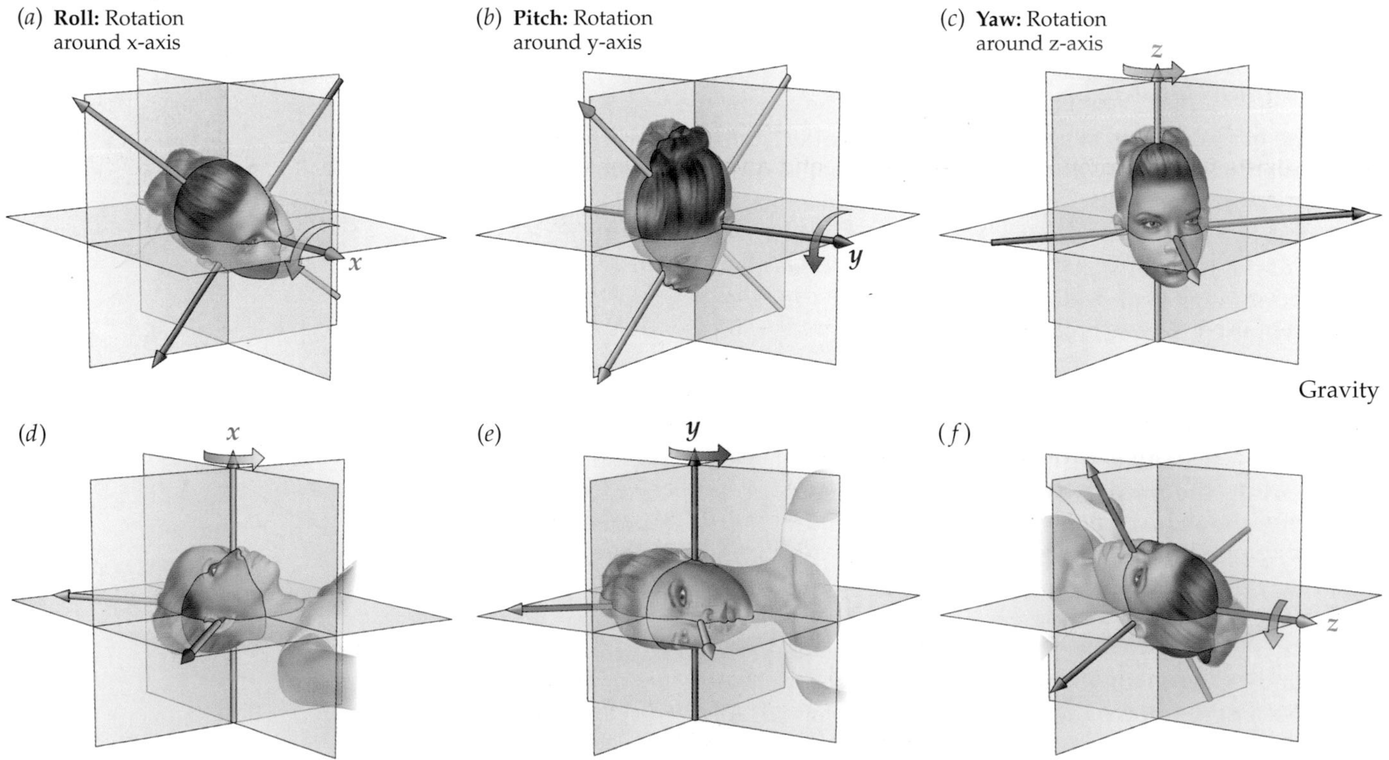

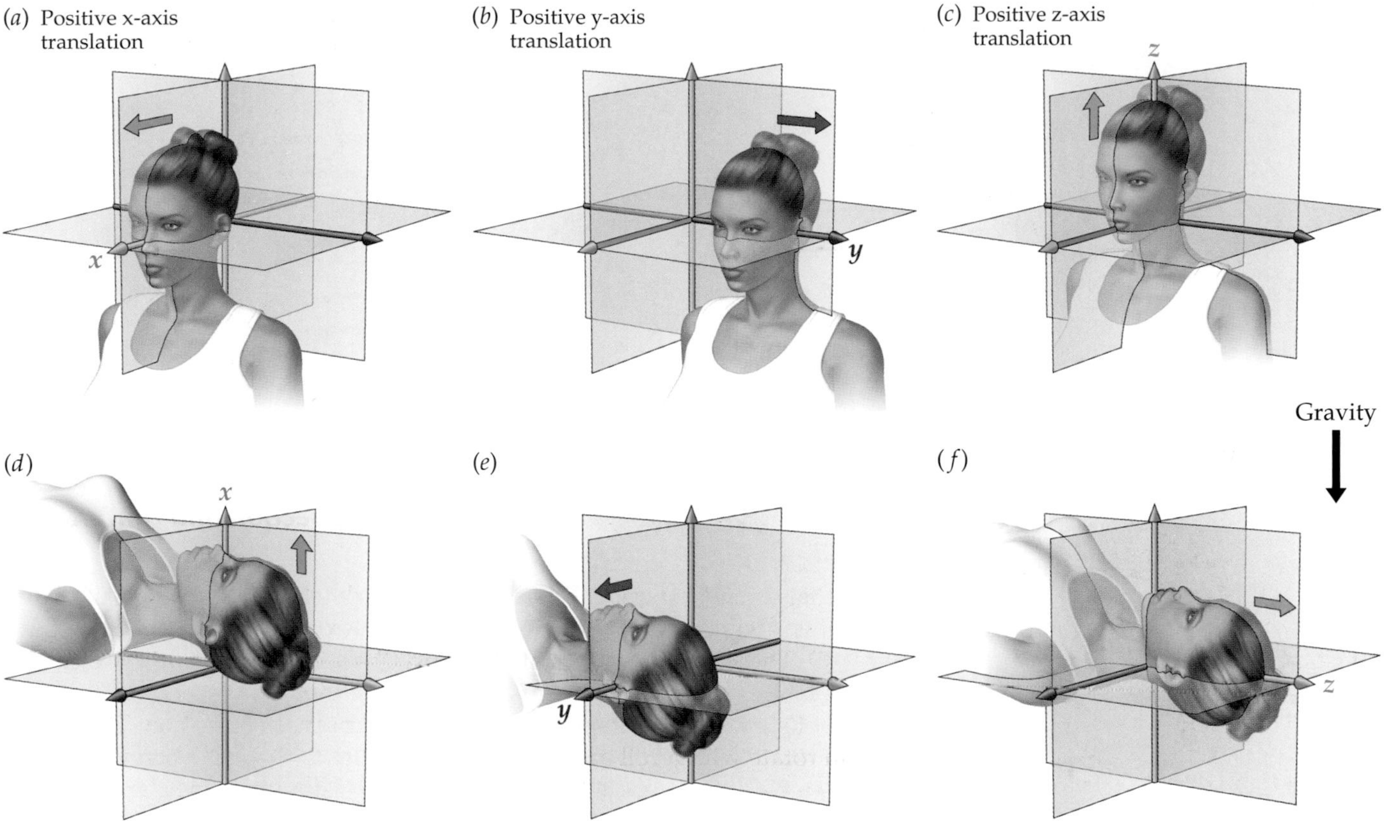

(*a*) Positive x-axis translation

(*b*) Positive y-axis translation

(*c*) Positive z-axis translation

(*d*)

(*e*)

(*f*)

Gravity

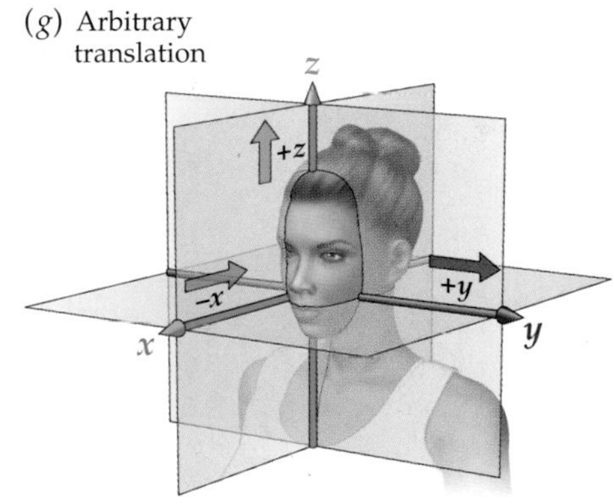

FIGURE 15.4 Translating bodies can move in three directions.The head can translate forward and backward along the x-axis (*a*, *d*), left and right along the y-axis (*b*, *e*), or along the z-axis (*c*, *f*). More generally, at any instant, the head can translate in any arbitrary direction composed of translations in each of the three directions (*g*).

15.3*e*), nodding "yes" yields a pitch angular velocity. More generally, a roll angular velocity exists for any rotation about the x-axis, a pitch angular velocity exists for any rotation about the y-axis, and a yaw angular velocity exists for any rotation about the z-axis.

Note that when you're on your side nodding "yes" (see Figure 15.3*e*), there is a pitch angular velocity but no change in the tilt of the head relative to gravity. The head always remains oriented with the right ear down in this example. In other words, roll, pitch, and yaw angular velocities do not tilt the head relative to gravity when the angular velocity is aligned with gravity. So, whenever the angular velocity is aligned with gravity, the head can have a roll (Figure 15.3*d*), pitch (Figure 15.3*e*), or yaw (Figure 15.3*c*) angular velocity without an accompanying roll, pitch, or yaw tilt with respect to gravity.

There are also three dimensions for linear motion. As for angular velocity, translations are defined relative to a coordinate system that moves with the head. Imagine (1) stepping forward or backward along the x-axis (**Figure 15.4***a*), (2) sliding from right to left along the y-axis (Figure 15.4*b*), or (3) translating up or down along the z-axis (Figure 15.4*c*). Translation along a straight line in any direction can be expressed as some amount of each of these three perpendicular translations (Figure 15.4*g*). For example, one can move forward and to the left while on an elevator that is simultaneously moving upward. Translations along the x-axis (Figure 15.4*d*), y-axis (Figure

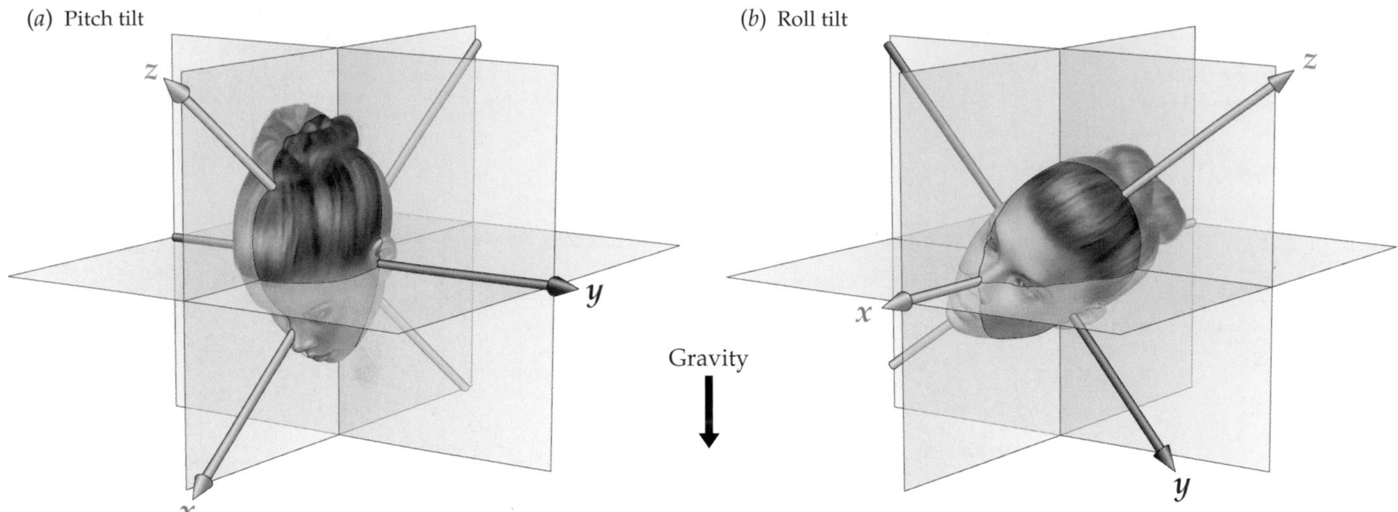

FIGURE 15.5 When you are initially upright with respect to gravity, there are two directions of tilt. You can pitch-tilt forward or backward (*a*), or you can roll-tilt to the left or right (*b*). For either tilt direction, the amplitude of the tilt can be small or large.

15.4*e*), and z-axis (Figure 15.4*f*) can also occur when the subject is lying down; recall that the xyz coordinate system moves with the head.

Finally, each orientation has two tilt directions. For example, when you are upright, you might experience a pitch tilt forward or backward (**Figure 15.5***a*). Or you might experience a roll tilt to the left or right (Figure 15.5*b*). What happened to the third dimension? The third rotation direction would be a yaw rotation, but this would not yield a change in the tilt of the head with respect to gravity (see Figure 15.3*c*). When head rotations align with gravity, there is no change in head tilt. So there are three directions for angular velocity (see Figure 15.3) and translation (see Figure 15.4), but only two directions for tilt.

AMPLITUDE The second quality of spatial orientation is amplitude. For linear motion we can perceive translation having high velocity (think of a car speeding along a freeway) or low velocity (think of the car in a crowded parking lot). Similarly, we can perceive rotation with a high amplitude (think of vigorously shaking your head) or a low amplitude. Finally, tilt amplitude is also important. Tilt amplitudes can be small (as when you nod your head) or large (as when you lie down or hang upside down).

Peripheral Structure of the Mammalian Vestibular System

To sense these various motions of the head, you need the sensors found in your vestibular system. The vestibular system's alternate name—"vestibular labyrinth"—reflects the anatomical complexity of the vestibular apparatus. It is about the size of a large pea or a small marble and can be found in the inner ear right next to the cochlea (**Figure 15.6**). The vestibular organs respond primarily to head motion—both linear and angular—and head tilt with respect to gravity. Each inner ear has one vestibular labyrinth, and each vestibular labyrinth includes five sense organs: three semicircular canals that sense rotational motion, and two otolith organs that sense gravity and linear acceleration. (See **Web Activity 15.1: A Guided Tour of the Vestibular System**.)

Hair Cells—Mechanical Transducers

hair cells Cells that support the stereocilia that transduce mechanical movement in the vestibular labyrinth into neural activity sent to the brain stem.

mechanoreceptors Sensory receptors that are responsive to mechanical stimulation (pressure, vibration, movement).

Like the hair cells involved in hearing, **hair cells** act as the **mechanoreceptors** in each of the five vestibular organs. As described in Chapter 9, pressure

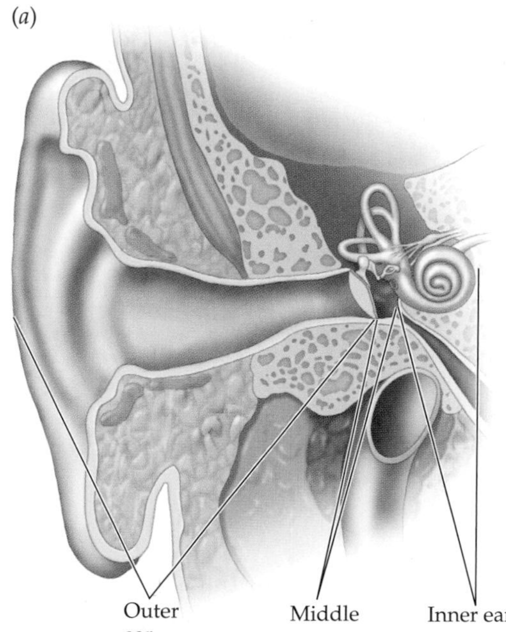

FIGURE 15.6 The vestibular apparatus is a membranous, fluid-filled sac that occupies a cavity in the temporal bone, near the cochlea, and is the nonhearing part of the inner ear. It consists of three semicircular canals—anterior, posterior, and horizontal—and two otolith organs—the utricle and saccule—on each side of the head.

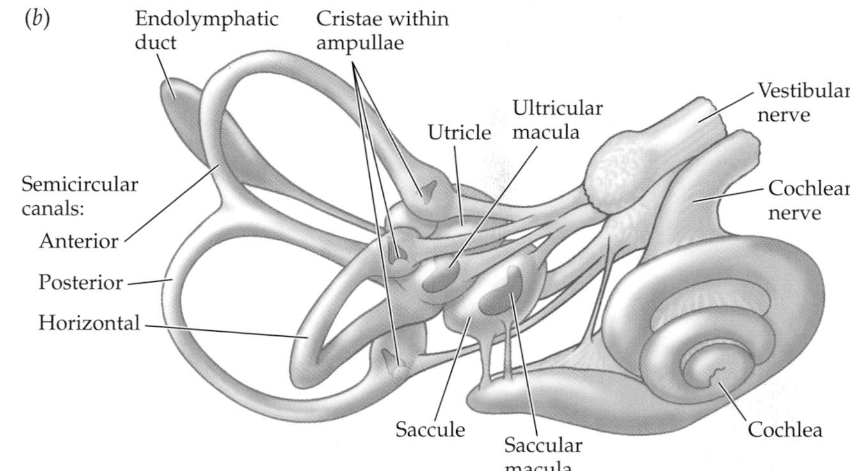

waves in the cochlea move cochlear membranes that, in turn, bend hair cell stereocilia. The process is similar for the vestibular organs, except that the hair cell motion is caused by head motion, which causes hair cell stereocilia to deflect. Stereocilia deflection causes a change in the hair cell voltage, which alters neurotransmitter release, which, in turn, evokes action potentials in those vestibular nerve fibers that have one or more dendritic synapses with the hair cell. These afferent neurons carry these action potentials to the brain.

Let's consider the hair cell responses in a bit more detail. In the absence of stimulation, the hair cells have a negative voltage and release neurotransmitter at a constant rate, evoking a constant rate of action potentials in the afferent neurons (**Figure 15.7***a*). Changes in hair cell voltage—called the **receptor potential**—are proportional to the bending of the hair cell bundles and control the rate at which hair cells release neurotransmitter to the afferent neurons. When a hair cell bends toward the tallest stereocilia (Figure 15.7*b* and *c*), the hair cell voltage becomes less negative. This voltage change is also called a depolarization because the hair cell becomes less polarized than the negative resting potential (Figure 15.7*a*). Through a series of bioelectrochemical reactions, the hair cell depolarization increases the release of neurotransmitter, causing an increase in the action potential rate (called excitation). On the other hand, if the hair cell is bent away from the tallest stereocilia, the cell potential becomes more negative (hyperpolarizes), causing a decrease in the release of neurotransmitter and a decrease in the action potential rate (called inhibition). In summary, the rate of action potentials transmitted by afferent neurons increases or decreases following the hair cell receptor potential. Thinking back to the fact that amplitude is one quality of our vestibular sense, we can begin to see how amplitude is encoded, since the rate of action potentials is proportional to the receptor potential, which, in turn, is proportional to the amount of hair cell deflection.

The fact that the hair cells respond oppositely for deflections in opposite directions (see Figure 15.7*a*) is crucial for the coding of vestibular stimuli. For example, as we'll discuss in detail in the following section, a yaw rotation to the left will increase the hair cell receptor potential of a horizontal

receptor potential The change in voltage of sensory receptor cells—hair cells for the vestibular system—in response to stimulation.

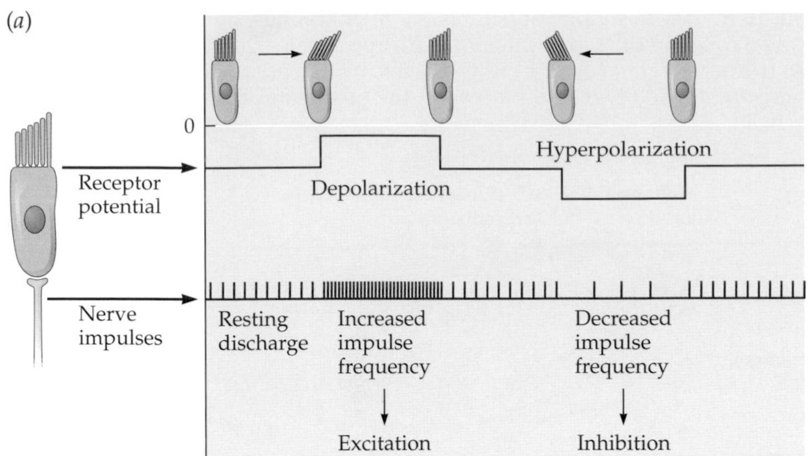

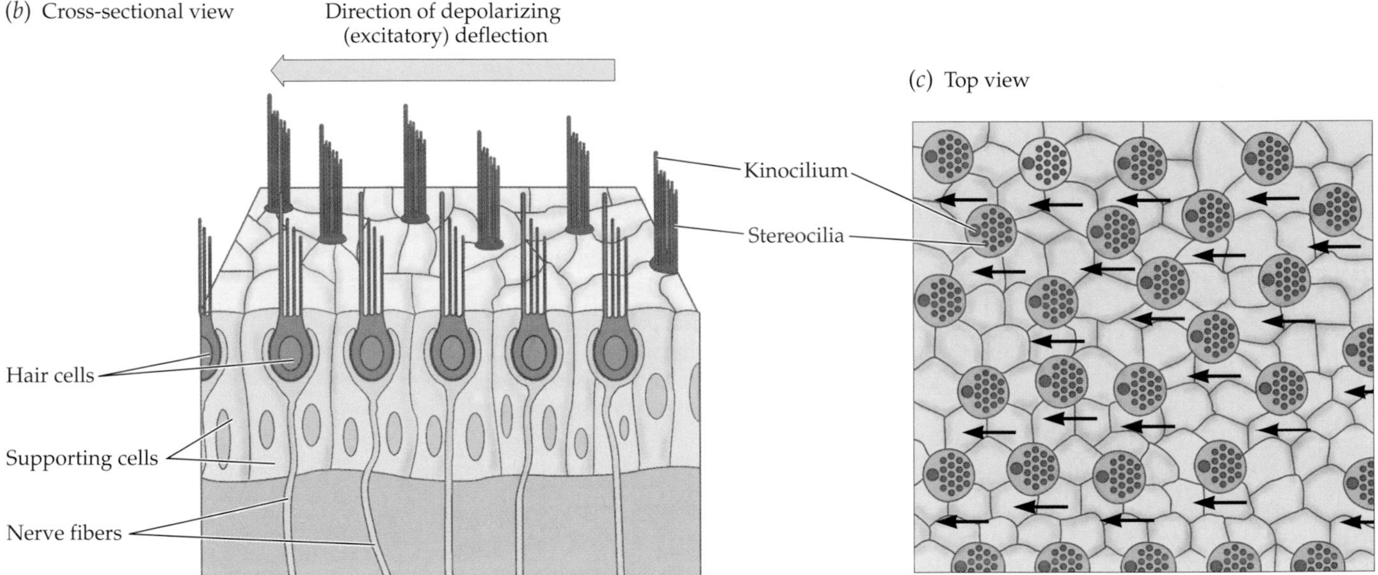

FIGURE 15.7 Hair cell responses. (*a*) In the absence of stimulation, the hair cells have a negative voltage and release neurotransmitter at a constant rate, evoking a constant rate of action potentials in the afferent nerves. When hair cell stereocilia bend toward the kinocilium and the tallest stereocilia, the hair cell voltage becomes less negative (depolarizes). When the stereocilia bend away from the kinocilium, the voltage becomes more negative (hyperpolarizes). These voltage changes control the rate at which hair cells release neurotransmitter. (*b*) A cross-sectional view of a hair cell array, showing the direction of deflection that causes depolarization. (*c*) A top view of a hair cell array.

canal located in the left ear, and a yaw rotation to the right will decrease the receptor potential for that same hair cell. A similar general principle applies for the otolith organs: acceleration in one direction yields increases in the receptor potentials of some hair cells, while acceleration in the opposite direction yields decreases in the receptor potentials for those same hair cells. This is an important part of how the other vestibular quality—direction—is transduced and encoded.

Semicircular Canals

The name *semicircular canal* roughly reflects the gross anatomy of this structure, which has the circular shape of a toroid or doughnut (**Figure 15.8**). About three-fourths of the toroid—hence the name *semi*circular—is formed by a tube about 15 millimeters (mm) long, with a cross section about 1.5 mm in diameter. This space—called the osseous (or bony) canal because it is a canal carved out of the mastoid bone—is filled with a fluid called perilymph. The remaining length of the toroid passes through the vestibule. A second, smaller toroid is found inside the larger toroid. This smaller toroid is

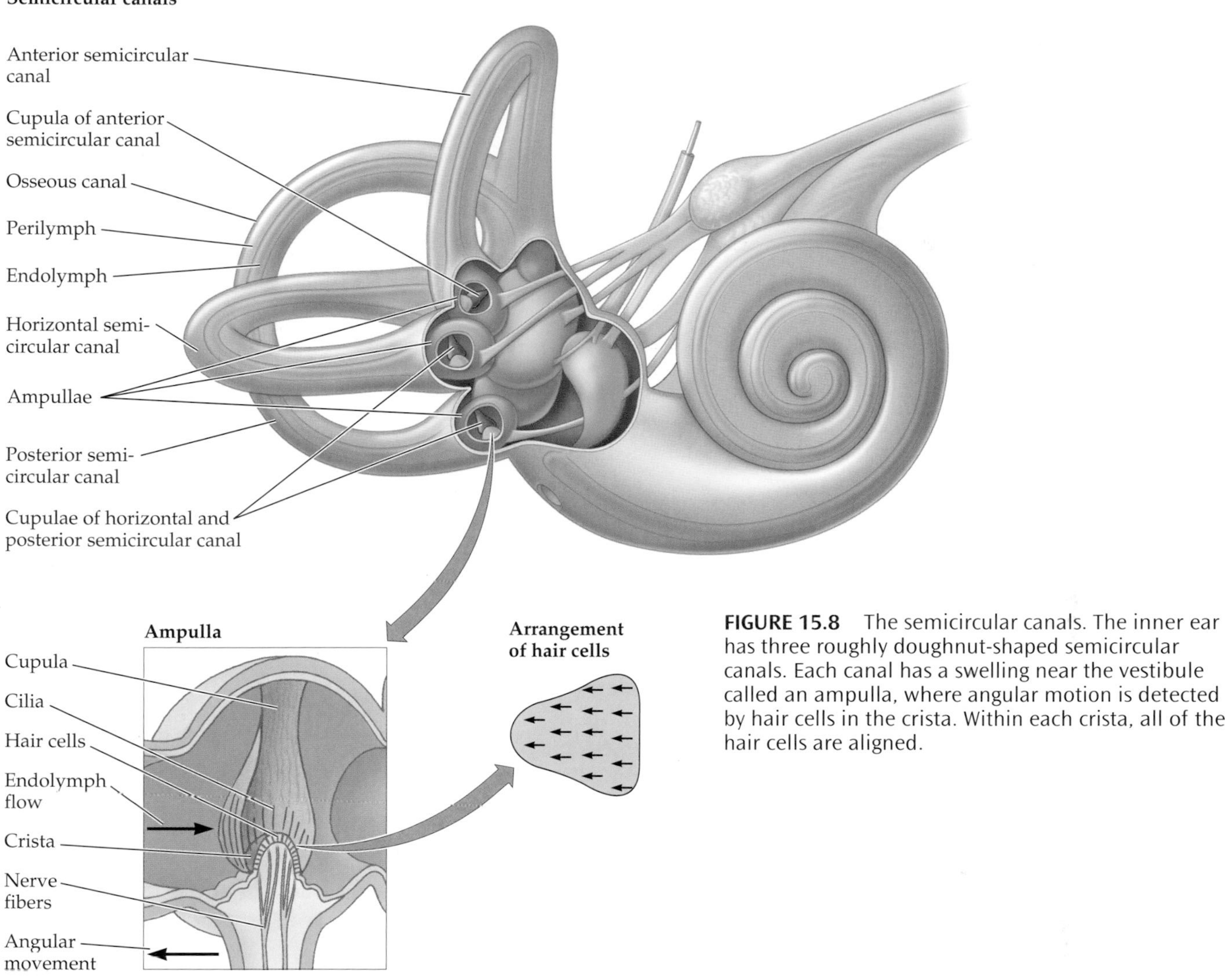

FIGURE 15.8 The semicircular canals. The inner ear has three roughly doughnut-shaped semicircular canals. Each canal has a swelling near the vestibule called an ampulla, where angular motion is detected by hair cells in the crista. Within each crista, all of the hair cells are aligned.

formed by a membrane filled with a fluid called endolymph, and in cross section it has a diameter of about 0.3 mm, which is just a little thicker than a very thick human hair.

The cross section for each canal swells substantially near where the canals join the vestibule. Each swelling is called an ampulla (plural *ampullae*) (see Figure 15.8). Within the endolymph space of each ampulla, the angular motion detectors are assembled into a sensory epithelium called the **crista** (plural *cristae*). Each crista consists of a small ridge, which has an epithelium made of about 7000 hair cells and associated supporting cells and nerve fibers. The cilia of the hair cells project into a jellylike cupula (plural *cupulae*) that forms an elastic dam extending to the opposite wall of the ampulla, with endolymph on both sides of the dam.

When the head rotates, the inertia of the endolymph causes it to lag behind the motion of the head, which leads to tiny deflections of the hair cells. As mentioned earlier, such deflections evoke voltage changes in the hair cells, which, in turn, cause changes in the firing rate of afferent neurons. For each individual semicircular canal, all of the hair cells are aligned (see Figure 15.8). Thus, rotations in one direction yield increases in the receptor potential

cristae The specialized detectors of angular motion located in each semicircular canal in a swelling called the ampulla.

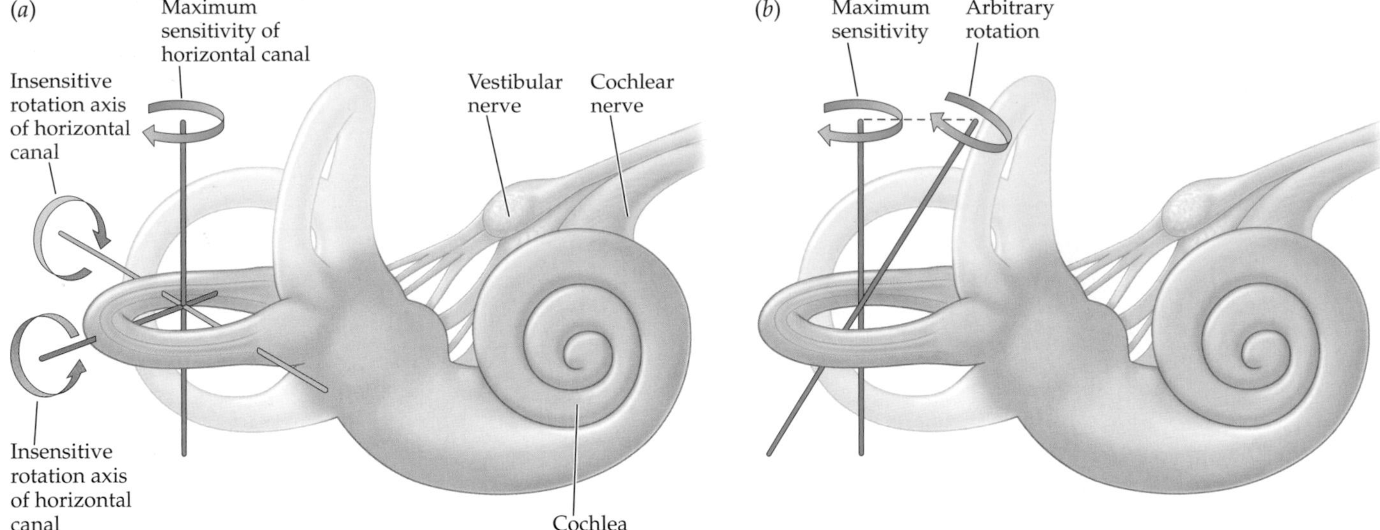

FIGURE 15.9 Each semicircular canal is maximally sensitive to rotations perpendicular to the canal plane. (*a*) Thinking of each semicircular canal as a wheel, we can see that the canals are maximally sensitive to rotations that align with the rotation axis (shown in green) and are insensitive to rotations that fall in the plane of the semicircular canal (e.g., purple and blue). (*b*) For any arbitrary rotation, we can find the component that aligns with the canal's maximum-sensitivity axis.

of all hair cells in that semicircular canal and concomitant increases in the action potential rate for all neurons that innervate that semicircular canal. Rotations in the opposite direction yield decreases in the hair cell receptor potentials and concomitant decreases in the rate of action potentials.

CODING OF DIRECTION IN THE SEMICIRCULAR CANALS Each inner ear has three semicircular canals—horizontal (or lateral), anterior (or superior), and posterior. The three canals are maximally sensitive to rotations in different planes, thus yielding part of the direction coding for head rotation.

Specifically, each canal is maximally sensitive to rotations around the axis perpendicular to it and insensitive to rotations about axes that fall in the plane of that canal (**Figure 15.9**). Think of the canal as a wheel that can spin about the center of the doughnut. The canal is maximally sensitive to rotations aligned with the wheel axle and insensitive to rotations perpendicular to the wheel axle.

We already considered the other part of direction coding—the fact that the hair cells and neurons for any individual canal increase their firing rate for rotations in one direction and decrease for rotations in the other direction. In fact, the semicircular canals are organized as functional pairs in what is called a push–pull arrangement. The two horizontal canals—one on the right side of the head and one on the left—lie in the same plane and form one of the three functional canal pairs (**Figure 15.10***a*). The horizontal-canal afferent neurons on the right all increase their firing rate for yaw head turns to the right (shaking "no"), and the horizontal-canal neurons on the left decrease their firing rate. For head turns to the left, the pattern is reversed, with left-canal afferent neurons increasing their firing rate and right-canal neurons decreasing their firing rate. The anterior and posterior canals are minimally sensitive to these yaw rotations.

In contrast to the horizontal-canal arrangement, the mirror symmetry of the semicircular canals in the left and right ears yields functional pairs that involve different vertical canals (Figure 15.10*b*); the maximum-sensitivity axis of the anterior semicircular canal on one side parallels the maximum-sensitivity axis of the posterior semicircular canal on the opposite side. So the right anterior and left posterior canals form one canal pair, as do the left anterior and right posterior canals. These canal pairs work in a push–pull manner like that previously described for the horizontal canals.

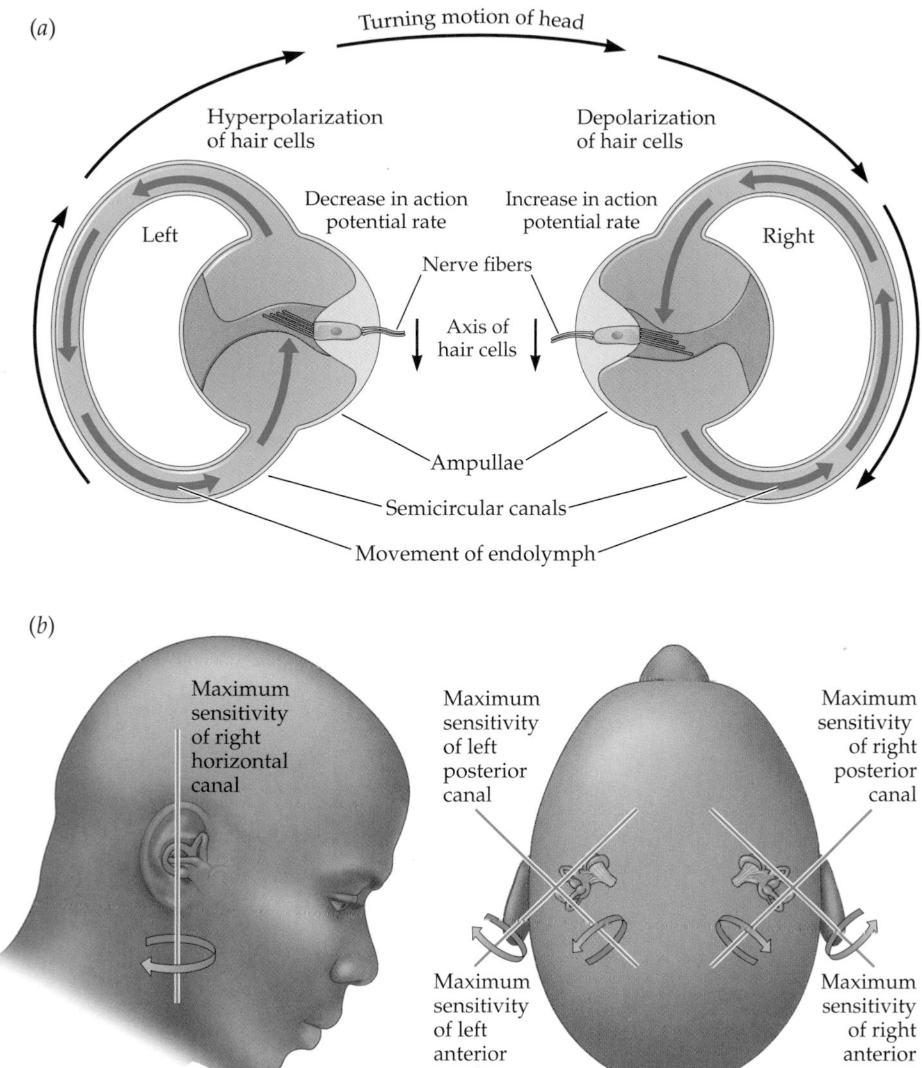

FIGURE 15.10 The semicircular canals function in pairs that have a push–pull relationship. (*a*) Bilateral stimulation of the horizontal semicircular canals as the head turns to the right (a yaw head rotation as shown in Figure 15.3*c*, but in the opposite direction). This yaw rotation produces relative movement of the endolymph in the horizontal semicircular canals on both sides of the head. The movement of the fluid bends the hair cells toward the tallest stereocilia on the right side, which depolarizes these hair cells and increases the rate of action potentials for neurons from the right side. The hair cells move away from the tallest stereocilia on the left, hyperpolarizing the hair cell voltage and decreasing the rate of action potentials for left-side neurons. This response—an increase on one side coupled with a response decrease on the other side—is often called a "push–pull response." (*b*) Arrangement of the canals in functional push–pull pairs. The two horizontal canals form one pair. The right anterior canal and the left posterior canal form another pair. Note that the maximum-sensitivity axes for the right anterior and left posterior canals are parallel. This means that they maximally respond to rotations around the same axis. The push–pull nature of this canal pair is a consequence of the opposite directions of their maximum-sensitivity rotations, as shown by the green arrows. The left anterior canal and the right posterior canal also form a similar push–pull canal pair.

CODING OF AMPLITUDE IN THE SEMICIRCULAR CANALS In the absence of any rotation, many afferent neurons from the semicircular canals respond with a nearly constant rate of action potentials; canal afferent firing rates at rest average about 100 action potentials ("spikes") per second, which is high relative to spontaneous rates for nerve fibers for other sensory systems. For comparison, recall that retinal ganglion cells fire spontaneously at a rate of about 1 spike per second in the dark. The relatively high spontaneous firing rate of vestibular afferent neurons allows these neurons to decrease the firing rate for rotations in one direction and increase the firing rate for rotations in the opposite direction.

The change in the firing rate is larger for large changes in the angular velocity of the head than for small changes in head velocity. Since the change in the firing rate is proportional to angular velocity, we can think of the canals as being somewhat similar to the speedometer in a car, but for the semicircular canals the change in neural activity is proportional to the angular velocity of the head. As a specific example, if the afferent neurons from a horizontal canal suddenly change their firing rate, we know that the rotation includes a component aligned with the sensitive axis of the horizontal canal.

(*a*)

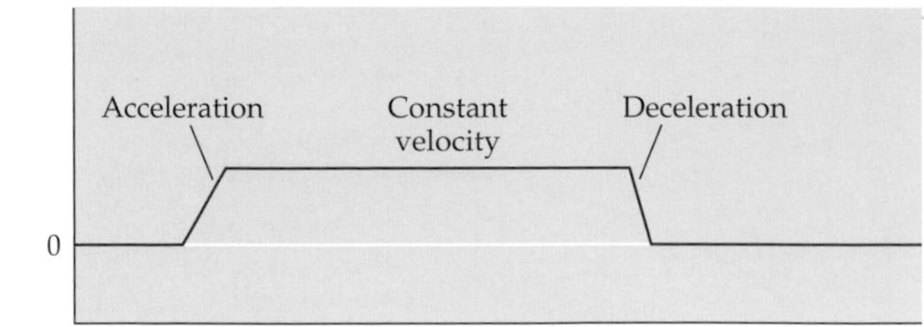

(*b*)

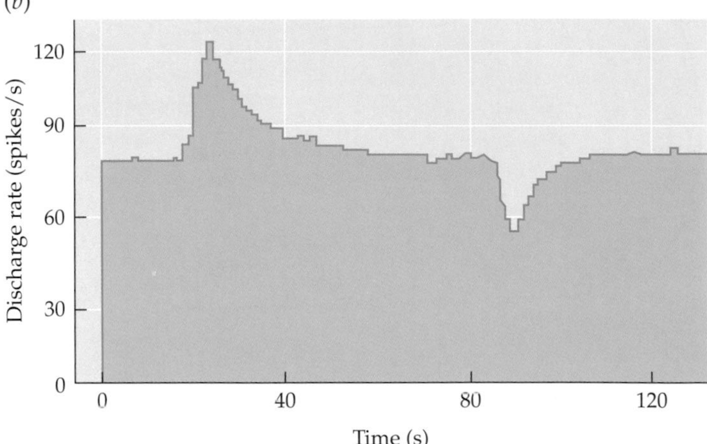

FIGURE 15.11 Response of a semicircular-canal neuron to rotation. (*a*) The stimulus is a rotation that first accelerates to a constant velocity, then maintains constant angular velocity, then decelerates the head to a stop. (*b*) During the initial acceleration, the cupula deflects, causing the neuron activity to increase. During the constant angular velocity, the cupula returns to its nondeflected position, so the neuron activity returns to the baseline rate after about 15 seconds of constant-velocity rotation. During deceleration, the cupula is deflected in the opposite direction, causing a transient decrease in the firing rate. (After Goldberg and Fernandez, 1971.)

More specifically, the change in the firing rate is proportional to the magnitude of the change in the angular-velocity component that aligns with that canal's sensitive axis. The same is true for all canals.

SEMICIRCULAR-CANAL DYNAMICS If you suddenly begin to rotate at a constant velocity, the semicircular canals sensitive to that rotation will respond with a sudden change in afferent activity. But as the rotation continues at a constant velocity, the afferent neural activity will decay back to near zero after about 15 seconds. If you then suddenly decelerate to a stop, the canals show a large response in the direction opposite of that first experienced (**Figure 15.11**). The afferent neural activity then decays with a time course similar to that during the constant-velocity rotation.

We will talk more about perception later, but for now, here's a simple example: if you are spun on a barstool in the dark at a nearly constant velocity, you will initially perceive an angular velocity that is roughly the same as the actual rotation. However, if the constant-velocity rotation lasts 20 seconds or so, you will perceive that you are slowing down. If the constant-velocity rotation continues for 30 to 60 seconds, you will perceive that you are no longer rotating. And what happens if you suddenly stop? You will perceive a rotation in the opposite direction; this illusory rotation also decays, typically lasting about 30 seconds. Many of us played with this illusion as children. (And some amusement park junkies still play with this illusion!) In any event, both the sensations described here and the neural responses shown in Figure 15.11 emphasize a very important characteristic of the semicircular canals: they are very good at sensing changes in angular velocity but bad at sensing constant-velocity rotations.

Figure 15.12 shows how the canal afferent response changes with head rotation frequency. As in audition, frequency is given in Hz—cycles per second—but the relevant frequencies are much lower. You do not want to shake your head at 4000 Hz (a fine auditory frequency). To experience a high-frequency head rotation, shake your head back and forth as if to emphatically say "no." When we try very hard, most of us can move the head back and

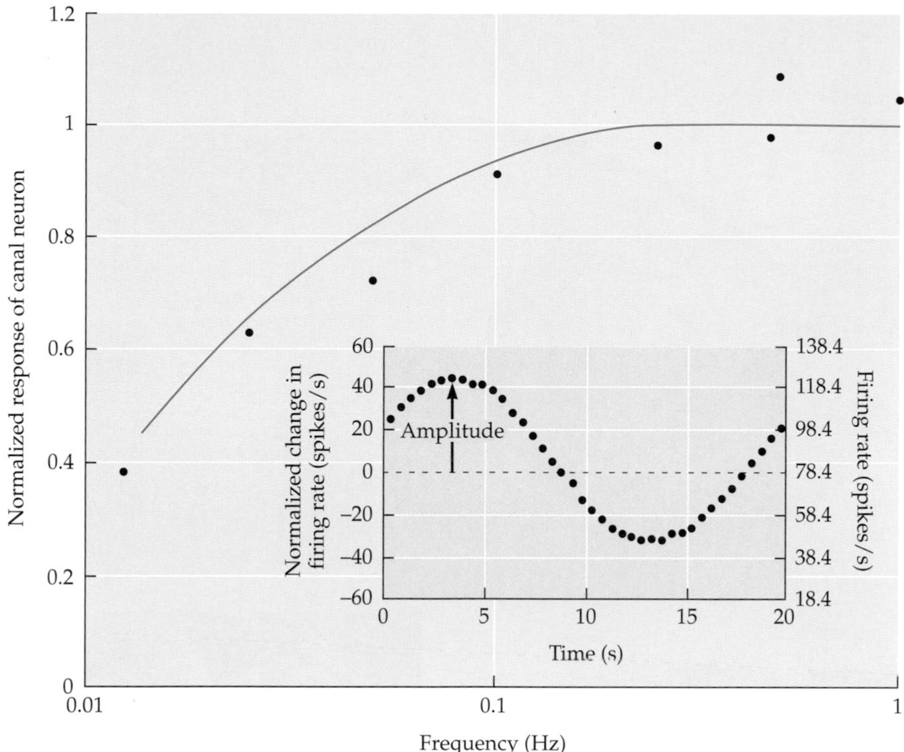

FIGURE 15.12 The semicircular canals have a nearly constant response at physiological frequencies: above about 0.1 Hz. The response decreases substantially for low frequencies: 0.03 Hz and below. The inset provides an example of the sinusoidal response at 0.05 Hz. Note that the change in the neural response amplitude is about 40 spikes per second. This change in the response amplitude is about 73% of the average change observed at the three highest frequencies. Data are normalized so that the average response at the three highest frequencies equals 1. (Data from Fernandez and Goldberg, 1971.)

forth in less than 1 second—a rotation frequency greater than 1 Hz. Figure 15.12 shows that the canal afferents respond maximally with a nearly constant response amplitude for high frequency rotations near 1 Hz, but that the canal afferents respond relatively poorly to very low rotation frequencies like 0.01 Hz (one cycle in 100 seconds). The amplitude of the canal responses decreases as the frequency decreases below 0.1 Hz (one cycle in 10 seconds). So, the canals transduce high-frequency responses appropriately, but they are not very good transducers at low frequencies—an effect that amusement park rides use to great advantage. (See **Web Essay 15.3: Amusement Park Rides—Vestibular Physics Is Fun.**)

Otolith Organs

As we mentioned before, the sensing of gravity and linear acceleration relies on two structures in each ear called the otolith organs—the **utricle** (or utriculus) and the **saccule** (or sacculus) (**Figure 15.13***a*). Each of these organs consists of a small, oval-shaped, fluid-filled sac that is about 3 mm long in the longest direction and includes an area called the **macula** (plural *maculae*) which is where actual sensory transduction occurs. Each macula is roughly planar and is sensitive primarily to shear forces, which are forces parallel with the macular plane. Forces perpendicular to the macular plane have little influence on neural response. The shear forces, which are due to gravity and/or linear acceleration, cause small movements parallel to the macular plane, which, in turn, deflect the hair cells and produce changes in the afferent firing rate.

Each human utricular macula contains about 30,000 hair cells; and each saccular macula, about 16,000. The hairs of the otolith hair cells are encased in a gelatinous structure (Figure 15.13*b*) that contains calcium carbonate crystals called **otoconia** (singular *otoconium*) (Figure 15.13*c*). These small stones give the otolith organs their name: *oto* means "ear," and *lithos* means

utricle One of the two otolith organs. A saclike structure that contains the utricular macula.

saccule One of the two otolith organs. A saclike structure that contains the saccular macula.

maculae The specialized detectors of linear acceleration and gravity found in each otolith organ.

otoconia Tiny calcium carbonate stones in the ear that provide inertial mass for the otolith organs, enabling them to sense gravity and linear acceleration.

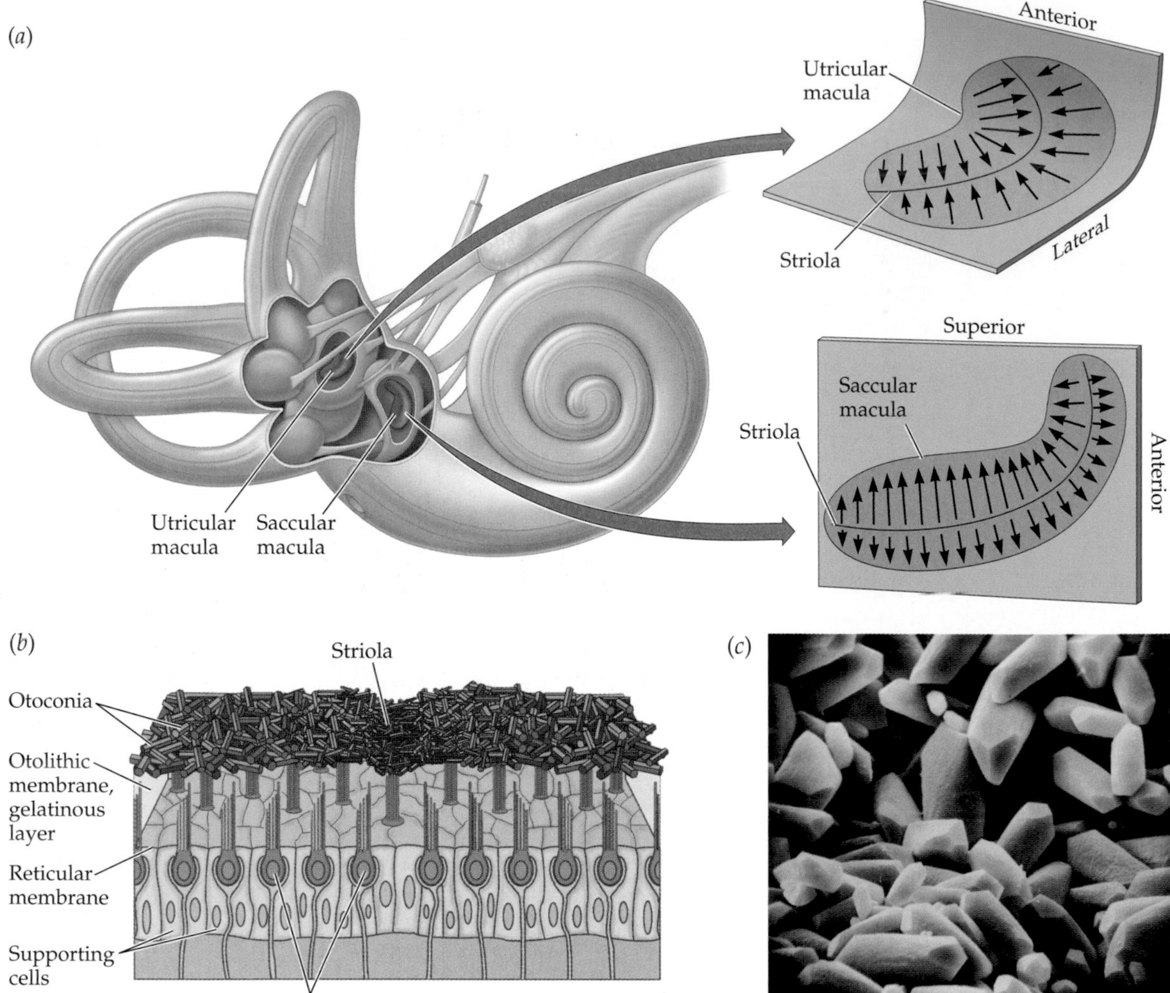

FIGURE 15.13 The otolith organs. (*a*) Orientation of the utricular and saccular maculae in the head. The saccules are oriented more or less vertically; and the utricles, more or less horizontally. The striola is a structural landmark consisting of small otoconia that divides each otolith organ. In the utricular macula, the tallest stereocilia are directed toward the striola. In the saccular macula, the tallest stereocilia point away from the striola. Arrows show the orientation of the tallest stereocilia. Because hair cells depolarize if stereocilia deflect toward the tallest stereocilia and hyperpolarize if deflection is away from the tallest, the arrows also show the movement direction that causes maximal neural excitation at each location on the maculae. Note that, given one utricle and saccule on each side of the body, there is a continuous representation of all directions for sensing gravity and linear acceleration. (*b*) Cross section of the utricular macula, showing hair bundles projecting into the gelatinous layer when the head is level. The structure of the saccular macula is very similar. (*c*) The otoconia shown in this scanning electron micrograph come from the utricular macula of a cat. Each crystal is about 50 millimeters long. (*c* from Lindeman, 1973.)

"stone" in Greek, so *otolith* translates as "ear stone." The otoconia are denser than the surrounding fluid. Like any dense object, they are pulled down by gravity and/or are moved whenever linear acceleration is present. The displacement of the otoconia drags the gelatinous layer, thereby moving the hair cell stereocilia, leading to changes in the hair cell receptor potential, which, in turn, cause changes in the rate of action potentials in the afferent neurons that convey information to the brain.

CODING OF DIRECTION IN THE OTOLITH ORGANS As with the semicircular canals, direction coding in the otolith organs arises, in part, from their anatomical orientation (see Figure 15.13*a*). The utricular macula is horizontal in the head; the saccular macula is oriented vertically in the head. Imagine the head in a standard upright orientation. Since these maculae are sensitive primarily to accelerations parallel to the plane of the macula and insensitive to accelerations perpendicular to the macula, the utricle will be sensitive primarily to forward–backward and/or side-to-side linear acceleration, as well as forward–backward pitch tilts and left–right roll tilts with respect to gravity (**Figure 15.14**). The saccule will be sensitive primarily to forward–backward and up–down linear accelerations, as well as forward–backward pitch tilts.

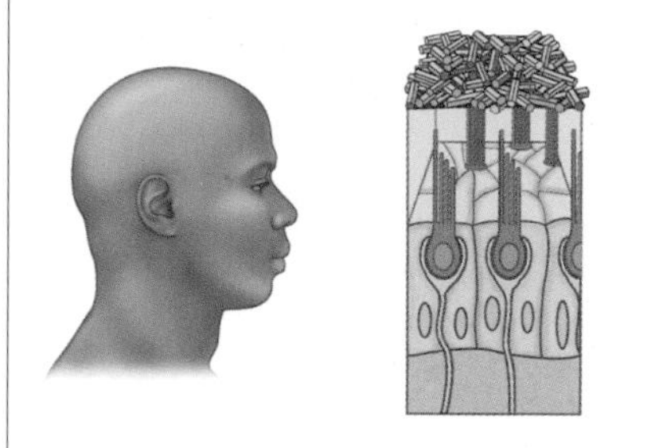

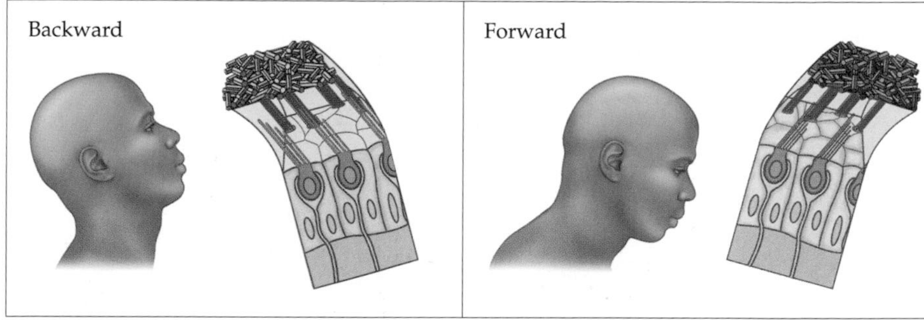

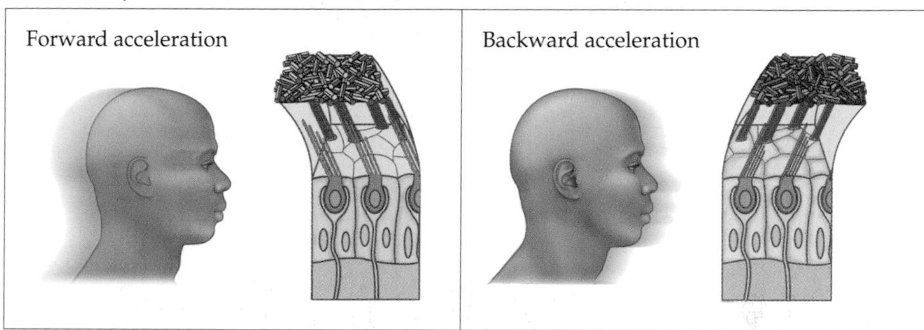

FIGURE 15.14 Forces acting on the head result in displacement of the otoconia. This example illustrates displacement of the utricular macula. For each of the head tilts and linear accelerations, some set of hair cells will be maximally excited, whereas another set will be maximally inhibited, according to the orientation of the hair cells. Note that head tilts and linear accelerations—when matched in direction and magnitude—produce similar otoconial movement, demonstrating that the otolith organs respond to both gravity and linear acceleration.

As in the semicircular canals, another aspect of the direction coding in the utricles and saccules can be found in the response of a single neuron or single hair cell. Recall that hair cell receptor potentials increase when hair bundle tips move toward the largest stereocilia, and receptor potentials decrease for movements in the opposite direction. Furthermore, the direction of rotation is coded by the brain's detection of excitation from a semicircular canal on one side and inhibition from the other side. This push–pull mechanism is incorporated into each macula in the otolith organs. Populations of hair cells on each macula have their stereocilia oriented in opposite directions (see Figure 15.13*a*). Both the utricle and the saccule include a central band called the striola. On opposite sides of the striola, hair cells are oriented in opposite directions. Remember that movement toward the tallest stereocilia produces excitation; movement in the opposite direction produces inhibition (see Figure 15.7). The same is true for otolith organ afferent neurons; tilts (or linear accelerations) in opposite directions cause opposite changes in firing rate (**Figure 15.15**). So an acceleration that maximally excites a hair cell and afferent neuron on one side of the striola will maximally inhibit a hair cell and afferent neuron on the opposite side. Given the variations in the orientation of the hair cells, cells in one region of the utricular macula will be maximally sensitive to forward–backward acceleration, while cells in another region will be maximally sensitive to side-to-side linear acceleration. In between, some cells will maximally respond to a linear acceleration that includes both forward–backward and side-to-side components.

CODING OF AMPLITUDE IN THE OTOLITH ORGANS Larger accelerations (or larger gravitational shear forces) move the otolith organs' otoconia more. This movement, in turn, leads to greater deflection of the hair cell bundles, which causes larger changes in the hair cell receptor potentials. The receptor potential evoked in an individual hair cell is proportional to the component of gravity or linear acceleration that is aligned with the sensitive axis of a

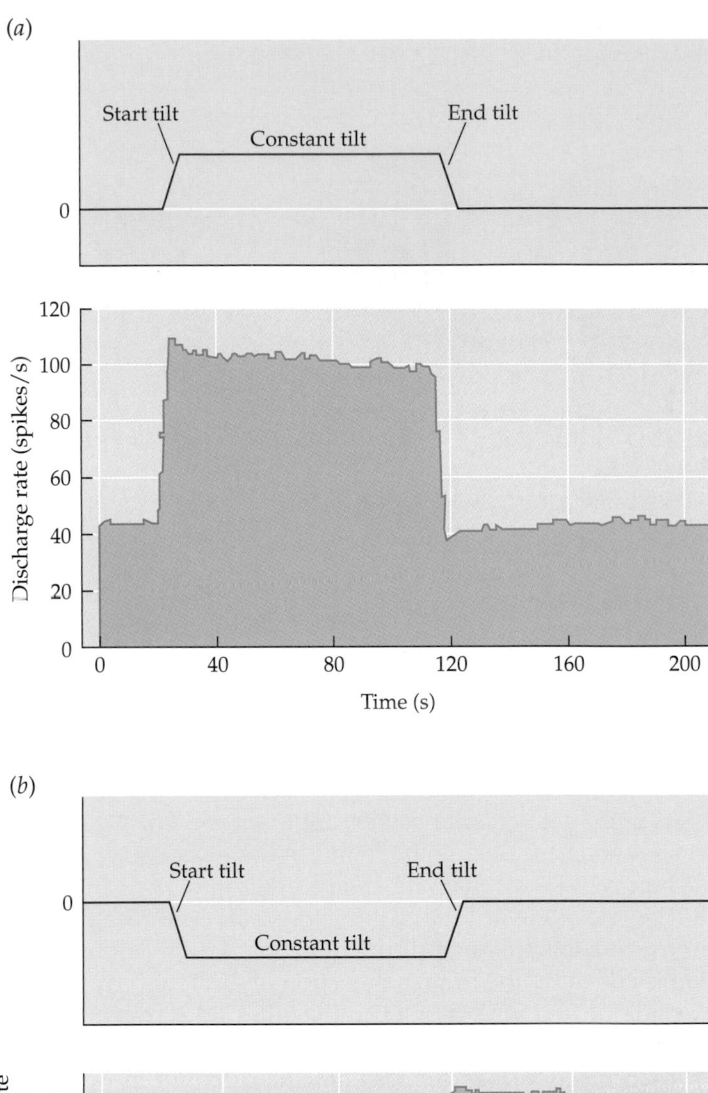

FIGURE 15.15 Activity of a vestibular nerve axon from the utricle (an otolith organ). (*a*) A change in head tilt is the stimulus (top). As shown in the histogram of the discharge rate (below), the neuron's activity increases in response to a tilt in a particular direction. (*b*) The same fiber decreases its activity in response to a tilt in the opposite direction. (After Goldberg and Fernandez, 1976.)

given hair cell. Larger changes in the hair cell receptor potential lead to larger changes in the rate of action potentials sent to the brain via afferent neurons.

Spatial Orientation Perception

Long after it was known that we see with our eyes and hear with our ears, the primary source for our perception of spatial orientation remained a mystery. In fact, in the eighteenth century, gross fluid shifts in the head were accepted as an explanation for the source of our sense of spatial orientation. Once it was established that this sense degrades when the vestibular system is damaged, it became clear that the vestibular system is a crucial source of information regarding spatial orientation. For example, when patients with vestibular loss are moved in the dark, they have a much more difficult time correctly detecting their motion than do people with normal vestibular function.

Today, three different techniques that you have encountered in measurements of the other senses are frequently used to investigate spatial orientation perception. These are threshold estimation, magnitude estimation, and matching methods. For example, we can ask, What is the minimum motion (the "threshold") required for correctly detecting the direction we are moved? Note that this is different from simply reporting *whether* we've moved, since vibration can provide a motion cue without informing about the direction of the motion. The vestibular system tells us more than whether motion is present or not; it actually informs us of the direction of motion—for example, whether we moved to the left or to the right.

In a magnitude estimation study, subjects might be asked to give verbal reports of how much they tilt, rotate, or translate using physical units like the number of degrees they rotated. Alternatively, magnitude estimation may utilize arbitrary scaling. For example, subjects may be trained to rotate a knob in proportion to their perceived velocity or provide a verbal indicator of their velocity on a scale of 1 to 10.

In a matching task, subjects might be asked to align a visual line with perceived Earth-vertical (which way is "down"). In such a task, the investigator could produce a vestibular stimulus by tilting the subject. That subject would be provided with a visible line in otherwise dark surroundings and with the ability to rotate the line to the perceived Earth-vertical. Alternatively, somatic sensation could be utilized instead of vision. For this technique, subjects might be asked to adjust a bar that they can feel but not see so that it is aligned with the perceived horizon.

Rotation Perception

When subjects are rotated in the dark (or with their eyes closed), they first feel a sense of motion consistent with their actual motion. If the actual rotation continues at a constant speed, however, the perceived motion changes—subjects feel as if they are slowing down (**Figure 15.16**). After about 30 seconds, subjects no longer feel that they are rotating. This description may remind you of the way the response of the semicircular canals decays during constant-velocity rotation (see Figure 15.11), but, interestingly, the time course of the perceptual decay is more gradual than that of the semicircular-canal signal sent to the brain. This effect is sometimes called "velocity storage" because the perception of rotation persists after the afferent signal from the

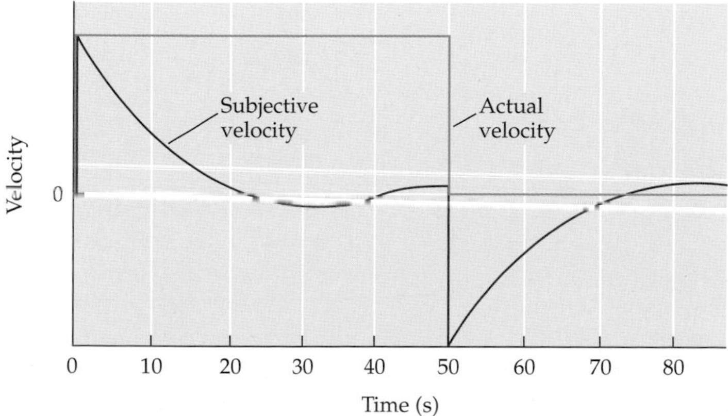

FIGURE 15.16 The green line on this graph shows the angular velocity of a person at rest, with eyes closed, who was suddenly rotated at a constant speed for 50 seconds, and then was abruptly returned to rest. Initially, the subject's estimate of angular velocity was accurate (purple line at time 0), but then the perceived velocity dropped to near 0 after about 20 seconds. When stopped, the subject perceived an abrupt velocity in the opposite direction, which mimicked the initial perception but in the opposite direction. (After Young, 1984.)

semicircular canals has dissipated. The velocity storage phenomenon is interesting and important because it shows that the brain has improved on the incoming sensory information to yield a rotation perception that—while far from perfect—is closer to the actual rotation than if the perception simply followed the time course of the semicircular-canal afferent signal.

Later, when subjects are abruptly brought to a stop, they perceive an angular velocity opposite that experienced when they were rotating. This rotation illusion is one that many of us played with as children when we would spin ourselves for a while and then suddenly stop spinning and try to stand or walk. The dizziness and imbalance that we experienced when we stopped rotating were due to the response of the semicircular canals, which causes an illusion of self-rotation.

One can develop an intuitive understanding of the cause of this illusion by considering an analogy with riding in a car. When you're riding at a constant velocity, you and the car are moving together. But when the car is suddenly stopped, you are thrown forward because you have momentum and keep moving even though the car has stopped. When you're rotating at a constant velocity, there is little or no hair cell deflection, because the endolymph and cupula are moving together. However, when the rotation is suddenly halted, the cupula stops moving quickly but the endolymph has momentum and tends to keep moving. Deflection of the hair cells results, and the direction of the hair cell response is opposite that measured when the constant-velocity rotation began.

How sensitive are we to vestibular stimuli? Direction detection thresholds for yaw rotation have been measured for rotational motion frequencies ranging from 0.05 Hz (one back-and-forth yaw rotation in 20 seconds) to 5 Hz (five back-and-forth yaw rotations in 1 second) with the subject's head roughly centered on the rotation axis. For frequencies of 0.5 Hz (one back-and-forth yaw rotation in 2 seconds) and above, the direction detection thresholds are roughly constant. Your head has to be moving at a speed of just a little below 1 degree per second. That is a rather slow turn of the head. It would take you 6 minutes to spin all the way around at that angular velocity of 1 degree per second. Clearly, we are very sensitive to rotation.

For frequencies below 0.2 Hz (one back-and-forth yaw rotation in 5 seconds), thresholds increase with decreasing frequency (**Figure 15.17**). Earlier we learned that the canals responded less and less as the frequency of rota-

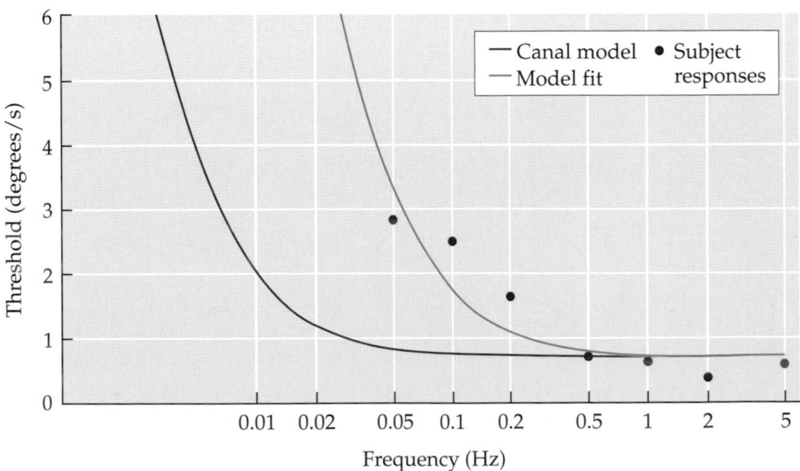

FIGURE 15.17 Mean velocity thresholds as a function of frequency for seven subjects. Threshold velocity was the peak velocity achieved during a single cycle of sinusoidal acceleration at which subjects correctly detected the direction of motion at least 79.4% of the time. The blue line shows a model fit to the data; the red line shows the theoretical threshold dynamics for the semicircular canals. Note that the measured threshold dynamics differ substantially from the response of the semicircular canals. This difference is probably due to central processing by the brain, but the exact mechanism and site are unknown. (After Grabherr et al., 2008.)

tion became smaller than 0.03 Hz. It is logical to consider that the change in the neural firing rate during rotation needs to exceed a certain amount for the rotation to be perceived. In this case, for very low frequency rotations, a larger-velocity rotation would be necessary to yield the same change in the canal firing rate. Thus, the direction detection threshold would increase for lower frequencies of rotation, as found experimentally.

These findings, however, cannot be explained entirely by the response dynamics of the semicircular canals, since the sensitivity of the canals begins to decrease at about 0.03 Hz—about one order of magnitude below the frequency at which the yaw rotation threshold begins to increase. Processing performed by the brain causes this difference.

Translation Perception

When subjects are passively translated short distances while seated on a chair in the dark and then asked, while still seated on the chair, to use a joystick to actively move the chair to reproduce the distance that they passively translated, they do so accurately. But even though not asked to do so, they also reproduce the velocity of the passive-motion trajectory (Berthoz et al., 1995). The unrequested replication of velocity suggests that the brain remembers and replicates the velocity trajectory. Earlier we said that the otolith organs transduce linear acceleration, which is the change in linear velocity. Therefore, replication of the velocity trajectory means that the brain also seems to mathematically integrate the acceleration signal provided by the otolith organs to yield a perception of linear velocity. This suggests that while otolith organs sense linear acceleration, our brains turn this into a perception of linear velocity.

Measured thresholds for detecting motion direction are also consistent with the idea that the brain integrates the linear acceleration transduced by the otolith organs to yield a perception of linear velocity. Data show that as long as linear acceleration is greater than about 5 cm/s^2, humans detect the direction of translation only when the linear velocity exceeds about 20 cm/s. For example, if a constant acceleration of 10 cm/s^2 were applied, it would take subjects about 2 seconds to determine the direction of motion—at which time they would be translating with a linear velocity of 20 cm/s. Data show that the direction of translation is detected correctly at an average velocity of about 20 cm/s for linear accelerations ranging between 5 and 60 cm/s^2.

Tilt Perception

How good we are at perceiving our tilt angle if we are positioned at a static orientation relative to gravity? For tilt angles of less than 90 degrees—that is, body orientations between standing up (0 degrees) and lying down (90 degrees)—we are quite good. This is true when any of the magnitude estimation techniques described earlier is used. Observers produce reliable answers if they indicate their perceived tilt verbally, or if they align a handheld probe with perceived vertical, or if they align a visible line with perceived vertical (**Figure 15.18**).

We are not perfect. Some consistent errors appear, especially in the subjective visual vertical task described earlier. Back in 1861, Aubert found that when he roll-tilted his head to the left or right while looking at a vertical streak of light, the vertical line appeared to tilt in the direction opposite his head tilt. For tilt angles less than 90 degrees, the illusory tilt error is typically about 10 degrees, but the apparent tilt of the visual line can be as large as 45

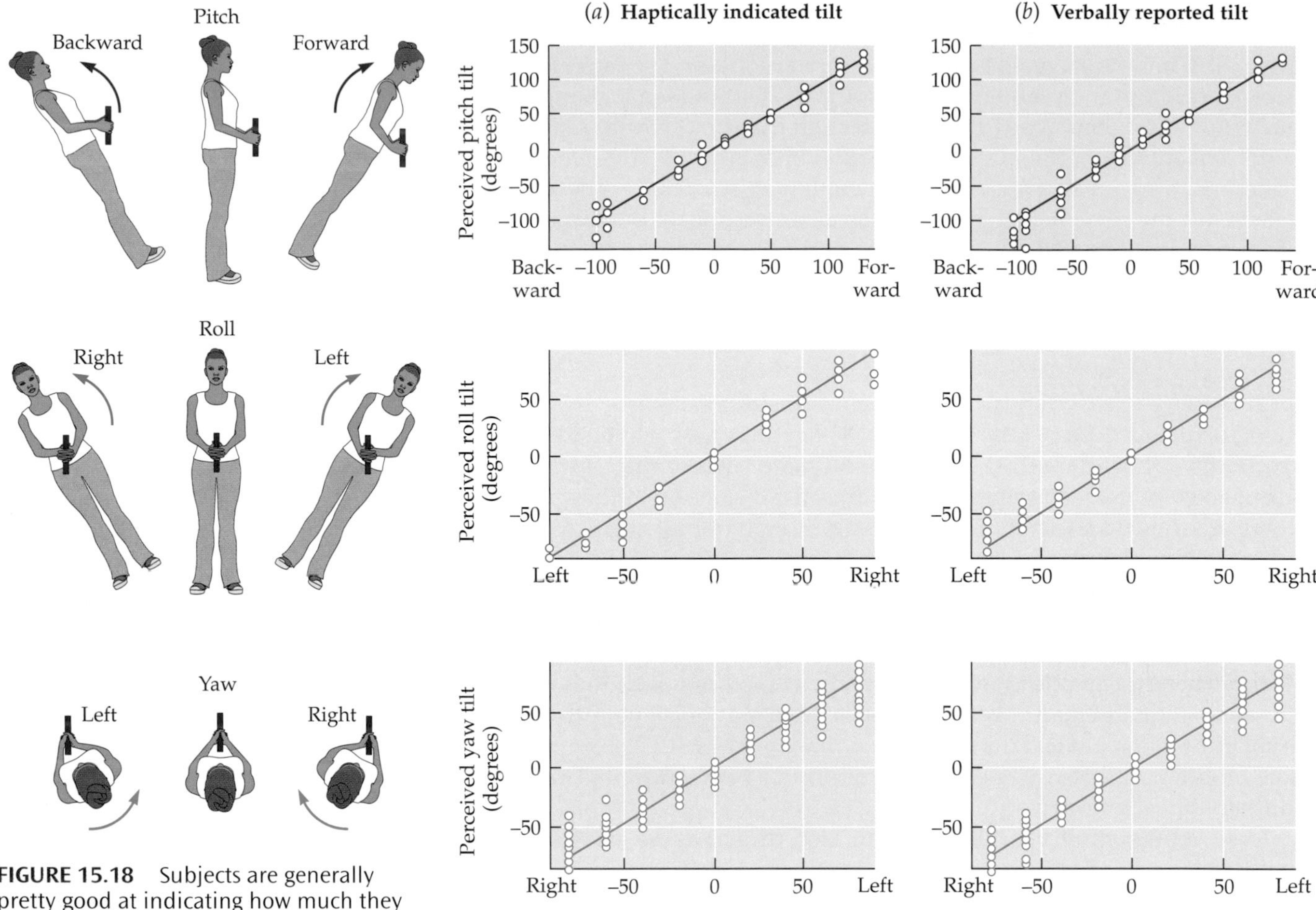

FIGURE 15.18 Subjects are generally pretty good at indicating how much they are tilted. Data (open circles) show tilt perception provided by subjects using a handheld haptic device (*a*) and verbally (*b*) for static pitch (top row), roll (middle row), and yaw (bottom row) tilts. Sketches at left define pitch, roll, and yaw and associated conventions. Perceived tilt roughly reflects the actual tilt (solid lines) for all three tilt directions. (After Bortolami et al., 2006.)

degrees when the head is tilted 135 degrees. You can investigate this illusion in a completely dark room by leaving the door open just a crack—just enough to see the line of light in the doorway without illuminating the room at all—while you hold your head at a tilted position. Does the line appear to tilt when your head is tilted? Does it move in the direction of your tilted head or in the opposite direction?

Thresholds for detection of the direction of tilt show that normal subjects correctly detect the direction of a static tilt when tilted just 2 degrees off vertical in the dark. This sensitivity serves our ability to stand upright, because standing up becomes more difficult the farther we are tilted from upright. For example, the amount of muscular effort required to maintain posture roughly doubles if we are tilted 4 degrees instead of 2 degrees, and just imagine the effort of trying to stand tilted even 15 degrees away from upright!

Sensory Integration

As we know, the senses do not operate independently. For example, visual cues influence sound localization—an effect utilized effectively by ventriloquists (this is related to the McGurk effect on speech perception discussed in Chapter 11). Vestibular signals combine with information from numerous sensory systems to provide us with an understanding of the position and movements of the head and body.

Visual–Vestibular Integration

Most of us have experienced illusions of self-motion caused by moving visual cues. Perhaps you have perceived self-motion while watching an IMAX movie. Or perhaps you've felt as if you were translating when you were stationary but the car (or train or bus) next to you began to move. Or perhaps you felt unsteady when standing on a bridge looking at the water flowing beneath. All of these situations can lead to perceptions of illusory self-motion called **vection**. Vection can be very compelling. For example, drivers stopped in traffic often press harder on the brake pedal when they perceive that they and their stopped car are moving, even though it is the cars around them that are moving.

vection An illusory sense of self motion produced when you are not, in fact, moving.

To consider the contributions of vection to spatial orientation, imagine a person standing upright while viewing the inside of a sphere rotating in roll (**Figure 15.19***a*). At first, subjective perceptions match reality; humans initially perceive that they are stationary and that the sphere is rotating. But if they continue to observe the rotating visual display for 10 seconds or so, they usually begin to perceive that they're rotating in the direction opposite the sphere rotation (Figure 15.19*b*). This illusory rotational vection demonstrates the crucial contributions of vision to our sense of self-rotation. In fact, retinal signals converge with the semicircular-canal signals in the vestibular nuclei, which is the first place in the brain that vestibular information reaches.

Paradoxically, subjects experiencing rotational vection like that described here almost never report that they are tumbling head over heels as they would if they truly were rotating to the extent that they perceive. In fact, subjects typically experience a simultaneous illusory sensation of tilt that gradually builds up to a relatively constant level (Figure 15.19*c*). These perceptions—experienced as a sensation of motion without getting anywhere—are contradictory, since we cannot be rotating relative to gravity (as suggested by the visual cues) while also maintaining a constant orientation with respect to gravity (as indicated by the otolith organs). In addition to exemplifying sensory integration, this sensation of motion without getting anywhere demonstrates that our sense of spatial orientation is not constrained to combinations of motion and orientation that are physically possible.

In this example, the role played by the vestibular system is to put the brakes on visually-induced vection. Patients suffering from severe vestibular damage generally report greater vection than do normal subjects. Astronauts

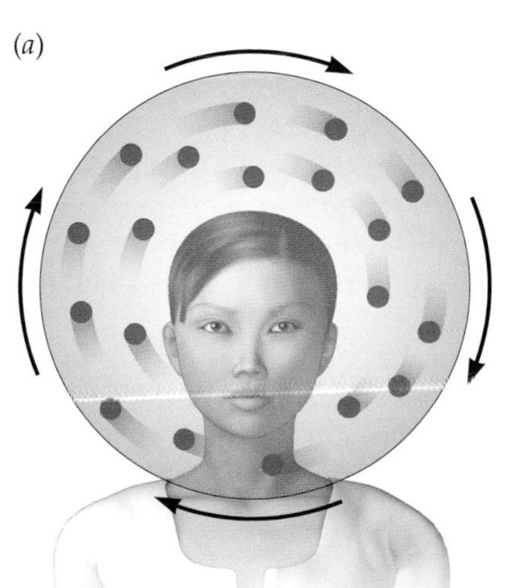

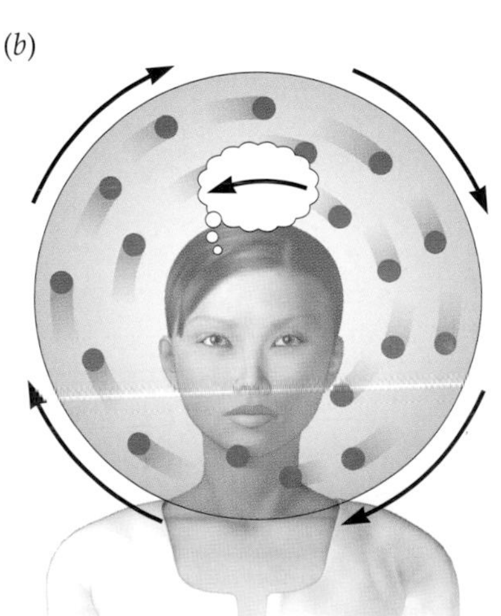

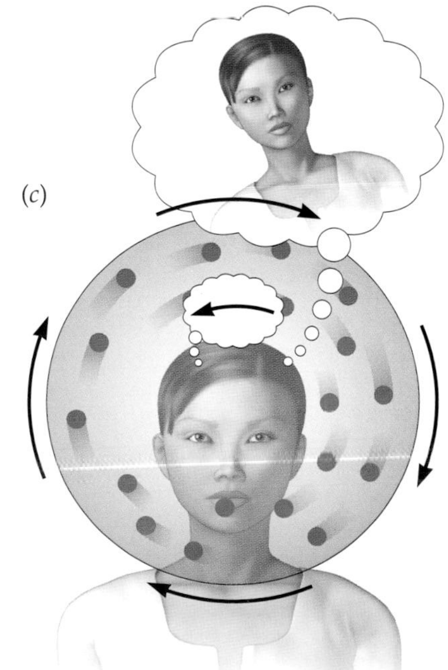

FIGURE 15.19 An illustration of rotational vection. (*a*) A subject views a visual display rotating in roll. For demonstration purposes, the visual display is shown here as transparent. Initially, subjects correctly sense that they are stationary and the visual display is rotating. (*b*) The subject begins to perceive that the motion of the display is slowing down, even though it is rotating at a constant velocity, and begins to experience vection—a sense of self-rotation in the direction opposite the rotation of the visual display. (*c*) Roll vection is often accompanied by an illusion of roll tilt that is induced by the perceived roll rotation. The direction of the perceived tilt is consistent with the tilt direction that would occur if the subject were truly rotating in roll. (After Young, Shelhamer, and Modestino, 1986.)

experiencing rotational vection in space—in the absence of gravitational signals—report a head-over-heels tumbling sensation that is absent on Earth. These findings are explained by the fact that neither the patients nor the astronauts receive normal gravitational cues from the otolith organs to contradict their visual rotational cues. (Web Essay 15.4: Space Motion Sickness discusses another aspect of spaceflight that many astronauts experience.) Since illusory motion is greater when there are no otolith cues to contradict the visual cues, we can infer that, under normal circumstances, information from the vestibular system is combined with visual information to yield a "consensus" about our sense of spatial orientation. Web Essay 15.5: Canal–Otolith Integration discusses a similar interaction of signals from the semicircular canals and otolith organs.

Reflexive Vestibular Responses

As mentioned earlier, some crucial contributions of the vestibular system are automatic, or reflexive, doing their work outside of conscious awareness. For example, there is a set of automatic responses called vestibulo-ocular reflexes—VORs for short. We started the chapter with one of these. Remember looking at your finger as you shook your head? (If not, now might be a good time to go back and try this demonstration again.) This task illustrated how the VOR contributes to visual stability by counterrotating the eyes in the head during head motion sensed by the vestibular system.

Then there is a set of vestibulo-autonomic reflexes that contribute to autonomic responses like those that regulate blood pressure and help maintain adequate blood flow to the brain. They also contribute to motion sickness. Finally, a set of vestibulo-spinal reflexes contributes to our balance or postural control. To demonstrate the vestibular contribution to your ability to stand upright, try standing on one foot with your eyes closed. (When you start to feel unsteady, immediately open your eyes and put both feet on the ground!) Most healthy people with normal vestibular function and a normal balance system can do this for at least 5 seconds and often much longer. Patients without vestibular function, however, cannot stand on one foot in the dark for more than a second or so.

Vestibulo-Ocular Responses

The most robust and well-studied vestibulo-ocular reflex is the angular VOR; the name derives from the fact that this eye movement helps compensate for *angular* rotations of the head. In fact, this reflex is so robust that it is a standard part of clinical examinations of vestibular function. The angular VOR is the compensatory eye rotation evoked by the semicircular canals when they sense head rotation. For example, when the head turns to the left, the reflex pathways cause the eye to rotate to the right with respect to the head, so as to compensate—at least in part—for the head turn. When observing the eye, we see this eye rotation as movement of the pupil to the right. Of course, since the eye is really a spherical eye*ball*, it is really rotating in the eye socket, not moving laterally.

Recall that six oculomotor muscles rotate the eyeball (see Chapter 7). Muscles can only pull; they cannot push. Muscles are paired to pull in opposite directions and are therefore called agonist–antagonist muscle pairs. For example, moving the left eye horizontally requires a coordination of the lateral rectus that pulls the eye to the left and the medial rectus that pulls the eye to the right. To make an eye movement to the right, the lateral rectus is inhibited and thus relaxes its pull, while the medial rectus is excited and

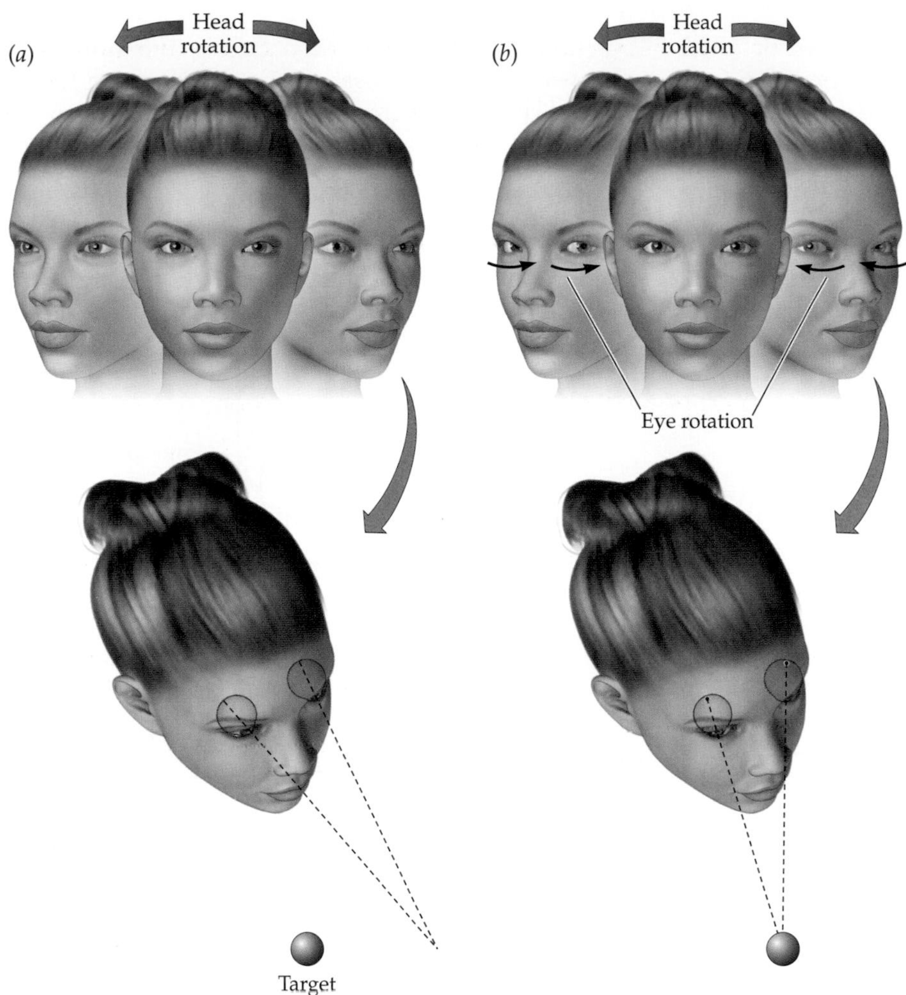

FIGURE 15.20 Contribution of the vestibulo-ocular reflex (VOR) to visual stability. (*a*) If the eyes rotate with the head, the image of the object is not foveated during a head rotation. (*b*) If the eye counterrotates during head rotation—with the amount of the eye rotation roughly equal to the amount of head rotation—then the image of an object can remain foveated even during head rotation. Note that the eyes continue to look at you in (*b*) but not in (*a*). This effect demonstrates how the VOR contributes to visual acuity, since this helps keep object images stationary on the retina, which reduces blurring.

thus increases its pull. The six oculomotor muscles are organized in three pairs that rotate the eye in each of three directions (see **Web Activity 15.2: Observing Torsional Eye Movement**). Eye movements result from a coordinated inhibition and excitation of the eye muscles.

When the vestibulo-ocular reflex is working effectively, it rotates the eye in the head such that, during head rotation, the eye rotates much less than the head. This smaller rotation of the eye with respect to the visual world helps stabilize the visual field on the retina (**Figure 15.20**). If the eyes do not counterrotate in the head, the retinal image tends to blur during head rotation. (Remember how your fingers blurred when you rapidly moved them back and forth?) The rotation of the eye in the head helps reduce this blur by reducing the motion of the image of an object across the retina.

The most direct neural path for the vestibulo-ocular reflexes consists of a chain of three neurons that yields reflexive eye responses with a latency of just 5 milliseconds. (That is really fast. Try doing anything else in 5 milliseconds.) The first of the three neurons is the afferent neuron that carries information from the vestibular periphery to the vestibular nuclei. There, the afferent neurons synapse with secondary neurons that then carry information to the ocular motor nuclei, where the secondary neurons synapse on oculomotor neurons that command the oculomotor muscles to rotate the eyeballs (**Figure 15.21**).

As you rotate your head from side to side, the angular VOR has properties similar to the characteristics that were discussed earlier for the semicircular

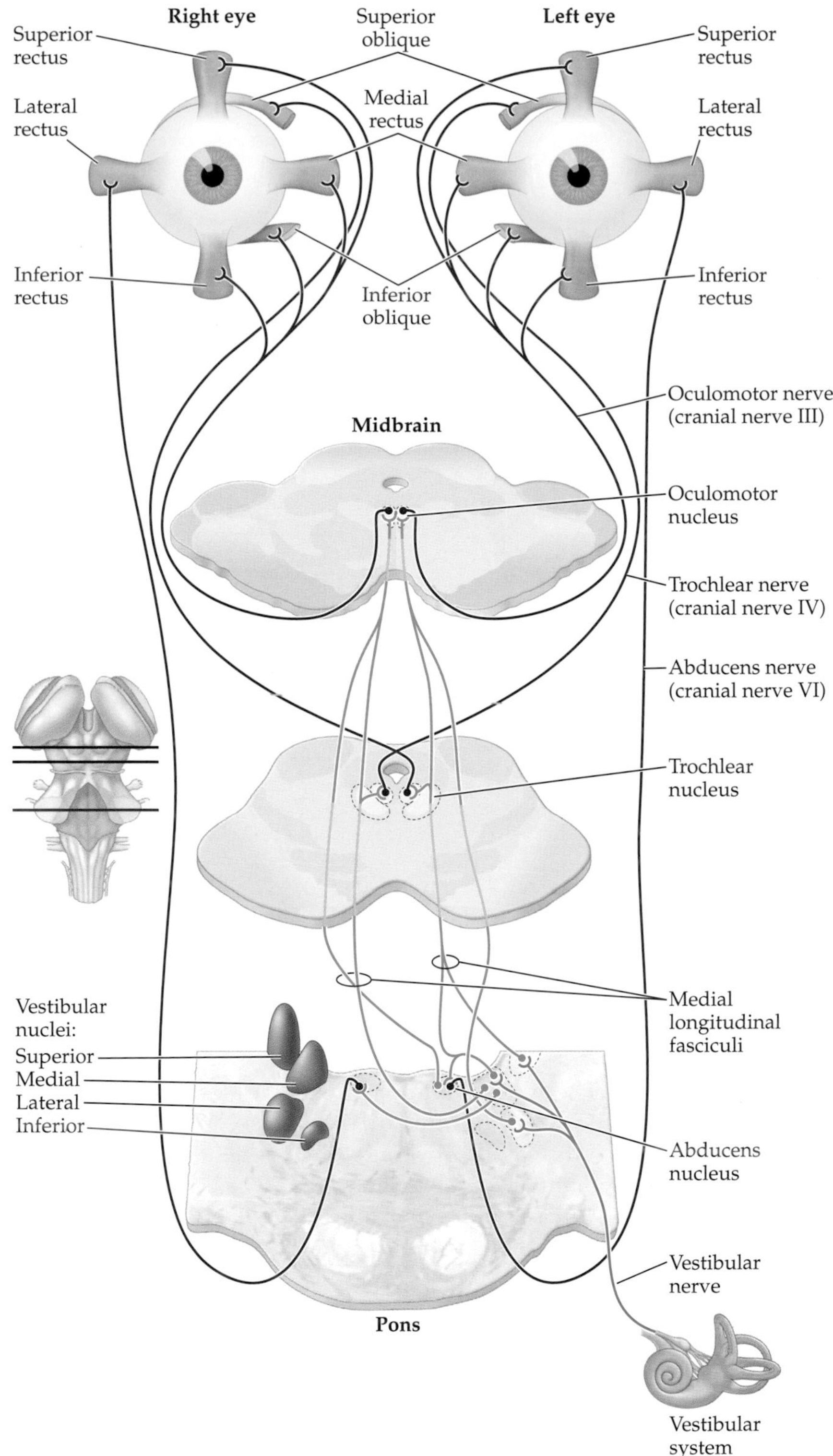

FIGURE 15.21 Neural pathways for the VOR. Most afferent neurons from the vestibular periphery first synapse on neurons in one of three vestibular nuclei: superior, medial, or lateral. Neurons from these vestibular nuclei then project to the three ocular motor nuclei: abducens, trochlear, and oculomotor. (Note that one of the three ocular motor nuclei is called the oculomotor nucleus.) Efferent neurons then project from these three ocular motor nuclei to the six oculomotor muscles: inferior oblique, superior oblique, inferior rectus, superior rectus, lateral rectus, and medial rectus. Vestibular afferent neurons are depicted here in blue. Oculomotor efferent neurons are red. Neurons that connect afferent and efferent neurons—called interneurons—are green.

canals. You can see this in **Figure 15.22**. The eye responses have a more or less constant, relatively high amplitude at high frequencies, but the VOR gets smaller and smaller as the frequency drops below about 0.01 Hz. Though the frequency characteristics of the VOR and canal afferents are qualitatively similar, there is an interesting difference. As you can see from the figure, the response of canal afferent neurons declines for frequencies below 0.03 Hz. In comparison, the VOR declines for frequencies below 0.01 Hz.

That difference is interesting because it means that, in some sense, the VOR is responding more accurately than a simple reading of its input signal

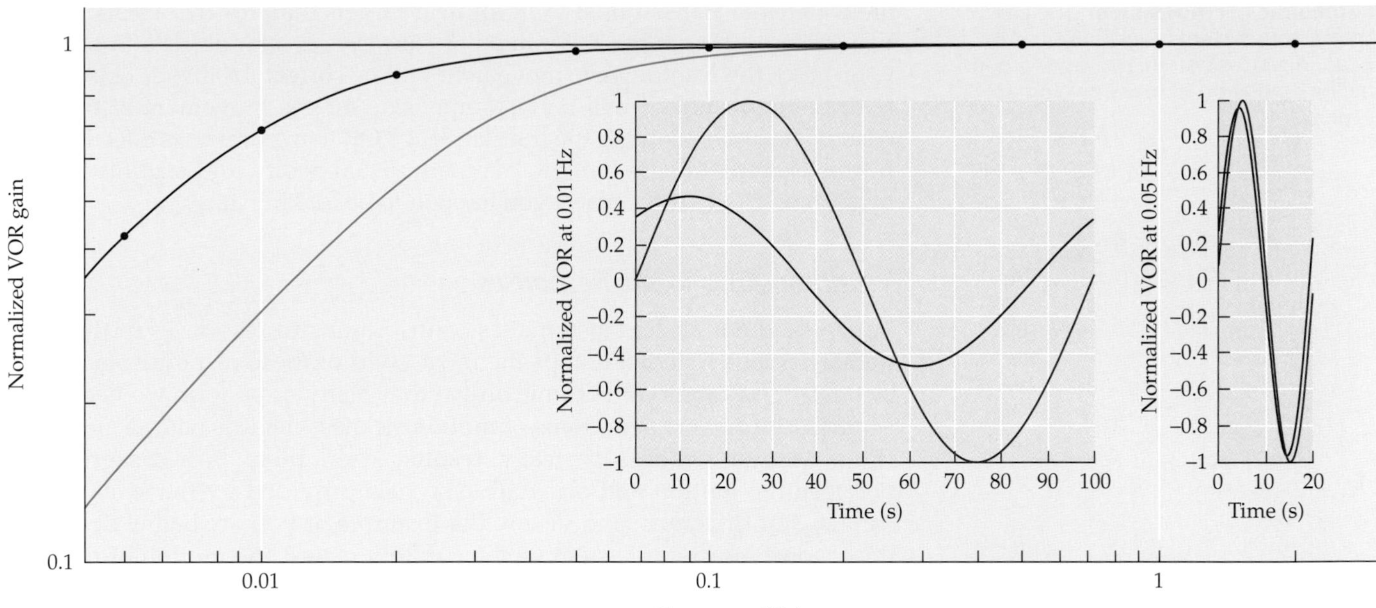

FIGURE 15.22 Dynamics of the VOR (shown in black) are such that the response has a nearly constant amplitude at frequencies between about 0.05 and 2 Hz. Below 0.05 Hz, the amplitude of the VOR response begins to decrease. For comparison, the normalized frequency response of the canals that we saw earlier is indicated by a blue line. The difference between the black and blue curves represents neural compensation performed by the brain that, in part, adjusts for the dynamics of the semicircular canals. Red represents the ideal VOR that precisely compensates for head rotation; data are normalized by the peak response so that the peak amplitude is 1. The inset furthest to the right shows the idealized normalized VOR (red) that would precisely compensate for rotation and the actual normalized VOR (black) at 0.05 Hz. The leftmost insert shows these at 0.01 Hz. The insets demonstrate changes in the amplitude of the sinusoidal VOR plotted against time as frequency changes.

would seem to permit. This effect, analogous to what we saw earlier for rotation perception (see Figure 15.16), is called velocity storage. It shows that the brain is not simply a relay station that passes sensory information to the muscles that yield the reflexive action. Instead the brain helps shape the reflexes to be as effective as possible, given the available sensory information. In this specific case, central processing can increase the frequency range over which the VOR works. This helps us to see more clearly at lower frequencies.

We also have a translational VOR that is evoked when the otolith organs sense head translation, especially high-frequency head translation. This translational VOR allows us to keep our eyes pointed at a single object while the head translates in one direction or the other. To demonstrate that the translational VOR can only track the relative movement of a single object, close one eye and extend your finger at arm's length between your eye and a more distant stationary object, like a doorknob. While holding your finger still, translate your head a few inches to the left and right. If you focus on your finger, you will notice that you can maintain gaze on your finger. At the same time, the far object will appear to move with your head. On the other hand, if you look at the far object, you can maintain gaze on the far object and your finger will appear to move in the direction opposite your head movement. For comparison, focus on your finger or the distant object while you rotate your head. This will evoke the angular VOR that was discussed earlier.

With the angular VOR, the relative movement between your finger and the distant object will be much less during head rotation than during head translation. Why is this? It is just geometry. Think about a line from eye to finger to doorknob. When you rotate your head, your eye moves only a little way from that line and the VOR eye rotation can compensate quite well for the movement of all visual targets—both near and far. Therefore, you see your finger and the distant target remaining more or less aligned during head rotation. However, when you translate your head, the eye moves well away from the finger–doorknob line and the eye rotation produced by the translational VOR can only compensate for the relative movement of one of the targets. This scaling of the eye movement with target distance occurs even in the dark. You

autonomic nervous system The part of the nervous system innervating glands, heart, digestive system, etc., and responsible for regulation of many involuntary actions.

have a greater translational VOR for near targets than for far targets, even if you can't see those targets. If you point your eyes at a far object and translate your head, the resulting eye movement will be correct for the far object even with the lights out. It will undercompensate for the movement of the near object. The brain is scaling the translational VOR to maximize its effectiveness. In this example it is helping to maintain visual acuity and stability during head translation for the object you happen to be looking at.

Vestibulo-Autonomic Responses

Your vestibular system also makes contributions to responses of the **autonomic nervous system**. Perhaps the most vivid of these responses is motion sickness, a vestibulo-autonomic ordeal that many of us wish we had never experienced. Severe symptoms of motion sickness include nausea and vomiting. Motion sickness typically results when there is a disagreement between the motion and orientation signals provided by the semicircular canals, otolith organs, and vision. For example, if you are below deck on a boat, your vestibular system will accurately record the motion of the boat while vision suggests no relative motion of the world, since you and the boat are moving together. What is this response good for? It may be a defense against some classes of poisons. If you have been poisoned, you want to get rid of the poison before it gets rid of you. But how do you know if you have been poisoned? If the poison is a neurotoxin, disruption of the sensory systems is a good hint. How do you know that your senses have been disrupted? One way is to check if senses that normally agree with one another have stopped doing so. Normally, if you move, your visual system and your vestibular system will both register that fact. If the vestibular system says one thing and the visual system says another, the digestive system may decide that it is time to rid the body of a possible cause of the disagreement. This could be a lifesaver if you just ate a bad mushroom. It is less desirable as a response to choppy weather at 35,000 ft.

Other vestibulo-autonomic responses are less spectacular and generally take the form of compensatory contributions. For example, consider the problem of regulating blood pressure. The heart pumps blood throughout the body, but maintaining oxygenation of the brain via blood flow is especially critical, because you will black out in just a few seconds if your brain does not receive adequate oxygen. Gravity pulls blood downward, so in the normal upright posture, your heart has to work to maintain blood flow to the brain. When you are lying down, it takes much less work to pump blood to the brain. Now, suppose that you rapidly stand up. The cardiovascular system has to suddenly change the regulation of blood flow to maintain adequate oxygen supply to the brain. If these mechanisms fail, you will experience light-headedness or, in extreme cases, blackout. By informing the relevant parts of the autonomic nervous system about the position and motion of the head, the vestibular system contributes to the regulation of blood flow to the brain. As a result, one consequence of destructive lesions of the vestibular labyrinth is that blood pressure regulation during whole-body tilts becomes much less stable (**Figure 15.23**).

FIGURE 15.23 Vestibular influences on blood pressure. (*a*) Trace shows blood pressure versus time in response to a nose-up tilt in a subject with a lesioned vestibular system. In the absence of vestibular contributions, a transient decrease in the blood pressure can be observed immediately after the tilt. (*b*) Change in blood pressure is much greater for the subject without a functional vestibular system (lesioned) than in the subject with a normal vestibular system. This demonstrates that the vestibular system helps maintain more constant blood pressure during whole-body tilts. (After Yates and Miller, 1998.)

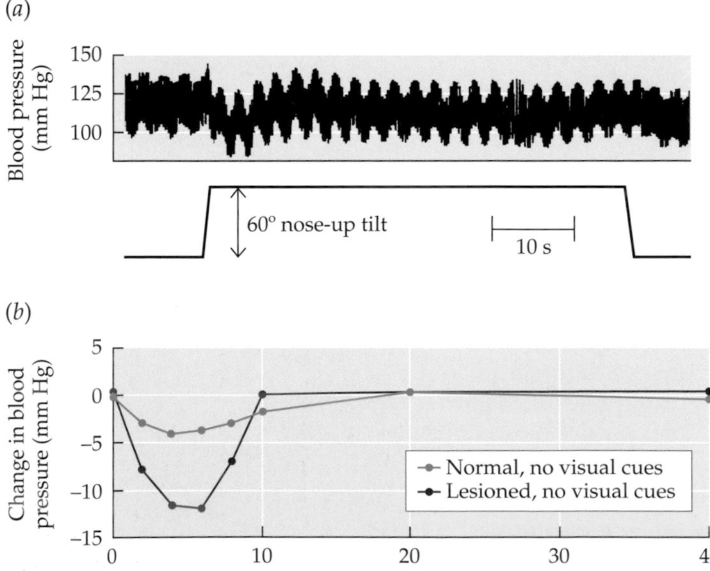

Vestibulo-Spinal Responses

Vestibular reflexes keep us from falling over. Without vestibulo-spinal reflexes our balance would be severely degraded. We would be unable to stand in the dark. Part of the reason is that when we stand, we are inherently unstable. As two-legged creatures, we can be thought of as being composed of a series of inverted pendulums—pendulums in which the mass is above the pivot point. Balancing a pencil or broom on your palm demonstrates a simple inverted pendulum. These challenging tasks can be mastered with practice, but imagine trying to stabilize a series of at least four brooms or pencils on top of one another. At its essence, this is the task faced by our balance system, which works to keep the head, torso, thighs, and calves—each an inverted pendulum—upright with respect to gravity.

A discussion of the dynamics of the entire posture control system is beyond the scope of this chapter. However, investigators have been able to simplify the dynamics experimentally by strapping the head and body to a rigid board that converts the complex multijoint body into a single inverted pendulum pitching forward and backward about the ankle joint. When the foot plate that the subject stands on is gently rocked forward and backward while the subject's eyes are closed, normal subjects demonstrate body sway that is less than the amplitude of the applied rocking movement (**Figure 15.24**), which means that the vestibular system is helping to compensate for the applied-movement disturbance. The vestibular system measures the movement of the head and sends commands to the postural control system that help reduce the amount of body sway. However, patients with complete vestibular loss demonstrate body sway that exceeds the amplitude of the disturbance. This difference between postural responses of people with normal vestibular function and patients with vestibular loss is a clear indication of the importance of the vestibular system and vestibulo-spinal reflexes to balance and posture control (see Figure 15.24). **Web Essay 15.6: Mal de Debarquement Syndrome** describes an unusual disorder that causes imbalance and/or spatial disorientation.

The vestibulo-spinal response can be thought of as a whole family of reflexes (**Figure 15.25**). In the vestibular nuclei, the primary afferent fibers

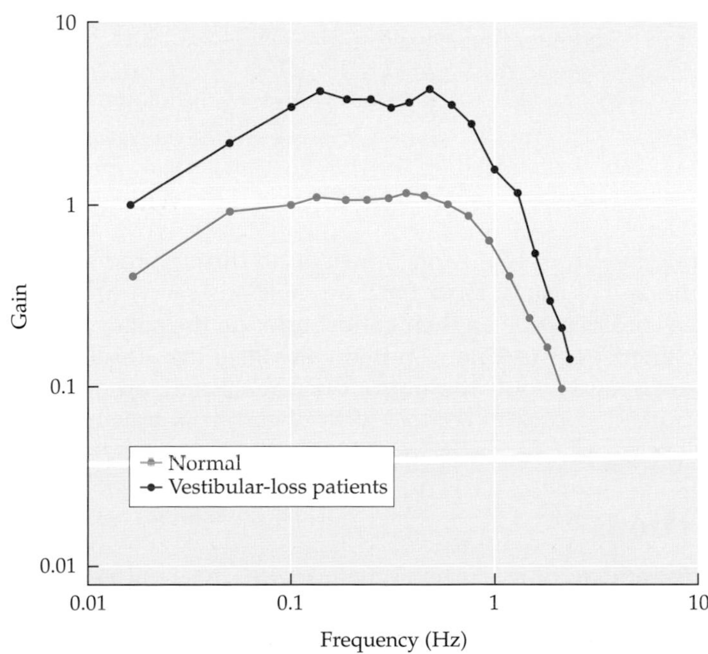

FIGURE 15.24 The contributions of the vestibular system to balance are demonstrated by the comparison of postural responses of subjects with normal vestibular function to responses of patients suffering severe bilateral vestibular loss. Subjects were asked to maintain themselves upright in the presence of small angular displacements of their feet that were designed to challenge their balance control. To simplify these experiments, which were performed with eyes closed, each subject's limbs, torso, and head were tethered to a back plate. The values on the y-axis (the "gain") represent the amplitude of the subject's response divided by the amplitude of displacement; therefore, a gain of 1 means that the response was equal to the displacement. Normal subjects responded to some of the disturbances with body sway that was less than the sway exhibited by vestibular-loss patients at all frequencies. In fact, the normal response gains were always near or below 1 for all frequencies, while patients had response gains that sometimes exceeded 1. The response difference between the patients and normal subjects clearly demonstrates the fundamental contributions of the vestibular system to balance control. (After Peterka, 2002.)

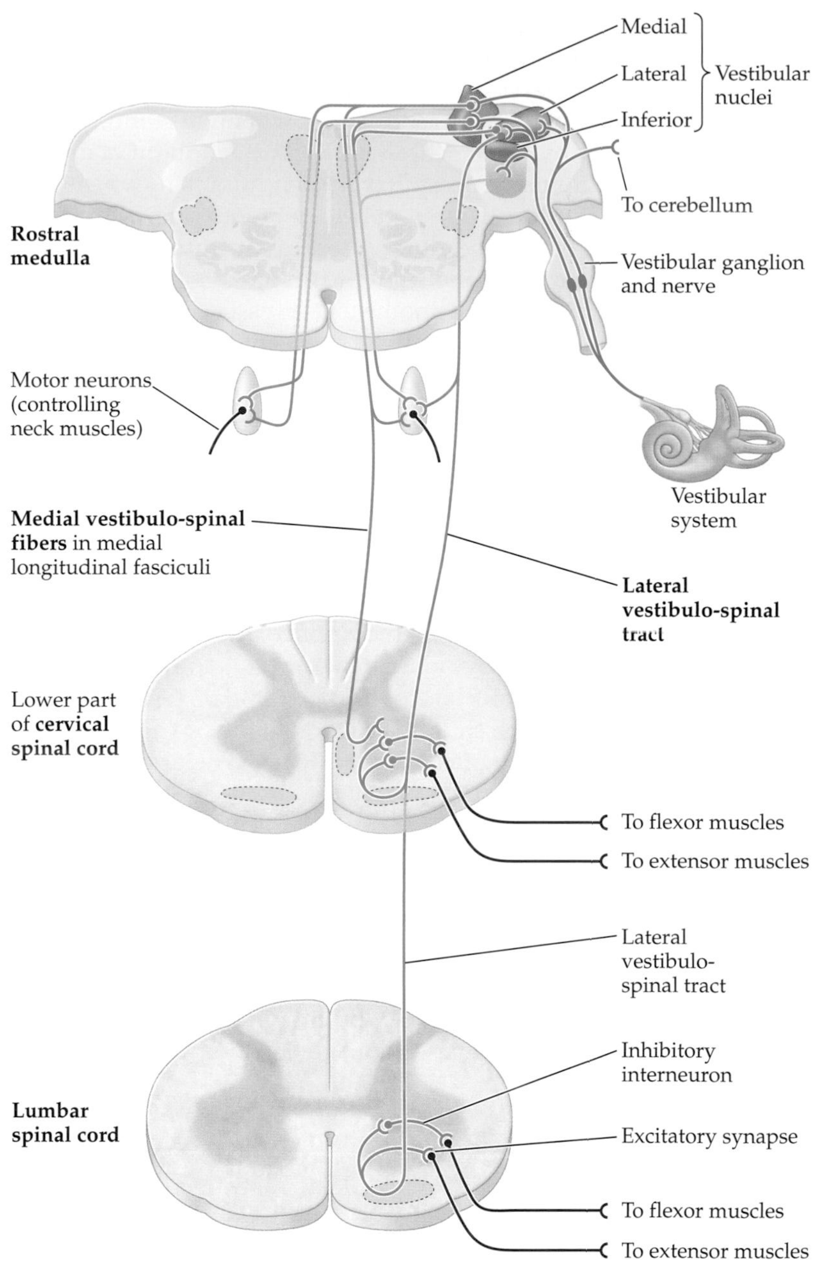

FIGURE 15.25 Neural pathways for vestibulo-spinal reflexes. Most vestibular afferent neurons (blue) synapse in one of the vestibular nuclei, but some project to the cerebellum. From the vestibular nuclei, descending interneurons (green) carry the information via vestibulo-spinal tracts downward through the brainstem and spinal cord until they synapse on efferent neurons (red) that activate the muscles that control balance. (After Netter, 1983.)

synapse on descending neurons that carry information through the lateral and medial vestibulo-spinal tracts. How far these neurons carry information down the spinal cord depends on their contribution to the balance system. If the neuron synapses onto a neuron that controls a leg muscle, the information is transmitted beyond the bottom of the spinal cord. If the information contributes to postural control of the head, it is transmitted only as far as the neck.

Cortical Projections

We have visual cortex and auditory cortex. What can we say about vestibular cortex? We can say that, unlike vision and hearing, there does not appear to be an exclusively vestibular cortex. There are areas of cortex that respond to vestibular input, but they tend to respond to visual input as well. Visuo-vestibular cortex is not shocking, since we learned earlier that perception of body motion and tilt result from multisensory convergence, including predominant contributions by the vestibular system and vision. But why don't we have pure vestibular cortex? One explanation is that the cortex simply lacks a good reason to process vestibular information without visual information if that visual information is available. The visual system is responsive to constant-velocity visual motion—like that experienced during rotation in the light as you see the room spin around you—while the vestibular system responds primarily to changes in velocity and is relatively insensitive to constant-velocity motion. For example, recall that when rotated at a constant velocity in the dark, humans perceive that they are not rotating after about 30 seconds (see Figure 15.16). Therefore, when rotating with a nearly constant velocity in the light, it seems reasonable that the brain would utilize the visual information indicating motion to better estimate self-motion. It thus makes sense that areas of the cortex related to the perception of tilt and self-motion demonstrate a convergence of visual and vestibular information.

Vestibular information reaches the cortex via what are called the thalamocortical pathways (**Figure 15.26**). This means simply that the vestibular information, like most other sensory information, reaches the cortex via the thalamus. Neurons from the vestibular nuclei carry vestibular information to the thalamus, where that information is processed and relayed to the cortex. Compare this, for example, to the visual system, where the retinal ganglion cells synapse in the lateral geniculate nucleus of the thalamus (see the section titled "The Lateral Geniculate Nucleus" in Chapter 3). There, the information is processed and passed on to visual cortex.

Evidence suggests that an area of the cortex called the multisensory parieto-insular cortex is involved in spatial orientation perception. This area of the cortex receives input from both the semicircular canals and the otolith organs. Furthermore, immediately after this part of the cortex is lesioned by a stroke, many patients report illusions of translation and illusory tilts of perceived vertical. Though more rare, rotational vertigo—an illusory sense of spinning—is reported by some of these patients.

The areas of the cortex that receive projections from the vestibular system also project back to the vestibular nuclei. The existence of these pathways suggests that feedback from the vestibular cortex likely modulates low-level vestibular processing in the brain stem. A specific role for these projections has not been proven, but it is known that higher cognitive knowledge can affect both perceptions and reflexive responses. For example, imagining whether an unseen visual target rotates with you or not alters the vestibulo-ocular reflex evoked by rotation. As is appropriate, the VOR is suppressed when subjects imagine that the target moves with them but is relatively large when subjects imagine that the target is Earth-fixed.

Another example of higher-order cortical influences is that knowledge of the motion capabilities of a specific device can influence motion perceptions. For example, if you were blindfolded and then taken to a merry-go-round that you had never ridden before, your perception of tilt and motion might differ from what you would experience if you were riding a familiar merry-go-round that you had ridden many times before. The vestibular stimuli would be the same but your knowledge and expectations—both of which are higher-level functions—would be different and could alter your spatial orientation perceptions.

There is also a vestibular pathway that leads to the hippocampus through the vestibular cortex, though more direct projections from the vestibular sys-

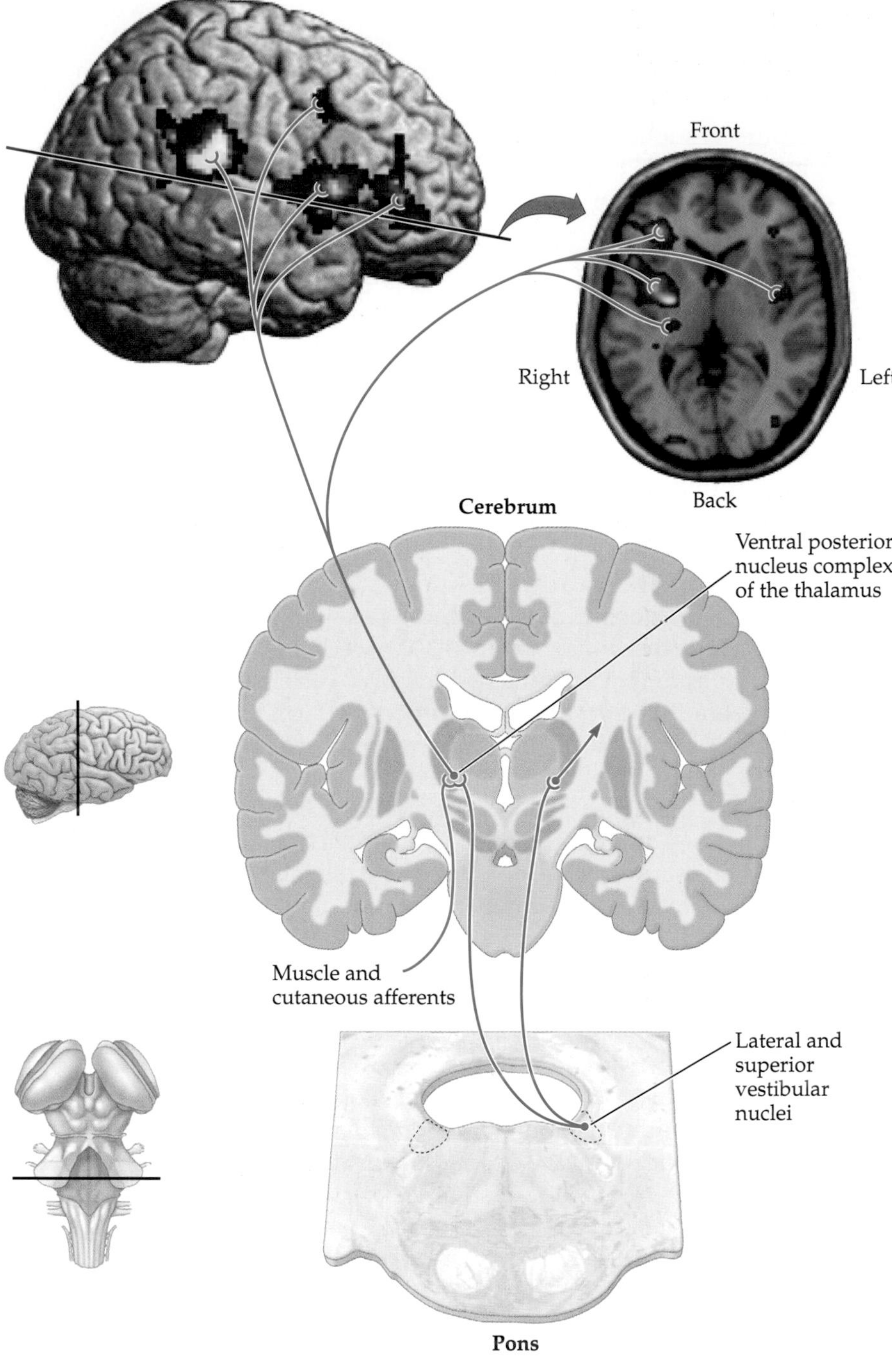

FIGURE 15.26 Ascending vestibular pathways pass from the vestibular nuclei to the posterolateral thalamus on their way to the temporo-insular cortex. Cortex activation patterns shown at the top are PET scans (positron emission tomography) obtained during stimulation of the vestibular system on the right side. Red and yellow indicate activation, which occurs in the temporo-parieto-insular areas of both hemispheres. Unlike most other sensory systems, much of the vestibular activation is not visible on the outermost surface of the cortex. (Brain images from Dieterich and Brandt, 2008; courtesy of Marianne Dieterich.)

tem may exist. Some neurons in the hippocampus respond to vestibular stimuli. These include a set of neurons called "direction cells" because they tend to spike vigorously when an animal's head is pointed toward a specific direction.

Compared to vision, our understanding of how and where vestibular information is processed in the cortex is immature. We are only beginning to learn how vestibular information is processed in the vestibular cortex.

Summary

1. The vestibular system is a set of sensory organs located in the inner ear that sense head motion and gravity and contribute to our sense of spatial orientation.
2. The vestibular system consists of three semicircular canals (horizontal, anterior, and posterior) that sense angular motion, and two otolith organs (utricle and saccule) that sense both gravity and linear acceleration.
3. Hair cells are the mechanoreceptors that convert both orientation with respect to gravity and head motion into signals that are sent to the brain.
4. Spatial orientation includes three sensory modalities: linear motion, angular motion, and tilt. Direction and amplitude are qualities that define each of these three sensory modalities.
5. The sense of spatial orientation results from a combination of information from multiple sensory systems. The vestibular and visual systems make predominant contributions to our sense of spatial orientation.
6. The sense of spatial orientation originates with the visual and vestibular sensory receptors, but the brain processes the information provided by these sensory organs to yield perceptions that may differ substantially from the responses found on the afferent neurons.
7. We are exquisitely sensitive to head motion. Thresholds to detect rotation direction in the dark are normally less than 1 degree per second. Thresholds to detect the direction of static tilt in the dark are as small as 2 degrees or so.
8. In addition to its contributions to spatial orientation perception, the vestibular system contributes to reflexive responses that include vestibulo-ocular, vestibulo-spinal, and vestibulo-autonomic reflexes.
9. No area of the cortex exclusively devoted to processing vestibular information has been identified. Areas of the cortex that respond to vestibular stimuli also respond to visual and other stimuli.

Refer to the **Sensation and Perception** website **(www.sinauer.com/wolfe2e)** for activities, essays, study questions, and other study aids.

Glossary

A

A-delta fiber An intermediate-sized, myelinated sensory nerve fiber that transmits pain and temperature signals. Compare *C fiber*.

A1 See *primary auditory cortex*.

abducens (VI) nerves The sixth pair of cranial nerves, which innervate the lateral rectus muscle of each eye.

absolute disparity A difference in the actual retinal coordinates in the left and right eyes of the image of a feature in a visual scene. Compare *relative disparity*.

absolute metrical depth cue A depth cue that provides absolute information about the distance in the third dimension (e.g., his nose sticks out 4 centimeters in front of his face). Compare *relative metrical depth cue*.

absolute threshold The minimum amount of stimulation necessary for a person to detect a stimulus 50% of the time.

absorb To take up light, noise, or energy and not transmit it at all.

ACC See *anterior cingulate cortex*.

accessory olfactory bulb (AOB) A smaller neural structure located behind the main olfactory bulb that receives input from the vomeronasal organ.

accidental viewpoint A viewing position that produces some regularity in the visual image that is not present in the world (e.g., the sides of two independent objects lining up perfectly). Compare *nonaccidental feature*.

accommodation The process by which the eye changes its focus (in which the lens gets fatter as gaze is directed toward nearer objects).

achromatopsia An inability to perceive colors that is caused by damage to the central nervous system. See *color-anomalous*.

acoustic reflex A reflex that protects the ear from intense sounds, via contraction of the stapedius and tensor tympani muscles.

acuity The smallest spatial detail that can be resolved.

adaptation A reduction in response caused by prior or continuing stimulation.

adapting stimulus A stimulus whose removal produces a change in visual perception or sensitivity.

additive color mixture A mixture of lights. If light A and light B are both reflected from a surface to the eye, in the perception of color the effects of those two lights add together. Compare *subtractive color mixture*.

aerial perspective A depth cue based on the implicit understanding that light is scattered by the atmosphere. More light is scattered when we look through more atmosphere. Thus, more distant objects are subject to more scatter and appear fainter, bluer, and less distinct. Also called *haze*.

afferent fiber A neuron that carries sensory information to the central nervous system. Compare *efferent fiber*.

afterimage A visual image seen after the stimulus has been removed.

agnosia A failure to recognize objects in spite of the ability to see them. Agnosia is typically due to brain damage. Compare *anomia*.

akinetopsia A rare neuropsychological disorder in which the affected individual has no perception of motion.

aliasing Misperception of a grating due to undersampling.

amacrine cells Retinal cells found in the inner synaptic layer that make synaptic contacts with bipolar cells, ganglion cells, and one another.

ambiguous figure A visual stimulus that gives rise to two or more interpretations of its identity or structure.

amblyopia A developmental disorder that is characterized by reduced spatial vision in an otherwise healthy eye, even with proper correction for refractive error. Often referred to as "lazy eye."

amplitude The magnitude of displacement (increase or decrease) of a sound pressure wave or of a head movement (e.g., angular velocity, linear acceleration, tilt).

amygdala–hippocampal complex The conjoined regions of the amygdala and hippocampus, which are key structures in the limbic system. This complex is critical for the unique emotional and associative properties of olfactory cognition.

analgesia Decreasing pain sensation during conscious experience.

anamorphic projection See *anamorphosis*.

anamorphosis (or anamorphic projection) Use of the rules of linear perspective to create a two-dimensional image so distorted that it looks correct only when viewed from a special angle or with a mirror that counters the distortion.

anomia An inability to name objects in spite of the ability to see and recognize them (as shown by usage). Anomia is typically due to brain damage. Compare *agnosia*.

anosmia The total inability to smell, most often resulting from sinus illness or head trauma.

anterior cingulate cortex (ACC) A region of the brain associated with the perceived unpleasantness of a pain sensation.

AOB See *accessory olfactory bulb.*

aperture problem The fact that when a moving object is viewed through an aperture (or a receptive field), the direction of motion of a local feature or part of the object may be ambiguous.

aperture An opening that allows only a partial view of the object.

apparent motion The (illusory) impression of smooth motion resulting from the rapid alternation of objects that appear in different locations in rapid succession.

aqueous humor The watery fluid in the anterior chamber of the eye. Compare *vitreous humor.*

area 17 See *primary visual cortex.*

articulation The act or manner of producing a speech sound using the vocal tract.

astigmatism A visual defect caused by the unequal curving of one or more of the refractive surfaces of the eye, usually the cornea.

attack The part of a sound during which amplitude increases (onset). Compare *decay.*

attention Any of the very large set of selective processes in the brain. To deal with the impossibility of handling all inputs at once, the nervous system has evolved mechanisms that are able to restrict processing to a subset of things, places, ideas, or moments in time.

attentional blink The difficulty in perceiving and responding to the second of two target stimuli amid a rapid stream of distracting stimuli if the observer has responded to the first target stimulus within 200 to 500 milliseconds before the second stimulus is presented.

audibility threshold The lowest sound pressure level that can be reliably detected at a given frequency.

auditory (VIII) nerves The eighth pair of cranial nerves, which connect the inner ear with the brain, transmitting impulses concerned with hearing and balance. The auditory nerve is composed of the cochlear nerve and the vestibular nerve and therefore is sometimes referred to as the "vestibulocochlear nerve."

auditory nerve fibers A collection of neurons that convey information from hair cells in the cochlea to (afferent) and from (efferent) the brain stem. This collection also includes neurons for the vestibular system.

auditory scene analysis See *source segregation.*

auditory stream segregation The perceptual organization of a complex acoustic signal into separate auditory events for which each stream is heard as a separate event.

autonomic nervous system The part of the nervous system innervating glands, heart, digestive system, etc., and responsible for regulation of many involuntary actions.

azimuth The angle of a sound source on the horizontal plane relative to a point in the center of the head between the ears. Azimuth is measured in degrees, with 0 degrees being straight ahead. The angle increases clockwise toward the right, with 180 degrees being directly behind.

B

basal cells One of the three types of cells in the olfactory epithelium. The basal cells are precursor cells to olfactory sensory neurons. Compare *olfactory sensory neurons* and *supporting cells.*

basic tastes The four taste qualities that are generally agreed to describe human taste experience: sweet, salty, sour, bitter.

basilar membrane A plate of fibers that forms the base of the cochlear partition and separates the middle and tympanic canals in the cochlea.

Bayesian approach A statistical model based on Reverend Thomas Bayes' insight that prior knowledge could influence our estimates of the probability of a current event.

belt area A region of cortex, directly adjacent to the primary auditory cortex (A1), with inputs from A1, where neurons respond to more complex characteristics of sounds. Compare *parabelt area.*

binding problem The challenge of tying different attributes of visual stimuli (e.g., color, orientation, motion), which are handled by different brain circuits, to the appropriate object so that we perceive a unified object (e.g., red, vertical, moving right).

binocular depth cue A depth cue that relies on information from both eyes. Stereopsis is the primary example in humans, but convergence and the ability of two eyes to see more of an object than one eye sees are also binocular depth cues. Compare *monocular depth cue.*

binocular disparity The differences between the two retinal images of the same scene. Disparity is the basis for stereopsis, a vivid perception of the three-dimensionality of the world that is not available with monocular vision.

binocular rivalry The competition between the two eyes for control of visual perception, which is evident when completely different stimuli are presented to the two eyes.

binocular summation The combination (or "summation") of signals from each eye in ways that make performance on many tasks better with both eyes than with either eye alone.

binocular vision See *correspondence problem.*

biological motion The pattern of movement of living beings (humans and animals).

bipolar cells Retinal cells that synapse with either rods or cones (not both) and with horizontal cells, and then pass the signals on to ganglion cells.

bitter The taste quality, generally considered unpleasant, produced by substances like quinine or caffeine.

body image The impression of our bodies in space.

brightness The distance from black (zero brightness) in color space. Compare *hue* and *saturation.*

C

C fiber A narrow-diameter, unmyelinated sensory nerve fiber that transmits pain and temperature signals. Compare *A-delta fiber.*

cataract Opacity of the crystalline lens.

CF See *characteristic frequency.*

change blindness The failure to notice a change between two scenes.

If the change does not alter the gist, or meaning, of the scene, quite large changes can pass unnoticed.

characteristic frequency (CF) The frequency to which a particular auditory nerve fiber is most sensitive.

chord A combination of three or more musical notes with different pitches played simultaneously.

chorda tympani The branch of cranial nerve VII (the facial nerve) that carries taste information from the anterior, mobile tongue (the part that can be stuck out). The chorda tympani nerve leaves the tongue with the lingual branch of the trigeminal nerve (cranial nerve V) and then passes through the middle ear on its way to the brain.

chromophore The light-catching part of the visual pigments of the retina.

cilia (s. cillium) Hairlike protrusions on the dendrites of olfactory sensory neurons. The receptor sites for odorant molecules are on the cilia, which are the first structures involved in olfactory signal transduction.

circumvallate papillae Circular structures that form an inverted *V* on the rear of the tongue (three to five on each side). Circumvallate papillae are moundlike structures surrounded by a trench (like a moat). These papillae are much larger than fungiform papillae.

CO See *cytochrome oxidase*.

coarticulation The phenomenon in speech whereby attributes of successive speech units overlap in articulatory or acoustic patterns.

cochlea A spiral structure of the inner ear containing the organ of Corti.

cochlear nucleus The first brain stem nucleus at which afferent auditory nerve fibers synapse.

cochlear partition The combined basilar membrane, tectorial membrane, and organ of Corti, which are together responsible for the transduction of sound waves into neural signals.

cognitive habituation The psychological process by which, after long-term exposure to an odorant, one is no longer able to detect that odorant or has very diminished detection ability.

cold fiber A sensory nerve fiber that fires when skin temperature decreases. Compare *warmth fiber*.

color constancy The tendency of a surface to appear the same color under a fairly wide range of illuminants.

color space The three-dimensional space, established because color perception is based on the outputs of three cone types, that describes the set of all colors.

color-anomalous A better term for what is usually called "color-blind." Most "color-blind" individuals can still make discriminations based on wavelength. Those discriminations are different from the normal—that is, *anomalous*.

color-opponent cell A neuron whose output is based on a difference between sets of cones.

column A vertical arrangement of neurons.

common region A Gestalt grouping rule stating that two features will tend to group together if they appear to be part of the same larger region.

comparator An area of the visual system that receives one copy of the order issued by the motor system when the eyes move (the other copy goes to the eye muscles). The comparator can compensate for the image changes caused by the eye movement.

complex cell A neuron whose receptive-field characteristics cannot be easily predicted by mapping with spots of light. Compare *simple cell*.

complex tone A sound wave consisting of more than one sinusoidal component of different frequencies. Compare *pure tone* and *sine wave*.

conductive hearing loss Hearing loss caused by problems with the bones of the middle ear.

cone monochromat An individual with only one cone type. Cone monochromats are truly color-blind. Compare *rod monochromat*.

cone of confusion A region of positions in space where all sounds produce the same time and level (intensity) differences (ITDs and ILDs).

cones Photoreceptors specialized for daylight vision, fine visual acuity, and color. Compare *rods*.

conjunction search Search for a target defined by the presence of two or more attributes (e.g., a *red, vertical* target among *red* horizontal and green *vertical* distractors). Compare *feature search*.

connectedness A Gestalt grouping rule stating that two items will tend to group together if they are connected.

continuity constraint In stereopsis, the observation that, except at the edges of objects, neighboring points in the world lie at similar distances from the viewer. This is one of several constraints that have been proposed to help solve the correspondence problem.

contralateral Referring to the opposite side of the body (or brain). Compare *ipsilateral*.

contralesional field The visual field on the side opposite a brain lesion (e.g., points to the left of fixation are contralesional to damage to the right hemisphere of the brain). Compare *ipsilesional field*.

contrast The difference in luminance between an object and the background, or between lighter and darker parts of the same object.

contrast-defined object See *texture-defined object*.

contrast sensitivity function (CSF) A function describing how the sensitivity to contrast (defined as the reciprocal of the contrast threshold) depends on the spatial frequency (size) of the stimulus.

contrast threshold The smallest amount of contrast required to detect a pattern.

convergence The ability of the two eyes to turn inward, often used in order to place the two images of a feature in the world on corresponding locations in the two retinal images (typically on the fovea of each eye). Convergence reduces the disparity of that feature to zero (or nearly zero). Compare *divergence*.

cornea The transparent "window" into the eyeball.

correspondence problem 1. In binocular vision, the problem of figuring out which bit of the image in the left eye should be matched with which bit in the right eye. The problem is particularly vexing when the images consist of thousands of similar features like dots in random dot stereograms. 2. In motion detection, the problem faced by the motion detection system of knowing which feature in frame 2 corresponds to a particular feature in frame 1.

corresponding retinal points A geometric concept stating that points on the retina of each eye where the monocular retinal images of a single object are formed are at the same distance from the fovea in each eye. The two foveas are also corresponding points.

cortical magnification The amount of cortical area (usually specified in millimeters) devoted to a specific region (e.g., 1 degree) in the visual field.

covert attentional shift A shift of attention in the absence of corresponding movements of the eyes. Compare *overt attentional shift*.

cranial nerves Twelve pairs of nerves (one for each side of the body) that originate in the brain stem and reach sense organs and muscles through openings in the skull.

cribriform plate A bony structure riddled with tiny holes, at the level of the eyebrows, that separates the nose from the brain. The axons from the olfactory sensory neurons pass through the tiny holes of the cribriform plate to enter the brain.

cristae (s. crista) The specialized detectors of angular motion located in each semicircular canal in a swelling called the ampulla.

critical bandwidth The range of frequencies conveyed within a channel in the auditory system.

critical period In the study of development, a period of time when the organism is particularly susceptible to developmental change. There are critical periods in the development of binocular vision, human language, and so on.

cross-adaptation The reduction in detection of an odorant following exposure to another odorant. Cross-adaptation is presumed to occur because the two odorants share one or more olfactory receptors for their transduction, but the order of odorant presentation also plays a role.

crossed disparity The sign of disparity created by objects in front of the plane of fixation (the horopter). The term *crossed* is used because images of objects located in front of the horopter appear to be displaced to the left in the right eye, and to the right in the left eye. Compare *uncrossed disparity*.

cross-modality matching The ability to match the intensities of sensations that come from different sensory modalities. This ability enables insight into sensory differences.

crystalline lens The lens inside the eye that enables changing focus.

CSF See *contrast sensitivity function*.

cue A stimulus that might indicate where (or what) a subsequent stimulus will be. Cues can be valid (correct information), invalid (incorrect), or neutral (uninformative).

cultural relativism In sensation and perception, the idea that basic perceptual experiences (e.g., color perception) may be determined in part by the cultural environment.

cycle For a grating, a pair consisting of one dark bar and one bright bar.

cycles per degree The number of dark and bright bars per degree of visual angle.

cyclopean Referring to stimuli that are defined by binocular disparity alone. Named after the one-eyed Cyclops of Homer's *Odyssey*.

cytochrome oxidase (CO) An enzyme used to reveal the regular array of "CO blobs," which are spaced about 0.5 millimeter apart in the primary visual cortex.

D

dB See *decibel*.

DCML pathway See *dorsal column–medial lemniscal pathway*.

decay The part of a sound during which amplitude decreases (offset). Compare *attack*.

decibel (dB) A unit of measure for the physical intensity of sound. Decibels define the difference between two sounds as the ratio between two sound pressures. Each 10:1 sound pressure ratio equals 20 dB, and a 100:1 ratio equals 40 dB.

depth cues Information about the third dimension (depth) of visual space. Depth cues may be monocular or binocular.

dermis The inner of two major layers of skin, consisting of nutritive and connective tissues, within which lie the mechanoreceptors.

deuteranope An individual who suffers from color blindness that is due to the absence of M-cones. Compare *protanope* and *tritanope*.

dichoptic Referring to the presentation of two stimuli, one to each eye. Different from *binocular* presentation, which could involve both eyes looking at a single stimulus.

difference threshold See *just noticeable difference*.

diffuse bipolar cells Bipolar retinal cells whose processes are spread out to receive input from multiple cones. Compare *midget bipolar cells*.

diplopia Double vision. If visible in both eyes, stimuli falling outside of Panum's fusional area will appear diplopic.

distractor In visual search, any stimulus other than the *target*.

divergence The ability of the two eyes to turn outward, often used in order to place the two images of a feature in the world on corresponding locations in the two retinal images (typically on the fovea of each eye). Divergence reduces the disparity of that feature to zero (or nearly zero). Compare *convergence*.

doctrine of specific nerve energies A doctrine formulated by Johannes Müller stating that the nature of a sensation depends on which sensory fibers are stimulated, not on how fibers are stimulated.

dorsal column–medial lemniscal (DCML) pathway The route from the spinal cord to the brain that carries signals from skin, muscles, tendons, and joints. Compare *spinothalamic pathway*.

dorsal horn A region at the rear of the spinal cord that receives inputs from receptors in the skin.

double dissociation The phenomenon in which one of two functions, such as hearing and sight, can be damaged without harm to the other, and vice versa.

dualism The idea that both mind and body exist.

duplex In reference to the retina, consisting of two parts: the rods and cones, which operate under different conditions.

E

ear canal The canal that conducts sound vibrations from the pinna to the tympanic membrane and prevents damage to the tympanic membrane.

eccentricity The distance between the retinal image and the fovea.

efferent fiber A neuron that carries information from the central nervous system to the periphery. Compare *afferent fiber*.

egocenter The center of a reference frame used to represent locations relative to the body.

emmetropia The condition in which there is no refractive error, because the refractive power of the eye is perfectly matched to the length of the eyeball.

empiricism The idea that experience from the senses is the only source of knowledge.

end stopping The process by which a cell in the cortex first increases its firing rate as the bar length increases to fill up its receptive field, and then decreases its firing rate as the bar is lengthened further.

endogenous opiates Chemicals released by the body that block the release or uptake of neurotransmitters necessary to transmit pain sensations to the brain.

endogenous spatial attention A form of top-down (knowledge-driven) control of spatial attention in which attention is voluntarily directed toward the site where the observer anticipates a stimulus will occur.

entorhinal cortex A phylogenetically old cortical region that provides the major sensory association input into the hippocampus. The entorhinal cortex also receives direct projections from olfactory regions.

entry-level category For an object, the label that comes to mind most quickly when we identify the object (e.g., *bird*). The object might be more specifically named; that's the "subordinate level" (e.g., *eagle*). The object might be more generally named; that's the "superordinate level" (e.g., *animal*).

epidermis The outer of two major layers of skin. Compare *dermis*.

equal-loudness curve A graph plotting sound pressure level (dB SPL) against the frequency for which a listener perceives constant loudness.

esotropia Strabismus in which one eye deviates inward.

Euclidean Referring to the geometry of the world, so named in honor of Euclid, the ancient Greek geometer of the third century BCE. In Euclidean geometry, parallel lines remain parallel as they are extended in space, objects maintain the same size and shape as they move around in space, the internal angles of a triangle always add to 180 degrees, and so forth.

exogenous spatial attention A form of bottom-up (stimulus-driven) spatial attention in which attention is reflexively directed toward the site at which a stimulus has abruptly appeared.

exotropia Strabismus in which one eye deviates outward.

exploratory procedure A stereotyped hand movement pattern used to contact objects in order to perceive their properties; each exploratory procedure is best for determining one (or more) object properties.

extinction In visual attention, the inability to perceive a stimulus to one side of the point of fixation (e.g., to the right) in the presence of another stimulus, typically in a comparable position in the other visual field (e.g., on the left side). Compare *neglect*.

extrastriate cortex The region of cortex bordering the primary visual cortex and containing multiple areas involved in visual processing.

F

familiar size A depth cue based on knowledge of the typical size of objects like humans or pennies.

feature integration theory Anne Treisman's theory of visual attention, which holds that a limited set of basic features can be processed in parallel preattentively, but that other properties, including the correct binding of features to objects, require attention. Compare *guided search theory*.

feature search Search for a target defined by a single attribute, such as a salient color or orientation. Compare *conjunction search*.

Fechner's law A principle describing the relationship between stimulus and resulting sensation such that the magnitude of subjective sensation increases proportionally to the logarithm of the stimulus intensity.

feed-forward process A process that carries out a computation (e.g., object recognition) one neural step after another, without need for feedback from a later stage to an earlier stage.

figure–ground assignment The process of determining that some regions of an image belong to a foreground object (figure) and other regions are part of the background (ground).

filiform papillae Small structures on the tongue that provide most of the bumpy appearance. Filiform papillae have no taste function.

filter An acoustic, electrical, electronic, or optical device, instrument, computer program, or neuron that allows the passage of some frequencies or digital elements and blocks the passage of others.

first-order motion The motion of an object that is defined by changes in luminance. Compare *second-order motion*.

flavor The combination of true taste (sweet, salty, sour, bitter) and retronasal olfaction.

focus of expansion The point in the center of the horizon from which, when we are in motion (e.g., driving on the highway), all points in the perspective image seem to emanate. The focus of expansion is one aspect of optic flow.

foliate papillae Folds of tissue containing taste buds. Foliate papillae are located on the rear of the tongue lateral to the circumvallate papillae, where the tongue attaches to the mouth.

formant A resonance of the vocal tract. Formants are specified by their center frequency and are denoted by integers that increase with relative frequency.

Fourier analysis A mathematical theorem by which any sound can be divided into a set of sine waves. Combining these sine waves will reproduce the original sound.

frame of reference The coordinate system used to define locations in space.

free fusion The technique of converging (crossing) or diverging the eyes in order to view a stereogram without a stereoscope.

frequency For sound, the number of times per second that a pattern of pressure change repeats.

fundamental frequency The lowest-frequency component of a complex periodic sound.

fundus (pl. fundi) The back layer of the retina—what the eye doctor sees through an ophthalmoscope.

fungiform papillae Mushroom-shaped structures (maximum diameter 1 millimeter) that are distributed most densely on the edges of the tongue, especially the tip. Taste buds (an average of six per papilla) are buried in the surface.

fusiform face area An area in the fusiform gyrus of human extrastriate cortex that responds preferentially to faces in fMRI studies. Compare *parahippocampal place area*.

G

G protein–coupled receptors (GPCRs) The class of receptors that are present on the surface of olfactory sensory neurons. All GPCRs are characterized by a common structural feature of seven membrane-spanning α-helices.

ganglion cells Retinal cells that receive visual information from photoreceptors via two intermediate neuron types (bipolar cells and amacrine cells) and transmit information to the brain and midbrain.

gate control theory A description of the system that transmits pain that incorporates modulating signals from the brain.

geons In Biederman's "recognition by components" model, the "geometric ions" out of which perceptual objects are built.

Gestalt grouping rules A set of rules describing which elements in an image will appear to group together. The original list was assembled by members of the Gestalt school of thought.

Gestalt In German, literally "form." In perception, the name of a school of thought stressing that the perceptual whole could be greater than the apparent sum of the parts.

gestation Fetal development during pregnancy.

global superiority effect The finding in various experiments that the properties of the whole object take precedence over the properties of parts of the object.

glomeruli (s. glomerulus) Spherical conglomerates containing the incoming axons of the olfactory sensory neurons. Each OSN converges onto two glomeruli (one medial, one lateral).

good continuation A Gestalt grouping rule stating that two elements will tend to group together if they seem to lie on the same contour.

GPCR See *G protein–coupled receptors*.

graded potential An electrical potential that can vary continuously in amplitude.

guided search Search in which attention can be restricted to a subset of possible items on the basis of information about the target item's basic features (e.g., its color). Compare *feature integration theory*.

gustation The sense of taste.

H

hair cells Cells that support the stereocilia that transduce mechanical movement in the cochlea and vestibular labyrinth into neural activity sent to the brain stem; some hair cells also receive inputs from the brain.

haptic perception Knowledge of the world that is derived from sensory receptors in skin, muscles, tendons, and joints, usually involving active exploration.

harmonic spectrum The spectrum of a complex sound in which energy is at integer multiples of the fundamental frequency.

haze See *aerial perspective*.

head-related transfer function (HRTF) A function that describes how the pinna, ear canal, head, and torso change the intensity of sounds with different frequencies that arrive at each ear from different locations in space (azimuth and elevation).

helicotrema The opening that connects the tympanic and vestibular canals at the apex of the cochlea.

hertz (Hz) A unit of measure for frequency. One hertz equals one cycle per second.

heuristic A mental shortcut.

high-spontaneous fibers Auditory nerve fibers with high rates (more than 30 per second) of spontaneous firing; high-spontaneous fibers increase their firing rate in response to relatively low levels of sound. Compare *low-spontaneous fibers* and *mid-spontaneous fibers*.

homologous regions Brain regions that appear to have the same function in different species.

homunculus (pl. homunculi) A map-like representation of regions of the body in the brain.

horizontal cells Specialized retinal cells that contact both photoreceptor and bipolar cells.

horopter The location of objects whose images lie on corresponding points. The surface of zero disparity. See also *Vieth-Müller circle*.

HRTF See *head-related transfer function*.

hue The chromatic (colorful) aspect of color (red, blue, green, yellow, and so on). Compare *brightness* and *saturation*.

hyperalgesia An increased or heightened response to a normally painful stimulus.

hypercolumn A 1-millimeter block of striate cortex containing two sets of columns, each covering every possible orientation (0–180 degrees), with one set preferring input from the left eye and one set preferring input from the right eye.

hyperopia A common condition in which light entering the eye is focused behind the retina. Compare *myopia*.

hyperpolarization An increase in membrane potential where the inner membrane surface becomes more negative than the outer membrane surface.

Hz See *hertz*.

I

ideal observer A theoretical observer with complete access to the best available information and the ability to combine different sources of information in the optimal manner. It can be useful to compare human performance to that of an ideal observer.

ILD See *interaural level difference*.

illuminant The light that illuminates a surface.

illusory conjunction An erroneous combination of two features in a visual scene—for example, seeing a red X when the display contains red letters and Xs but no red Xs.

illusory contour A contour that is perceived, even though nothing changes from one side of the contour to the other in the image.

image A picture or likeness.

incus The middle ossicle. The incus connects the *malleus* and the *stapes*.

inferior colliculus A midbrain nucleus in the auditory pathway.

inferotemporal (IT) cortex Part of the cerebral cortex in the lower portion of the temporal lobe, important in object recognition.

inner ear A hollow cavity in the temporal bone of the skull, and the structures within this cavity: the cochlea and vestibular canals.

inner segment The part of a photoreceptor that lies between the outer segment and the cell nucleus. Compare *outer segment*.

insular cortex The primary cortical processing area for taste—the part of the cortex that first receives taste information.

intensity The amount of sound energy falling on a unit area (such as a square centimeter).

interaural level difference (ILD) The difference in level (intensity) between a sound arriving at one ear versus the other. Compare *interaural time difference*.

interaural time difference (ITD) The difference in time between a sound arriving at one ear versus the other. Compare *interaural level difference*.

interocular transfer The transfer of an effect (such as adaptation) from one eye to the other.

inverse-square law A principle stating that as distance from a source increases, intensity decreases faster such that decrease in intensity is the distance squared. This general law also applies to optics and other forms of energy.

ipsilateral Referring to the same side of the body (or brain). Compare *contralateral*.

ipsilesional field The visual field on the same side as a brain lesion. Compare *contralesional field*.

iris The colored part of the eye, consisting of a muscular diaphragm surrounding the pupil and regulating the light entering the eye by expanding and contracting the pupil.

isointensity curve A map plotting the firing rate of an auditory nerve fiber against varying frequencies at varying intensities.

IT See *inferotemporal cortex*.

ITD See *interaural time difference*.

J

JND See *just noticeable difference*.

just noticeable difference (JND) (or difference threshold) The smallest detectable difference between two stimuli, or the minimum change in a stimulus that enables it to be correctly judged as different from a reference stimulus.

K

kinesthesis The perception of the position and movement of our limbs in space.

kinesthetic Referring to perception involving sensory mechanoreceptors in muscles, tendons, and joints.

L

L-cone A cone that is preferentially sensitive to long wavelengths; colloquially (but not entirely accurately) known as a "red cone." Compare *S-cone* and *M-cone*.

labeled lines A theory of taste coding in which each taste nerve fiber carries a particular taste quality. For example, the quality evoked from a sucrose-best fiber is sweet, that from an NaCl-best fiber is salty, and so on.

lateral geniculate nucleus (LGN) A structure in the thalamus, part of the midbrain, that receives input from the retinal ganglion cells and has input and output connections to the visual cortex.

lateral inhibition Antagonistic neural interaction between adjacent regions of the retina.

lateral superior olive (LSO) A relay station in the brain stem where inputs from both ears contribute to the detection of the interaural level difference. Compare *medial superior olive*.

learned taste aversion The avoidance of a novel flavor after it has been paired with gastric illness. The smell, not the taste, of the substance is key for the learned aversion response in humans.

lesion In neuropsychology: 1. (n) A region of damaged brain. 2. (v) To destroy a section of the brain.

LGN See *lateral geniculate nucleus*.

limbic system The encompassing group of neural structures that includes the olfactory cortex, the amygdala, the hippocampus, the piriform cortex, and the entorhinal cortex. The limbic system is involved in many aspects of emotion and memory. Olfaction is unique among the senses for its direct and intimate connection to the limbic system.

linear perspective A depth cue based on the fact that lines that are parallel in the three-dimensional world will appear to converge in a two-dimensional image.

lordosis The position that a sow needs to assume in order to be impregnated. It involves the inward curving of the spinal column and exposure of the genitals.

loudness The psychological aspect of sound related to perceived intensity or magnitude.

low-spontaneous fibers Auditory nerve fibers with low rates (less than 10 per second) of spontaneous firing; low-spontaneous fibers require relatively intense sound before firing at higher rates. Compare *high-spontaneous fibers* and *mid-spontaneous fibers*.

LSO See *lateral superior olive*.

luminance-defined object An object that is delineated by changes in reflected light.

M

M-cone A cone that is preferentially sensitive to middle wavelengths; colloquially (but not entirely accurately) known as a "green cone." Compare *S-cone* and *L-cone*.

M ganglion cells Ganglion cells resembling little umbrellas that receive excitatory input from diffuse bipolar cells and feed the magnocellular layer of the lateral geniculate nucleus. Compare *P ganglion cells.*

maculae (s. macula) The specialized detectors of linear acceleration and gravity found in each otolith organ.

MAE See *motion aftereffect.*

magnitude estimation A psychophysical method in which the participant assigns values according to perceived magnitudes of the stimuli.

magnocellular layers The neurons in the bottom two layers of the lateral geniculate nucleus, which are physically larger than those in the top four layers. Compare *parvocellular layers.*

main olfactory bulb (MOB) The olfactory bulb; the blueberry-sized extension of the brain just above the nose; the first region of the brain where smells are processed. In humans we simply refer to "olfactory bulb(s)," but in animals with accessory olfactory bulbs, we distinguish between "main" and "accessory."

malleus One of the ossicles. The malleus receives vibration from the tympanic membrane and is attached to the incus. See also *incus* and *stapes.*

masking Using a second sound, frequently noise, to make the detection of another sound more difficult.

materialism The idea that physical matter is the only reality, and everything including the mind can be explained in terms of matter and physical phenomena. Materialism is a type of monism.

mechanoreceptors Sensory receptors that are responsive to mechanical stimulation (pressure, vibration, movement).

medial geniculate nucleus The part of the thalamus that relays auditory signals to the temporal cortex and receives input from the auditory cortex.

medial superior olive (MSO) A relay station in the brain stem where inputs from both ears contribute to detection of the interaural time difference. Compare *lateral superior olive.*

Meissner corpuscle A specialized nerve ending associated with fast-adapting (FA I) fibers that have small receptive fields.

melody An arrangement of notes or chords in succession.

mentalism The idea that the mind is the true reality and objects exist only as aspects of the mind's awareness. Mentalism is a type of monism.

Merkel cell neurite complex A specialized nerve ending associated with slow-adapting (SA I) fibers that have small receptive fields.

mesopic Light intensities in a middle range that will stimulate both rod and cone photoreceptors. Compare *photopic* and *scotopic.*

metamers Different mixtures of wavelengths that look identical. More generally, any pair of stimuli that are perceived as identical in spite of physical differences.

method of adjustment The method of limits for which the subject controls the change in the stimulus.

method of constant stimuli A psychophysical method in which many stimuli, ranging from rarely to almost always perceivable (or rarely to almost always perceivably different from a reference stimulus), are presented one at a time. Participants respond to each presentation: "yes/no," "same/different," and so on.

method of limits A psychophysical method in which the particular dimension of a stimulus, or the difference between two stimuli, is varied incrementally until the participant responds differently.

metrical depth cue A depth cue that provides quantitative information about distance in the third dimension. Compare *nonmetrical depth cue.*

microvilli (s. microvillus) Slender projections on the tips of some taste bud cells that extend into the taste pore.

middle (midlevel) vision A loosely defined stage of visual processing that comes after basic features have been extracted from the image (early vision) and before object recognition and scene understanding (high-level vision).

middle canal One of three fluid-filled passages in the cochlea. The middle canal is sandwiched between the tympanic and vestibular canals and contains the cochlear partition. Also called *scala media.*

middle ear An air-filled chamber containing the middle bones, or ossicles. The middle ear conveys and amplifies vibration from the tympanic membrane to the oval window.

middle temporal lobe (MT) An area of the brain thought to be important in the perception of motion.

midget bipolar cells Small cone bipolar cells in the central retina that receive input from a single cone. Compare *diffuse bipolar cells.*

midlevel vision See *middle vision.*

mid-spontaneous fibers Auditory nerve fibers with medium rates (10–30 per second) of spontaneous firing. The characteristics of mid-spontaneous fibers are intermediate between *low-spontaneous fibers* and *high-spontaneous fibers.*

mind–body dualism Originated by René Descartes, the idea positing the existence of two distinct principles of being in the universe: spirit/soul and matter/body.

mitral cells The main projective output neurons in the olfactory bulbs. Compare *tufted cells.*

MOB See *main olfactory bulb.*

monism The idea that mind and matter are formed from, or reducible to, a single ultimate substance or principle of being.

monocular With one eye. Compare *binocular.*

monocular depth cue A depth cue that is available even when the world is viewed with one eye alone. Compare *binocular depth cue.*

monosodium glutamate (MSG) The sodium salt of glutamic acid (an amino acid).

motion aftereffect (MAE) The illusion of motion of a stationary object that occurs after prolonged exposure to a moving object.

motion parallax An important depth cue that is based on head movement. The geometric information obtained from an eye in two different positions at two different times is similar to the information from two eyes in different positions in the head at the same time. See *stereopsis.*

MSG See *monosodium glutamate.*

MSO See *medial superior olive.*

MT See *middle temporal lobe.*

muscle spindle A sensory receptor located in a muscle that senses its tension.

myopia A common condition in which light entering the eye is focused in front of the retina and distant objects cannot be seen sharply. Compare *hyperopia*.

N

naïve template theory The proposal that the visual system recognizes objects by matching the neural representation of the image with a stored representation of the same "shape" in the brain.

nativism The idea that the mind produces ideas that are not derived from external sources, and that we have abilities that are innate and not learned.

Necker cube An outline that is perceptually bi-stable. Unlike the situation with most stimuli, two interpretations continually battle for perceptual dominance.

negative afterimage An afterimage whose polarity is the opposite of the original stimulus. Light stimuli produce dark negative afterimages. Colors are complementary; for example, red produces green; yellow produces blue.

neglect In visual attention, the inability to attend to or respond to stimuli in the contralesional visual field (typically, neglect of the left field after right parietal damage). Also, neglect of half of the body or half of an object. Compare *extinction*.

neural plasticity The ability of neural circuits to undergo changes in function or organization as a result of previous activity.

neurotransmitter A chemical substance used in neuronal communication at synapses.

neutral point The point at which an opponent color mechanism is generating no signal. If red–green and blue–yellow mechanisms are at their neutral points, a stimulus will appear achromatic. (The black–white process has no neutral point.)

nociceptors Sensory receptors that transmit information about noxious (painful) stimulation that causes damage or potential damage to the skin.

nonaccidental feature A feature of an object that is not dependent on the exact (or accidental) viewing position of the observer. Compare *accidental viewpoint*.

nonmetrical depth cue A depth cue that provides information about the depth order (relative depth) but not depth magnitude (e.g., his nose is in front of his face). Compare *metrical depth cue*.

nontaster of PTC/PROP An individual born with two recessive alleles for the *Tas2r38* gene and unable to taste the compounds phenylthiocarbamide or propylthiouracil. Compare *taster of PTC/PROP* and *supertaster*.

O

occlusion A cue to relative depth order in which, for example, one object obstructs the view of part of another object.

octave The interval between two sound frequencies having a ratio of 2:1.

ocular dominance The property of the receptive fields of striate cortex neurons by which they demonstrate a preference, responding somewhat more rapidly when a stimulus is presented in one eye than when it is presented in the other.

oculomotor (III) nerves The third pair of cranial nerves, which innervate all the extrinsic muscles of the eye except the lateral rectus and the superior oblique muscles, and which innervate the elevator muscle of the upper eyelid, the ciliary muscle, and the sphincter muscle of the pupil.

odor hedonics The liking dimension of odor perception, typically measured with scales pertaining to an odorant's perceived pleasantness, familiarity, and intensity.

odor A general smell sensation of a particular quality. For example, "The cake had a chocolate *odor*." By contrast, when referring to a specific chemical entity, the term *odorant* should be used.

odorant Any specific aromatic chemical. For example, "You were given the *odorant* menthol to smell." Compare *odor*.

OFF bipolar cells Bipolar cells that respond to a decrease in light captured by the cones. Compare *ON bipolar cells*.

OFF-center cell A cell that depolarizes in response to a decrease in light intensity in its receptive field center. Compare *ON-center cell*.

olfaction The sense of smell.

olfactory (I) nerves The first pair of cranial nerves. The axons of the olfactory sensory neurons bundle together after passing through the cribriform plate to form the olfactory nerve.

olfactory bulb The blueberry-sized extension of the brain just above the nose, where olfactory information is first processed. There are two olfactory bulbs, one in each brain hemisphere, corresponding to the right and left nostrils.

olfactory cleft A narrow space at the back of the nose into which air flows, where the main olfactory epithelium is located.

olfactory epithelium A secretory mucosa in the human nose whose primary function is to detect odorants in the inspired air. Located on both sides of the upper portion of the nasal cavity and the olfactory clefts, the olfactory epithelium contains three types of cells: olfactory sensory neurons, basal cells, and supporting cells.

olfactory receptor (OR) The region on the cilia of olfactory sensory neurons where odorant molecules bind.

olfactory sensory neurons (OSNs) The main cell type in the olfactory epithelium. OSNs are small neurons located beneath a watery mucous layer in the epithelium. The cilia on the OSN dendrites contain the receptor sites for odorant molecules. Compare *basal cells* and *supporting cells*.

ON bipolar cells Bipolar cells that respond to an increase in light captured by the cones. Compare *OFF bipolar cells*.

ON-center cell A cell that depolarizes in response to an increase in light intensity in its receptive field center. Compare *OFF-center cell*.

opponent color theory The theory that perception of color is based on the output of three mechanisms, each of them based on an opponency between two colors: red–green, blue–yellow, and black–white.

optic (II) nerves The second pair of cranial nerves, which arise from the retina and carry visual information to the thalamus and other parts of the brain.

optic array The collection of light rays that interact with objects in the world in front of a viewer. Term coined by J. J. Gibson.

optic flow The changing angular positions of points in a perspective image that we experience as we move through the world.

optical isomers See *stereoisomers.*

OR See *olfactory receptor.*

orbitofrontal cortex The part of the frontal lobe of the cortex that lies above the bone (orbit) containing the eyes. The orbitofrontal cortex is responsible for processing olfaction. It is also the area of the brain critical for assigning affective value to stimuli—in other words, determining hedonic meaning.

organ of Corti A structure on the basilar membrane of the cochlea that is composed of hair cells and dendrites of auditory nerve fibers.

orientation tuning The tendency of neurons in striate cortex to respond optimally to certain orientations, and less to others.

OSN See *olfactory sensory neurons.*

ossicles Three tiny bones of the middle ear: malleus, incus, and stapes.

otitis media Inflammation of the middle ear, commonly in children as a result of infection.

otoconia (s. otoconium) Tiny calcium carbonate stones in the ear that provide inertial mass for the otolith organs, enabling them to sense gravity and linear acceleration.

otolith organs The mechanical structures in the vestibular system that sense both linear acceleration and gravity.

otosclerosis Abnormal growth of the middle-ear bones that causes hearing loss.

ototoxic Producing adverse effects on organs or nerves involved in hearing or balance.

outer ear The external sound-gathering portion of the ear, consisting of the pinna and the ear canal.

outer segment The part of a photoreceptor that contains photopigment molecules. Compare *inner segment.*

oval window The flexible opening to the cochlea through which the stapes transmits vibration to the fluid inside.

overt attentional shift A shift of attention accompanied by corresponding movements of the eyes. Compare *covert attentional shift.*

P

P ganglion cells Small ganglion cells that receive excitatory input from single midget bipolar cells in the central retina and feed the parvocellular layer of the lateral geniculate nucleus. Compare *M ganglion cells.*

Pacinian corpuscle A specialized nerve ending associated with fast-adapting (FA II) fibers that have large receptive fields.

panpsychism The idea that all matter has consciousness.

Panum's fusional area The region of space, in front of and behind the horopter, within which binocular single vision is possible. See also *diplopia.*

papillae (s. papilla) Structures that give the tongue its bumpy appearance. From smallest to largest, the papillae types that contain taste buds are fungiform, foliate, and circumvallate; filiform papillae, which do not contain taste buds, are the smallest and most numerous.

parabelt area A region of cortex, lateral and adjacent to the belt area, where neurons respond to more complex characteristics of sounds, as well as to input from other senses. Compare *belt area.*

parahippocampal place area A region of cortex in the temporal lobe of humans that appears to respond with particular strength to images of places (as opposed to isolated objects). Compare *fusiform face area.*

parallel In visual attention, referring to the processing of multiple stimuli at the same time.

parallelism A rule for figure–ground assignment stating that parallel contours are likely to belong to the same figure.

parietal lobe In each cerebral hemisphere, a lobe that lies toward the top of the brain between the frontal and occipital lobes.

parvocellular layers The neurons in the top four layers of the LGN, which are physically smaller than those in the bottom two layers. Compare *magnocellular layers.*

period The time (or space) required for one cycle of a repeating waveform.

phantom limb Sensation perceived from a physically amputated limb of the body.

phase locking Firing of a single neuron at one distinct point in the period (cycle) of a sound wave at a given frequency. (The neuron need not fire on every cycle, but each firing will occur at the same point in the cycle.)

phase In vision, the relative position of a grating. In hearing, the relative position of two or more sine waves. For sounds, the *phase* is the relative position in time.

pheromone A chemical emitted by one member of a species that triggers a physiological or behavioral response in another member of the same species. Pheromones are signals for chemical communication and do not need to have any smell.

photoactivation Activation by light.

photon A quantum of visible light or other form of electromagnetic radiation demonstrating both particle and wave properties.

photopic Light intensities that are bright enough to stimulate the cone photoreceptors and bright enough to "saturate" the rod photoreceptors (i.e., drive them to their maximum responses). Compare *scotopic* and *mesopic.*

photoreceptors Light-sensitive receptors in the retina.

pictorial depth cue A cue to distance or depth used by artists to depict three-dimensional depth in two-dimensional pictures. Compare *monocular depth cue.*

pinna (pl. pinnae) The outer, funnel-like part of the ear.

pitch The psychological aspect of sound related mainly to the fundamental frequency.

place code Tuning of different parts of the cochlea to different frequencies, in which information about the particular frequency of an incoming sound wave is coded by the place along the cochlear partition that has the greatest mechanical displacement. Compare *temporal code.*

polysensory Blending multiple sensory systems.

positivism A philosophical position arguing that all we really have to go on is the evidence of the senses, so the world might be nothing more than an elaborate hallucination. Compare *realism*.

preattentive stage The processing of a stimulus that occurs before selective attention is deployed to that stimulus.

prefrontal cortex A region of the brain concerned with cognition and executive control.

presbyopia Literally "old sight." The loss of near vision because of insufficient accommodation.

primary auditory cortex (A1) The first area within the temporal lobes of the brain responsible for processing acoustic information.

primary olfactory cortex The neural area where olfactory information is first processed, which includes the amygdala–hippocampal complex and the entorhinal cortex.

primary visual cortex (V1) The area of the cerebral cortex of the brain that receives direct inputs from the lateral geniculate nucleus, as well as feedback from other brain areas, and is responsible for processing visual information. Also called *area 17* or *striate cortex*.

primer pheromone A pheromone that triggers a physiological (often hormonal) change among conspecifics. This effect usually involves prolonged pheromone exposure.

problem of univariance The fact that an infinite set of different wavelength–intensity combinations can elicit exactly the same response from a single type of photoreceptor. One photoreceptor type cannot make color discriminations based on wavelength.

projective geometry For purposes of studying perception of the three-dimensional world, the geometry that describes the transformations that occur when the three-dimensional world is *projected* onto a two-dimensional surface. For example, parallel lines do not converge in the world, but they do in the two-dimensional projection.

proprioception Perception mediated by kinesthetic and vestibular receptors.

prosopagnosia An inability to recognize faces.

protanope An individual who suffers from color blindness that is due to the absence of L-cones. Compare *deuteranope* and *tritanope*.

proximity A Gestalt grouping rule stating that the tendency of two features to group together will increase as the distance between them decreases.

psychoacoustics The study of the psychological correlates of the physical dimensions of acoustics; a branch of psychophysics.

psychophysics The science of defining quantitative relationships between physical and psychological (subjective) events.

pupil The dark circular opening at the center of the iris in the eye, where light enters the eye.

pure tone See *sine wave*.

R

random dot stereogram (RDS) A stereogram made of a large number (often in the thousands) of randomly placed dots. Random dot stereograms contain no monocular cues to depth. Stimuli visible stereoscopically in random dot stereograms are cyclopean stimuli.

rapid serial visual presentation (RSVP) An experimental procedure in which stimuli appear in a stream at one location (typically the point of fixation) at a rapid rate (typically about eight per second).

rate saturation The point at which a nerve fiber is firing as rapidly as possible and further stimulation is incapable of increasing the firing rate.

rate–intensity function A map plotting the firing rate of an auditory nerve fiber in response to a sound of constant frequency at increasing intensities.

RDS See *random dot stereogram*.

reaction time (RT) A measure of the time from the onset of a stimulus to a response.

realism A philosophical position arguing that there is a real world to sense. Compare *positivism*.

receiver operating characteristics (ROC) curve In studies of signal detection, the graphical plot of the hit rate as a function of the false alarm rate. If these are the same, points fall on the diagonal, indicating that the observer cannot tell the difference between the presence and absence of the signal. As the observer's sensitivity increases, the curve bows upward toward the upper left corner. That point represents a perfect ability to distinguish signal from noise (100% hits, 0% false alarms).

receptive field The region on the retina in which visual stimuli influence a neuron's firing rate.

receptor adaptation The biochemical phenomenon that occurs after continuous exposure to an odorant, whereby the receptors stop responding to the odorant and detection ceases.

receptor potential The change in voltage of sensory receptor cells—e.g., hair cells for the vestibular system—in response to stimulation.

"recognition by components" model Biederman's model of object recognition, which holds that objects are recognized by the identities and relationships of their component parts. See also *geons*.

reflect To redirect something that strikes a surface—especially light, sound, or heat—usually back toward its point of origin.

reflectance The percentage of light hitting a surface that is reflected and not absorbed into the surface. Typically reflectance is given as a function of wavelength.

reflexive eye movement A movement of the eye that is automatic and involuntary.

refract 1. To alter the course of a wave of energy that passes into something from another medium, as water does to light entering it from the air. 2. To measure the degree of refraction in a lens or eye.

Reissner's membrane A thin sheath of tissue separating the vestibular and middle canals in the cochlea.

relatability The degree to which two line segments appear to be part of the same contour.

related color A color, such as brown or gray, that is seen only in relation to other colors. A "gray" patch in complete darkness appears white. Compare *unrelated color*.

relative disparity The difference in absolute disparities of two elements in a visual scene. Compare *absolute disparity*.

relative height As a depth cue, the observation that objects at different distances from the viewer on the ground plane will form images at different heights in the retinal image. Objects farther away will be seen as higher in the image.

relative metrical depth cue A depth cue that could specify, for example, that object A was twice as far away as object B without providing information about the absolute distance to either A or B. Compare *absolute metrical depth cue*.

relative size A comparison of size between items without knowing the absolute size of either one.

releaser pheromone A pheromone that triggers an immediate behavioral response among conspecifics.

repetition blindness A failure to detect the second occurrence of a letter, word, or picture in a rapidly presented stream of stimuli when the second occurrence falls within 200 to 500 milliseconds of the first.

response enhancement An effect of attention on the response of a neuron in which the neuron responding to an attended stimulus gives a bigger response.

retina A light-sensitive membrane in the back of the eye that contains rods and cones, which receive an image from the lens and send it to the brain through the optic nerve.

retinitis pigmentosa (RP) A progressive degeneration of the retina that affects night vision and peripheral vision. RP commonly runs in families and can be caused by defects in a number of different genes that have recently been identified.

retronasal olfactory sensation The sensation of an odor that is perceived when chewing and swallowing force an odorant in the mouth up behind the palate into the nose. Such odor sensations are perceived as originating from the mouth, even though the actual contact of odorant and receptor occurs at the olfactory mucosa.

reverse staircase method See *staircase method*.

rhodopsin The visual pigment found in rods.

ROC curve See *receiver operating characteristics curve*.

rod monochromat An individual with no cones of any type. In addition to being truly color-blind, rod monochromats are badly visually impaired in bright light. Compare *cone monochromat*.

rods Photoreceptors specialized for night vision. Compare *cones*.

round window A soft area of tissue at the base of the tympanic canal that releases excess pressure remaining from extremely intense sounds.

RP See *retinitis pigmentosa*.

RSVP See *rapid serial visual presentation*.

RT See *reaction time*.

Ruffini ending A specialized nerve ending associated with slow-adapting (SA II) fibers that have large receptive fields.

S

S-cone A cone that is preferentially sensitive to short wavelengths; colloquially (but not entirely accurately) known as a "blue cone." Compare *M-cone* and *L-cone*.

S1 See *somatosensory area 1*.

S2 See *somatosensory area 2*.

saccade A rapid movement of the eyes that changes fixation from one object or location to another. Compare *smooth pursuit* and *vergence*.

saccadic suppression The reduction of visual sensitivity that occurs when we make saccadic eye movements. Saccadic suppression eliminates the smear from retinal image motion during an eye movement.

saccule One of the two otolith organs. A saclike structure that contains the saccular macula.

salience The vividness of a stimulus relative to its neighbors.

salty The taste quality produced by the cations of salts (e.g., the sodium in sodium chloride produces the salty taste). Some cations also produce other taste qualities (e.g., potassium tastes bitter as well as salty). The purest salty taste is produced by sodium chloride (NaCl), common table salt.

saturation The chromatic strength of a hue. White has zero saturation, pink is more saturated, and red is fully saturated. Compare *brightness* and *hue*.

scala media See *middle canal*.

scala tympani See *tympanic canal*.

scala vestibuli See *vestibular canal*.

scatter To disperse light in an irregular fashion.

scotopic Light intensities that are bright enough to stimulate the rod photoreceptors but too dim to stimulate the cone photoreceptors. Compare *photopic* and *mesopic*.

second-order motion The motion of an object that is defined by changes in contrast or texture, but not by luminance. Compare *first-order motion*.

selective attention The form of attention involved when processing is restricted to a subset of the possible stimuli.

semicircular canals The three toroidal tubes in the vestibular system that sense angular motion.

sense of angular motion The spatial orientation modality that senses motion resulting from rotation.

sense of linear motion The spatial orientation modality that senses translation.

sense of tilt The spatial orientation modality that senses head inclination with respect to gravity.

sensitivity 1. The ability to perceive via the sense organs. 2. Extreme responsiveness to radiation, especially to light of a specific wavelength. 3. The ability to respond to transmitted signals.

sensorineural hearing loss Hearing loss due to defects in the cochlea or auditory nerve.

sensory transducer A receptor that converts physical energy from the environment into neural activity.

serial self-terminating search A search from item to item, ending when a target is found.

set size The number of items in a visual display.

shape-pattern theory The current dominant biochemical theory for how chemicals come to be perceived as specific odorants. Shape-pattern theory contends that different scents—as a function of odorant-shape to OR-shape fit—activate different arrays of olfactory receptors in the olfactory epithelia. These various arrays produce specific firing patterns of neurons in the olfactory bulb, which then determine the particular scent we perceive. Compare *vibration theory*.

sharper tuning An effect of attention on the response of a neuron in which the neuron responds more precisely. For example, a neuron that responds to lines with orientations from –20° to +20° might come to respond to ±10-degree lines.

signal detection theory A psychophysical theory that quantifies the response of an observer to the presentation of a signal in the presence of noise. Measures attained from a series of presentations are sensitivity (*d′*) and criterion of the observer.

similarity A Gestalt grouping rule stating that the tendency of two features to group together will increase as the similarity between them increases.

simple cell A cortical neuron with clearly defined excitatory and inhibitory regions. Compare *complex cell*.

simultagnosia An inability to perceive more than one object at a time. Simultagnosia is a consequence of bilateral damage to the parietal lobes (Balint syndrome).

sine wave The waveform for which variation as a function of time is a sine function. Also called *pure tone*. Compare to *complex tone*.

sine wave grating A grating with a sinusoidal luminance profile.

smooth pursuit A type of eye movement in which the eyes move smoothly to follow a moving object. Compare to *saccade* and *vergence*.

SOA See *stimulus onset asynchrony*.

somatosensation A collective term for sensory signals from the body.

somatosensory area 1 (S1) The primary receiving area for touch in the cortex.

somatosensory area 2 (S2) The secondary receiving area for touch in the cortex.

somatotopic Spatially mapped in the somatosensory cortex in correspondence to spatial events on the skin.

sour The taste quality produced by the hydrogen ion in acids.

source segregation Processing an auditory scene consisting of multiple sound sources into separate sound images. Also called *auditory scene analysis*.

spatial frequency The number of cycles of a grating per unit of visual angle (usually specified in degrees).

spatial layout The description of the structure of a scene (e.g., enclosed, open, rough, smooth) without reference to the identity of specific objects in the scene.

spatial orientation A sense comprised of three interacting sensory modalities: our senses of linear motion, angular motion, and tilt.

spatial-frequency channel A pattern analyzer, implemented by an ensemble of cortical neurons, in which each set of neurons is tuned to a limited range of spatial frequencies.

specific anosmia The inability to smell one specific compound amid otherwise normal smell perception.

specific hungers theory The idea that deficiency of a given nutrient produces craving (a specific hunger) for that nutrient. Curt Richter first proposed this idea and demonstrated that cravings for salty or for sweet are associated with deficiencies in those substances. However, the idea proved wrong for other nutrients (e.g., vitamins).

spectral power distribution The physical energy in a light as a function of wavelength.

spectral reflectance function The function relating the wavelength of light to the percentage of that wavelength that is reflected from a surface.

spectrogram A pattern for sound analysis that provides a three-dimensional display plotting time on the horizontal axis, frequency on the vertical axis, and intensity on a color or gray scale.

spectrum (pl. spectra) A representation of the relative energy (intensity) present at each frequency.

spinothalamic pathway The route from the spinal cord to the brain that carries most of the information about skin temperature and pain. Compare *dorsal column–medial lemniscal pathway*.

staircase method A psychophysical method for determining the concentration of a stimulus required for detection at the threshold level. A stimulus (e.g., odorant) is presented in an ascending concentration sequence until detection is indicated, and then the concentration is shifted to a descending sequence until the response changes to "no detection." This ascending and descending sequence is typically repeated several times, and the concentrations at which reversals occur are averaged to determine the threshold detection level of that odorant for a given individual. Also called *reverse staircase method*.

stapedius The muscle attached to the stapes; tensing the stapedius decreases vibration.

stapes One of the ossicles. Connected to the incus on one end, the stapes presses against the oval window of the cochlea on the other end. See also *incus* and *malleus*.

stereoacuity A measure of the smallest binocular disparity that can generate a sensation of depth.

stereoblindness An inability to make use of binocular disparity as a depth cue. This term is typically used to describe individuals with vision in both eyes. Someone who has lost one (or both) eyes is not typically described as "stereoblind."

stereocilia (s. stereocilium) Hairlike extensions on the tips of hair cells in the cochlea that initiate the release of neurotransmitters when they are flexed.

stereoisomers Isomers (molecules that can exist in different structural forms) in which the spatial arrangement of the atoms are mirror-image rotations of one another, like a right and left hand. Also called *optical isomers*.

stereopsis The ability to use binocular disparity as a cue to depth. Compare *monocular*.

stereoscope A device for presenting one image to one eye and another image to the other eye. Stereoscopes can be used to present dichoptic stimuli for stereopsis and binocular rivalry.

Stevens' power law A principle describing the relationship between stimulus and resulting sensation, such that the magnitude of subjective sensation is proportional to the stimulus magnitude raised to an exponent.

stimulus onset asynchrony (SOA) The time between the onset of one stimulus and the onset of another.

strabismus A misalignment of the two eyes such that a single object in space is imaged on the fovea of one eye, and on a nonfoveal area of the other (turned) eye.

striate cortex See *primary visual cortex*.

structural description A description of an object in terms of the nature of its constituent parts and the relationships between those parts.

structuralism A school of thought believing that complex objects or perceptions could be understood by analysis of the components. Compare *Gestalt*.

substantia gelatinosa A jellylike region of interconnecting neurons in the dorsal horn of the spinal cord.

subtractive color mixture A mixture of pigments. If pigments A and B mix, some of the light shining on the surface will be subtracted by A, and some by B. Only the remainder contributes to the perception of color. Compare *additive color mixture*.

superior colliculus A structure in the midbrain that is important in initiating and guiding eye movements.

superior olive An early brain stem region in the auditory pathway where inputs from both ears converge.

supertaster An individual who perceives the most intense taste sensations. A variety of factors may contribute to this heightened perception; among the most important is the density of fungiform papillae. Compare *nontaster of PTC/PROP* and *taster of PTC/PROP*.

supporting cells One of the three types of cells in the olfactory epithelium. This cell type provides metabolic and physical support for the OSNs. Compare *basal cells* and *olfactory sensory neurons*.

suppression In vision, the inhibition of an unwanted image. Suppression occurs frequently in persons with strabismus.

surroundedness A rule for figure–ground assignment stating that if one region is entirely surrounded by another, it is likely that the surrounded region is the figure.

sweet The taste quality produced by some sugars, such as glucose, fructose, and sucrose. These three sugars are particularly biologically useful to us, and our sweet receptors are tuned to them. Some other compounds (e.g., saccharin, aspartame), are also sweet.

symmetry A rule for figure–ground assignment stating that symmetrical regions are more likely to be seen as figure.

synapse The junction between neurons that permits information transfer.

synaptic terminal The location where axons terminate at the synapse for transmission of information by release of a chemical transmitter.

T

tactile agnosia The inability to identify objects by touch.

Tadoma A method by which those who are both deaf and blind can perceive speech in real time using their hands.

target The goal of a visual search. Compare *distractor*.

tastant Any stimulus that can be tasted.

taste buds Globular clusters of cells that have the function of creating the neural signals conveyed to the brain by taste nerves. Some of the cells (see *taste receptor cells*) in the taste bud have specialized sites on their apical projections (see *microvilli*) that interact with taste stimuli. Some of the cells form synapses with taste nerve fibers. Current research is just revealing the complex events within taste buds that result in neural signals.

taste receptor cells Cells within the taste bud that contain sites on their apical projections that can interact with taste stimuli. These sites fall into two major categories: those interacting with charged particles (e.g., sodium and hydrogen ions), and those interacting with specific chemical structures.

taster of PTC/PROP An individual born with one or both dominant alleles for the *Tas2r38* gene and able to taste the compounds phenylthiocarbamide and propylthiouracil. Tasters of PTC/PROP who also have a high density of fungiform papillae are supertasters. Compare *nontaster of PTC/PROP* and *supertaster*.

tau (τ) Information in the optic flow that could signal TTC (time to collision) without the necessity of estimating either absolute distances or rates. The ratio of the retinal image size at any moment to the rate at which the image is expanding is tau, and TTC is proportional to tau.

tectorial membrane A gelatinous structure, attached on one end, that extends into the middle canal of the ear, floating above inner hair cells and touching outer hair cells.

tempo The perceived speed of the presentation of sounds.

temporal code Tuning of different parts of the cochlea to different frequencies, in which information about the particular frequency of an incoming sound wave is coded by the timing of neural firing as it relates to the period of the sound. Compare *place code*.

temporal integration The process by which a sound at a constant level is perceived as being louder when it is of greater duration. The term also applies to perceived brightness, which depends on the duration of light.

tensor tympani The muscle attached to the malleus; tensing the tensor tympani decreases vibration.

texture gradient A depth cue based on the geometric fact that items of the same size form smaller images when they are farther away. An array of items that change in size across the image will appear to form a surface in depth.

texture segmentation Carving an image into regions of common texture properties.

texture-defined (contrast-defined) object An object that is defined by changes in contrast or texture, but not by luminance.

thermoreceptors Sensory receptors that signal information about changes in skin temperature.

threshold tuning curve A map plotting the thresholds of a neuron or fiber in response to sine waves with varying frequencies at the lowest intensity that will give rise to a response.

tilt aftereffect The perceptual illusion of tilt, produced by adaptation to a pattern of a given orientation.

timbre The psychological sensation by which a listener can judge that two sounds with the same loudness and pitch are dissimilar. Timbre quality is conveyed by harmonics and other high frequencies.

time to collision (TTC) The time required for a moving object (such as a cricket ball) to hit a stationary object (such as a batsman's head). TTC = distance/rate.

tip link A tiny filament that stretches from the tip of a stereocilium to the side of its neighbor.

tip-of-the-nose phenomenon The inability to name an odorant, even though it is very familiar. Contrary to the tip-of-the-tongue phenomenon, one has no lexical access to the name of the odorant, such as first letter, rhyme, number of syllables, and so on, when in the tip-of-the-nose state. This is one example of how language and olfactory perception are deeply disconnected.

tone chroma A sound quality shared by tones that have the same octave interval.

tone height A sound quality corresponding to the level of pitch. Tone height is monotonically related to frequency.

tonotopic organization An arrangement in which neurons that respond to different frequencies are organized anatomically in order of frequency.

topographical mapping The orderly mapping of the world in the lateral geniculate nucleus and the visual cortex.

transduced Referring to the conversion from one form of energy (e.g., light) to another (e.g., electricity).

transmit To convey something (e.g., light) from one place or thing to another.

transparent Allowing light to pass through with no interruption so that objects on the other side can be clearly seen.

triangle test A test in which a participant is given three odors to smell, of which two are the same and one is different. The participant is required to state which is the odd odor out. The order of the three odors given (e.g., same, same, different; different, same, same; same, different, same) is typically manipulated and the test repeated several times for greater accuracy.

trichromacy See *trichromatic theory of color vision*.

trichromatic theory of color vision The theory that the color of any light is defined in our visual system by the relationships of three numbers, the outputs of three receptor types now known to be the three cones. Also known as *trichromacy* or the *Young–Helmholtz theory*.

trigeminal (V) nerves The fifth pair of cranial nerves, which transmit information about the 'feel' of an odorant (e.g., menthol feels cool, and cinnamon feels warm), as well as pain and irritation sensations (e.g., ammonia feels burning).

tritanope An individual who suffers from color blindness that is due to the absence of S-cones. Compare *deuteranope* and *protanope*.

trochlear (IV) nerves The fourth pair of cranial nerves, which innervate the superior oblique muscles of the eyeballs.

TTC See *time to collision*.

tufted cells A secondary class of output neurons in the olfactory bulbs. Compare *mitral cells*.

two-point touch threshold The minimum distance at which two stimuli (e.g., two simultaneous touches) are just perceptible as separate.

two-tone suppression A decrease in the firing rate of one auditory nerve fiber due to one tone, when a second tone is presented at the same time.

tympanic canal One of three fluid-filled passages in the cochlea. The tympanic canal extends from the round window at the base of the cochlea to the helicotrema at the apex. Also called *scala tympani*. See also *middle canal* and *vestibular canal*.

tympanic membrane The eardrum; a thin sheet of skin at the end of the outer ear canal. The tympanic membrane vibrates in response to sound.

U

umami The taste sensation evoked by monosodium glutamate.

uncrossed disparity The sign of disparity created by objects behind the plane of fixation (the horopter). The term *uncrossed* is used because images of objects located behind the horopter will appear to be displaced to the right in the right eye, and to the left in the left eye. Compare *crossed disparity*.

unique blue A blue that has no red or green tint.

unique hue Any of four colors that can be described with only a single color term: red, yellow, green, blue. Other colors (e.g., purple or orange) can be described as compounds (reddish blue, reddish yellow).

uniqueness constraint In stereopsis, the observation that a feature in the world is represented exactly once in each retinal image. This constraint simplifies the correspondence problem.

unrelated color A color that can be experienced in isolation. Compare *related color*.

utricle One of the two otolith organs. A saclike structure that contains the utricular macula.

V

V1 See *primary visual cortex*.

vanishing point The apparent point at which parallel lines receding in depth converge. See also *Euclidean* and *linear perspective*.

vection An illusory sense of self motion produced when you are not, in fact, moving.

vergence A type of eye movement in which the two eyes move in opposite directions—for example, both eyes turn toward the nose (convergence) or away from the nose (divergence). Compare *saccade* and *smooth pursuit*.

vestibular canal One of three fluid-filled passages in the cochlea. The vestibular canal extends from the oval window at the base of the cochlea to the helicotrema at the apex. Also called *scala vestibuli*. See also *middle canal* and *tympanic canal*.

vestibular system The set of five organs—three semicircular canals and two otolith organs—located in each inner ear that sense head motion and head orientation with respect to gravity. Also called *vestibular labyrinth*.

vestibulocochlear nerve See *auditory (VIII) nerves*.

vibration theory An alternative to *shape-pattern theory*, describing how olfaction works; most recently championed by Luca Turin. Vibration theory proposes that every perceived smell has a different vibrational frequency, and that molecules that produce the same vibrational frequencies will smell the same. Compare *shape-pattern theory*.

Vieth–Müller circle The location of objects whose images fall on geometrically corresponding points in the two retinas. If life were simple, this circle would be the horopter, but life is not simple.

viewpoint invariance 1. A property of an object that does not change when observer viewpoint changes. 2. A class of theories of object recognition that proposes representations of objects that do not change when viewpoint changes.

virtual haptic environment A synthetic world that may be experienced haptically by operation of an electromechanical device that delivers forces to the hand of the user.

visual acuity A measure of the finest detail that can be resolved by the eyes.

visual angle The angle subtended by an object at the retina.

visual search Looking for a target in a display containing distracting elements.

visual-field defect A portion of the visual field with no vision or with abnormal vision, typically resulting from damage to the visual nervous system.

vitalism The idea that "vital forces" are active within living organisms, and these forces cannot be explained by physical processes of matter more generally.

vitreous humor The transparent fluid that fills the vitreous chamber in the posterior part of the eye. Compare *aqueous humor*.

VNO See *vomeronasal organ*.

vocal tract The airway above the larynx used for the production of speech. The vocal tract includes the oral tract and nasal tract.

volley principle An idea stating that multiple neurons can provide a temporal code for frequency if each neuron fires at a distinct point in the period of a sound wave but does not fire on every period.

vomeronasal organ (VNO) A chemical sensing organ at the base of the nasal cavity with a curved tubular shape. The VNO evolved to detect chemicals that cannot be processed by the olfactory epithelium, such as large and/or aqueous molecules—the types of molecules that constitute pheromones.

W

warmth fiber A sensory nerve fiber that fires when skin temperature increases. Compare *cold fiber*.

wave An oscillation that travels through a medium by transferring energy from one particle or point to another without causing any permanent displacement of the medium.

Weber fraction The constant of proportionality in Weber's law.

Weber's law The principle that the just noticeable difference (JND) is a constant fraction of the comparison stimulus.

white noise Noise consisting of all audible frequencies in equal amounts. White noise in hearing is analogous to white light in vision, for which all wavelengths are present.

Y

Young–Helmholtz theory See *trichromatic theory of color vision*.

References

Ackerman, D. (1990). *A Natural History of the Senses.* New York: Random House.

Addams, R. (1834). An account of a peculiar optical phenomenon seen after having looked at a moving body, etc. *Lond Edinb Philos Mag J Sci* 5: 373–374.

Adelson, E. H. (1993). Perceptual organization and the judgment of brightness. *Science* 262: 2042–2044.

Adelson, E. H., and Bergen, J. R. (1985). Spatiotemporal energy models perception of motion. *J Opt Soc Am A* 2: 284–299.

Ahissar, M., and Hochstein, S. (2004). The reverse hierarchy theory of visual perceptual learning. *Trends Cogn Sci* 8: 457–464.

Alais, D., and Blake, R. (2005). *Binocular Rivalry and Perceptual Ambiguity.* Cambridge, MA: MIT Press.

Alpern, M., Kitahara, K., and Krantz, D. H. (1983). Classical tritanopia. *J Physiol* 335: 655–681.

American Standards Association. (1960). *Acoustical Terminology SI, 1-1960.* New York: American Standards Association.

Anderson, J. A., Silverstein, J. W., Ritz, S. A., and Jones, R. S. (1977). Distinctive features, categorical perception, and probability learning: Some applications of a neural model. *Psychol Rev* 84: 413–451.

Anderson, J. S., Lampl, I., Gillespie, D. C., and Ferster, D. (2000). Contribution of noise to contrast invariance of orientation tuning in cat visual cortex. *Science* 290: 1968–1972.

Attneave, F., and Olson, R. K. (1971). Pitch as a medium: A new approach to psychophysical scaling. *Am J Psychol* 84: 147–166.

Aubert, H. (1886). Die Bewegungsempfindung. *Arch Ges Physiol* 39: 347–370.

Ayabe-Kanamura, S., Schicker, I., Laska, M., Hudson, R., Distel, H., Kobabyakaw, T., and Saito, S. (1998). Differences in perception of everyday odors: A Japanese-German cross-cultural study. *Chem Senses* 23: 31–38.

Bachem, A. (1950). Tone height and tone chroma as two different pitch qualities. *Acta Psychol* 7: 80–88.

Bahill, A. T., and Stark, L. (1979). The trajectories of saccadic eye movements. *Sci Am* 240(1): 108–117.

Banks, M. S., Aslin, R. N., and Letson, R. D. (1975). Sensitive period for the development of human binocular vision. *Science* 190: 675–677.

Barclay, C. D., Cutting, J. E., and Kozlowski, L. T. (1978). Temporal and spatial factors in gait perception that influence gender recognition. *Percept Psychophys* 23: 145–152.

Baringa, M. (2002). How the brain's clock gets daily enlightenment. *Science* 295: 955–957.

Barlow, H. B. (1972). Single units and sensation: A neuron doctrine for perceptual psychology. *Perception* 1: 371–394.

Barlow, H. (1995). The neuron doctrine in perception. In M. S. Gazzaniga (Ed.), *The Cognitive Neurosciences* (pp. 415–435). Cambridge, MA: MIT Press.

Barlow, H. B., Blakemore, C., and Pettigrew, J. D. (1967). The neural mechanism of binocular depth discrimination. *J Physiol* 193: 327–342.

Barlow, H. B., and Levick, W. R. (1965). The mechanism of directionally selective units in rabbit's retina. *J Physiol* 178: 477–504.

Bartoshuk, L. M. (1979). Bitter taste of saccharin: Related to the genetic ability to taste the bitter substance 6-*n*-propylthiouracil (PROP). *Science* 205: 934–935.

Bartoshuk, L. M. (1991). Taste, smell and pleasure. In R. C. Bolles (Ed.), *The Hedonics of Taste* (pp. 15–28). Hillsdale, NJ: Erlbaum.

Bartoshuk, L. M., Fast, K., and Snyder, D. (2005). Differences in our sensory worlds: Invalid comparisons with labeled scales. *Curr Dir Psychol Sci* 14: 122–125.

Bartoshuk, L. M., and Wolfe, J. M. (1990). Conditioned taste aversions in humans: Are the olfactory aversions? *Chem Senses* 15: 551.

Bashford, J. A., and Warren, R. M. (1987). Multiple phonemic restorations follow the rules for auditory induction. *Percept Psychophys* 42: 114–121.

Basson, M. D., Bartoshuk, L. M., Dichello, S. Z., Panzini, L., Weiffenbach, J. M., and Duffy, V. B. (2005). Association between 6-*n*-propylthiouracil (PROP) bitterness and colonic neoplasms. *Dig Dis Sci* 50: 483–489.

Beale, J. M., and Keele, F. C. (1995). Categorical effects in the perception of faces. *Cognition* 57: 217–239.

Beck, J. (1982). Textural segmentation. In J. Beck (Ed.), *Organization and Representation in Perception* (pp. 285–317). Hillsdale, NJ: Erlbaum.

Bergen, J. R., and Adelson, E. H. (1988). Early vision and texture perception. *Nature* 333: 363–364.

Berger, A., Henderson, M., Nadoolman, W., Duffy, V. B., Cooper, D., Saberski, L., and Bartoshuk, L. (1995). Oral capsaicin provides temporary relief for oral mucositis pain secondary to chemotherapy/radiation therapy. *J Pain Symptom Manage* 10: 243–248.

Berkeley, G. (1837). *The Works of George Berkeley.* London: Tegg. (Original works published in 1709, 1710, 1713.)

Berlin, B., and Kay, P. (1969). *Basic Color Terms: Their Universality and Evolution.* Berkeley: University of California Berkeley.

Bernstein, I. L. (1978). Learned taste aversions in children receiving chemotherapy. *Science* 200: 1302–1303.

Berthoz, A., Israel, I., Georges-Francois, P., Grasso, R., and Tsuzuku, T. (1995). Spatial memory of body linear displacement: What is being stored? *Science* 269: 95–98.

Bertino, M., Beauchamp, G. K., and Engelman, K. (1982). Long-term reduction in dietary sodium alters the taste of salt. *Am J Clin Nutr* 36: 1134–1144.

Bialystok, E., and Hakuta, K. (1994). *In Other Words: The Science and Psychology of Second-Language Acquisition.* New York: Basic Books.

Biederman, I. (1987). Recognition-by-components: A theory of human image understanding. *Psychol Rev* 94: 115–147.

Binder, J. R. (2000). The neuroanatomy of speech perception (Editorial). *Brain* 123: 2371–2372.

Binder, J. R., Rao, S. M., Hammeke, T. A., Yetkin, F. Z., Jesmanowicz, A., Bandettini, P. A., Wong, E. C., Estkowski, L. D., Goldstein, M. D., Haughton, V. M., and Hyde, J. S. (1994). Functional magnetic resonance imaging of human auditory cortex. *Ann Neurol* 35: 662–672.

Birch, E. E. (1993). Stereopsis in infants and it's developmental relation to visual acuity. In K. Simons (Ed.), *Early Visual Development Normal and Abnormal* (pp. 224–234). New York: Oxford University Press.

Birch, E., and Petrig, B. (1996). FPL and VEP measures of fusion, stereopsis and stereoacuity in normal infants. *Vision Res* 36: 1321–1326.

Blake, R. (1988). Cat spatial vision. *Trends Neurosci* 11: 78–83.

Blake, R., and Logothetis, N. K. (2002). Visual competition. *Nat Rev Neurosci* 3: 13–21.

Blakemore, C., and Campbell, F. W. (1969). On the existence of neurons in the human visual system selectively sensitive to the orientation and size of images. *J Physiol* 203: 237–260.

Blakemore, S.-J., Wolpert, D. M., and Frith, C. D. (1998). Central cancellation of self-produced tickle sensation. *Nat Neurosci* 1: 635–640.

Bloj, M. G., Kersten, D., and Hurlbert, A. C. (1999). Perception of three-dimensional shape influences colour perception through mutual illumination. *Nature* 402: 877–880.

Blood, A. J., and Zatorre, R. J. (2001). Intensely pleasurable responses to music correlate with activity in brain regions implicated in reward and emotion. *Proc Natl Acad Sci USA* 98: 11818–11823.

Bloom, P. (2004). *Descartes' Baby: How the Science of Child Development Explains What Makes Us Human.* New York: Basic Books.

Blumenfeld, H. (2002). *Neuroanatomy through Clinical Cases.* Sunderland, MA: Sinauer.

Blundell, J., and Hill, A. J. (1986). Paradoxical effects of an intense sweetener (aspartame) on appetite. *Lancet* 1: 1092–1093.

Bolton, T. L. (1894). Rhythm. *Am J Psychol* 6: 145–238.

Boothe, R. G., Dobson, V., and Teller, D. Y. (1985). Postnatal development of vision in human and non-human primates. *Annu Rev Neurosci* 8: 495–545.

Boring, E. G. (1950). *A History of Experimental Psychology* (2nd ed.). New York: Appleton-Century-Crofts.

Bortolami, S. B., Pierobon, A., DiZio, P., and Lackner, J. R. (2006). Localization of the subjective vertical during roll, pitch, and recumbent yaw body tilt. *Exp Brain Res* 173: 364–373.

Bouvrie, J. V., and Sinha, P. (2007). Observations in congenitally blind children and a computational model. *Neurocomputing* 70: 2218–2233.

Boycott, B. B., and Dowling, J. E. (1969). Organization of the primate retina: Light microscopy. *Philos Trans R Soc Lond B Biol Sci* 255: 109–176.

Brady, T. F., Konkle, T., Alvarez, G. A., and Oliva , A. (2008). Visual long-term memory has a massive storage capacity for object details. *Proc Natl Acad Sci USA* 105: 14325–14329.

Brand, A., Behrend, O., Marquardt, T., McAlpine, D., and Grothe, B. (2002). Precise inhibition is essential for microsecond interaural time difference coding. *Nature* 417: 543–547.

Breedlove, S. M., Rosenzweig, M. R., and Watson, N. V. (2007). *Biology Psychology: An Introduction to Behavioral, Cognitive, and Clinical Neuroscience* (5th ed.). Sunderland, MA: Sinauer.

Brefczynski, J. A., and DeYoe, E. A. (1999). A physiological correlate of the "spotlight" of visual attention. *Nat Neurosci* 2: 370–374.

Bregman, A. S., and Campbell, J. (1971). Primary auditory stream segregation and perception of order in rapid sequences of tones. *J Exp Psychol* 89: 244–249.

Brugge, J. F., and Howard, M. A. (2002). Hearing. In V. S. Ramachandran (Ed.), *Encyclopedia of The Human Brain* (pp. 429–448). New York: Academic Press.

Brungart, D. S., Durlach, N. I., and Rabinowitz, W. M. (1999). Auditory localization of nearby sources. II. Localization of a broadband source. *J Acoust Soc Am* 106: 1956–1968.

Buchsbaum, G., and Gottschalk, A. (1983). Trichromacy, opponent colours coding and optimum colour information transmission in the retina. *Proc R Soc Lond B Biol Sci* 220: 89–113.

Buck, L., and Axel, R. (1991). A novel multigene family may encode odorant receptors: A molecular basis for odor recognition. *Cell* 65: 175–187.

Bufe, B., Hofmann, T., Krautwurst, D., Raguse, J.-D., and Meyerhof, W. (2002). The human TAS2R16 receptor mediates bitter taste in response to B-glucopyranosides. *Nat Genet* 32: 397–401.

Busey, T. A., Tunnicliff, J., Loftus, G. R., and Loftus, E. F. (2000). Accounts of the confidence-accuracy relation in recognition memory. *Psychon Bull Rev* 7: 26–48.

Cain, W. S., and Engen, T. (1969). Olfactory adaptation and the scaling of odor intensity. In C. Pfaffmann (Ed.), *Olfaction and Taste III* (pp. 127–141). New York: Rockefeller University Press.

Cain, W. S., and Johnson, F., Jr. (1978). Lability of odor pleasantness: Influence of mere exposure. *Perception* 7: 459–465.

Calder, A. J., Young, A. W., Perrett, D. I., Etcoff, N. L., and Rowland, D. (1996). Categorical perception of morphed facial expressions. *Vis Cogn* 3: 81–117.

Calvert, G. A., Bullmore, E. T., Brammer, M. J., Campbell, R., Williams, S. C. R., McGuire, P. K., Woodruff, P. W. R., Iversen, S. D., and David, A. S. (1997). Activation of auditory cortex during silent lipreading. *Science* 276: 593–596.

Cameron, E. L. (2007). Measures of human olfactory perception during pregnancy. *Chem Senses* 32: 775–782.

Campbell, F. W., and Green, D. G. (1965). Optical and retinal factors affecting visual resolution. *J Physiol* 181: 576–593.

Campbell, F. W., and Robson, J. G. (1968). Application of Fourier analysis to the visibility of gratings. *J Physiol* 197: 551–556.

Campbell, R., Pascalis, O., Coleman, M., Wallace, B., and Benson, P. J. (1997). Are faces of different species perceived categorically by human observers? *Proc R Soc Lond B Biol Sci* 264: 1429–1434.

Carskadon, M., and Herz, R. S. (2004). Minimal olfactory perception during sleep: Why odor alarms will not work for humans. *Sleep* 27: 402–405.

Carskadon, M. A., Wyatt, J., Etgen, G., and Rosekind, M. R. (1989). Nonvisual sensory experiences in dreams of college students. *Sleep Res* 18: 159.

Cavanagh, P., and Leclerc, Y. G. (1989). Shape from shadows. *J Exp Psychol Hum Percept Perform* 15: 3–27.

Cave, K. R., and Bichot, N. P. (1999). Visuospatial attention: Beyond a spotlight model. *Psychon Bull Rev* 6: 204–223.

Changizi, M. A., Zhang, Q., and Shimojo, S. (2006). Bare skin, blood and the evolution of primate colour vision. *Biol Lett* 2: 217–221.

Chaudhari, N., Landin, A. M., and Roper, S. D. (2000). A metabotropic glutamate receptor variant functions as a taste receptor. *Nat Neurosci* 3: 113–119.

Chino, Y. M., Smith, E. L., III, Hatta, S., and Cheng, H. (1997). Postnatal development of binocular disparity sensitivity in neurons of the primate visual cortex. *J Neurosci* 17: 296–307.

Chun, M. M. (1997). Types and tokens in visual processing: A double dissociation between the attentional blink and repetition blindness. *J Exp Psychol Hum Percept Perform* 23: 738–755.

Chun, M. M., and Potter, M. C. (1995). A two-stage model for multiple target detection in RSVP. *J Exp Psychol Hum Percept Perform* 21: 109–127.

Clark, F. J., and Horch, K. W. (1986). Kinesthesia. In K. R. Boff, L. Kaufman, and J. P. Thomas (Eds.), *Handbook of Perception & Human Performance*, Vol. 1: *Sensory Processes and Perception* (pp. 13-1 to 13-62). New York: Wiley.

Classen, C., Howes, D., and Synnott, A. (1994). *Aroma: The Cultural History of Smell.* London: Routledge.

Coady, J. A., Kluender, K. R., and Rhode, W. S. (2003). Effects of contrast between onsets of speech and other complex spectra. *J Acoust Soc Am* 114: 2225–2235.

Coan, J. A., Schaefer, H. S., and Davidson, R. J. (2006). Lending a hand: Social regulation of the natural response to threat. *Psychol Sci* 17: 1032–1039.

Cole, J. (1991). *Pride and a Daily Marathon.* Boston: MIT Press.

Conway, B. R., Kitaoka, A., Yazdanbakhsh, A., Pack, C. C., and Livingstone, M. S. (2005). Neural basis for a powerful static motion illusion. *J Neurosci* 25: 5651–5656.

Cornsweet, T. N. (1970). *Visual Perception.* New York: Academic Press.

Coss, R. G., Gusé, K. L., Poran, N. S., and Smith, D. (1993). Development of antisnake defense in California ground squirrels (*Sperophilus beecheyi*). II. Microevolutionary effects of relaxed selection from rattlesnakes. *Behavior* 124: 137–165.

Craig, J. C., and Johnson, K. O. (2000). The two-point threshold: Not a measure of tactile spatial resolution. *Curr Dir Psychol Sci* 9: 29–32.

Cronin, T. W., Jarvilehto, M., Weckstrom, M., and Lall, A. B. (2000). Tuning of photoreceptor spectral sensitivity in fireflies (Coleoptera: Lampyridae). *J Comp Physiol [A]* 186: 1–12.

Crystal, S. R., and Bernstein, I. L. (1995). Morning sickness: Impact on offspring salt preference. *Appetite* 25: 231–240.

Cumming, B. G., and Parker, A. J. (1999). Binocular neurons in V1 of awake monkeys are selective for absolute, not relative, disparity. *J Neurosci* 19: 5602–5618.

Curcio, C. A., Sloan, K. R., Kalina, R. E., and Hendrickson, A. E. (1990). Human photoreceptor topography. *J Comp Neurol* 292: 497–523.

Dalton, P. (1996). Odor perception and beliefs about risk. *Chem Senses* 21: 447–458.

Dalton, P. (2002). Olfaction. In H. Pashler, S. Yantis, D. Medin, R. Gallistel, and J. Wixted (Eds.), *Stevens' Handbook of Experimental Psychology* (3rd ed.), Vol. 1: *Sensation and Perception* (pp. 691–746). New York: Wiley.

Dalton, P., Doolittle, N., and Breslin, P. A. S. (2002). Gender-specific induction of enhanced sensitivity to odors. *Nat Neurosci* 5: 199–200.

Dalton, P., Wysocki, C. J., Brody, M. J., and Lawley, H. J. (1997). Perceived odor, irritation and health symptoms following short-term exposure to acetone. *Am J Ind Med* 31: 558–569.

Damper, R. I., and Harnad, S. R. (2000). Neural network models of categorical perception. *Percept Psychophys* 62: 843–867.

Darwin, C. (1859). *The Origin of Species, by Means of Natural Selection or the Preservation of Favoured Races in the Struggle for Life.* New York: New York American Library.

Darwin, C. (1871). *The Descent of Man, and Selection in Relation to Sex.* New York: Burt.

Darwin, C. J. (1984). Perceiving vowels in the presence of another sound: Constraints on formant perception. *J Acoust Soc Am* 76: 1636–1647.

Davidoff, J., Davies, I., and Roberson, D. (1999). Is colour categorisation universal? New evidence from a stone-age culture. *Nature* 398: 203–204.

Davidson, R. J., Putnam, K. M., and Larson, C. L. (2000). Dysfunction in the neural circuitry of emotion regulation—A possible prelude to violence. *Science* 289: 591–594.

Davidson, T. L., and Swithers, S. E. (2004). A Pavlovian approach to the problem of obesity. *Int J Obes Relat Metab Disord* 28: 933–935.

Davis, C. M. (1928). Self selection of diet by newly weaned infants: An experimental study. *Am J Dis Child* 36: 651–679.

Davis, M. and Whalen, P. J. (2001). The amygdala: Vigilance and emotion. *Mol Psychiatry* 6: 13–34.

DeCasper, A. J., and Fifer, W. P. (1980). Of human bonding: Newborns prefer their mother's voices. *Science* 208: 1174–1176.

DeCasper, A. J., and Spence, M. J. (1986). Prenatal maternal speech influences newborns' perception of speech sounds. *Infant Behav Dev* 9: 133–150.

De Gelder, B., Teunisse, J. P., and Benson, P. J. (1997). Categorical perception of facial expressions: Categories and their internal structure. *Cogn Emol* 11: 1–23.

Derrington, A. M., Krauskopf, J., and Lennie, P. (1984). Chromatic mechanisms in lateral geniculate nucleus of macaque. *J Physiol* 357: 241–265.

Descartes, R. (1664). *Le Monde.* Paris: Jacques Le Gras.

De Valois, R., Abramov, I., and Jacobs, G. (1966). Analysis of response patterns of LGN cells. *J Opt Soc Am A* 56: 966–977.

De Valois, R. L., Albrecht, D. G., and Thorell, L. G. (1982). Spatial frequency selectivity of cells in macaque visual cortex. *Vision Res* 22: 545–559.

De Valois, R. L., Yund, E. W., and Hepler, N. (1982). The orientation and direction selectivity of cells in macaque visual cortex. *Vision Res* 22: 531–544.

Diamond, J., Dalton, P., Doolittle, N., and Breslin, P. A. (2005). Gender-specific olfactory sensitization: Hormonal and cognitive influences. *Chem Senses* Suppl.1: i224–i225.

DiCarlo, J. J., and Cox, D. D. (2007). Untangling invariant object recognition. *Trends Cogn Sci* 11: 333–341.

DiCarlo, J. J., and Maunsell, J. H. (2003). Anterior inferotemporal neurons of monkeys engaged in object recognition can be highly sensitive to object retinal position. *J Neurophysiol* 89: 3264–3278.

Dieterich, M., and Brandt, T. (2008). Functional brain imaging of peripheral and central vestibular disorders. *Brain* [Epub ahead of print].

Dijkerman, C., and de Haan, E. (2007). Somatosensory processes subserving perception and action. *Behav Brain Sci* 30: 189–239.

Dilks, D. D., Dalton, P., and Beauchamp, G. K. (1999). Cross-cultural variation in responses to malodors. *Chem Senses* 24: 599.

Di Lollo, V., Enns, J. T., and Rensink, R. A. (2000). Competition for consciousness among visual events: The psychophysics of reentrant visual pathways. *J Exp Psychol Gen* 129: 481–507.

DiLorenzo, P. M., and Monroe, S. (1995). Corticofugal influence on taste responses in the nucleus of the solitary tract in the rat. *J Neurophysiol* 74: 258–272.

Dittman, A., and Quinn, T. (1996). Homing in Pacific salmon: Mechanisms and ecological basis. *J Exp Biol* 199(Pt 1): 83–91.

Dobb, E. (1989). The scents around us. *Sciences* 29(6): 46–53.

Dorr, S., and Neumeyer, C. (1996). The goldfish—A colour-constant animal. *Perception* 25: 243–250.

Downing, P., Liu, J., and Kanwisher, N. (2001). Testing cognitive models of visual attention with fMRI and MEG. *Neuropsychologia* 39: 1329–1342.

Driver, J. (1998). The neuropsychology of spatial attention. In H. Pashler (Ed.), *Attention* (pp. 297–340). Hove, East Sussex, UK: Psychology Press.

Duffy, V. B., Bartoshuk, L. M., Striegel-Moore, R., and Rodin, J. (1998). Taste changes across pregnancy. In C. Murphy (Ed.), *Olfaction and Taste XIX: An Interna-*

tional Symposium (Vol. 855, pp. 805–809). New York: Annals of the New York Academy of Sciences.

Duffy, V. B., Davidson, A. C., Kidd, J. R., Kidd, K. K., Speed, W. C., Pakstis, A. J., Reed, D. R., Snyder, D. J., and Bartoshuk, L. M. (2004). Bitter receptor gene (TAS2R38), 6-*n*-propylthiouracil (PROP) bitterness and alcohol intake. *Alcohol Clin Exp Res* 28: 1629–1637.

Duffy, V. B., Lucchina, L. A., and Bartoshuk, L. M. (2004). Genetic variation in taste: Potential biomarker for cardiovascular disease risk? In J. Prescott and B. J. Tepper (Eds.), *Genetic Variations in Taste Sensitivity: Measurement, Significance and Implications* (pp. 195–228). New York: Dekker.

Durgin, F. H., Proffitt, D. R., Olson, T. J., and Reinke, K. S. (1995). Comparing depth from motion with depth from binocular disparity. *J Exp Psychol Hum Percept Perform* 21: 679–699.

Ehrsson, H. H. (2007). The experimental induction of out-of-body experiences. *Science* 317: 1048.

Eich, E. (1995). Mood as a mediator of place dependent memory. *J Exp Psychol* 124: 293–308.

Engen, T. (1982). *The Perception of Odors.* Toronto: Academic Press.

Engen, T. (1991). *Odor Sensation and Memory.* New York: Praeger.

Engen, T., Kuisma, J. E., and Eimas, P. D. (1973). Short-term memory of odors. *J Exp Psychol* 99: 222–225.

Engen, T., and Ross, B. M. (1973). Long-term memory odours with and verbal descriptions. *J Exp Psychol* 100: 221–227.

Enns, J. T., and Rensink, R. A. (1990). Scene based properties influence visual search. *Science* 247: 721–723.

Enroth-Cugell, C., and Robson, J. G. (1984). Functional characteristics and diversity of cat retinal ganglion cells: Basic characteristics and quantitative description. *Invest Ophthalmol Vis Sci* 25: 250–267.

Epstein, R., Harris, A., Stanley, D., and Kanwisher, N. (1999). The parahippocampal place area: Recognition, navigation, or encoding? *Neuron* 23: 115–125.

Epstein, R., and Kanwisher, N. (1998). A cortical representation of the local visual environment. *Nature* 392: 598–601.

Ernst, M. O., and Banks, M. S. (2002). Humans integrate visual and haptic information in a statistically optimal fashion. *Nature* 415: 429–433.

Eskew, R. T., Jr. (2008). Chromatic detection and discrimination. In R. H. Masland and T. D. Albright (Eds.), *The Senses: A Comprehensive Reference*, Vol. 2: *Vision II* (pp. 101–117). New York: Academic Press.

Etcoff, N. L., and Magee, J. J. (1992). Categorical perception of facial expressions. *Cognition* 44: 227–240.

Evers, S., and Suhr, B. (2000). Changes of the neurotransmitter serotonin but not of hormones during short time music perception. *Eur Arch Psychiatry Clin Neurosci* 250: 144–147.

Fahle, M. (1982). Binocular rivalry: Suppression depends on orientation and spatial frequency. *Vision Res* 22: 787–800.

Farah, M. (1992). Is an object an object an object? Cognitive and neurospychological investigations of domain specificity in visual object recognition. *Curr Dir Psychol Sci* 1: 165–169.

Fast, K. (2004). *Developing a Scale to Measure Just About Anything: Comparisons across Groups and Individuals.* New Haven, CT: Yale University School of Medicine.

Fedderson, W. E., Sandel, T. T., Teas, D. C., and Jeffress, L. A. (1957). Localization of high frequency tones. *J Acoust Soc Am* 29: 988–991.

Fernandez, C., and Goldberg, J. (1971). Physiology of peripheral neurons innervating semicircular canals of the squirrel monkey. II. Response to sinusoidal stimulation and dynamics of peripheral vestibular system. *J Neurophysiol* 34: 661–675.

Fettiplace, R., and Hackney, C. M. (2006). The sensory and motor roles of auditory hair cells. *Nature* 7: 19–29.

Field, D. J., Hayes, A., and Hess, R. F. (1992). Contour integration by the human visual system: Evidence for a local "association field." *Vision Res* 33: 173–193.

Fine, I., Wade, A. R., Brewer, A. A., May, M. G., Goodman, D. F., Boynton, G. M., Wandell, B. A., and MacLeod, D. I. (2003). Long-term deprivation affects visual perception and cortex. *Nat Neurosci* 6: 915–916.

Firestein, S. (2001). How the olfactory system makes sense of scents. *Nature* 413: 211–218.

Fischer, R., and Griffin, F. (1964). Pharmacogenetic aspects of gustation. *Drug Res* 14: 673–686.

Fisher, S. K., and Ciuffreda, K. J. (1988). Accommodation and apparent distance. *Perception* 17: 609–621.

Flege, J. E., Bohn, O. S., and Jang, S. (1997). Effects of experience on non-native speakers' production and perception of English vowels. *J Phon* 25: 437–470.

Fletcher, H. (1940). Auditory patterns. *Rev Mod Phys* 12: 47–65.

Fletcher, H., and Galt, R. H. (1950). The perception of speech and its relation to telephony. *J Acoust Soc Am* 22: 89–151.

Fowler, C. A., Best, C. T., and McRoberts, G. W. (1990). Young infants' perception of liquid coarticulatory influences on following stop consonants. *Percept Psychophys* 48: 559–570.

Fox, A. L. (1931). Six in ten "tasteblind" to bitter chemical. *Sci News Lett* 9: 249.

Fox, R., and Blake, R. R. (1971). Stereoscopic vision in the cat. *Nature* 233: 55–56.

Francis, S. T., Rolls, E. T., Bowtell, R., McGlone, F., O'Doherty, J. O., Browning, A., Clare, S., and Smith, E. (1999). The representation of pleasant touch in the brain and its relationship with taste and olfactory areas. *Neuroreport* 10: 453–459.

Frank, M. (1973). An analysis of hamster afferent taste nerve response functions. *J Gen Physiol* 61: 588–618.

Freedman, D. J., Riesenhuber, M., Poggio, T., and Miller, E. K. (2001). Categorical perception of visual stimuli in the primate prefrontal cortex. *Science* 291: 312–316.

Freire, A., Lewis, T. L., Maurer, D., and Blake, R. (2006). The development of sensitivity to biological motion in noise. *Perception* 35: 647–657.

Friedman-Hill, S. R., Robertson, L. C., and Treisman, A. (1995). Parietal contributions to visual feature binding: Evidence from a patient with bilateral lesions. *Science* 269: 853–855.

Friesen, C. K., Ristic, J., and Kingstone, A. (2004). Attentional effects of counterpredictive gaze and arrow cues. *J Exp Psychol Hum Percept Perform* 30: 319–329.

Frisby, J. P. (1980). *Seeing: Illusion, Brain and Mind.* Oxford, UK: Oxford University Press.

Galanter, E. (1962). Direct measurement of utility and subjective probability. *Am J Psychol* 75: 208–220.

Gandhi, S. P., Heeger, D. J., and Boynton, G. M. (1998). Spatial attention affects brain activity in human primary visual cortex. *Proc Natl Acad Sci USA* 96: 3314–3319.

Gauthier, I., Behrmann, M., and Tarr, M. J. (1999). Can face recognition really be dissociated from object recognition? *J Cogn Neurosci* 11: 349–370.

Gauthier, I., Williams, P., Tarr, M. J., and Tanaka, J. (1998). Training "greeble" experts: A framework for studying expert object recognition processes. *Vision Res* 38: 2401–2428.

Gegenfurtner, K. R. (2003). Cortical mechanisms of colour vision. *Nat Rev Neurosci* 4: 563–572.

Geisler, C. D. (1998). *From Sound to Synapse: Physiology of the Mammalian Ear.* New York: Oxford University Press.

Geisler, W. S. (1989). Sequential ideal-observer analysis of visual discriminations. *Psychol Rev* 96: 267–314.

Geldard, F. A. (1972). *The Human Senses* (2nd ed.). New York: Wiley.

Gescheider, G. A. (1974). *Temporal Relations in Cutaneous Stimulation* (Conference on Cutaneous Communication Systems and Devices). Oxford, UK: Psychonomic Society.

Gibson, J. J. (1957). Optical motions and transformations as stimuli for visual perception. *Psychol Rev* 64: 288–295.

Gilad, Y., Wiebe, V., Przeworski, M., Lancet, D., and Paabo, S. (2004). Loss of olfactory receptors genes coincides with the acquisition of full trichromatic vision in primates. *PLoS Biol* 2: 120–125.

Gillam, B. (1980). Geometrical illusions. *Sci Am* 242(1): 102–111.

Goldberg, J. (2008). The quivering bundles that let us hear: The goal: Extreme sensitivity and speed. *Seeing, Hearing, and Smelling the World: A Report from the Howard Hughes Medical Institute.* www.hhmi.org/senses/c120.html.

Goldberg, J. M., and Fernandez, C. (1971) Physiology of peripheral neurons innervating semicircular canals of the squirrel monkey, Parts 1, 2, 3. *J Neurophysiol* 34: 635–684.

Goldberg, J. M., and Fernandez, C. (1976). Physiology of peripheral neurons innervating otolith organs of the squirrel monkey, Parts 1, 2, 3. *J Neurophysiol* 39: 970–1008.

Govardovskii, V. I. (1983). On the role of oil drops in colour vision. *Vision Res* 23: 1739–1740.

Goycoolea, M. V., Goycoolea, H. G., Farfan, C. R., Rodriguez, L. G., Martinez, G. C., and Vidal, R. (1986). Effect of life in industrialized societies on hearing in natives of Easter Island. *Laryngoscope* 96: 1391–1396.

Grabherr, L., Nicoucar, K., Mast, F. W., and Merfeld, D. M. (2008). Direction detection thresholds for yaw rotation about an earth-vertical axis as a function of frequency. *Exp Brain Res* 186: 677–681.

Graham, N., and Nachmias, J. (1971). Detection of grating patterns containing two spatial frequencies: A comparison of single-channel and multiple-channel models. *Vision Res* 11: 251–259.

Green, B. G. (1993). Evidence that removal of capsaicin accelerates desensitization on the tongue. *Neurosci Lett* 150: 44–48.

Green, C. S., and Bavelier, D. (2003). Action video game modifies visual attention. *Nature* 423: 534–537.

Green, D. M., and Swets, J. (1966). *Signal Detection Theory and Psychophysics.* New York: Wiley.

Gregory, R. L. (1966). *Eye and Brain.* New York: World University Library.

Gregory, R. L. (1970). *The Intelligent Eye.* London: Weidenfeld and Nicolson.

Gregory, R. L., and Wallace, J. G. (1963). *Recovery from Early Blindness: A Case Study* (Experimental Psychology Society Monograph, no. 2). Cambridge, UK: Experimental Psychology Society.

Grill-Spector, K., and Malach, R. (2004). The human visual cortex. *Annu Rev Neurosci* 27: 649–677.

Gross, C. G., Rocha-Miranda, C. E., and Bender, D. B. (1972). Visual properties of neurons in inferotemporal cortex of the macaque. *J Neurophysiol* 35: 96–111.

Grushka, M., and Bartoshuk, L. M. (2000). Burning mouth syndrome and oral dysesthesias. *Can J Diagn* 17: 99–109.

Guyton, A. C. (1991). *Textbook of Medical Physiology* (8th ed). Philadelphia: Saunders.

Haenny, P. E., and Schiller, P. H. (1988). State dependent activity in monkey visual cortex. I. Single cell activity in V1 and V4 on visual tasks. *Exp Brain Res* 69: 225–244.

Haggard, P., Newman, C., Blundell, J., and Andrew, H. (2000). The perceived position of the hand in space. *Percept Psychophys* 68: 363–377.

Haller, R., Rummel, C., Henneberg, S., Pollmer, U. and Koster, E. P. (1999). The influence of early experience with vanillin on food preference in later life. *Chem Senses* 24: 465–467.

Handel, S. (1989). *Listening: An Introduction to the Perception of Auditory Events.* Cambridge, MA: MIT Press.

Handel, S., and Oshinsky, J. S. (1981). The meter of syncopated auditory polyrhythms. *Percept Psychophys* 30: 1–9.

Harkness, L. (1977). Chameleons use accommodation cues to judge distance. *Nature* 267: 346–349.

Hartline, H. K. (1940). The nerve messages in the fibers of the visual pathway. *J Opt Soc Am* 30: 239–247.

Hayes, J. E., Bartoshuk, L. M., Kidd, J. R., and Duffy, V. B. (2008). Supertasting and PROP bitterness depends on more than the *Tas2r38* gene. *Chem Senses* 33: 255–265.

Hayward, W. G., and Williams, P. (2000). Viewpoint dependence and object discriminability. *Psychol Sci* 11: 7–12.

Heider, E. R. (1972). Universals in color naming and memory. *J Exp Psychol* 93: 10–20.

Heise, G. A., and Miller, G. A. (1951). An experimental study of auditory patterns. *Am J Psychol* 64: 68–77.

Helmholtz, H. von. (1863/1954). *On the Sensations of Tone as a Physiological Basis for the Theory of Music.* Repr. New York: Dover.

Helmholtz, H. von. (1924). *Helmholtz's Treatise on Physiological Optics* (translated from the 3rd German ed.; edited by J. P. C. Southall). Rochester, NY: Optical Society of America.

Hering, E. (1878). *Zur Lehre vom Lichtsinn.* Vienna: Gerold.

Herness, S., Zhao, F.-L., Kaya, N., Shen, T., Lu, S.-G., and Cao, Y. (2005). Communication routes within the taste bud by neurotransmitters and neuropeptides. *Chem Senses* 30(Suppl.1): i37–i38.

Herz, R. S. (1997). Emotion experienced during encoding enhances odor retrieval cue effectiveness. *Am J Psychol* 110: 489–505.

Herz, R. S. (1998). Are odors the best cues to memory? A cross-modal comparison of associative memory stimuli. *Ann NY Acad Sci* 855: 670–674.

Herz, R. S. (2000). Scents of time. *Sciences* 40(4): 34–39.

Herz, R. S. (2001). Ah, sweet skunk: Why we like or dislike what we smell. *Cerebrum* 3(4): 31–47.

Herz, R. S. (2004). A comparison of autobiographical memories triggered by olfactory, visual and auditory stimuli. *Chem Senses* 29: 217–224.

Herz, R. (2007). *The Scent of Desire: Discovering Our Enigmatic Sense of Smell.* New York: Morrow.

Herz, R. S., Beland, S. L., and Hellerstein, M. (2004). Changing odor hedonic perception through emotional associations in humans. *Int J Comp Psychol* 17: 315–339.

Herz, R. S., and Cupchik, G. C. (1995). The emotional distinctiveness of odor-evoked memories. *Chem Senses* 20: 517–528.

Herz, R. S., Eliassen, J. C., Beland, S. L., and T. Souza. (2003). Neuroimaging evidence for the emotional potency of odor-evoked memory. *Neuropsychologia* 42: 371–378.

Hillis, J., Watt, S., Landy, M., and Banks, M. (2004). Slant from texture and disparity cues: Optimal cue combination. *J Vis* 4: 967–992.

Hobbes, T. (1651/1914). *Leviathan.* Repr. London: J. M. Dent & Sons Ltd.

Hoffman, D. D., and Richards, W. A. (1984). Parts of recognition. *Cognition* 18: 65–96.

Hofman, P. M., Van Riswick, J. G. A., and Van Opsal, A. J. (1998). Relearning sound localization with new ears. *Nat Neurosci* 1: 417–421.

Hohmann A., and Creutzfeldt, O. D. (1975). Squint and the development of binocularity in humans. *Nature* 254: 613–614.

Hollingworth, A., and Henderson, J. M. (2002). Accurate visual memory for previously attended objects in natural scenes. *J Exp Psychol Hum Percept Perform* 28: 113–136.

Hollins, M. (2002). Touch and haptics. In H. Pashler and S. Yantis (Eds.), *Stevens Handbook of Experimental Psychology* (3rd ed.), Vol. 1: *Sensation and Perception* (pp. 585–618). New York: Wiley.

Hollins, M., Bensmaïa, S., and Washburn, S. (2001). Vibrotactile adaptation impairs discrimination of fine, but not coarse, textures. *Somatosens Mot Res* 18: 253–262.

Horton, J. C., and Hocking, D. R. (1996). An adult-like pattern of ocular dominance columns in striate cortex of newborn monkeys prior to visual experience. *J Neurosci* 16: 1791–1807.

Horton, J. C., and Trobe, J. D. (1999). Akinetopsia from nefazodone toxicity. *Am J Ophthalmol* 128: 530–531.

Howard, I. P., and Rogers, B. J. (1995). *Binocular Vision and Stereopsis.* New York: Oxford University Press

Howard, I. P., and Rogers, B. J. (2001). *Seeing in Depth.* Toronto: Porteous.

Hubel, D. H. (1982). Exploration of the primary visual cortex, 1955–78. *Nature* 299: 515–524.

Hubel, D. H. (1988). *Eye, Brain, and Vision.* New York: Scientific American Library.

Hubel, D. H., and Wiesel, T. N. (1962). Receptive fields, binocular interaction and functional architecture in the cat's visual cortex. *J Physiol* 160: 106–154.

Hubel, D. H., and Wiesel, T. N. (1973). A re-examination of stereoscopic mechanisms in area 17 of the cat. *J Physiol* 232: 29P–30P.

Hubel, D. H., Wiesel, T. N., and Stryker, M. P. (1978). Anatomical demonstration of orientation columns in macaque monkey. *J Comp Neurol* 177: 361–380.

Hudspeth, A. J. (1997). How hearing happens. *Neuron* 19: 947–950.

Hughes, A. (1977). The topography of vision in mammals of contrasting life styles: Comparative optics and retinal organization. In F. Crescitelli (Ed.), *Handbook of Sensory Physiology*, Vol. VII/5: *The Visual System in Vertebrates* (pp. 613–756). New York: Springer.

Huk, A. C., Ress, D., and Heeger, D. J. (2001). Neuronal basis of the motion aftereffect reconsidered. *Neuron* 32: 161–172.

Hummel, T., Kobel, G., Gudziol, H., and Mackay-Sim, A. (2007). Normative data for the "Sniffin' Sticks" including tests of odor identification, odor discrimination, and olfactory thresholds: An upgrade based on a group of more than 3,000 subjects. *Eur Arch Otorhinolaryngol* 264: 237–243.

Hummel, T., von Mering, R., Huch, R., and Kolble, N. (2002). Olfactory modulation of nausea during early pregnancy? *BJOG* 109: 1394–1397.

Hurvich, L., and Jameson, D. (1957). An opponent process theory of color vision. *Psychol Rev* 64: 384–404.

Imai, S., Flege, J., and Wayland, R. (2002). Perception of cross-language vowel differences: A longitudinal study of native Spanish learners of English. *J Acoust Soc Am* 111: 2364–2364.

Ingle, D. J. (1985). The goldfish as a retinex animal. *Science* 227: 651–654.

Intraub, H. (1981). Rapid conceptual identification of sequentially presented pictures. *J Exp Psychol Hum Learn Mem* 7: 604–610.

Iriki, A., Tanaka, M., and Iwamura, Y. (1996). Coding of modified body schema during tool use by macaque postcentral neurons. *Neuroreport* 7: 2325–2330.

Irwin, D. E. (1996). Integrating information across saccadic eye movements. *Curr Dir Psychol Sci* 5: 94–100.

Irwin, D. E., Yantis, S., and Jonides, J. (1983). Evidence against visual integration across saccadic eye movements. *Percept Psychophys* 34: 49–57.

Irwin, D. E., Zacks, J. L., and Brown, J. S. (1990). Visual memory and the perception of a stable visual environment. *Percept Psychophys* 47: 35–46.

Jacob, S., Hayreh, D. J. S, and McClintock, M. (2001). Context-dependent effects of steroid chemosignals on human physiology and mood. *Physiol Behav* 74: 15–27.

James, W. (1890). *The Principles of Psychology* (2 vols.). New York: Holt.

Johansson, G. (1975). Visual motion perception. *Sci Am* 232(6): 76–88.

Johansson, R. S., and Vallbo, A. B. (1983). Tactile sensory coding in the glabrous skin of the human hand. *Trends Neurosci* 6: 27–32.

Johnson, K. O. (2002). Neural basis of haptic perception. In H. Pashler and S. Yantis (Eds.), *Stevens Handbook of Experimental Psychology* (3rd ed.), Vol. 1: *Sensation and Perception* (pp 537–583). New York: Wiley.

Jolicoeur, P., Gluck, M. A., and Kosslyn, S. M. (1984). Pictures and names: Making the connection. *Cogn Psychol* 16: 243–275.

Jones, L. A. (1999). Somatic senses 3: Proprioception. In H. Cohen (Ed.), *Neuroscience for Rehabilitation* (2nd ed.), pp. 111–130. Lippincott, Williams & Wilkins.

Jones, R. K., and Lee, D. N. (1981). Why two eyes are better than one: The two views of binocular vision. *J Exp Psychol Hum Percept Perform* 7: 30–40.

Judd, D., and Kelly, K. (1939). Method of designating colors. *J Res Natl Bur Stand* 23: 355.

Julesz, B. (1964). Binocular depth perception without familiarity cues. *Science* 45: 356–362.

Julesz, B. (1971). *Foundations of Cyclopean Perception.* Chicago: University of Chicago Press.

Kadohisa, M., and Wilson, D. A. (2006). Olfactory cortical adaptation facilitates detection of odors against background. *J Neurophysiol* 95: 1888–1896.

Kanwisher, N. (1987). Repetition blindness: Type recognition without token individuation. *Cognition* 27: 117–143.

Kanwisher, N., McDermott, J., and Chun, M. M. (1997). The fusiform face area: A module in human extrastriate cortex specialized for face perception. *J Neurosci* 17: 4302–4311.

Kapfer, C., Seidl, A. H., Schweizer, H., and Grothe, B. (2002). Experience-dependent refinement of inhibitory inputs to auditory coincidence-detector neurons. *Nat Neurosci* 5: 247–253.

Kappers, S. (2007). Haptic space perception. *Can J Exp Psychol* 61: 208–218.

Kay, K. N., Naselaris, T., Prenger, R. J., and Gallant, J. L. (2008). Identifying natural images from human brain activity. *Nature* 452: 352–355.

Keller, A., and Vosshall, L. B. (2004). A psychophysical test of the vibration theory of olfaction. *Nat Neurosci* 7: 337–338.

Keller, A., Zhuang, H., Chi, Q., Vosshall, L. B., and Matsunami, H. (2007). Genetic variation in a human odorant receptor alters odour perception. *Nature* 449: 468–472.

Kellman, P. (1998). An update on gestalt psychology. In *Perception, Cognition, and Language: Essays in Honor of Henry and Lila Gleitman* (pp. 157–190). Cambridge, MA: MIT Press.

Kellman, P. J., and Shipley, T. F. (1991). A theory of visual interpolation in object perception. *Cogn Psychol* 23: 141–221.

Kepecs, A., Uchida, N., and Mainen, Z. F. (2007). Rapid and precise control of sniffing during olfactory discrimination in rats. *J Neurophysiol* 98: 205–213.

Kern, R. C., Conley, D. B., Haines, G. K., and Robinson, A. M. (2004). Pathology of the olfactory mucosa: Implications for the treatment of olfactory dysfunction. *Laryngoscope* 114: 279–285.

Kessel, R. G., and Kardon, R. H. (1979). *Tissues and Organs: A Text-Atlas of Scanning Electron Microscopy.* San Francisco: Freeman.

Khan, R. M., Luk, C. H., Flinker, A., Aggarwal, A., Lapid, H., Haddad, R., and Sobel, N. (2007). Predicting odor pleasantness from odorant structure: Pleasantness as a reflection of the physical world. *J Neurosci* 27: 1–9.

Kiefte, M., and Kluender, K. R. (2005). The relative importance of spectral tilt in monopthongs and diphthongs. *J Acoust Soc Am* 117: 1395–1404.

Kiefte, M., and Kluender, K. R. (2008). Absorption of reliable spectral characteristics in auditory perception. *J Acoust Soc Am* 123: 366–376.

Kim, U. K., Jorgenson, E., Coon, H., Leppert, M., Risch, N., and Drayna, D. (2003). Positional cloning of the human quantitative trait locus underlying taste sensitivity to phenylthiocarbamide. *Science* 299: 1221–1225.

Kistler, D. J., and Wightman, F. L. (1992). The dominant role of low-frequency interaural time differences in sound localization. *J Acoust Soc Am* 91: 1648–1661.

Klatzky, R. L., Lederman, S. J., and Metzger, V. (1985). Identifying objects by touch: An "expert system." *Percept Psychophys* 37: 299–302.

Kluender, K. R., and Alexander, J. M. (2008). Perception of speech sounds. In A. I. Basbaum, A. Kaneko, G. M. Shepard, and G. Westheimer (Eds.), *The Senses: A Comprehensive Reference*, Vol. 3: *Audition* (P. Dallos and D. Oertel, Eds.) (pp. 829–860). San Diego: Academic Press.

Kluender, K. R., Diehl, R. L., and Killeen, P. R. (1987). Japanese quail can learn phonetic categories. *Science* 237: 1195–1197.

Kluender, K. R., and Jenison, R. L. (1992). Effects of glide slope, noise intensity, and noise duration on the extrapolation of FM glides through noise. *Percept Psychophys* 51: 231–238.

Kluender, K. R., Lotto, A. J., and Holt, L. L. (2005). Contributions of nonhuman animal models to understanding human speech perception. In S. Greenberg and W. Ainsworth (Eds.), *Listening to Speech: An Auditory Perspective* (pp. 203–220). Mahwah, NJ: Erlbaum.

Kluender, K. R. Lotto, A. J., Holt, L. L., and Bloedel, S. L. (1998). Role of experience for language-specific functional mapping of vowel sounds. *J Acoust Soc Am* 104: 3596–3582.

Klumpp, R. G., and Eady, H. R. (1956). Some measurements of interaural time-difference thresholds. *J Acoust Soc Am* 28: 859–860.

Klüver, H., and Bucy, P. C. (1938). An analysis of certain effects of bilateral temporal lobectomy in the rhesus monkey, with special reference to "psychic blindness." *J Psychol* 5: 33–54.

Klüver, H., and Bucy, P. C. (1939). Preliminary analysis of functions of the temporal lobes in monkeys. *Arch Neurol Psychiatry* 42: 979–1000.

Koenigsberger, L. (1906/1965). *Hermann von Helmholtz* (translated by F. A. Welby). Repr. New York: Dover.

Konen, C. S., and Kastner, S. (2008). Two hierarchically organized neural systems for object information in human visual cortex. *Nat Neurosci* 11: 224–231.

Kosslyn, S. M., Thompson, W. L., Kim, I. J., and Alpert, A. M. (1995). Topographic representations of mental images in primary visual cortex. *Nature* 378: 496–498.

Kovacs, I., and Julesz, B. (1993). A closed curve is much more than an incomplete one: Effect of closure in figure-ground segmentation. *Proc Natl Acad Sci USA* 90: 7495–7497.

Krauskopf, J., Williams, D. R., and Heeley, D. W. (1982). Cardinal directions of color space. *Vision Res* 22: 1123–1131.

Krestel, D., Passe, D., Smith, J. C., and Jonsson, L. (1984). Behavioral determinants of olfactory thresholds to amyl acetate in dogs. *Neurosci Biobehav Rev* 8: 169–174.

Kubovy, M., and Cohen, D. J. (2001). What boundaries tell us about binding. *Trends Cogn Sci* 5: 93–95.

Kuffler, S. W. (1953). Discharge patterns and functional organization of mammalian retina. *J Neurophysiol* 16: 37–68.

Kuhl, P. K. (1981). Discrimination of speech by nonhuman animals: Basic sensitivities conducive to the perception of speech sound categories. *J Acoust Soc Am* 70: 340–349.

Kuhl, P. K., and Miller, J. D. (1978). Speech perception by the chinchilla: Identification functions for synthetic VOT stimuli. *J Acoust Soc Am* 63: 905–917.

Kuhl, P. K., Williams, K. A., Lacerda, F., Stevens, K. N., and Lindblom, B. (1992). Linguistic experience alters phonetic perception in infants six months of age. *Science* 255: 606–608.

Kumagami, T., Zhang, B., Smith, E. L., III, and Chino, Y. M. (2000). Effect of onset age of strabismus on the binocular responses of neurons in the monkey visual cortex. *Invest Ophthalmol Vis Sci* 41: 948–954.

Kwok, R. H. M. (1968). Chinese-restaurant syndrome. *N Engl J Med* 278: 796.

Laing, D. G., and Francis, G. W. (1989). The capacity of humans to identify odors in mixtures. *Physiol Behav* 46: 809–814.

Laing, D. G., and Glemarec, A. (1992). Selective attention and the perceptual analysis of odor mixtures. *Physiol Behav* 33: 309–319.

La Mettrie, J. O. (1912). *Man a machine.* La Salle, IL: Open Court. (Original published in French, 1747.)

LaMotte, R. H., and Srinivasan, M. A. (1991). Surface microgeometry: Tactile perception and neural encoding. In O. Franzen and J. Westman (Eds.), *Information Processing in the Somatosensory System* (pp. 49–58). London: Macmillan.

Laska, M., Koch, B., Heid, B., and Hudson, R. (1996). Failure to demonstrate systematic changes in olfactory perception in the course of pregnancy: A longitudinal study. *Chem Senses* 21: 567–571.

Lawless, H., and Engen, T. (1977). Associations to odors: Interference, mnemonics, and verbal labelling. *J Exp Psychol* 3: 52–59.

Lecanuet, J. P., Granier-Deferre, C., Cohen, C., Le Houezec, R., and Busnel, M. C. (1986). Fetal responses to acoustic stimulation depend on heart rate variability pattern stimulus intensity and repetition. *Early Hum Dev* 13: 269–283.

Lederman, S. J., and Klatzky, R. L. (1987). Hand movements: A window into haptic object recognition. *Cogn Psychol* 19: 342–368.

Lederman, S. J., and Klatzky, R. L. (1997). Relative availability of surface and object properties during early haptic processing. *J Exp Psychol Hum Percept Perform* 23: 1680–1707.

Lederman, S., Klatzky, R., Chataway, C., and Summers, C. (1990). Visual mediation and the haptic recognition of two-dimensional pictures of common objects. *Percept Psychophys* 47: 54–64.

Lederman, S. J., Thorne, G., and Jones, B. (1986). The perception of texture by vision and touch: Multidimensionality and intersensory integration. *J Exp Psychol Hum Percept Perform* 12: 169–180.

Ledgeway, T. (1994). Adaptation to second-order motion results in a motion aftereffect for directionally-ambiguous test stimuli. *Vision Res* 34: 2879–2889.

Ledgeway, T., and Smith, A. T. (1994). The duration of the motion aftereffect following adaptation to first-order and second-order motion. *Perception* 23: 1211–1219.

Lee, D. N. (1976). A theory of visual control of braking based on information about time-to-collision. *Perception* 5: 437–459.

Lee, S.-H., and Blake, R. (1999). Visual form created solely from temporal structure. *Science* 284: 1165–1168.

Lehman, C. D., Bartoshuk, L. M., Catalanotto, F. C., Kveton, J. F., and Lowlicht, R. A. (1995). The effect of anesthesia of the chorda tympani nerve on taste perception in humans. *Physiol Behav* 57: 943–951.

LeVay, S., Hubel, D. H., and Wiesel, T. N. (1975). The pattern of ocular dominance columns in macaque visual cortex revealed by a reduced silver stain. *J Comp Neurol* 159: 559–576.

Levi, D. M. (2008). Crowding—An essential bottleneck for object recognition: A mini-review. *Vision Res* 48: 635–654.

Levi, D. M., Klein, S. A., and Aitsebaomo, A. P. (1985). Vernier acuity, crowding and cortical magnification. *Vision Res* 25: 963–977.

Levine, M. W. (2000). *Levine & Shefner's Fundamentals of Sensation and Perception* (3rd ed.). Oxford, UK: Oxford University Press.

Li, B., Peterson, M. R., and Freeman, R. D. (2003). Oblique effect: A neural basis in the visual cortex. *J Neurophysiol* 90: 204–217.

Liberman, A. M., Cooper, F. S., Shankweiler, D. P., and Studdert Kennedy, M. (1967). Perception of the speech code. *Psychol Rev* 74: 431–461.

Liberman, A. M., and Mattingly, I. G. (1985). The motor theory of speech perception revised. *Cognition* 21: 1–36.

Liebenthal, E., Binder, J. R., Spitzer, S. M., Possing, E. T., and Medler, D. A. (2005). Neural substrates of phonemic perception. *Cereb Cortex* 15(10): 162–163.

Lieberman, P. (1984). *The Biology and Evolution of Language.* Cambridge, MA: Harvard University Press.

Liem, D. G., and Mennella, J. A. (2003). Heightened sour preferences during childhood. *Chem Senses* 28: 173–180.

Lindeman, H. H. (1973) Anatomy of the otolith organs. *Adv Otorhinolaryngol* 20: 404–433.

Lindsey, D. T., and Brown, A. M. (2006). Universality of color names. *Proc Natl Acad Sci USA* 103: 16608–16613.

Lisker, L. (1978). Rapid versus rabid: A catalogue of acoustical features that may cue the distinction. *Haskins Lab Status Rep Speech Res* SR 54: 127–132.

Livingstone, M., and Hubel, D. (1988). Segregation of form, color, movement, and depth: Anatomy, physiology, and perception. *Science* 240: 740–749.

Loftus, G. R., and Mackworth, N. H. (1978). Cognitive determinants of fixation location during picture viewing. *J Exp Psychol Hum Percept Perform* 4: 565–576.

Löfvenberg, J., and Johansson, R. S. (1984). Regional differences and interindiviudal variability in sensitivity to vibration in the glabrous skin of the human hand. *Brain Res* 301: 65–72.

Logothetis, N. K., Pauls, J., and Poggio, T. (1995). Shape representation in the inferior temporal cortex of monkeys. *Curr Biol* 5: 552–563.

Loomis, J. M. (1981). On the tangibility of letters and braille. *Percept Psychophys* 29: 37–46.

Loomis, J. M. (1990). A model of character recognition and legibility. *J Exp Psychol Hum Percept Perform* 16: 106–120.

Lorig, T. (1999). On the similarity of odor and language perception. *Neurosci Biobehav Rev* 23: 391–398.

Lotto, A. J., Kluender, K. R., and Holt, L. L. (1997). Perceptual compensation for coarticulation by Japanese quail (*Coturnix coturnix japonica*). *J Acoust Soc Am* 102: 1134–1140.

Lowe, D. G. (1985). *Perceptual Organization and Visual Recognition.* Boston: Kluwer.

Lu, Z.-L., and Dosher, B. A. (1998). External noise distinguishes attention mechanisms. *Vision Res* 38: 1183–1198.

Lundstrom, J. N., and Olsson, M. J. (2005). Subthreshold amounts of a social odorant affect mood, but not behavior, in heterosexual women when tested by a male, but not a female experimenter. *Biol Psychol* 60: 197–204.

Lynch, M. P., and Eilers, R. E. (1990). Innateness, experience, and music perception. *Psychol Sci* 1: 272–276.

MacLeod, D. I., and Lennie, P. (1976). Red-green blindness confined to one eye. *Vision Res* 16: 691–702.

Macmillan, N. A., and Creelman, C. D. (2005). *Detection Theory.* Mahwah, NJ: Erlbaum.

Maddieson, I. (1984). *Patterns of Sound.* Cambridge, UK: Cambridge University Press.

Maffei, L., and Fiorentini, A. (1973). The visual cortex as a spatial frequency analyzer. *Vision Res* 13: 1255–1267.

Malik, J., and Perona, P. (1990). Preattentive texture discrimination with early vision mechanisms. *J Opt Soc Am A* 7: 923–932.

Maloney, L. T. (1986). Evaluation of linear models of surface spectral reflectance with small numbers of parameters. *J Opt Soc Am A* 3: 1673–1683.

Maquet, P., Peters, J., Aerts, J., Delfiore, G., Degueldre, C., Luxen, A., and Franck, G. (1996). Functional neuroanatomy of human rapid-eye-movement sleep and dreaming. *Nature* 383: 163–166.

Maresh, A., Gil, D. R., Whitman, M. C., and Greer, C. A. (2008). Principles of glomerular organization in the human olfactory bulb—Implications for odor processing. *PLoS ONE* 3: 1–6.

Marks, L. E., Stevens, J. C., Bartoshuk, L. M., Gent, J. G., Rifkin, B., and Stone, V. K. (1988). Magnitude matching: The measurement of taste and smell. *Chem Senses* 13: 63–87.

Marr, D., and Nishihara, H. K. (1977). Representation and recognition of the spatial organization of three-dimensional shapes. *Proc R Soc Lond B Biol Sci* 200: 269–294.

Marr, D., and Poggio, T. (1979). A computational theory of human stereo vision. *Proc R Soc Lond B Biol Sci* 204: 301–328.

Martinez, A., Anllo-Vento, L., Sereno, M. I., Frank, L. R., Buxton, R. B., Dubowitz, D. J., Wong, E. C., Hinrichs, H., Heinze, H. J., and Hillyard, S. A. (1999). Involvement of striate and extrastriate visual cortical areas in spatial attention. *Nat Neurosci* 2: 364–369.

Maruniak, J. A., Silver, W. L., and Moulton, D. G. (1983). Olfactory receptors respond to blood-borne odorants. *Brain Res* 265: 312–316.

Mather, G., and Murdoch, L. (1994). Gender discrimination in biological motion displays based on dynamic cues. *Proc R Soc Lond B Biol Sci* 258: 273–279.

Matin, L., Picoult, E., Stevens, J. K., Edwards, M. W., Jr., Young, D., and MacArthur, R. (1982). Oculoparalytic illusion: Visual-field dependent spatial mislocalizations by humans partially paralyzed with curare. *Science* 216: 198–201.

Maurer, D., Lewis, T. L., Brent, H. P., and Levin, A. V. (1999). Rapid improvement in the acuity of infants after visual input. *Science* 286: 108–110.

Mays, L. E., and Sparks, D. L. (1980). Dissociation of visual and saccade-related responses in superior colliculus neurons. *J Neurophysiol* 43: 207–232.

McCann, J. J., McKee, S. P., and Taylor, T. H. (1976). Quantitative studies in retinex theory. A comparison between theoretical predictions and observer responses to the "color mondrian" experiments. *Vision Res* 16: 445–458.

McConkie, G. W., and Currie, C. (1996). Visual stability across saccades while viewing complex pictures. *J Exp Psychol Hum Percept Perform* 22: 563–581.

McGlone, F., Vallbo, A. B., Olausson, H., Loken, L. S., and Wessberg, J. (2007). Discriminative touch and emotional touch. *Can J Exp Psychol* 61: 173–183.

McGurk, H., and MacDonald, J. (1976). Hearing lips and seeing voices. *Nature* 264: 746–748.

McMains, S. A., and Somers, D. C. (2004). Multiple spotlights of attentional selection in human visual cortex. *Neuron* 42: 677–686.

Mehler, J., Jusczyk, P., Lambertz, C., Halsted, N., Bertoncini, J., and Amiel-Tison, C. (1988). A precursor of language acquisition in young infants. *Cognition* 29: 143–178.

Melzack, R., and Wall, P. D. (1973). *The Puzzle of Pain.* Harmondsworth, UK: Penguin Education.

Melzack, R., and Wall, P. D. (1988). *The Challenge of Pain.* London: Penguin.

Menashe, I., Man, O., Lancet, D., and Gilad, Y. (2003). Different noses for different people. *Nat Genet* 34: 143–144.

Mennella, J. A., and Beauchamp, G. K. (1991). The transfer of alcohol to human milk: Effects on flavor and the infant's behavior. *N Engl J Med* 325: 981–985.

Mennella, J. A., and Beauchamp, G. K. (1993). The effects of repeated exposure to garlic-flavored milk on the nursling's behavior. *Pediatr Res* 34: 805–808.

Mennella, J. A., Johnson, A., and Beauchamp, G. K. (1995). Garlic ingestion by pregnant women alters the odor of amniotic fluid. *Chem Senses* 20: 207–209.

Miller, G., Tybur, J. M., and Jornda, B. D. (2007). Ovulatory cycle effects on tip earnings by lap dancers: Economic evidence for human estrus? *Evol Hum Behav* 28: 375–381.

Miller, G. A., and Heise, G. A. (1950). The trill threshold. *J Acoust Soc Am* 22: 637–638.

Ming, D., Ninomiya, Y., and Margolskee, R. F. (1999). Blocking taste receptor activation of gustducin inhibits gustatory responses to bitter compounds. *Proc Natl Acad Sci USA* 96: 9903–9908.

Mombaerts, P., Wang, F., Dulac, C., Chao, S. K., Nemes, A., Mendelsohn, M., Edmondson, J., and Axel, R. (1996). Visualizing an olfactory sensory map. *Cell* 87: 675–686.

Moncrieff, R. W. (1966). *Odour Preferences.* New York: Wiley.

Moore, B. C. J. (2003). *An Introduction to the Psychology of Hearing* (5th ed.). London: Academic Press.

Moran, J., and Desimone, R. (1985). Selective attention gates visual processing in the extrastriate cortex. *Science* 229: 782–784.

Moskowitz, H. R., Dravnieks, A., and Klarman, L. A. (1976). Odor intensity and pleasantness for a diverse set of odorants. *Percept Psychophys* 19: 122–128.

Motohashi, K., and Umino, M. (2001). Heterotopic painful stimulation decreases the late component of somatosensory evoked potentials induced by electrical tooth stimulation. *Brain Res Cogn Brain Res* 11: 39–46.

Mounts, J. R. (2000). Evidence for suppressive mechanisms in attentional selection: Feature singletons produce inhibitory surrounds. *Percept Psychophys* 62: 969–983.

Mozer, M. C. (1991). *The Perception of Multiple Objects: A Connectionist Approach.* Cambridge, MA: MIT Press.

Mueller, K. L., Hoon, M. A., Erlenbach, I., Chandrashekar, J., Zuker, C. S., and Ryba, N. J. (2005). The receptors and coding logic for bitter taste. *Nature* 434: 225–229.

Müller, J. (1838/1912). *Handbook of Physiology* (translation from B. Rand [1912], *The Classical Psychologists*). Repr. Boston: Houghton-Mifflin.

Murphy, C., Cain, W. S., Gilmore, M. M., and Skinner, R. B. (1991). Sensory and semantic factors in recognition memory for odors and graphic stimuli: Elderly versus young persons. *Am J Psychol* 104: 161–192.

Nagy, A. L., MacLeod, D. I., Heyneman, N. E., and Eisner, A. (1981). Four cone pigments in women heterozygous for color deficiency. *J Opt Soc Am* 71: 719–722.

Nathans, J. (1986). Molecular genetics of inherited variation in human color vision. *Science* 232: 203–210.

Nathans, J., Thomas, D., and Hogness, D. S. (1986). Molecular genetics of human color vision: The genes encoding blue, green, and red pigments. *Science* 232: 193–202.

Nauhaus, I., Benucci, A., Carandini, M., and Ringach, D. L. (2008). Neuronal selectivity and local map structure in visual cortex. *Neuron* 57: 673–679.

Navon, D. (1977). Forest before the trees: The precedence of global features in visual perception. *Cogn Psychol* 9: 353–383.

Neitz, J., Geist, T., and Jacobs, G. H. (1989). Color vision in the dog. *Vis Neurosci* 3: 119–125.

Nerger, J. L., Volbrecht, V. J., and Ayde, C. J. (1995). Unique hue judgments as a function of test size in the fovea and at 20-deg temporal eccentricity. *J Opt Soc Am A Opt Image Sci Vis* 12: 1225–1232.

Neri, P., Luu, J. Y., and Levi, D. M. (2006). Meaningful interactions can enhance visual discrimination of human agents. *Nat Neurosci* 9: 1186–1192.

Neri, P., Morrone, M. C., and Burr, D. C. (1998). Seeing biological motion. *Nature* 395: 894–896.

Newcombe, F., and de Haan, E. H. F. (1994). Category specificity in visual recognition. In M. J. Farah and G. Ratcliff (Eds.), *The Neuropsychology of High-Level Vision: Collected Tutorial Essays* (Carnegie Mellon Symposia on Cognition) (pp. 103–132). Hillsdale, NJ: Erlbaum.

Newell, F. N., Ernst, M. O., Tjan, B. S., and Bulthoff, H. (2001). Viewpoint dependence in visual and haptic object recognition. *Psychol Sci* 12: 37–42.

Newsome, W. T., and Pare, E. B. (1988). A selective impairment of motion perception following lesions of the middle temporal visual area (MT). *J Neurosci* 8: 2201–2211.

Noble, A. C. (1996). Taste-aroma interactions. *Trends Food Sci Technol* 7: 439–444.

Norcia, A. M., Tyler, C. W., and Hamer, R. D. (1990). Development of contrast sensitivity in the human infant. *Vision Res* 30: 1475–1486.

Nothdurft, H. C., and Li, C. Y. (1984). Representation of spatial details in textured patterns by cells of the cat striate cortex. *Exp Brain Res* 57: 9–21.

O'Craven, K. M., and Kanwisher, N. (2000). Mental imagery of faces and places activates corresponding stiimulus-specific brain regions. *J Cogn Neurosci* 12: 1013–1023.

O'Dell, C., and Boothe, R. G. (1997). The development of stereoacuity in infant rhesus monkeys. *Vision Res* 37: 2675–2684.

Ohzawa, I., and Freeman, R. D. (1986a). The binocular organization of simple cells in the cat's visual cortex. *J Neurophysiol* 56: 221–242.

Ohzawa, I., and Freeman, R. D. (1986b). The binocular organization of complex cells in the cat's visual cortex. *J Neurophysiol* 56: 243–259.

Okano, T., Fukada, Y., and Yoshizawa, T. (1995). Molecular basis for tetrachromatic color vision. *Comp Biochem Physiol B* 112: 405–414.

Oliva, A., and Torralba, A. (2001). Modeling the shape of the scene: A holistic representation of the spatial envelope. *Int J Comput Vis* 42: 145–175.

Olney, J. W., and Sharpe, L. G. (1969). Brain lesions in an infant rhesus monkey treated with monosodium glutamate. *Science* 166: 386–388.

O'Regan, K. (1992). Solving the "real" mysteries of visual perception: The world as an outside memory. *Can J Psychol* 46: 461–488.

Ostrovsky, Y., Andalman, A., and Sinha, P. (2006). Vision following extended congenital blindness. *Psychol Sci* 17: 1009–1014.

Owens, D. A. (1987). Oculomotor information and perception of three-dimensional space. In H. Heuer and A. F. Sanders (Eds.), *Perspectives on Perception and Action* (pp. 215–248. Hillside, NJ: Erlbaum.

Oxbury, J. M., Oxbury, S. M., and Humphrey, N. K. (1969). Varieties of colour anomia. *Brain* 92: 847–860.

Oyster, C. W. (1999). *The Human Eye: Structure and Function.* Sunderland, MA: Sinauer.

Palmer, S. E. (1992). Common region: A new principle of perceptual grouping. *Cogn Psychol* 24: 436–447.

Palmer, S. E., and Ghose, T. (2008). Extremal edges: A powerful cue to depth perception and figure-ground organization. *Psychol Sci* 19: 77–84.

Palmeri, T. J., and Gauthier, I. (2004). Visual object understanding. *Nat Rev Neurosci* 5: 291–303.

Panum, P. L. (1940). *Physiological Investigations Concerning Vision with Two Eyes* (translated from German by C. Hubscher). Hanover, NH: Dartmouth Eye Institute. (Original work published 1858.)

Parker, A. J. (2007). Binocular depth perception and the cerebral cortex. *Nat Rev Neurosci* 8: 379–391.

Parrish, E. E., Giaschi, D. E., Boden, C., and Dougherty, R. (2005). The maturation of form and motion perception in school age children. *Vision Res* 45: 827–837.

Pascual-Leone, A., and Hamilton, R. (2001). The metamodal organization of the brain. *Prog Brain Res* 134: 427–445.

Patterson, R. D., and Johnsrude, I. S. (2008). Functional imaging of the auditory processing applied to speech sounds. *Philos Trans R Soc B Biol Sci* 363: 1023–1035.

Pause, B. M., Miranda, A., Goder, R., Aldenhoff, J. B., and Ferstl, R. (2001). Reduced olfactory performance in patients with major depression. *J Psychiatr Res* 35: 271–277.

Penfield, W., and Rasmussen, T. (1950). *The Cerebral Cortex of Man: A Clinical Study of Localization of Function.* New York: Macmillan.

Perlman, M., and Krumhansl, C. L. (1996). An experimental study of internal interval standards in Javanese and Western musicians. *Music Percept* 14: 95–116.

Perrett, D. I., Hietanen, J. K., Oram, M. W., and Benson, P. J. (1992). Organization and functions of cells responsive to faces in the temporal cortex. *Philos Trans R Soc Lond B Biol Sci* 335: 23–30.

Perrett, D. I., Rolls, E. T., and Caan, W. (1982). Visual neurones responsive to faces in the monkey temporal cortex. *Exp Brain Res* 47: 329–342.

Perrett, D. I., Smith, P. A., Potter, D. D., Mistlin, A. J., Head, A. S., Milner, A. D., and Jeeves, M. A. (1984). Neurones responsive to faces in the temporal cortex: Studies of functional organization, sensitivity to identity and relation to perception. *Hum Neurobiol* 3: 197–208.

Pessoa, L. (1996). Mach bands: How many models are possible? Recent experimental findings and modeling attempts. *Vision Res* 36: 3205–3227.

Peterhans, E., von der Heydt, R., Baumgartner, G., Pettigrew, J. D., Sanderson, K. J., and Levick, W. R. (1986). Neuronal responses to illusory contour stimuli reveal stages of visual cortical processing. In J. D. Pettigrew, K. J. Sanderson, and W. R. Levick (Eds.), *Visual Neuroscience* (pp. 343–351). Cambridge, UK: Cambridge University Press.

Peterka, R. J. (2002). Sensorimotor integration in human postural control. *J Neurophysiol* 88: 1097–1118.

Peterson, M. A., and Rhodes, G. (Eds.). (2003). *Analytic and Holistic Processes.* London: Oxford University Press.

Peterson, M. A., and Skow, E. (2008). Inhibitory competition between shape properties in figure-ground perception. *J Exp Psychol Hum Percept Perform* 34: 251–267.

Pettigrew, J. D., Nikara, T., and Bishop, P. O. (1968). Binocular interaction on single units in cat striate cortex: Simultaneous stimulation by single moving slit with receptive fields in correspondence. *Exp Brain Res* 6: 391–410.

Pfaffmann, C. (1941). Gustatory afferent impulses. *J Cell Comp Physiol* 17: 243–258.

Pfaffmann, C. (1960). The pleasures of sensation. *Psychol Rev* 67: 253–268.

Pierce, J. D., Jr., Wysocki, C. J., Aronov, E. V., Webb, J. B., and Boden, R. M. (1996). The role of perceptual and structural similarity in cross-adaptation. *Chem Senses* 21: 223–237.

Pignatiello, M. F., Camp, C. J., and Rasar, L. A. (1986). Musical mood induction: An alternative to the Velten technique. *J Abnorm Psychol* 95: 295–297.

Plailly, J., Howard, J. D., Gitelman, D. R., and Gottfried, J. A. (2008). Attention to odor modulates thalamocortical connectivity in the human brain. *J Neurosci* 28: 5257–5267.

Plomp, R. (1976). *Aspects of Tone Sensation—A Psychophysical Study.* New York: Academic Press.

Poggio, G. F., and Talbot, W. H. (1981). Mechanisms of static and dynamic stereopsis in foveal cortex of the rhesus monkey. *J Physiol* 315: 469–492.

Polat, U., and Sagi, D. (1993). Lateral interactions between spatial channels: Suppression and facilitation revealed by lateral masking experiments. *Vision Res* 33: 993–999.

Ponzo, M. (1913). Rapports entre quelque illusions visuelles de contraste angulaire et l'appreciation de grandeur astres a l'horizon. *Arch Ital Biol* 58: 327–329.

Poran N. S., and Coss, R. G. (1990). Development of antisnake defenses in California ground squirrels (*Spermaphilus beecheyi*): I. Behavioral and immunological relationships. *Behavior* 112: 222–245.

Porter, J., Carven, B., Khan, R. M., Chang, S. J., Kang, I., Judkewicz, B., Volpe, J., Settles, G., and Sobel, N. (2007). Mechanisms of scent-tracking in humans. *Nat Neurosci* 10: 27–29.

Posner, M. I. (1980). Orienting of attention. *Q J Exp Psychol* 32: 3–25.

Potter, M. C. (1975). Meaning in visual search. *Science* 187: 965–966.

Potter, M. C. (1976). Short-term conceptual memory for pictures. *J Exp Psychol Hum Learn Mem* 2: 509–522.

Prescott, J. (2004). Effects of added glutamate on liking for novel flavors. *Appetite* 42: 143–150.

Price, D. D. (2000). Psychological and neural mechanisms of the affective dimension of pain. *Science* 288: 1769–1772.

Price, D. D., Wu, J. W., Dubner, R., and Gracely, R. H. (1977). Peripheral suppression of first pain and central summation of second pain evoked by noxious heat pulses. *Pain* 3: 57–68.

Prinzmetal, W., and Beck, D. M. (2001). The tilt-constancy theory of visual illusions. *J Exp Psychol Hum Percept Perform* 27: 206–217.

Prinzmetal, W., Shimamura, A. P., and Mikolinski, M. (2001). The Ponzo illusion and the perception of orientation. *Percept Psychophys* 63: 99–114.

Pritchard, T. C., and Norgren, R. (2004). Gustatory system. In G. Paxinos and J. K. Mai (Eds.), *The Human Nervous System* (2nd ed., pp. 1171–1196). Amsterdam: Elsevier.

Pugh, M. C., Ringach, D. L., Shapley, R., and Shelley, M. J. (2000). Computational modeling of orientation tuning dynamics in monkey primary visual cortex. *J Comput Neurosci* 8: 143–159.

Purves, D., Augustine, G. J., Fitzpatrick, D., Hall, W. C., LaMantia, A.-S., McNamara, J. O., and White, L. E. (Eds.). (2008). *Neuroscience* (4th ed.). Sunderland, MA: Sinauer.

Quiroga, R. Q., Kreiman, G., Koch, C., and Fried, I. (2008). Sparse but not 'grandmother-cell' coding in the medial temporal lobe. *Trends Cogn Sci* 12: 87–91.

Quiroga, R. Q., Reddy, L., Kreiman, G., Koch, C., and Fried, I. (2005). Invariant visual representation by single neurons in the human brain. *Nature* 435: 1102–1107.

Rabin, M. D., and Cain, W. S. (1984). Odor recognition, familiarity, identifiability and encoding consistency. *J Exp Psychol Learn Mem Cogn* 10: 316–325.

Rainville, P., Duncan, G. H., Price, D. D., Carrier, B., and Bushnell, M. C. (1997). Pain affect encoded in human anterior cingulate but not somatosensory cortex. *Science* 277: 968–971.

Ramachandran, V. S. (1993). Behavioral and magnetoencephalographic correlates of plasticity in the adult human brain. *Proc Natl Acad Sci USA* 90: 10413–10420.

Rasch, B., Buchel, C., Gais, S., and Born, J. (2007). Odor cues during slow-wave sleep prompt declarative memory consolidations. *Science* 315: 1426–1429.

Rasch, R. A. (1978). The perception of simultaneous notes such as in polyphonic music. *Acustica* 40: 1–72.

Raymond, J. E. (1993). Complete interocular transfer of motion adaptation effects on motion coherence thresholds. *Vision Res* 33: 1865–1870.

Rayner, K. (1978). Eye movements in reading and information processing. *Psychol Bull* 85: 618–660.

Rayner, K., Liversedge, S. P., White, S. J., and Vergilino-Perez, D. (2003). Reading disappearing text: Cognitive control of eye movements. *Psychol Sci* 14: 385–388.

Reed, C. L., and Caselli, R. J. (1994). The nature of tactile agnosia: A case study. *Neuropsychologia* 32: 527–539.

Reed, C. L., Caselli, R. J., and Farah, M. J. (1996). Tactile agnosia: Underlying impairment and implications for normal tactile object recognition. *Brain* 119: 875–888.

Reed, C. L., Klatzky, R. L., and Halgren, E. (2005). What versus where in touch: An fMRI study. *Neuroimage* 25: 718–726.

Reed, C. L., Shoham, S., and Halgren, E. (2004). Neural substrates of tactile object recognition: A fMRI study. *Hum Brain Mapp* 21: 236–246.

Regan, D. (1991). Depth from motion and motion in depth. In D. Regan (Ed.), *Binocular Vision* (pp. 137–169). London: Macmillan.

Reichardt, W. (1986). Processing of optical information by the visual system of the fly. *Vision Res* 26: 113–126.

Rensink, R. A., O'Regan, J. K., and Clark, J. J. (1997). To see or not to see: The need for attention to perceive changes in scenes. *Psychol Sci* 8: 368–373.

Reynolds, J. H., and Chelazzi, L. (2004). Attentional modulation of visual processing. *Annu Rev Neurosci* 27: 611–647.

Rhode, W. S., and Cooper, N. P. (1993). Two-tone suppression and distortion production on the basilar membrane in the hook region of the cat and guinea pig cochleae. *Hear Res* 66: 31–45.

Riecke, L., van Opstal, A. J., Goebel, R., and Formisano, E. (2007). Hearing illusory sounds in noise: Sensory-perceptual transformations in primary auditory cortex. *J Neurosci* 27: 12684–12689.

Rind, F. C., and Simmons, P. J. (1999). Seeing what is coming: Building collision-sensitive neurones. *Trends Neurosci* 22: 215–220.

Robson, J., and Campbell, F. (1997). A quick demonstration of your own contrast sensitivity function. In D. G. Pelli and A. M. Torres, *Thresholds: Limits of Perception*. New York: NY Arts Magazine.

Rock, I., and Victor, J. (1964) Vision and touch: An experimentally created conflict between the two senses. *Science* 143: 594–596.

Rodieck, R. W. (1998). *The First Steps in Seeing*. Sunderland, MA: Sinauer.

Rogers, B. J., and Collett, T. S. (1989). The appearance of surfaces specified by motion parallax and binocular disparity. *Q J Exp Psychol A* 41: 697–717.

Rollman, G. B. (1991). Pain responsiveness. In M. A. Heller and W. Schiff (Eds.), *The Psychology of Touch* (pp. 91–114). Hillsdale, NJ: Erlbaum.

Rolls, E. T., O'Doherty, J. O., Kringelbach, M. L, Francis, S., Bowtell, R., and McGlone, F. (2003). Representations of pleasant and painful touch in the human orbitofrontal and cingulate cortex. *Cereb Cortex* 13: 308–317.

Roorda, A., and Williams, D. R. (1999). The arrangement of the three cone classes in the living human eye. *Nature* 397: 520–522.

Roper, S. D. (2006). Cell communication in taste buds. *Cell Mol Life Sci* 63: 1494–1500.

Rosenzweig, M. R., Breedlove, S. M., and Watson, N. V. (2005). *Biological Psychology: An Introduction to Behavioral and Cognitive Neuroscience* (4th ed.). Sunderland, MA: Sinauer.

Rossetti, Y., Rode, G., and Boisson, D. (1995). Implicit processing of somaesthetic information: A dissociation between where and how? *Neuroreport* 15: 506–510.

Royden, C. S., Banks, M. S., and Crowell, J. A. (1992). The perception of heading during eye movements. *Nature* 360: 583–585.

Royet, J.-P, and Plailly, J. (2004). Lateralization of olfactory processes. *Chem Senses* 29: 731–745.

Rozin, P. (Ed.). (1967). *Thiamin Specific Hunger* (Vol. 1). Washington, DC: American Physiological Society.

Rushton, W. (1972). Visual pigments in man. In H. Dartnall (Ed.), *Photochemistry of Vision* (Vol. VII/1, pp. 364–394). New York: Springer.

Sachse, S., Rueckert, E., Keller, A., Okada, R., Tanaka, N. K., Ito, K., and Vosshall, L. B. (2007). Activity dependent plasticity in an olfactory circuit. *Neuron* 56: 838–850.

Sacks, O. (1993, May 10). To see and not see. *New Yorker*, 59–73.

Sacks, O. (2006, June 19). A neurologist's notebook: "Stereo Sue." *New Yorker*, 64.

Saffran, J. R. (2001). Words in a sea of sounds: The output of statistical learning. *Cognition* 81: 149–169.

Saffran, J. R. (2002). Constraints on statistical language learning. *J Mem Lang* 47: 172–196.

Saffran, J. R., Aslin, R. N., and Newport, E. L. (1996). Statistical learning by 8-month-old infants. *Science* 274: 1926–1928.

Saffran, J. R., Johnson, E. K., Aslin, R. N., and Newport, E. L. (1999). Statistical learning of tone sequences by human infants and adults. *Cognition* 70: 27–52.

Saffran, J. R., Loman, M. M., and Robertson, R. R. W. (2000). Infant memory for musical experiences. *Cognition* 77: B15–B23.

Salzman, C. D., Britten, K. H., and Newsome, W. T. (1990). Cortical microstimulation influences perceptual judgements of motion direction. *Nature* 346: 174–177.

Sasaki, T. (1980). Sound restoration and temporal localization of noise in speech and music sounds. *Tohoku Psychol Folia* 39: 79–88.

Sato, M., Ogawa, H., and Yamashita, S. (1975). Response properties of macaque monkey chorda tympani fibers. *J Gen Physiol* 66: 781–810.

Sceniak, M. P., Ringach, D. L., Hawken, M. J., and Shapley, R. (1999). Contrast's effect on spatial summation by macaque V1 neurons. *Nat Neurosci* 2: 733–739.

Schaal, B., Marlier, L., and Soussignan, R. (1995). Responsiveness to the odor of amniotic fluid in the human neonate. *Biol Neonate* 671: 397–406.

Schaal, B., Marlier, L., and Soussignan, R. (1998). Olfactory function in the human fetus: Evidence from selective neonatal responsiveness to the odor of amniotic fluid. *Behav Neurosci* 112: 1438–1449.

Schild, D. and Restrepo, D. (1998). Transduction mechanism in vertebrate olfactory receptor cells. *Physiol Rev* 37: 369–375.

Schiller, P. H., and Sandell, J. H. (1983). Interactions between visually and electrically elicited saccades before and after superior colliculus and frontal eye field ablations in the rhesus monkey. *Exp Brain Res* 49: 381–392.

Schleidt, M., Hold, B., and Attila, G. (1981). A cross-cultural study on the attitude towards personal odors. *J Chem Ecol* 7: 19–31.

Schmelz, M., Schmidt, R., Bickel, A., Handwerker, H. O., and Torebjork, H. E. (1997). Specific 0043-receptors for itch in human skin. *J Neurosci* 17: 8003–8008.

Schnapf, J. L., Kraft, T. W., and Baylor, D. A. (1987). Spectral sensitivity of human cone photoreceptors. *Nature* 325: 439–441.

Scholz, J., and Woolf, C. J. (2002). Can we conquer pain? *Nat Neurosci* 5 Suppl.: 1062–1067.

Schoonevelt, G. P., and Moore, B. C. J. (1989). Comodulation masking release (CMR) as a function of masker bandwidth, modulator bandwidth, and signal duration. *J Acoust Soc Am* 85: 273–281.

Scott, S. K., Blank, C. C., Rosen, S., and Wise, R. J. S. (2000). Identification of a pathway for intelligible speech in the left temporal lobe. *Brain* 123: 2400–2406.

Seay, C. F. (1975). *First Thoughts on a Theology of Music from the Psalter.* Dallas, TX: Dallas Theological Seminary.

Selfridge, O. G. (1959). Pandemonium: A paradigm for learning. In D. V. Blake and A. M. Uttley (Eds.), *Proceedings of the Symposium on the Mechanisation of Thought Processes* (pp. 511–529). London: Her Majesty's Stationery Office.

Serre, T., Oliva, A., and Poggio, T. (2007). A feedforward architecture accounts for rapid categorization. *Proc Natl Acad Sci USA* 104: 6424–6429.

Shapiro, K. L. (1994). The attentional blink: The brain's eyeblink. *Curr Dir Psychol Sci* 3: 86–89.

Shepard, R. N. (1967). Recognition memory for words, sentences, and pictures. *J Verbal Learn Verbal Behav* 6: 156–163.

Sherrick C., and Cholewiak, R. (1986). Cutaneous sensitivity. In K. R. Boff, L. Kaufman, and J. P. Thomas (Eds.), *Handbook of Perception and Human Performance* (Vol 1., pp. 12-1 to 12-58). New York: Wiley.

Shevell, S. K. (2003). Color appearance. In S. K. Shevell (Ed.), *The Science of Color* (2nd ed., pp. 149–190). Oxford, UK: Elsevier.

Simons, D. J., and Levin, D. T. (1997). Change blindness. *Trends Cogn Sci* 1: 261–267.

Sipiora, M. L., Murtaugh, M. A., Gregoire, M. B., and Duffy, V. B. (2000). Bitter taste perception and severe vomiting during pregnancy. *Physiol Behav* 69: 259–267.

Sloboda, J. A. (1999). Music: Where cognition and emotion meet. *Psychologist* 12: 450–455.

Smith, J. D., Kemler Nelson, D. G., Grohskopf, L. A., and Appleton, T. (1994). What child is this? What interval was that? Familiar tunes and music perception in novice listeners. *Cognition* 52: 23–54.

Smithson, H. E. (2005). Sensory, computational and cognitive components of human colour constancy. *Philos Trans R Soc Lond B Biol Sci* 360: 1329–1346.

Snyder, D. J., Davidson, A. C., Kidd, J. R., Kidd, K. K., Speed, W. C., Pakstis, A. J., Cubells, J. F., O'Malley, S. S., and Bartoshuk, L. M. (2005). *Oral Sensation Influences Tobacco Use: Genetic and Psychophysical Evidence.* Paper presented at the Society for Research on Nicotine and Tobacco, Prague, Czech Republic.

Snyder, D. J., Dwivedi, N., Mramor, A., Bartoshuk, L. M., and Duffy, V. B. (2001). *Taste and Touch May Contribute to the Localization of Retronasal Olfaction: Unilateral and Bilateral Anesthesia of Cranial Nerves V/VII.* Paper presented at the Society of Neuroscience Abstract, San Diego, CA.

Snyder, J. S., and Alain, C. (2007). Toward a neurophysiological theory of auditory stream segregation. *Psychol Bull* 133, 780–799.

Sollberger, B., Reber, R., and Eckstein, D. (2003). Musical chords as affective priming context in a word-evaluation task. *Music Percept* 20: 263–283.

Spence, C., Nicholls, M. E. R., and Driver, J. (2001). The cost of expecting events in the wrong sensory modality. *Percept Psychophys* 63: 330–336.

Spence, C., Pavani, F., and Driver, J. (2000). Crossmodal links between vision and touch in covert endogenous spatial attention. *J Exp Psychol Hum Percept Perform* 26: 1298–1319.

Spencer, N. A., McClintock, M. K., Sellergren, S. A., Bullivant, S., Jacob, S., and Mennella, J. A. (2004). Social chemosignals from breastfeeding women increase sexual motivation. *Hum Behav* 46: 362–370.

Sperling, G., and Weichselgartner, E. (1995). Episodic theory of the dynamics of spatial attention. *Psychol Rev* 102: 503–532.

Stabell, B., and Stabell, U. (2002). Effects of rod activity on color perception with light adaptation. *J Opt Soc Am A Opt Image Sci Vis* 19: 1249–1258.

Stager, D. R., and Birch, E. (1986). Preferential-looking acuity and stereopsis in infantile esotropia. *J Pediatr Ophthalmol Strabismus* 23: 160–165.

Standing, L. (1973). Learning 10,000 pictures. *Q J Exp Psychol* 25: 207–222.

Standing, L., Conezio, J., and Haber, R. N. (1970). Perception and memory for pictures: Single trial learning of 2500 visual stimuli. *Psychon Sci* 19: 73–74.

Stein, L. J., Cowart, B. J., Epstein, A. N., Pilot, L. J., Laskin, C. R., and Beauchamp, G. K. (1996). Increased liking for salty foods in adolescents exposed during infancy to a chloride-deficient feeding formula. *Appetite* 27: 65–77.

Stein, M., Ottenberg, M. D., and Roulet, N. (1958). A study of the development of olfactory preferences. *Arch Neurol Psychiatry* 80: 264–266.

Steiner, J. E. (1973). The gustofacial response: Observation on normal and anencephalic newborn infants. In J. F. Bosma (Ed.), *Development in the Fetus and Infant* (pp. 254–278). Washington, DC: U.S. Government Printing Office.

Stellman, S. D., and Garfinkel, L. (1986). Artificial sweetener use and one-year weight change among women. *Prev Med* 15: 195–202.

Stevens, J. C. (1959). Cross-modality validation of subjective scales for loudness, vibration, and electric shock. *J Exp Psychol* 57: 201–209.

Stevens, J. C., and Cain, W. S. (1987). Old-age deficits in the sense of smell as gauged by thresholds, magnitude matching and odor identification. *Psychol Aging* 2: 36–42.

Stevens, J. C., Plantinga, A., and Cain, W. S. (1982). Reduction of odor and nasal pungency associated with aging. *Neurobiol Aging* 3: 125–132.

Stevens, S. S. (1961). To honor Fechner and repeal his law. *Science* 133: 80–86.

Stevens, S. S. (1962). The surprising simplicity of sensory metrics. *Am Psychol* 17: 29–39.

Stevens, S. S. (1975). *Psychophysics.* New York: Academic Press.

Stevens, S. S., and Galanter, E. H. (1957). Ratio scales and category scales for a dozen perceptual continua. *J Exp Psychol* 54: 377–411.

Stryker, M. P., and, Schiller, P. H. (1975). Eye and head movements evoked by electrical stimulation of monkey superior colliculus. *Exp Brain Res* 23: 103–112.

Sugase, Y., Yamane, S., Ueno, S., and Kawano, K. (1999). Global and local information coded by single neurons in the temporal visual cortex. *Nature* 400: 869–873.

Sugita, Y. (1997). Neuronal correlates of auditory induction in the cat cortex. *Neuroreport* 8: 1155–1159.

Sugita, Y. (1999). Grouping of image fragments in primary visual cortex. *Nature* 401: 269–272.

Sulmont, C., Issanchou, S., and Koster, E. P. (2002). Selection of odorants for memory tests on the basis of familiarity, perceived complexity, pleasantness, similarity and identification. *Chem Senses* 27: 307–317.

Svaetichin, G., and Macnichol, E. F., Jr. (1959). Retinal mechanisms for chromatic and achromatic vision. *Ann NY Acad Sci* 74: 385–404.

Tan, H. Z., Durlach, N. I., Reed, C. M., and Rabinowitz, W. M. (1999). Information transmission with a multifinger tactual display. *Percept Psychophys* 61: 993–1008.

Tanaka, J. W., and Taylor, M. (1991). Object categories and expertise: Is the basic level in the eye of the beholder? *Cogn Psychol* 23: 457–482.

Tarr, M. J., and Pinker, S. (1990). When does human object recognition use a viewer-centered reference frame? *Psychol Sci* 1: 253–256.

Teller, D. Y., and Movshon, J. A. (1986). Visual development. *Vision Res* 26: 1483–1506.

Temussi, P. (2007). The sweet taste receptor: A single receptor with multiple sites and modes of interaction. In S. Taylor (Ed.), *Advances in Food and Nutrition Research* (Vol. 53, pp. 199–239). Elsevier, New York.

Thomas, O. M., Cumming, B. G., and Parker, A. J. (2002). A specialization for relative disparity in V2. *Nat Neurosci* 5: 472–478.

Thompson, P. (1980). Margaret Thatcher: A new illusion. *Perception* 9: 482–484.

Thorpe, S., Fize, D., and Marlot, C. (1996). Speed of processing in the human visual system. *Nature* 381: 520–552.

Tipper, S. P., and Behrmann, M. (1996). Object-centered not scene-based visual neglect. *J Exp Psychol Hum Percept Perform* 22: 1261–1278.

Treisman, A. (1986a). Features and objects in visual processing. *Sci Am* 255(5): 114–125.

Treisman, A. (1986b). Properties, parts, and objects. In K. R. Boff, L. Kaufmann, and J. P. Thomas (Eds.), *Handbook of Perception and Human Performance*, Vol. 2: *Cognitive Processes and Performance* (pp. 35.31–35.70). New York: Wiley.

Treisman, A. (1996). The binding problem. *Curr Opin Neurobiol* 6: 171–178.

Treisman, A., and Gelade, G. (1980). A feature-integration theory of attention. *Cogn Psychol* 12. 97–136.

Treisman, A. M., and Schmidt, H. (1982). Illusory conjunctions in the perception of objects. *Cogn Psychol* 14: 107–141.

Tresilian, J. R. (1999). Visually timed action: Time-out for "tau"? *Trends Cogn Sci* 3: 301–310.

Treue, S., and Trujillo, J. C. M. (1999). Feature-based attention influences motion processing gain in macaque visual cortex. *Nature* 399: 575–579.

Tsotsos, J. K. (1990). Analyzing vision at the complexity level. *Behav Brain Sci* 13: 423–469.

Turin, L. (1996). A spectroscopic mechanism for primary olfactory reception. *Chem Senses* 21: 773–791.

Tyler, C. W. (1991). Cyclopean vision. In D. Regan (Ed.), *Binocular Vision* (Vol. 9, pp. 38–74). Boca Raton, FL: CRC Press.

Uppenkamp, S., Johnsrude, I. S., Norris, D., Marslen-Wilson, W., and Patterson, R. D. (2006). Locating the initial stages of speech-sound processing in human temporal cortex. *Neuroimage* 31: 1284–1296.

Vaina, L. M., and Cowey, A. (1996). Impairment of the perception of second order motion but not first order motion in a patient with unilateral focal brain damage. *Proc R Soc Lond B Biol Sci* 263: 1225–1232.

Vaina, L. M., Makris, N., Kennedy, D., and Cowey, A. (1998). The selective impairment of the perception of first-order motion by unilateral cortical brain damage. *Vis Neurosci* 15: 333–348.

van Noorden, L. P. A. S. (1975). *Temporal Coherence in the Perception of Tone Sequences.* PhD diss., Technical University, Eindhoven, Netherlands.

Verhagen, J. V., Wesson, D. W., Netoff, T. I., White, J. A., and Wachowiak, M. (2007). Sniffing controls an adaptive filter of sensory input to the olfactory bulb. *Nat Neurosci* 10: 631–639.

Verrillo, R. T. (1963). Effect of contactor area on the vibrotactile threshold. *J Acoust Soc Am* 35: 1962–1966.

Vishwanath, D., Girshik, A. R., and Banks, M. (2005). Why pictures look right when viewed from the wrong place. *Nat Neurosci* 8: 1401–1410.

von der Heydt, R., Peterhans, E., and Baumgartner, G. (1984). Illusory contours and cortical neuron responses. *Science* 224: 1260–1262.

von der Malsburg, C. (1981). *The Correlation Theory of Brain Function.* Göttingen, Germany: Max-Planck-Institute for Biophysical Chemistry.

Walker, R., and Lupien, J. R. (2000). The safety evaluation of monosodium glutamate. *J Nutr* 130(4S Suppl.): 1049S–1052S.

Walla, P., Hufnagl, B., Lehern, J., Mayer, D., Lindinger, G., Imhof, H., Deeke, L., and Lang, W. (2003). Olfaction and depth of word processing: A magnetoencephalographic study. *Neuroimage* 18: 104–116.

Wallach, H. (1940). The role of head movements and vestibular and visual clues in sound localization. *J Exp Psychol* 27: 339–368.

Wang, Y., and Frost, B. J. (1992). Time to collision is signalled by neurons in the nucleus rotundus of pigeons. *Nature* 356: 236–238.

Ward, W. D. (1954). Subjective musical pitch. *J Acoust Soc Am* 26: 369–380.

Warren, R. M. (1984). Perceptual restoration of obliterated sounds. *Psychol Rev* 96: 371–385.

Warren, R. M., and Obusek, C. J. (1971). Speech perception and phonemic restorations. *Percept Psychophys* 9: 358–362.

Warren, R. M., and Sherman, G. L. (1974). Phonemic restorations based on subsequent context. *Percept Psychophys* 16: 150–156.

Warren, W. H., Jr., and Hannon, D. J. (1990). Eye movements and optical flow. *J Opt Soc Am A* 7: 160–169.

Warren, W. H., Jr., Morris, M. W., and Kalish, M. (1988). Perception of translational heading from optical flow. *J Exp Psychol Hum Percept Perform* 14: 646–660.

Warren, W. H., Jr., and Saunders, J. A. (1995). Perceiving heading in the presence of moving objects. *Perception* 24: 315–331.

Warren, W. H., Jr., and Verbrugge, R. R. (1984). Auditory perception of breaking and bouncing events: A case study in ecological acoustics. *J Exp Psychol Hum Percept Perform* 10: 704–712.

Wasserman, E. A., and Zentall, T. R. (2006). *Comparative Cognition: Experimental Explorations of Animal Intelligence.* New York: Oxford University Press.

Weinstein, S. (1968). Intensive and extensive aspects of tactile sensitivity as a function of body part, sex, and laterality. In D. R. Kenshalo (Ed.), *The Skin Senses* (pp. 195–222). Springfield, IL: Thomas.

Werker, J. F., and Tees, R. C. (1984). Phonemic and phonetic factors in adult cross-language speech perception. *J Acoust Soc Am* 75: 1866–1878.

Werner, A., Menzel, R., and Wehrhahn, C. (1988). Color constancy in the honeybee. *J Neurosci* 8: 156–159.

Werner, J. S., Peterzell, D. H., and Scheetz, A. J. (1990). Light, vision, and aging. *Optom Vision Sci* 67: 214–229.

Wessel, D. L. (1979). Timbre space as a musical control structure. *Comput Music J* 3: 45–52.

Westling, G., and Johannson R. S. (1984). Factors influencing the force control during precision grip. *Exp Brain Res* 53: 277–284.

Wever, E. G. (1949). *Theory of Hearing*. New York: Wiley.

Wheatstone, C. (1852). Some remarkable and hitherto unobserved phenomena of binocular vision: Part two. *Philos Mag* 4: 504–523.

Wiesel, T. N. (1982). Postnatal development of the visual cortex and the influence of environment. *Nature* 299: 583–591.

Wightman, F. L., and Jenison, R. (1995). Auditory spatial layout. In W. Epstein and S. Rogers (Eds.), *Perception of Space and Motion* (pp. 365–400). San Diego, CA: Academic Press.

Wightman, F., and Kistler, D. (1998). Of Vulcan ears, human ears and "earprints." *Nat Neurosci* 1: 337–339.

Wilkins, L., and Richter, C. P. (1940). A great craving for salt by a child with cortico-adrenal insufficiency. *J Am Med Assoc* 114: 866–868.

Willis, C. M., Church, S. M., Guest, C. M., Cook, W. A., McCarthy, N., Bransbury, A. J., Church, M. R. T., and Church J. C. T. (2004). Olfactory detection of human bladder cancer by dogs: Proof of principle study. *Br Med J* 329: 712–714.

Winawer, J., Witthoft, N., Frank, M. C., Wu, L., Wade, A. R., and Boroditsky, L. (2007). Russian blues reveal effects of language on color discrimination. *Proc Natl Acad Sci USA* 104: 7780–7785.

Winberg, J., and Porter, R. H. (1998). Olfaction and human neonatal behaviour: Clinical implications. *Acta Paediatr* 87: 6–10.

Wolfe, J. M. (1994). Guided Search 2.0: A revised model of visual search. *Psychon Bull Rev* 1: 202–238.

Wolfe, J. M., Cave, K. R., and Franzel, S. L. (1989). Guided Search: An alternative to the Feature Integration model for visual search. *J Exp Psychol Hum Percept Perform* 15: 419–433.

Wolfe, J. M., and Held, R. (1981). A purely binocular mechanism in human vision. *Vision Res* 21: 1755–1759.

Wolfe, J. M., and Horowitz, T. S. (2004). What attributes guide the deployment of visual attention and how do they do it? *Nat Rev Neurosci* 5: 495–501.

Wolfe, J. M., Reinecke, A., and Brawn, P. (2006). Why don't we see changes? The role of attentional bottlenecks and limited visual memory. *Vis Cogn* 14: 749–780.

Womelsdorf, T., Anton-Erxleben, K., Pieper, F., and Treue, S. (2006). Dynamic shifts of visual receptive fields in cortical area MT by spatial attention. *Nat Neurosci* 9: 1156–1160.

Woodrow, H. (1909). A quantitative study of rhythm. *Arch Psychol* 14: 1–66.

Wrzesniewski, A., McCauley, C., and Rozin, P. (1999). Odor and affect: Individual differences in the impact of odor on liking for places, things and people. *Chem Senses* 24: 713–721.

Wyert, C., Webster, W. W., Chen, J. H., Wilson, S. R., McClary, A., Khan, R. M., and Sobel, N. (2007). Smelling a single component of male sweat alters levels of cortisol in women. *J Neurosci* 27: 1261–1265.

Wysocki, C. J., Dalton, P., Brody, M. J., and Lawley, H. J. (1997). Acetone odor and irritation thresholds obtained from acetone-exposed factory workers and from control (occupationally non-exposed) subjects. *Am Ind Hyg Assoc J* 58: 704–712.

Wysocki, C. J., Dorries, K. M., and Beauchamp, G. K. (1989). Ability to perceive androstenone can be acquired by ostensibly anosmic people. *Proc Natl Acad Sci USA* 86: 7976–7978.

Yantis, S. (1993). Stimulus-driven attentional capture. *Curr Dir Psychol Sci* 2: 156–161.

Yarbus, A. L. (1967). *Eye Movements and Vision.* New York: Plenum.

Yates, B., and Miller, A. (1998). Physiological evidence that the vestibular system participates in autonomic and respiratory control. *J Vestib Res* 8: 17–26.

Yin, C., Kellman, P. J., and Shipley, T. F. (1997). Surface completion complements boundary interpolation in the visual integration of partly occluded objects. *Perception* 26: 1459–1479.

Yin, T. C. T., and Chan, J. C. L. (1990). Interaural time sensitivity in medial superior olive of cat. *J Neurophysiol* 65: 465–488.

Yonas, A., Craton, L. G., and Thompson, W. B. (1987). Relative motion: Kinetic information for the order of depth at an edge. *Percept Psychophys* 41: 53–59.

Young, L. (1984). Perception of the body in space: Mechanisms," in I. Darian-Smith (Ed.), *Handbook of Physiology—The Nervous System*, Vol. 3(2) (pp. 1023–1066). Bethesda, MD: American Physiological Society.

Young, L. R., Shelhamer, M., and Modestino, S. (1986) M.I.T./Canadian vestibular experiments on the Spacelab-1 mission. 2. Visual vestibular tilt interaction in weightlessness. *Exp Brain Res* 64: 299–307.

Yu, K., and Blake, R. (1992). Do recognizable figures enjoy an advantage in binocular rivalry? *J Exp Psychol Hum Percept Perform* 18: 1158–1173.

Yuille, A., and Kersten, D. (2006). Vision as Bayesian inference: Analysis by synthesis? *Trends Cogn Sci* 10: 301–308.

Yuodelis, C., and Hendrickson, A. (1986). A qualitative and quantitative analysis of the human fovea during development. *Vision Res* 26: 847–855.

Zadra, A., Nielsen, T. A., and Donderi, D. C. (1998). Prevalence of auditory, olfactory, and gustatory experiences in home dreams. *Percept Mot Skills* 87: 819–826.

Zahorik, P. (2002). Assessing auditory distance perception using virtual acoustics. *J Acoust Soc Am* 111: 1832–1846.

Zaidi, Q. (1997). Decorrelation of L- and M-cone signals. *J Opt Soc Am A Opt Image Sci Vis* 14: 3430–3431.

Zatorre, R. J. (2001). Do you see what I'm saying? Interactions between auditory and visual cortices in cochlear implant users. *Neuron* 1: 13–14.

Zatorre, R. J., and Binder, J. (2000). Functional and structural imaging of the human auditory system. In A. Toga and J. Mazziotta (Eds.), *Brain Mapping the Systems* (pp. 365–402). San Diego: Academic Press.

Zeki, S. M. (1978). Functional specialisation in the visual cortex of the rhesus monkey. *Nature* 274: 423–428.

Zeki, S. (1990). A century of cerebral achromatopsia. *Brain* 113(Pt 6): 1721–1777.

Zelano, C., Bensafi, M., Porter, J., Mainland, J., Johnson, B., Bremner, E., Telles, C., Khan, R., and Sobel, N. (2005). Attentional modulation in human primary olfactory cortex. *Nat Neurosci* 8: 114–120.

Zhang, B., Zheng, J., Watanabe, I., Maruko, I., Bi, H., Smith, E. L., III, and Chino, Y. (2005). Delayed maturation of receptive field center/surround mechanisms in V2. *Proc Natl Acad Sci USA* 102: 5862–5867.

Zhao, G. Q., Zhang, Y., Hoon, M. A., Chandrashekar, J., Erlenbach, I., Ryba, N. J., and Zuker, C. S. (2003). The receptors for mammalian sweet and umami taste. *Cell* 115: 255–266.

Zheng, J., Zhang, B., Bi, H., Maruko, I., Watanabe, I., Nakatsuka, C., Smith, E. L., III, and Chino, Y. M. (2007). Development of temporal response properties and contrast sensitivity of V1 and V2 neurons in macaque monkeys. *J Neurophysiol* 97: 3905–3916.

Zipser, K., Lamme, V. A., and Schiller, P. H. (1996). Contextual modulation in primary visual cortex. *J Neurosci* 16: 7376–7389.

Zotterman, Y. (1939). Touch, pain and tickling: An electrophysiological investigation on cutaneous sensory nerves. *J Physiol* 95: 1–28.

Zou, Z., Li, F., and Buck, L. B. (2005). Odor maps in the olfactory cortex. *Proc Natl Acad Sci USA* 102: 7724–7729.

Photo Credits

CHAPTER 1 1.1: © Warner Brothers. 1.4: © Zigmund Lezczynski/Animals Animals/Photolibrary. 1.5*a, c*: Photos by David McIntyre. 1.5*b, d*: © Gerry Ellis/DigitalVision. 1.28: Neuroscience History Archives, Brain Research Institute, University of California, Los Angeles. 1.30: Courtesy Österreichische Gesellschaft für Zeitgeschichte, Wien—Bildarchiv.

CHAPTER 3 3.30: Photo by David McIntyre.

CHAPTER 4 4.1*a, c*: Courtesy of Leslie Smith and Walter K. Boas. 4.13*a, b*: © Asther Lau Choon Siew/ShutterStock. 4.13*c*: © Miles Boyer/ShutterStock. 4.16: Courtesy of Paul Philippon/The Duck-Rabbit Craft Brewery. 4.27 *Aniston alone*: Stills from *Picture Perfect* © 3 Art Entertainment. 4.27 *Aniston and Pitt*: © Allstar Picture Library/Alamy. 4.27 *Linney*: Still from *The Truman Show* © Paramount Pictures. 4.27 *spider*: © John Bell/ShutterStock. 4.27 *Sydney Opera*: Courtesy of Christian Mehlführer. 4.27 *Leaning Tower*: © Lawrence Sawyer/istockphoto.com. 4.27 *Eiffel Tower*: © S. Greg Panosian/istockphoto.com. 4.33*a*: © William Leaman/Alamy. 4.33*b*: © SuperStock/Alamy. 4.33*c*: © Gerry Ellis/DigitalVision. 4.33*d*: © Gerry Ellis/DigitalVision.

CHAPTER 5 5.3: Courtesy of John Bortniak, NOAA. 5.22: Courtesy of Amy Bedell. 5.24: © Franco Deriu/Fotolia.com. 5.25: Photo by David McIntyre. 5.26: Courtesy of Tom Eisner. 5.27*a*: © Carol Buchanan/Painet, Inc. 5.27*b*: © Gerry Ellis/DigitalVision. 5.27*c*: © Dynamic Graphics Group/Creatas/Alamy.

CHAPTER 6 6.6: Photo by David McIntyre. 6.14: Courtesy of Jeremy Wolfe. 6.19*a*: © Lewis Whyld/PA Wire URN:5419221 (Press Association via AP Images). 6.19*b*: © Lewis Whyld/PA Wire URN:5249592 (Press Association via AP Images). 6.22–6.26: Photos by David McIntyre. 6.29*a*: © Jupiter Images/Brand X/Alamy. 6.29*b*, 6.31: Courtesy of the Library of Congress. 6.41 *Colonnade*: © xyno/istockphoto.com.

CHAPTER 7 7.2: Courtesy of Frans A. J. Verstraten. 7.12*a*: © Tim Kiusalaas /Masterfile www.masterfile.com. 7.13: © Associated Press.

CHAPTER 8 8.2: From *Where's Waldo?* © Martin Handford 2005. 8.5: © Stephane Tougard/ShutterStock. 8.9: © Oleksiy Maksymenko/Alamy. 8.17: *face*: Courtesy of Jennifer Basil; *house*: Courtesy of Nancy and Marc Desrosiers. 8.18: *left*: From Downing, Liu, and Kanwisher, 2001. *right*: Courtesy of Jennifer Basil. 8.20: From Womelsdorf et al. 2006. 8.21: Images courtesy of Lynn Robertson and Krista Schendel. 8.25 and 8.26 *pigs, children, pears, grapes, scientist*: courtesy of the USDA; *stairway, market women, waterfall, butterfly, churches, cacti, frigate bird, stained glass*: Andrew D. Sinauer; *kangaroo, tawny frogmouth, penguins, wolf, giraffes*: © Gerry Ellis/DigitalVision; *tree, snail shells, water lily, cat*: David McIntyre. 8.27: Modified from *Les Tres Riches Heures du Duc de Berry*. 8.29: David Hockney, 1985, "Place Furstenberg, Paris, August 7, 8, 9, 1985." Photographic collage, edition: 2. 43 1/2 x 61 3/8" © David Hockney.

CHAPTER 9 9.9 *human*: Courtesy of Alex Scudder. 9.9 *capybara*: © John de la Bastide/ShutterStock. 9.9 *sealion*: Courtesy of Andrew D. Sinauer. 9.9 *rabbit*: © Heather Craig/istockphoto.com. 9.9 *possums*: © Stuart Elflett/ShutterStock. 9.9 *elephant*: © Gerry Ellis/DigitalVision. 9.9 *chimp*: © Holger Ehlers/ShutterStock. 9.13: Courtesy of A. J. Hudspeth. 9.27: Courtesy of Cochlear.

CHAPTER 10 10.9 *top left*: © image100/Alamy. 10.9 *others*: courtesy of Rosemary Cole, David McIntyre, Alex Scudder, Richard Cole, and Jennifer Basil. 10.12: Courtesy of Jennifer Basil.

CHAPTER 11 11.15*b*: Photo by David McIntyre, courtesy of Annie Huyler, Pioneer Valley Chinchillas. 11.16 *monkey*: © DigitalVision/PictureQuest. 11.16 *cow*: Courtesy of Scott Bauer/USDA. 11.19: Courtesy of Nancy Asai and Joanne Delphia.

CHAPTER 12 12.1: Photo by David McIntyre. 12.10: From Rainville et al., 1997.

CHAPTER 13 13.7*b*, 13.13: Photos by David McIntyre. 13.15: Photo by David McIntyre and Nancy Asai. 13.16*a*: Courtesy of the U. S. Fish and Wildlife Service. 13.16*b*: © John Bell/ShutterStock.

CHAPTER 14 14.3: Courtesy of Linda Bartoshuk and the Bartoshuk Lab. 14.10*a*: © Image Source/Alamy. 14.10*b*: © Profimedia.CZ s.r.o./Alamy. 14.11, 14.16: Photos by David McIntyre.

Index

Numbers in *italic* refer to information in an illustration or table.

A

D

E

Q

R

T

U

V

About the Book

Editor: Graig Donini

Production Editor: Laura Green

Copyeditor: Stephanie Hiebert

Indexer: Grant Hackett

Production Manager: Christopher Small

Book Design and Production: Jefferson Johnson

Illustration Program: Dragonfly Media Group